Neurobiology of
Acetylcholine

Neurobiology of Acetylcholine

Edited by

Nae J. Dun

Loyola University Stritch School of Medicine
Maywood, Illinois

and

Robert L. Perlman

University of Illinois College of Medicine
Chicago, Illinois

Plenum Press • New York and London

Library of Congress Cataloging in Publication Data

Neurobiology of acetylcholine.

Proceedings of a symposium held in honor of Alexander G. Karczmar June 5–7,
1985, in Maywood, Ill.
Includes bibliographies and index.
1. Acetylcholine—Congresses. 2. Cholinergic receptors—Congresses. 3. Nervous
system, Parasympathetic—Congresses. 4. Karczmar, A. G. (Alexander George),
1918–   —Congresses. I. Dun, Nae J. II. Perlman, Robert L. III. Karczmar, A. G.
(Alexander George), 1918–   . [DNLM: 1. Acetylcholine—congresses. QV 122
N494 1985]
QP364.7.N44   1987   612'.814   87-2467
ISBN 0-306-42493-2

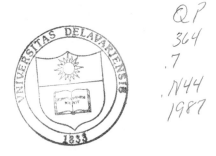

QP
364
.7
.N44
1987

Proceedings of symposium on Neurobiology of Acetylcholine,
held in honor of Dr. Alexander G. Karczmar, June 5–7, 1985,
in Maywood, Illinois.

© 1987 Plenum Press, New York
A Division of Plenum Publishing Corporation
233 Spring Street, New York, N.Y. 10013

Printed in the United States of America

PREFACE

This Festschrift volume in honor of Professor Alexander Karczmar is the outcome of a three-day symposium entitled "Neurobiology of Acetylcholine" held at Loyola University Medical Center from June 3 to 5, 1985. This volume serves two purposes. It expresses the respect and admiration of the contributors to Alex Karczmar, and it provides a forum for detailing recent advances in the cholinergic field which has attracted the undivided and untiring attention of Dr. Karczmar over some 40 years. During this period, the cholinergic system has grown from its infancy to become one of the most studied and understood transmitter systems today.

Dr. Karczmar's interest in cholinergic system is appropriately reflected by the range of topics, molecular, cellular, developmental, behavioral and toxicological, that were discussed here. A detailed synopsis of Dr. Karczmar's research and his contributions to the field of cholinergic systems can be found in the following chapter by his close friend and colleague, Dr. George Koelle.

We would like to take this opportunity to thank the enthusiastic responses of the participants making this Festschrift a memorable event. Also, we are greatly indebted to the following organizations for their generous financial support which made this meeting possible: American Critical Care Division, American Hospital Corporation; American Cyanamid Company; Bristol-Myers Company; Burroughs Wellcome Company; Hoffmann-LaRoche, Inc.; Lilly Research Laboratories, Division of Eli Lilly and Company; Marion Laboratories, Inc.; G. B. Searle; Sterling Drug Inc.; Syntex Research, Division of Syntex, Inc.; Travenol Laboratories, Inc.; Upjohn Company; United States Army Medical Research and Development Command; and Loyola University Stritch School of Medicine.

Lastly, the assistance of Mrs. Dee Miller in every phase of the meeting and of Jackie Greer in preparing the manuscripts is gratefully acknowledged.

Nae J. Dun
Maywood, IL
and
Robert L. Perlman
Chicago, IL

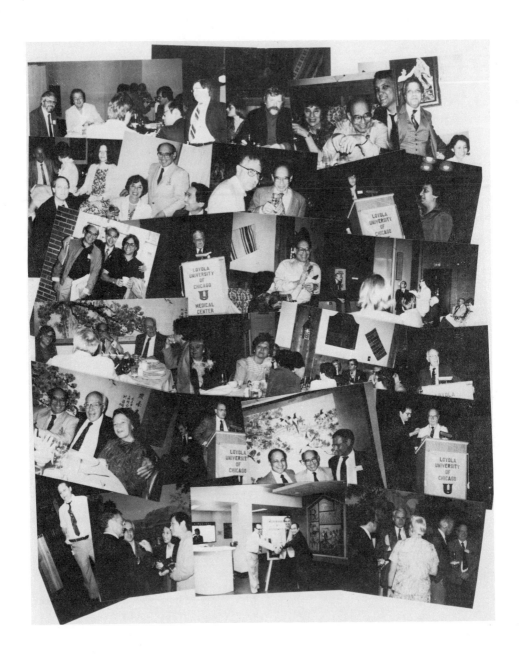

A TRIBUTE TO ALEXANDER G. KARCZMAR

George B. Koelle

Department of Pharmacology
University of Pennsylvania
School of Medicine
Philadelphia, Pennsylvania   19104

It is most fitting that a symposium on the Neurobiology of Acetylcholine should mark Alexander George (Nicky) Karczmar's twenty-nine years
of service at Stritch School of Medicine, Loyola University, as Professor
and Chairman of the Department of Pharmacology. In the years subsequent
to his arrival at Stritch, he has acquired a number of additional titles
and responsibilities, including Senior Director of the Institute of Mind,
Drugs and Behavior, Associate Dean, Loyola University Stritch School of
Medicine Research and Graduate Training, and Associate Director Research
Services. Fifteen years ago Nicky organized a somewhat similar symposium
at Stritch which was edited and published in collaboration with Sir John
Eccles (Brain and Human Behavior, Springer, 1972), who is also among the
present attendees.

Before coming to Stritch, and throughout his tenure there, Nicky's
primary investigative interest has focused on acetylcholine, the enzymes
that synthesize and destroy it, and the drugs that simulate or block its
actions. I know of no one who has addressed the functions of acetylcholine at so many levels as has Nicky: molecular, biochemical, developmental, electrophysiological, pharmacological, toxicological, and behavioral. All these aspects are included appropriately in the present
Symposium. In spite of his continually increasing administrative responsibilities, Nicky has been able (how, I do not know) to continue his
investigative work on acetylcholine with the collaboration of a great
number of associates at all levels.

There is no doubt that much of Nicky's success can be attributed to
the support and encouragement he has received from his remarkable family.
Marian, his wife, has worked in all phases of the theater, as an actress,
playwright, and director. Their older son, Gregory, who looks like Nicky,
is a molecular biologist. Their younger son, Christopher, who features
are a masculine counterpart of Marian's, is an actor. Surely this family
portrait could provide the basis for an interesting socio-genetic study.

To note a few of the highlights in Nicky's adventures with acetylcholine, in the early 1950's while at Georgetown he and the late Theodore
Koppanyi published a series of classical papers on the effects of anticholinesterase agents on the developmental and early behavioral patterns
of embryo newts. Subsequently, in collaboration with Al Lands at Ster-
ling-Winthrop, he played the major role in introducing ambenonium for the

treatment of myasthenia gravis. During his years at Stritch his investigations on acetylcholine and related drugs (as well as on monoamines, peptides, and other agents) blossomed forth in many directions: comparative and developmental pharmacology (in collaboration with Charles Scudder, Raji Srinivasan and Joseph Bernsohn), electrophysiology (in collaboration with Kwang Kim, Kyozo Koketsu, Syogoro Nishi, Les Blaber, Bob Jacobs, Joel Gallagher, Nae J. Dun, Kozue Kaibara, Takashi Akasu, Yuko Ohta, Hiroshi Hasuo, and Tashihiko Nishimura), toxicology, therapy of myasthenia gravis, (with Joel Brumlik), and behavioral (with Frank Cann, Priscilla Bourgault and also with Scudder). (I apologize to his many collaborators whose names have been omitted--the list is long!) One of the most unique approaches in the behavioral category was the establishment of Mouse City. This consisted of an isolated room in which a number of free-roaming mice were given access to houses, playgrounds, and perhaps even supermarkets, which permitted observation of their reactions and interactions to various psychopharmacological agents in a practically normal environment. But, as I mentioned at the Symposium, the experiment was terminated when the time came to elect a mayor of Mouse City, and Nicky discovered a nefarious situation of vote fraud.

Nicky has served on a great number of national and international committees and editorial boards. I mention only that he was a founding fellow of the American College of Neuropsychopharmacology, an organization he has always held in particular affection. I shall not attempt to list the others or his honorary degrees, medals, and lectureships; they can be found in his CV.

Beyond his scientific, teaching, and administrative accomplishments, Alexander Karczmar is truly a man for all seasons. His knowledge of history, American and European literature, art, music, and science beyond pharmacology is overwhelming. He speaks fluently at least eight languages.

The esteem in which Nicky is held by so many people is evidenced by the attendance at the present symposium. It has attracted distinguished scientists from all parts of North America, and from across the Atlantic and Pacific Oceans. Their presentations recorded here make this a memorable and invaluable monograph.

On a personal note, I thank Nae Dun for the opportunity to write this tribute, for Win and I consider Marian and Nicky among our closest friends. Let me add that this consideration has in no way influenced the foregoing objective account.

CONTENTS

ELECTROPHYSIOLOGY

FUNCTIONAL ASPECTS OF CHOLINERGIC SYSTEM

TOXICOLOGY

ALEXANDER G. KARCZMAR, CONCLUDING REMARKS:
PAST, PRESENT AND FUTURE OF CHOLINERGIC RESEARCH

MORPHOLOGICAL AND DEVELOPMENTAL STUDIES

DISTRIBUTION OF CHOLINERGIC NEURONS IN HUMAN BRAIN

P. L. McGeer, E. G. McGeer, K. Mizukawa, H. Tago and J. H. Peng

Kinsmen Laboratory of Neurological Research
Department of Psychiatry
University of British Columbia
Vancouver, B. C., Canada, V6T 1W5

INTRODUCTION

Acetylcholine (ACh) was the first neurotransmitter to be identified, ushering in the modern concept of chemical transmission in the nervous system. Nevertheless, for many years information regarding cholinergic pathways, particularly in the central nervous system, lagged behind several other neurotransmitters because of technical difficulties in cellular localization of cholinergic structures. Initial information came from measurements of the effects of various lesions on the levels of ACh or its specific synthesizing enzyme, choline acetyltransferase (ChAT), and from histochemical studies on the degrading enzyme, acetylcholinesterase (AChE)[1]. The best early application of the latter method was in the papers of Shute and Lewis [2],[3]. Unfortunately, although AChE has a relatively high concentration in known cholinergic structures[4-8], it also occurs in non-cholinergic cells[8-9]. Suppression of AChE with DFP has done much to separate cholinergic from non-cholinergic AChE-containing cells[5],[10]; but, since some of the latter contain anomalously high concentrations of AChE, the method cannot be relied upon as a definitive method for identifying cholinergic structures. Moreover, the DFP pretreatment suppresses fiber staining, thus reducing the potential for tracing pathways. A more definitive method depends upon immunohistochemical staining using antibodies to the selective enzyme, ChAT[11]. Although the purification of ChAT has been fraught with difficulty and many of the antibodies prepared are of relatively low titer, the method has allowed much to be learned about ChAT-containing structures in the brain. Much fundamental information remains to be elicited and a number of controversies have developed around existing reports, but the data already available have permitted new insights into cholinergic pharmacology and the relationship between a number of disease processes and cholinergic systems.

This paper will emphasize the distribution of cholinergic cells in human brain. This has been particularly difficult to define because of the inability to use the DFP-AChE histochemical method and the problems in using ChAT immunohistochemistry in postmortem tissue. But it is also of particular interest because of the possible involvement of cholinergic systems in a number of disease states, including Alzheimer's disease[12-13], Huntington's disease[1], amyotrophic lateral sclerosis[14], Parkinson dementia[15], pol-

3

iomyelitis[16] and, possibly, epilepsy[17], dystonia[18], Guillain Barré syndrome[19] and some forms of mental illness[20].

ChAT-POSITIVE CHOLINERGIC STRUCTURES

The cholinergic systems of the brain have now been described in several species using the technique of ChAT immunohistochemistry. Maps of varying completeness have been produced for the cat[21], rat[8-9],[22-27], monkey[28-30], baboon[31] and human[32]. There may be some minor species differences but the general pattern is similar. There are relatively few major cholinergic cell groups in the brain. They can be thought of as five major systems, plus a few minor ones located mainly in the brain stem. The five major cholinergic systems (Figure 1) are: the neostriatal-nucleus accumbens, the medial basal forebrain, the parabrachial, the reticular, and the cranial motor[11]. The minor systems include some nuclei associated with VIII nerve function such as the superior olive and some vestibular nuclei[11]. Some small ChAT-positive cells have been reported in the rat cortex, hippocampus and medial habenula[22-23],[26-27],[33] and in the rat and cat red nucleus[21],[24],[34] but such neurons have not yet been identified in the human.

Neostriatal-Nucleus Accumbens Interneurons

It has long been known from lesions studies that internal systems of cholinergic neurons exist in the neostriatum and nucleus accumbens. Giant cells within these nuclei stain positively for ChAT in all species so far studied[21-24],[31-32]. They constitute a surprisingly small percentage (< 5%) of the total neurons in these nuclei considering the extremely high levels

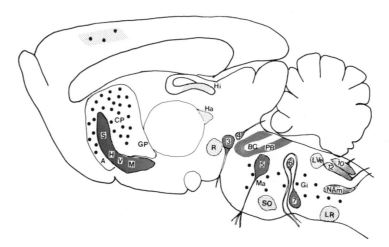

Fig. 1. Sagittal view of rat brain illustrating ChAT-containing neurons. Major systems are indicated by black dots or heavy stippling, minor ones by light stippling. (From McGeer et al.[11]). Abbreviations: A, Nucleus accumbens; Am, Amygdala; BC, Brachium conjunctivum; CP, Caudate-putamen; Gi, Gigantocellular division of the reticular formation; GP, Globus pallidus; H, Horizontal limb of diagonal band; Ha, Habenula; Hi, Hippocampus; IC, Inferior colliculus; IP, Interpeduncular nucleus; LR. Lateral reticular nucleus; LVe, Lateral vestibular nucleus; M, Nucleus basalis of Maynert; Ma, Magnocellular division of the reticular formation; NAm, Nucleus ambiguus; PB, Parabrachial complex; R, Red nucleus; S, Medial septum; SN, Substantia nigra; SO, Superior olive; V, Vertical limb of diagonal band.

of ACh, ChAT and AChE found by biochemical measurement. Smaller cholinergic cells have also been reported in the striatum of the rat[22],[35] and, while the giant cells are certainly the most prominent ones, they may not be the entire cholinergic population.

The Medial Forebrain Complex

This is a more or less continuous sheet of giant cholinergic cells which starts anteriorly on the medial surface of the cortex and extends in a caudolateral direction, always maintaining its position close to the medial and ventral surfaces of the brain, and terminating towards the caudal aspect of the lentiform nucleus. The names usually given to the various sub-regions of this complex from rostral to caudal order are the following: medial septal nucleus, nucleus of the vertical limb of the diagonal band of Broca, nucleus of the horizontal limb of the diagonal band of Broca, and the nucleus basalis of Meynert (S,V,H and M in Figure 1) or substantia innominata. This complex has been extensively studied in a number of species and has been shown to provide cholinergic innervation to the hippocampus, amygdala, interpeduncular nucleus and all neocortical areas[1],[11]. The horizontal portion of this complex has been mapped in the human by both ChAT immunohistochemistry[36-38] (Figure 2a) and AChE histochemistry[39]. All the giant cells in this region are positive for ChAT[12]. The number of such cells appears to decrease with normal aging[12],[38] and, more profoundly, in Alzheimer's disease[12-13],[37-38]. Figures 2c and 2d show a comparison of the ChAT staining in this region in postmortem brains of a normal and a person with Alzheimer's disease. In our hands, the number of cholinergic cells counted in this region correlates well with the average value obtained by biochemical assay of ChAT in seven cortical regions (Figure 2b).

The Parabrachial System

This system is the most intense and concentrated cholinergic cell group in the brain stem. It surrounds the brachium conjunctivum commencing in the most rostral aspects of the pons and follows the direction of the brachium conjunctivum (superior cerebellar peduncles) in a caudodorsal direction. Various subnuclei are separately identified in this particular region and the nomenclature varies somewhat from species to species. The most commonly described nucleus is the pedunculopontine tegmental nucleus in the lateral aspect at the most rostral portion of the complex (Figures 3a and 3b). In the human staining was also seen in the medial and lateral parabrachial nuclei and in the nucleus tegmentalis peduncuolopontinus. A few ChAT-positive cells were also found in the human in the lateral lemniscus and these may be related either to this parabrachial complex or to a cholinergic system associated with VIIIth nerve function.

Projections from the nuclei of this complex have been reported to the cortex, various thalamic nuclei, the hypothalamus, amygdala and substantia nigra, as well as some descending projections. Some of the ascending projections seem to be partly cholinergic and some have been reported to contain substance P as a cotransmitter. Much, however, remains to be learned about the cholinergic tracts arising in this complex.

The Reticular System

This is composed of a scattered collection of very large cells extending throughout the gigantocellular and magnocellular tegmental fields of the reticular formation (Gi and Ma in Figure 1). Caudally the giganto and magnocellular ChAT-containing neurons are gradually aggregated medially towards the granular layer of the raphe and ventrally to the area near the inferior olivary nucleus. Thus, these cells extend continuously from the rostral pons into the caudal medulla as a longitudinally oriented cluster. In the human, positively staining nuclei of this system include the reticularis pontis oralis and caudalis, reticularis tegmenti pontis, reticularis gigantocellularis, reticularis lateralis and the formatio reticularis centralis (medulla). Figures 4a and 4b are photomicrographs of some of the ChAT-positive gigantocellular neurons.

The cholinergic projections are largely unknown but probably include some to the spinal cord and cerebellum as well as ascending fibers to the thalamus and other rostral nuclei.

Motor Nuclei of the Peripheral Nerves

All motor nuclei of the cranial nerves (III-VII and IX-XII), as well as the nucleus supraspinalis, are ChAT-positive in the human as well as other species. These are the counterparts of the cells in the anterior and later-al horns of the spinal cord which are also cholinergic. Figure 4c shows typical staining of cholinergic neurons in such a motor nucleus in the human.

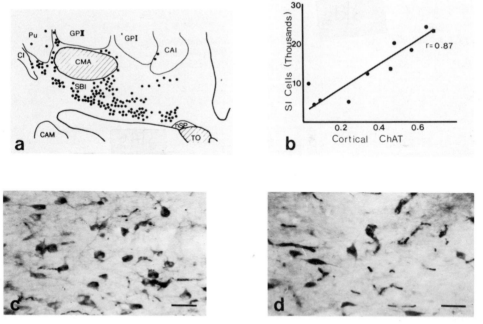

Fig. 2. a) A coronal diagram of human brain showing the location of cholinergic, neurons at the mid-sagittal level of the substantia innominata (SBI). Other abbreviations: Pu, putamen; CMA, anterior commissure; Cl, claustrum; CAM, amygdala; GPpl, globus pallidus pars lateralis; GPpm, globus pallidus pars medialis; CA1, internal capsule;
nSP, supraoptic nucleus; TO, optic tract.   b) Plot of number of
cholinergic cells in the SI in individual human brains against the
average ChAT activities measured in 7 cortical areas.
    c and d) Examples of ChAT-positive staining seen in a typical
normal and SDAT case, respectively. Bars = 100 μm.

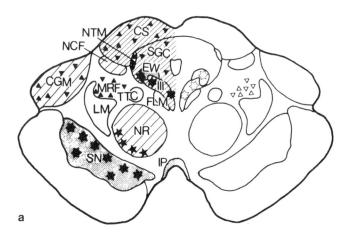

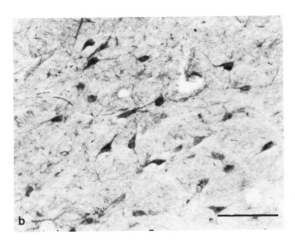

Fig. 3. a) One of eight cross-sectional maps of human brain stem from Mizukawa et al.[32] indicating AChE-containing structures (left side) and
ChAT-containing structures (right side). Abbreviations are: CGM,
corpus geniculatum medialis; CS, superior colliculus; EW, n. access-
orius nervi oculomotorii; FLM, fasciculus longitudinalis medialis;
IP, n. interpeduncularis; LM, medial lemniscus; MRF, mesencephalic
reticular formation; NCF, n. cuneiformis; NR, n. ruber; NTM, n.
mesencephalicus nervi trigemini; SGC, substantia grisea centralis;
SN, substantia nigra; TTC, tractus tegmentalis centralis; III, n.
nervi oculomotorii. Symbols: ☆ large, intensely ChAT-positive cells
with prominent processes; ★ large, intensely AChE-positive cells
with prominent processes; ★ large, AChE-positive cells with less
prominent processes; △ or ▲ small or medium size, AChE- or ChAT-
positive cells with less prominent processes; ▨ intense AChE
fiber staining;▥ moderate AChE fiber staining; // light AChE
fiber staining. b) ChAT staining of the nucleus tegmentalis
pedunculopontinus showing medium size, multipolar cells with some
prominent processes. Bar = 50 μm.

7

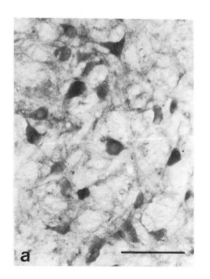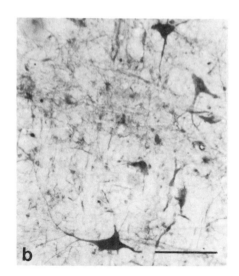

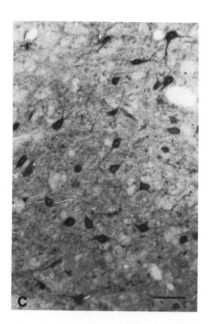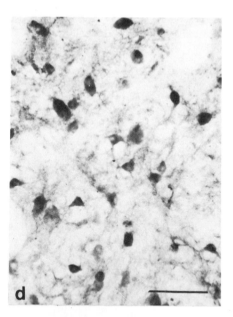

Fig. 4. a) ChAT-positive cells in the nucleus gigantocellularis demonstrating few processes. These tend to occur in clusters. b) Isolated
cells in the same nucleus with very prominent processes. c) ChAT-
positive staining of cells of the nucleus motorius nervi trigemini.
d) ChAT-positive staining of the nucleus vestibularis. The cells
are relatively weakly stained and do not demonstrate prominent
processes. Bars = 50 μm

The Vestibular System

As previously reported for the cat[21] and rat[24], minor staining of cells for ChAT has been found in the human in components of the vestibular (and possibly auditory) system. These include cells in the nucleus vestibularis lateralis and nuclei olivaris superioris medialis and lateralis (Figure 4d).

The Red Nucleus

Magnocellular neurons of the red nucleus have been reported to stain positively for ChAT in the cat[21] and rat[24,34] and to accumulate radioactive choline by retrograde flow from the spinal cord[40]. This would suggest that the rubrospinal tract may be partially cholinergic. In the human, however, we have not seen strongly ChAT-positive cells in this area although there were strongly AChE-positive cells. It is not known whether this is a species difference or a relative insensitivity of the ChAT immunohistochemical method in human tissue

USEFULNESS OF ACHE HISTOCHEMISTRY

In the forebrain, AChE histochemistry, particularly after pretreatment of animals with DFP, seems to be a very useful tool for the detection of most cholinergic neurons[10]. AChE histochemistry, without DFP pretreatment, is useful in identifying cholinergic neurons of the medial basal forebrain complex but the cholinergic neurons of the neostriatum and nucleus accumbens are generally obscured by the dense staining of the neuropile.

In the brain stem, AChE histochemistry, even with DFP pretreatment, is not very useful in identifying cholinergic neurons because so many non-cholinergic neurons are AChE-intensive. These include, for example, the catecholamine and serotonin neurons of the substantia nigra, locus coeruleus and raphe. In the human, of course, pretreatment with DFP is not possible. The AChE-positive structures of human hindbrain have been mapped using a highly sensitive modification of the Karnovsky and Roots[41] procedure. The type of staining obtained is exemplified in Figures 5a and 5b. Under these conditions, all ChAT-positive cells are also AChE-positive (Figure 5a). In

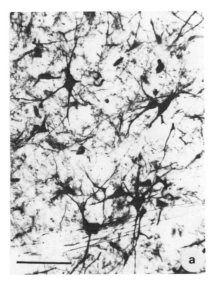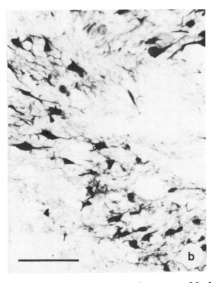

Fig. 5. a) AChE-positive staining of cells of the nucleus gigantocellularis (compare with Figs. 4a,b). b) AChE-positive staining of cells of the nucleus gracilis. Bars = 50 μm.

addition, however, as exemplified in Figures 3a and 5b, many ChAT-negative neurons stain for AChE. Besides the previously mentioned catecholamine and serotonin neurons, such cells were noted in several sensory systems, including the nuclei gracilis and cuneatus, all of the sensory nuclei of the Vth nerve, the tractus solitarius and the auditory and vestibular sensory nuclei, cells and fibers in the inferior and superior colliculi, as well as the nucleus intercollicularis . Also staining for AChE were cells in the pontine gray matter and arcuate nucleus. The inferior olive and the dorsal and medial olivary nuclei showed some AChE staining.

The significance of the AChE-positive staining in most of these structures remains to be determined. It may be that the cells are cholinoceptive, as many of them were so defined in the map of the cat brain[21]. That would mean that afferent AChE-containing fibers to these structures represent terminal fields for true cholinergic neurons. Future studies with more refined techniques will be necessary to define these details in the human and in other mammalian species.

The conditions necessary for AChE staining are far less exacting than those for ChAT. The high sensitivity of the method of Tago et al. (personal communication) for identifying AChE-positive structures, and particularly for AChE-positive fiber systems, may be especially useful in following changes associated with aging and disease in humans. Many of the appropriate associations between AChE-positive structures and true cholinergic cells have been revealed by the correlative study of ChAT- and AChE-positive staining[32]. It will be important to establish more exact connections in the future.

CHOLINERGIC PHARMACOLOGY AND PATHOLOGY

The cholinergic systems presented in Figure 1 are far from complete but they nevertheless suggest reasons why cholinergic agents possess their characteristic constellation of effects and why diseases affecting certain cholinergic systems may produce particular signs and symptoms.

Associating some of the known physiological actions of cholinergic stimulants and blockers with particular cell groups ignores the multiplicity of cholinergic receptors and the possible contribution of more than a single group or system to a given physiological action. Thus it must be regarded as no more than a rough indication of the possible division of cholinergic activity.

Cortical Cholinergic Pharmacology

The medial basal forebrain cholinergic system is associated with cortical function. It has long been recognized in animal work that cholinergic blockers produce memory deficits and confusion and that cholinergic agonists or cholinesterase inhibitors reverse the effect[42-46]. A clinical correlation is provided in Alzheimer's disease. In this disease, ChAT levels in the cortex and hippocampus are sharply decreased[46-49]. There is a concomitant loss of memory and cognition. More recently it has been shown that the decreases in ChAT are accompanied by a loss of cholinergic cells in the medial basal forebrain complex but not of muscarinic cholinergic receptors in postsynaptic areas of the cerebral cortex[12-13],[37-38],[50-54]. There also seems to be a loss of these cells during the normal aging process. Thus, the substantia innominata of a young individual will contain in excess of 450,000 cholinergic neurons. This declines to about 150,000 in the elderly, while Alzheimer's cases have less than 100,000 such cells[12],[38]. The dropout of cells during aging may help to explain the increasing incidence of Alzheimer's disease with age[55], as well as the increasing effects on memory

of cholinergic blockade. For example, young dystonia muscularum deformans
cases can tolerate far higher doses of Artane than elderly Parkinsonians
before memory deficit occurs[18]. Cholinergic stimulants or AChE inhibitors
may be of some benefit in Alzheimer's disease[46,56].

Extrapyramidal Cholinergic Pharmacology

Cholinergic stimulation induces tremor while cholinergic blockade partially overcomes the akinesia, rigidity and tremor of Parkinson's disease
and drug-induced Parkinsonism[57]. The existence of a cholinergic-dopaminergic balance in the extrapyramidal system was postulated over twenty years
ago[58], well before the existence of striatal cholinergic interneurons was
established through the technique of chemical lesioning[59]. The actual visualization of these interneurons by immunohistochemistry was thus anticipated. However, much is yet to be learned about the nature of intrastriatal
cholinergic cells, and the exact manner in which they contribute to extrapyramidal function.

Parabrachial Cholinergic Pharmacology

Only sketchy knowledge of this aspect of cholinergic pharmacology is
available, but it can be anticipated that it will grow substantially now
that the existence of such a prominent cholinergic cell complex is known.
The anatomical connections from the mixed neuronal population of this area
are mainly to rostral structures[60-61], such as the amygdala, diencephalon
and medial basal forebrain areas. The information carried from this part
of the nervous system is at least partially associated with gustatory function[62]. Descending connections also exist[63], which appear to be associated,
amongst other activities, with coordination of respiration[64-65] and regulation of blood pressure[66]. It is possible that this complex acts as a central parasympathetic ganglion in much the same way that the locus coeruleus
has been postulated to act as a central sympathetic ganglion. However, the
existence of connections from the dorsal pedunculopontine area to the midline thalamic nuclei is suggestive of a role in the recruiting mechanisms
associated with those thalamic areas. Characteristically, cholinergic agonists produce EEG desynchronization, corresponding to mental arousal and the
learning state[67]. This cholinergic group, along with the medial basal forebrain and reticular formation groups, could also represent the cholinergic
arousal mechanisms. Connections to the substantia nigra and subthalamic
nucleus are consistent with a role in movement[68]. Obviously this is a
fruitful area for future research.

Reticular Formation Cholinergic Pharmacology

Four cholinergic functions may be partially associated with the magnocellular and gigantocellular neurons of this region: antinociception, induction of REM sleep, cortical arousal and respiratory coordination. Descending connections from the reticular formation to the lamina of the posterior horn could be related to the pronounced antinociceptive action of
cholinomimetic agents[67,69-72]. The action of cholinergic agonists in promoting REM sleep when administered peripherally[67] can be mimicked by their
administration into the pontine gigantocellular reticular formation[73-75].
The effects of cholinergic agents on respiration could be related to centers
in the parabrachial, nucleus ambiguus or reticular formation regions. The
nature and location of brain stem respiratory centers is somewhat complicated[65] but maximal inspiratory responses have been obtained from stimulating
the gigantocellular reticular formation[76].

Poliomyelitis is a viral infection which attacks primarily anterior
horn cells. The bulbar form is frequently fatal, attacking primarily cholinergic cells from cranial nerve nuclei in the brain stem as well as the

reticular formation[16]. Respiratory complications are amongst the most severe of the deficits that develop, possibly due to the involvement of cells in the respiratory centers in the parabrachial and reticular areas as well as in the direct cholinergic motor systems.

Motor Nuclei Cholinergic Pharmacology

The concentration of large cholinergic neurons in cranial nerve nuclei found by immunohistochemistry was also anticipated in many historic studies of the cranial nerves themselves and the muscles and ganglia which they innervate. Nonetheless, the confirmation of these cellular groupings completes our knowledge of the direct cholinergic linkages between the CNS and the periphery and consolidates pharmacological information on peripheral cholinergic effects.

Vestibular Olivary Cholinergic Pharmacology

Cholinergic stimulation produces nausea and vomiting, while cholinergic blockade, as for example with scopolamine[77], combats motion sickness. While some of this effect is undoubtedly due to peripheral action, a central mechanism is suggested by the presence of cholinergic neurons in the vestibulo-olivary complex.

Cholinergic Function and Behavior

An intriguing aspect of cholinergic function that cannot yet be addressed from an anatomical point of view is that relating to behavior. Mood is down regulated by cholinergic stimulation. Manic patients have decreased symptoms following DFP[79] or physostigmine[20] administration. Normal persons experience depression, and depressed patients increased severity of symptoms. Atropine counteracts the effect[20,78-79]. While it has been suggested that cholinergic stimulation might improve schizophrenia[80], the situation is much less clear than with mood[20,79]. Presumably limbic cholinergic pathways are involved in these effects but no convincing pathology has been found in mental illness.

CONCLUSIONS

Immunohistochemical methods based on antibodies to ChAT have been used to define the main outlines of central cholinergic structures in several species, including humans. In turn, this information has permitted new interpretations of Alzheimer's and other diseases of the nervous system and has provided better insights into the pharmacology of cholinergic agents.

ACKNOWLEDGEMENTS

The authors wish to acknowledge the expert technical assistance of Joane Suzuki and Ronald Walker, as well as the help of the U.B.C. Department of Pathology and Mrs. M. Craig. This research was supported by the Medical Research Council of Canada, the Mr. and Mrs. P.A. Woodward's Foundation and the B.C. Medical Services Foundation.

REFERENCES

1. P. L. McGeer and E. G. McGeer, Cholinergic systems and cholinergic pathology, in: "Handbook of Neurochemistry, 2nd edition, Vol. 6," A. Lajtha, ed., Plenum Press, New York, 1984, pp. 379-410.
2. C. C. D. Shute and P. R. Lewis, Cholinesterase-containing systems of

the brain of the rat, Nature 199:1160 (1963)

3. P. R. Lewis and C. C. D. Shute, The cholinergic limbic system: Projections to the hippocampal formation, medial cortex, nuclei of the ascending cholinergic reticular system, and the subfornical organ and supraoptic crest, Brain 90:521 (1967).

4. V. Bigl, N. J. Woolf and L. L. Butcher, Cholinergic projections from the basal forebrain to frontal, parietal, temporal, occipital, and cingulate cortices: A combined fluorescent tracer and acetylcholinesterase analysis, Brain Res. Bull. 8:727 (1982).

5. L. L. Butcher, R. Marchand, A. Parent and L. J. Poirier, Morphological characteristics of acetylcholinesterase-containing neurons in the CNS of DFP-treated monkeys. Part 3. Brain stem and spinal cord, J. Neurol. Sci. 32:169 (1977).

6. A. Parent, L. J. Poirier, R. Boucher and L. L. Butcher, Morphological characteristics of acetylcholinesterase containing neurons in the CNS of DFP-treated monkeys. Part 2. Diencephalic and medial telencephalic structures, J. Neurol. Sci. 32:9 (1977).

7. L. J. Poirier, A. Parent, R. Marchand and L. L. Butcher, Morphological characteristics of acetylcholinesterase containing neurons in the CNS of DFP-treated monkeys. Part 1. Extrapyramidal and related structures, J. Neurol. Sci. 31:181 (1977).

8. K. Satoh, D. M. Armstrong and H. C. Fibiger, A comparison of the distribution of central cholinergic neurons as demonstrated by acetylcholinesterase pharmacohistochemistry and choline acetyltransferase immunohistochemistry, Brain. Res. Bull. 11:693 (1983).

9. F. Eckenstein and M. V. Sofroniew, Identification of central cholinergic neurons containing both choline acetyltransferase and acetylcholinesterase and of central neurons containing only acetylcholinesterase, J. Neurosci. 3:2286 (1983).

10. J. Lehmann and H. C. Fibiger, Minireview: Acetylcholinesterase and the cholinergic neuron, Life Sci. 25:1939 (1979).

11. P. L. McGeer, E. G. McGeer and J. H. Peng, Choline acetyltransferase purification and immunohistochemical localization, Life Sci. 34:2319 (1984).

12. P. L. McGeer, E. G. McGeer, J. Suzuki, C. E. Dolman and T. Nagai, Aging, Alzheimer's disease and the cholinergic system of the basal forebrain, Neurology, 34:741 (1984).

13. P. J. Whitehouse, D. L. Price, R. G. Struble, A. W. Clark, J. T. Coyle and M. R. DeLong, Alzheimer's disease and senile dementia: loss of neurons in the basal forebrain, Science 215:1237 (1982).

14. Y. Nagata, M. Okuya, R. Watanabe and M. Honda, Regional distribution of cholinergic neurons in human spinal cord transections in the patients with and without motor neuron disease, Brain Res. 244:223 (1982).

15. P. J. Whitehouse, J. C. Hedreen, C. L. White and D. L. Price, Basal forebrain neurons in the dementia of Parkinson disease, Ann. Neurol. 13:143 (1983).

16. D. Bodian, in: "Pathology of the Nervous System," J. Minckler (ed), McGraw Hill, New York (1972) pp 2323-2344.

17. H. Kimura, Y. Kaneko and J. A. Wada, Catecholamine and cholinergic systems and amygdala kindling, in: "Kindling 2," J.A. Wada, ed., Raven Press, New York (1981) pp. 265-287.

18. S. Fahn, High dosage anticholinergic therapy in dystonia, Neurology, 33:1255 (1983).

19. S. Guibaud, A. Simplot and A. Mercatello, CSF acetylcholinesterase in Guillain-Barré syndrome, Lancet 2:1456 (1982).

20. D. S. Janowsky and S. C. Risch, Cholinomimetic and anticholinergic drugs used to investigate an acetylcholine hypothesis of affective disorders and stress, Drug Develop. Res. 4:125 (1984).

21. H. Kimura, P. L. McGeer, J. H. Peng and E. G. McGeer, The central cholinergic system studied by choline acetyltransferase immunohistochemistry in the cat, J. Comp. Neurol. 200:151 (1981).

22. D. M. Armstrong, C. B. Saper, A. I. Levey, B. H. Wainer and R. D. Terry, Distribution of cholinergic neurons in rat brain: Demonstrated by the immunocytochemical localization of choline acetyltransferase, J. Comp. Neurol. 216:53 (1983).

23. C. R. Houser, G. D. Crawford, R. P. Barber, P. M. Salvaterra and J. E. Vaughn, Organization and morphological characterstics of cholinergic neurons: An immunocytochemical study with a monoclonal antibody to choline acetyltransferase, Brain Res. 266:97 (1983).

24. H. Kimura, P. L. McGeer and J. H. Peng, Choline acetyltransferase-containing neurons in the rat brain, in: "Handbook of Chemical Neuroanatomy, Vol. 3," A. Bjorklund, T. Hokfelt and M.J. Kuhar, eds., Elsevier Scientific Publishing Co., Amsterdam (1984) pp. 51-67.

25. A. I. Levey, B. H. Wainer, E. J. Mufson and M. M. Mesulam, Colocalization of acetylcholinesterase and choline acetyltransferase in the rat cerebrum, Neuroscience 9:9 (1983).

26. M. V. Sofroniew, F. Eckenstein, H. Thoenen and A. C. Cuello, Topography of choline acetyltransferase-containing neurons in the forebrain of the rat, Neurosci. Lett. 33:7 (1982).

27. C. R. Houser, G. D. Crawford, P. M. Salvaterra and J. E. Vaughn, Immunocytochemical localization of choline acetyltransferase in rat cerebral cortex: A study of cholinergic neurons and synapses, J. Comp. Neurol. 234:17 (1985).

28. J. C. Hedreen, S. J. Bacon, L. C. Cork, C. A. Kitt, G. D. Crawford, P. M. Salvaterra and D. L. Price, Immunocytochemical identification of cholinergic neurons in the monkey central nervous system using monoclonal antibodies against choline acetyltransferase, Neurosci. Lett. 43:173 (1983).

29. M. M. Mesulam, E. J. Mufson, A. I. Levey and B. H. Wainer, Cholinergic innervation of cortex by the basal forebrain: cytochemistry and cortical connections of the septal area, diagonal band nuclei, nucleus basalis (substantia innominata) and hypothalamus in the rhesus monkey, J. Comp. Neurol. 214:170 (1983).

30. M. M. Mesulam, E. J. Mufson, A. I. Levey and B. H. Wainer, Atlas of cholinergic neurons in the forebrain and upper brainstem of the macque based on monoclonal choline acetyltransferse immunohistochemistry and acetylcholinesterase histochemistry, Neuroscience 12:669 (1984).

31. K. Satoh and H. C. Fibiger, Distribution of central cholinergic neurons in the baboon (Papio papio). I. General morphology, J. Comp. Neurol. 236:197 (1985).

32. K. Mizukawa, P. L. McGeer, H. Tago, J. H. Peng, E. G. McGeer and H. Kimura, The cholinergic system of the human hindbrain studied by choline acetyltransferase immunohistochemistry and acetylcholinesterase histochemistry, Brain Res. (in press).

33. D. A. Matthews, P. M. Salvaterra, G. D. Crawford, C. R. Houser and J. E. Vaughn, Distribution of choline acetyltransferase positive neurons and terminals in hippocampus, Soc. Neurosci. Abstrs. 9:79 (1983).

34. M. V. Sofroniew, F. Eckstein, H. Thoenen and A.C. Cuello, Immunohistochemistry of choline acetyltransferase in the rat brain, Soc. Neurosci. Abstrs 8:516 (1982).

35. T. Hattori, E. G. McGeer, V. K. Singh and P. L. McGeer, Cholinergic synapse of the interpeduncular nucleus, Exp. Neurol. 55:666 (1977).

36. T. Nagai, T. Pearson, J. H. Peng, E. G. McGeer and P. L. McGeer, Immunohistochemical staining of the human forebrain with monoclonal antibody to human choline acetyltransferase, Brain Res. 265:300 (1983).

37. T. Nagai, P. L. McGeer, J. H. Peng, E. G. McGeer and C. E. Dolman, Choline acetyltransferase immunohistochemistry in brains of Alzheimer's disease patients and controls, Neurosci. Lett. 36:195 (1983).

38. P. L. McGeer, Aging, Alzheimer's disease and the cholinergic system, Can. J. Physiol. Pharmacol. 52:741 (1984).

39. J. C. Hedreen, R. G. Struble, P. J. Whitehouse and D.P. Price, Topography of the magnocellular basal forebrain system in human brain, J.

Neuropath. Exp. Neurol. 43:1 (1984).

40. M. F. Pare, B. E. Jones and A. Beaudet, Application of a selective retrograde labeling technique to the identification of acetylcholine subcortispinal neurons, Soc. Neurosci. Abstrs. 8:517 (1982).

41. M. J. Karnovsky and L. Roots, A 'direct-coloring' thiocholine method for cholinesterase, J. Histochem. Cytochem. 12:219 (1964).

42. D. A. Drachman and J. Leavitt, Human memory and the cholinergic system: a relationship to aging? Arch. Neurol. 30:113 (1974).

43. D. J. Safer and R. P. Allen, The central effects of scopolamine in man, Biol. Psychiatry 3:347 (1971).

44. J. A. Deutsch, The cholinergic synapse and the site of memory, Science 174:788 (1971).

45. K. L. Davis, R. C. Mohs and J. R. Tinklenberg, Enhancement of memory by physostigmine, New Eng. J. Med. 301:946 (1979).

46. R. T. Bartus, R. L. Dean, B. Beer and A. S. Lippa, The cholinergic hypothesis of geriatric memory dysfunction, Science 217:408 (1979).

47. D. M. Bowen, C. B. Smith, P. White and A. N. Davison, Neurotransmitter-related enzymes and indices of hypoxia in senile dementia and other abiotrophies, Brain 99:459 (1976).

48. P. Davies and A. J. R. Maloney, Selective loss of central cholinergic neurons in Alzheimer's disease, Lancet 1976ii:1403.

49. E. K. Perry, R. H. Perry, G. Blessed and B. E. Tomlinson, Necropsy evidence of central cholinergic deficits in senile dementia, Lancet 1977i:189.

50. P. J. Whitehouse, D. L. Price, A. W. Clark, J. T. Coyle and M. R. Delong, Alzheimer's disease: evidence for selective loss of cholinergic neurons in the nucleus basalis, Ann. Neurol. 10:122 (1981).

51. P. Davies and A. H. Verth, Regional distribution of muscarinic acetylcholine receptor in normal and Alzheimer's type dementia brains, Brain Res. 138:385 (1978).

52. W. Lang and H. Henke, Cholinergic receptor binding and autoradiography in brains of non-neurological and senile dementia of Alzheimer's type patients, Brain Res. 267:271 (1983).

53. J. M. Palacios, Autoradiographic localization of muscarinic cholinergic receptors in the hippocampus of patients with senile dementia, Brain Res. 243:173 (1982).

54. P. White, M .J. Goodhardt, J. P. Kent, C. R. Hiley, L. H. Carrasco, I. E. Williams and D. M. Bowen, Neocortical cholinergic neurons in elderly people, Lancet 1977i:668.

55. D. W. Kay, K. Bergman, E. M. Foster, A. A. McKechnie and M. Roth, Mental illness and hospital usage in the elderly: a random sample followed up, Compr. Psychiat. 11:26 (1970).

56. J. E. Christie, A. Shering, J. Ferguson and A. I. Glen, Physostigmine and arecoline: effects of intravenous infusions in Alzheimer presenile dementia, Br. J. Psychiatry 138:46 (1981).

57. P. L. McGeer, J. C. Boulding, W. C. Gibson and R. G. Foulkes, Drug-induced extrapyramidal reactions, J. Am. Med. Assoc. 177:665 (1961).

58. P. L. McGeer, Central amines and extrapyramidal functions, J. Neuropsych. 4:247 (1963).

59. P. L. McGeer, E. G. McGeer, H. C. Fibiger and V. Wickson, Neostriatal choline acetylase and cholinesterase following selective brain lesions, Brain Res. 35:308 (1971).

60. K. Voshart and D. van der Kooy, The organization of the efferent projections of the parabrachial nucleus to the forebrain in the rat: a retrograde fluorescent study, Brain Res. 212:271 (1981).

61. S. Nomura, N. Mizuno, K. Itoh, K. Matsuda, T. Sugimoto and Y. Nsksmurs, Localization of parabrachial nucleus neurons projecting to the thalamus or the amygdala in the cat using horseradish peroxidase, Exp. Neurol. 64: 375 (1979).

62. R. Norgren, Taste pathways to the hypothalamus and amygdala, J. Comp. Neurol. 166:17 (1976).

63. M. B. Carpenter and J. Sutin, "Human Neuroanatomy, 8th edition," Williams and Wilkins, Baltimore (1983) p. 291, 296, 334, 372.

64. F. Bertrand and A. Hugelin, Respiratory synchronizing function of nucleus parabrachialis medialis: pneumotaxic mechanisms, J. Neurophysiol. 34:189 (1971).

65. E. K. Bystrzycka, Afferent projections to the dorsal and ventral respiratory nuclei in the medulla oblongata of the cat studied by the horseradish peroxidase technique, Brain Res. 185:59 (1971).

66. S. Mraovitch, M. Kumada and D. J. Reis, Role of the nucleus parabrachialis in cardiovascular regulation in cat, Brain Res. 232:57 (1982).

67. A. G. Karczmar, Basic phenomena underlying novel use of cholinergic agents, anticholinesterases and precursors in neurological including peripheral and psychiatric disease, Adv. Behav. Biol. 25:853 (1981).

68. E. G. McGeer, W. A. Staines and P. L. McGeer. Neurotransmitters in the basal ganglia, Can. J. Neurol. Sci. 11:89 (1984).

69. S. Flodmark and T. Wramner, The analgetic action of morphine, eserine and prostigmine studied by a modified Hardy-Wolff-Goodell method, Acta Physiol. Scand. 9:88 (1945).

70. D. Slaughter and E. G. Gross, Some new aspects of morphine action. Effect on intestine and blood pressure; toxicity studies, J. Pharmacol. Exp. Ther. 68:96 (1940).

71. G. L. Koehn, G. Henderson and A. G. Karczmar, Diisopropyl phosphorfluoridate-induced antinociception: possible role of endogenous opioids, Eur. J. Pharmacol. 61:167 (1980).

72. N. W. Pedigo and W. L. Dewey, Acetylcholine induced antinociception: comparisons to opiate analgesia, Adv. Behav. Biol. 25:795 (1981).

73. J. A. Hobson, M. Goldberg, E. Vivadi and D. Riew, Enhancement of desynchronized sleep signs after pontine microinjection of the muscarinic agonist bethanechol, Brain Res. 275:127 (1983).

74. M. Jouvet, Telencephalic and rhombencephalic sleep in the cat, in: "The Nature of Sleep," G. E. W. Wolstenholme and M. O'Connor, eds. J.A. Churchill, London (1961) pp. 188-208,.

75. N. Sitaram, R. J. Wyatt, S. Dawson and J. C. Gillin, REM sleep induction by physostigmine infusion during sleep, Science 191:1281 (1976).

76. A. Torvik and A. Brodal, The origin of reticulospinal fibers in the cat, Anat. Rec. 128:113 (1957).

77. L. S. Goodman and A. Gilman, "The Pharmacological Basis of Therapeutics," 4th edition, Macmillan, New York (1970) p. 541.

78. D. W. Rowntree, S. Nevin and A. Wilson, Effects of diisopropylfluorophonate in schizophrenia and manic depressive psychosis, J. Neurol. Neurosurg. Psychiat. 13:47 (1950).

79. K. L. Davis, P. A. Berger, L. E. Hollister and J. D. Barchas, Minireview: Cholinergic involvement in mental disorders, Life Sci. 22:1865 (1978).

80. C. C. Pfeiffer and E. H. Jenney, The inhibition of the conditioned response and the counteraction of schizophrenia by muscarinic stimulation of the brain, Ann. N.Y. Acad. Sci. 66:753 (1957).

DEVELOPMENT OF THE ACETYLCHOLINE RECEPTOR CLUSTERS

INDUCED BY BASIC POLYPEPTIDES IN CULTURED MUSCLE CELLS

H. Benjamin Peng

Department of Anatomy, University of Illinois at Chicago
Present Address: Dept. of Anatomy, Laboratories for Cell
Biology, Univ. of North Carolina, Chapel Hill, N.C. 27514

INTRODUCTION

Vertebrate neuromuscular junction is marked by a concentration of acetylcholine receptors (AChR) in the postsynaptic membrane. From studies using electron-microscopic (EM) autoradiography, it has been estimated that there are over ten thousand AChR per square micron within the AChR cluster (1). This concentration of AChR is essential for the efficiency of the synaptic transmission and is the key event in the development of the postjunctional membrane. Tissue culture of neurons and muscle cells has provided a simple and convenient system to study this process. In monolayer cultures, the growth of the neurons and the establishment of the synaptic connection can be followed with high-resolution light microscopy and electron microscopy. The ease of being able to manipulate the preparation also gives it tremendous advantage in physiological and pharmacological studies over the in vivo systems.

During innervation, processes from the motoneurons grow to the muscle and induce the formation of the AChR clusters (2, 3). It is generally thought that the nerve terminal may release certain trophic molecules which induce the clustering process. Extracts from the brain or the spinal cord have been shown to increase the number of AChR clusters in cultured muscle cells (4-7). On the other hand, the molecules which induce AChR clustering may reside on the surface of neurites. Thus, the neuromuscular contact may cause a local perturbation of the muscle membrane and this may trigger the mechanism of AChR clustering. Such a pertubation may be mediated, for example, by an adhesion between the nerve and the muscle.

To test this hypothesis, we examined the effect of local application of highly adhesive molecules on the formation of AChR clusters in cultured muscle cells. Such surface is produced by coating latex spheres with positively charged polypeptide molecules, such as polylysine and polyornithine. Our results (8, 9) have shown that these molecules can induce a postsynaptic-type differentiation similar to that observed at the developing neuromuscular junction.

MATERIALS AND METHODS

Cell Cultures

Myotomal muscle cells were isolated from Xenopus laevis embryos according to the published methods (10, 11). In short, the dorsal part of the embryo, including the myotomes, the neural tube and the notochord, was cut out. The parts were dissociated with collagenase and each was further dissociated into single cells with Ca^{2+}, Mg^{2+}-free medium. For nerve-muscle cocultures, the collagenase dissociation step can be omitted. Muscle cultures were maintained at 15-22° up to a month. Since these cells carry their endogenous nutrient supply in the form of yolk platelets, they can be kept in culture with a simple medium. The one we routinely use is composed of Steinberg's solution (60 mM NaCl, 0.67 mM KCl, 0.34 mM $Ca(NO_3)_2$, 0.83 mM $MgSO_4$, and 10 mM HEPES buffer, pH 7.4), supplemented with 10% L-15 (Leibovitz) medium and 1% fetal bovine serum.

Visulization of AChR Clusters

Tetramethylrhodamine-conjugated α-bungarotoxin (R-BTX) was used to label the AChR. The preparation of this label followed that published by Ravdin and Axelrod (12). The cultures were labeled with R-BTX for 30 min at room temperature, fixed with 95% ethanol at -20°C and mounted on slide. The location of the AChR clusters, as evidenced by rhodamine fluorescence, and their position on the cell were examined with fluorescence and phase-contrast microscopy.

Preparation of Coated Latex Beads

Polystyrene latex beads with a diameter of 1-10 μm were coated with polypeptide molecules by absorption. The beads were incubated in a solution containing the peptide overnight at 4°C. They were then washed in phosphate-buffered saline (PBS) by repeated centrifugation and resuspension using a microcentrifuge. These beads can be stored in PBS at 4°C up to 4 weeks.

Electron Microscopy

Both thin-section and freeze-fracture electron microscopy were used in this study. The methods can be found in our previous publications (9, 11).

RESULTS

Formation of AChR Clusters Induced by Coated Latex Beads

When muscle cells treated with basic polypeptide-coated latex beads were examined with R-BTX fluorescence microscopy, a striking colocalization of the AChR clusters and the beads was observed. An example of the polyornithine bead-induced AChR clusters is shown in Fig. 1. These clusters are formed discretely at the bead-muscle contacts. The size of the clusters as well as their number can be controlled by varying the size and the number of the beads applied to the cell. For example, 4.5 μm beads cause the formation of clusters with a mean diameter of 8.4 ± 4.2 μm^2, whereas 10 μm beads cause the formation of clusters with a mean diameter of 17.9 ± 8.0 μm^2. Figure 2 shows that the number of bead-induced clusters is linearly related to the number of bead-muscle contacts. In this example, nearly every contact resulted in AChR clustering. On the average, one can expect 60-70% of the bead-muscle contacts to be associated with AChR clusters.

These bead-induced AChR clusters can also be easily studied in freeze-fracture replicas. As shown in Fig. 3, AChR, represented by 11-12 nm intramembranous particles, form aggregates at the bead-muscle contact. The entire cluster at the contact is composed of many such aggregates. This pattern is similar to the AChR cluster at the postsynaptic membrane, which is also composed of smaller subclusters.

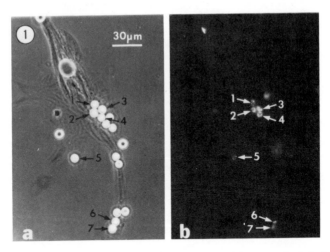

Fig. 1. AChR cluster induced by polyornithine-coated latex beads. a, phase-contrast micrograph showing the bead-muscle contacts; b, fluorescence micrograph showing the positions of the AChR clusters. The culture was labeled with tetramethyl rhodamine-conjugated α-bungarotoxin. The numbers in a and b indicate the correspondence in the positions of the beads and the AChR clusters.

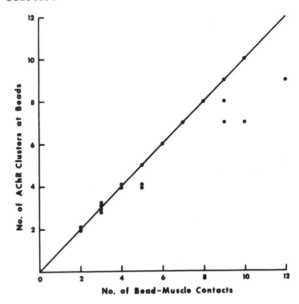

Fig. 2. A simple quantitation of effect of latex bead-induced AChR clustering. The ordinate shows the number of bead-induced AChR clusters. The abscissa shows the number of bead-muscle contacts. Each point represents one cell. In this culture, almost all the contacts are cluster-positive.

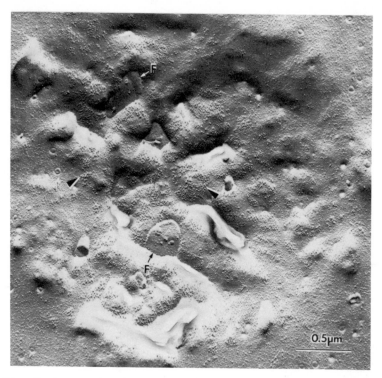

Fig. 3. Image of a bead-induced AChR cluster revealed with the
freeze-fracture technique. This is the protoplasmic face (P-
face) of the muscle cell. The bead has been fractured away,
leaving behind a shallow depression on the membrane. AChR
clusters appear as aggregates of 11-12 nm intramembranous
particles (arrowheads). A few membrane infoldings (F) can also
be observed. Areas between clusters are devoid of AChR
particles.

We have tested the effectiveness of a number of polypeptides on the
AChR clustering. The results are summarized in Table I. It can be seen
that basic polypeptides, including polylysine, polyornithine and
polyarginine, can all induce the formation of AChR clusters. Acidic
polypeptides, including polyglutamic acid and polyaspartic acid, are
ineffective. Neurotensin, which has arginine residues at positions 8-9,
is as effective as polyarginine. Uncoated beads are ineffective in
causing AChR clustering, although they do adhere to the cells. This
indicates that this phenomenon is not simply caused by a mechanical
perturbation.

Development of Other Postsynaptic Specializations

In addition to AChR clusters, the postsynaptic membrane at the
neuromuscular junction is marked a set of elaborate ultrastructural
specializations. These include the postsynaptic density, membrane
infoldings and the basement membrane. To understand whether the latex
beads can also induce these specializations, EM studies were conducted.
As shown in Fig. 4, all these structures characteristic of the
postsynaptic membrane were also formed at the bead-muscle contact. This
suggests that the process for the formation of AChR clusters is coupled
with the process for the development of these specializations.

Table I

Effects of Peptides on the Formation of AChR Clusters

Molecule[a]	% Beads associated with AChR clusters[b]
Poly-L-α-ornithine	62.7 ± 4.4
Poly-L-lysine (M.W. 3,000)	66.4 ± 4.4
Poly-L-lysine (M.W. 80,000)	62.6 ± 7.0
Poly-L-arginine	37.9 ± 3.9
Poly-L-aspartic acid	5.1 ± 2.5
Poly-L-glutamic acid	8.6 ± 3.2
Neurotensin	37.3 ± 3.5

[a]The peptide molecules were adsorbed onto polystyrene latex beads and applied to the muscle cultures. After a coculture period of 24 hr, the cultures were labeled with R-BTX and the relationship between the AChR clusters and the bead-muscle contacts was assayed with fluorescence and phase-contrast microscopy.

[b]Results from 20 cells in each culture were calculated. They are expressed as mean±S.E.M..

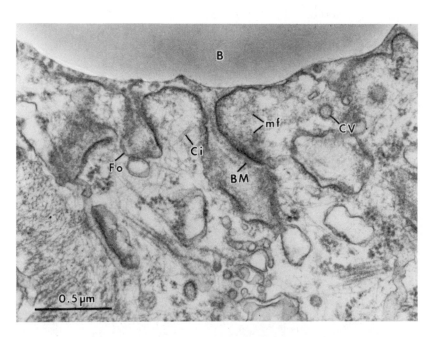

Fig. 4. Postsynaptic specializations at the AChR cluster induced by the basic polypeptide-coated latex bead. These include a membrane-associated cytoplasmic density, a meshwork of thin filaments (mf), basement membrane (BM), and membrane infoldings (Fo). Ci, smooth membrane cistern; CV, coated vesicle; B, bead.

The Cellular Mechanisms of AChR Clustering

Since the formation of AChR clusters can be induced by the beads at premarked location on the cell and at precisely controlled time, it offers a convenient system to examine the cellular mechanisms of AChR clustering. Two questions were asked: what is the signal for the AChR clustering and what is cellular machinery?

Involvement of Ca^{2+}. We hypothesize that the effect of the beads is mediated by an ionic mechanism triggered by a change in the membrane conductance resulting from the contact of the highly positive substrate with the cell membrane. Calcium, being the most important regulatory ion, may play a role in this process. Thus, we tested its involvement with Ca^{2+} antagonists. Our results showed that divalent cations Co^{2+}, Ni^{2+} at concentrations of 1-5 mM or organic compounds verapamil and D-600 at concentrations of 0.1-0.5 mM reversibly inhibit the formation of the bead-induced AChR clustering (13). Furthermore, calmodulin inhibitors such as trifluoperazine and W-7 at concentrations of 1-20 μM also inhibit this process (13). These results suggest that a local Ca^{2+} and calmodulin-mediated process may be involved in activating the clustering process.

Cellular Machinery. To understand the machinery of AChR clustering, we conducted EM studies at different times after the addition of the beads to determine which structure is related to the clustering process. Our studies show that the onset of the clustering process follows immediately the addition of the beads (14). Thus, the structures which may serve as the machinery should be detectable at equally early time. Our EM studies were thus concentrated on early (<1 hr) bead-muscle cocultures. As shown in Fig. 5, the earliest specialization at the bead-muscle contact is a meshwork of thin filaments. These filaments have a diameter of 5-6 nm and are identical to the actin filaments in myofibrils. Other organelles, except a system of smooth endoplasmic reticulum similar to the sarcoplasmic reticulum, are excluded from the cell cortex occupied by this meshwork. This suggests that this actin-containing cytoskeletal meshwork is assembled prior to the formation of the AChR clusters. Studies are underway to elucidate the function of this meshwork as related to the formation of the AChR clusters.

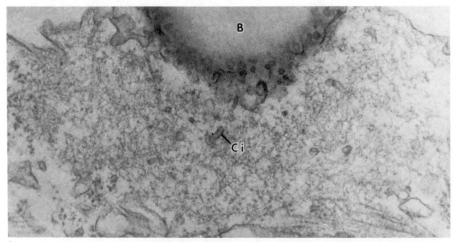

Fig. 5. A meshwork of thin filaments at the bead-muscle contact at 1 hr after the addition of the beads to the culture. B, bead; Ci, smooth endoplasmic reticulum. This micrograph is at the same magnification as Fig. 4.

DISCUSSION

This study demonstrates the usefulness of a simple model system involving coated latex beads and cultured muscle cells for the study of the neuromuscular junction development. Although this paper only discusses the postsynaptic development, our recent studies have shown that these beads can also induce the presynaptic differentiation in the form of an aggregation of synaptic vesicles when applied to spinal cord explants from Xenopus embryos. Thus, this approach can be used to study the entire synaptogenesis at the neuromuscular junction. Previous studies have also demonstrated its potential in understanding synaptogenesis in central nervous system (15).

These results clearly showed that the muscle cell is equipped with the machinery for the postsynaptic differentiation. Nerve contact seems merely to dictate the position of this process. It also suggests that the trophic molecule used in this process may be a basic peptide molecule. In this respect, it is interesting to note that the basic neuropeptide neurotensin is also effective in inducing the clustering process. Neuropeptides have been shown to function as neurotransmitters or modulators. To that list, one may soon add its role as a trophic molecule as this study suggests. Our present method of coating the latex beads is via a simple adsorption of ligands to the beads. In future studies, we plan to link the ligands and the beads covalently. This should greatly increase the versatility of this method.

The data presented in this paper suggest the involvement of Ca^{2+} and calmodulin in the activation of the AChR clustering process. We envision that the latex bead, because of its charged surface, may cause a perturbation of the membrane and and this may lead to an influx of Ca^{2+} into the cell. The resultant increase in the local calcium concentration may trigger the clustering process. This hypothesis is schematically represented in Fig. 6. The machinery, represented by the distribution of the calmodulin molecules, appears to be uniformly distributed in the cell as our recent data suggest (13). It may be locally activated by the latex bead or by the nerve.

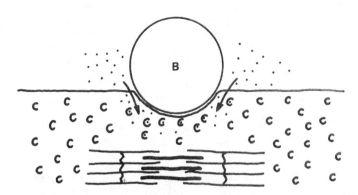

Fig. 6. Model of the bead muscle interaction. The contact of the basic polypeptide-coated bead (B) is thought to induce a local influx of calcium (represented by dots) into the cell. This elevates the local concentration of this ion, which binds to the calmodulin molecule (C) and activates the clustering process.

The machinery for the formation of the AChR clusters seems to involve the cytoskeleton. However, the nature of the interaction between the AChR and the cytoskeleton is not yet known. AChR-rich postsynaptic membranes isolated from Torpedo electric organ contains a number of other proteins in addition to the receptors (16). One of these proteins with a molecular weight of 43K has been found to colocalize with the cytoplasmic side of AChR clusters in Torpedo and in skeletal muscle (17). Our recent study has shown that this protein is also associated with the new AChR clusters induced by the latex beads (18). Thus, this postsynaptic 43K protein may be involved in mediating the interaction between the AChR and the cytoskeleton. By utilizing this model system as described in this paper, we hope to understand the principle of the postsynaptic differentiation at the neuromuscular junction.

ACKNOWLEDGEMENT

The author gratefully acknowledges the support of NIH (grant no. NS-16259) and the Muscular Dystrophy Association on this project.

REFERENCES

1. Fertuck, H.C., and M.M. Salpeter. 1976. Quantitation of junctional and extrajunctional acetylcholine receptors by electron microscope autoradiography after ^{125}I-α-bungarotoxin binding at mouse neuromuscular junctions. J. Cell Biol. 69:144-158.
2. Anderson, M.J., and M.W. Cohen. 1977. Nerve-induced and spontaneous redistribution of acetylcholine receptors on cultured muscle cells. J. Physiol. (Lond.). 268:757-773.
3. Frank, E., and G.D. Fischbach. 1979. Early events in neuromuscular junction formation in vitro. J. Cell Biol. 83:143-158.
4. Podleski, T.R., D. Axelrod, P. Ravdin, I. Greenberg, M.M. Johnson, and M.M. Salpeter. 1978. Nerve extract induces increase and redistribution of acetylcholine receptors on cultured muscle cells. Proc. Natl. Acad. Sci. USA. 75:2035-2039.
5. Jessell, T.M., R.E. Siegel, and G.D. Fischbach. 1979. Induction of acetylcholine receptors on cultured skeletal muscle by a factor extracted from brain and spinal cord. Proc. Natl. Acad. Sci. USA. 76:5397-5401.
6. Christian, C.N., M.P. Daniels, H. Sugiyama, Z. Vogel, L. Jacques, and P.G. Nelson. 1978. A factor from neurons increases the number of acetylcholine receptor aggregates on cultured muscle cells. Proc. Natl. Acad. Sci. USA. 75:4011-4015.
7. Schaffner, A.E., and M.P. Daniels. 1982. Conditioned medium from cultures of embryonic neurons contains a high molecular weight factor which induces acetylcholine receptor aggregation on cultured myotubes. J. Neurosci. 2:623-632.
8. Peng, H. B., P.-C. Cheng, and P. W. Luther. 1981. Formation of ACh receptor clusters induced by positively charged latex beads. Nature. 292:831-834.
9. Peng, H. B., and P.-C. Cheng. 1982. Formation of postsynaptic specializations induced by latex beads in cultured muscle cells. J. Neurosci. 2:1760-1774.
10. Anderson, M.J., M.W. Cohen, and E. Zorychta. 1977. Effects of innervation on the distribution of acetylcholine receptors on cultured muscle cells. J. Physiol. (Lond.). 268:731-756.
11. Peng, H.B., and Y. Nakajima. 1978. Membrane particle aggregates in innervated and noninnervated cultures of Xenopus embryonic muscle cells. Proc. Natl. Acad. Sci. USA. 75:500-504.
12. Ravdin, P., and D. Axelrod. 1977. Fluorescent tetramethyl rhodamine derivatives of α-bungarotoxin: preparation, separation and charaterization. Anal. Biochem. 80:585-592.

13. Peng, H.B. 1984. Participation of calcium and calmodulin in the formation of acetylcholine receptor clusters. J. Cell Biol. 98:550-557.
14. Peng, H.B., and K.A. Phelan. 1984. Early cytoplasmic specialization at the presumptive acetylcholine receptor cluster: a meshwork of thin filaments. J. Cell Biol. 99:344-349.
15. Burry, R.W., D.A. Kniss, and L.R. Scribner. 1984. Mechanisms of synapse formation and maturation. In "Current topics in research on synapses", Ed. E.G.Jones. Vol. 1, pp. 1-51. Allan R. Liss, Inc., New York.
16. Froehner, S.C. 1984. Peripheral proteins of postsynaptic membranes from Torpedo electric organ identified with monoclonal antibodies. J. Cell Biol. 99:88-96.
17. Froehner, S.C., V. Gulbrandsen, C. Hyman, A.Y. Jeng, R.R. Neubig, and J. B. Cohen. 1981. Immunofluorescence localization at the mammalian neuromuscular junction of the M_r 43,000 protein of Torpedo post-synaptic membranes. Proc. Natl. Acad. Sci. USA. 78:5230-5234.
18. Peng, H.B., and S.C. Froehner. 1985. Association of the postsynaptic 43K protein with newly formed acetylcholine receptor clusters in cultured muscle cells. J. Cell Biol. 100:1698-1795.

CHARACTERISTICS OF CHOLINERGIC SYNAPSES

IN NEUROBLASTOMA MYOTUBE CO-CULTURES

Michael Adler[1], Sharon Reutter[1], Sharad S. Deshpande[2],
C. Sue Hudson[2] and Margaret G. Filbert[1]

[1]Neurotoxicology Branch, U. S. Army Medical Research
Institute of Chemical Defense, Aberdeen Proving Ground
MD 21010-5425; [2]Department of Pharmacology and
Experimental Therapeutics, University of Maryland
School of Medicine, Baltimore, MD 21201

INTRODUCTION

Cultures of continuous cell lines have proved useful for studying excitation-secretion coupling. Such cell lines enable the investigator to perform
both biochemical and electrophysiological experiments on a relatively homogeneous cell population and to manipulate the state of cellular differentiation
by suitable alterations of culture conditions. Among the better characterized cell lines are those derived from the C-1300 neuroblastoma tumor
(Augusti-Tocco and Sato, 1969). A number of cholinergic and adrenergic
clones have been isolated from this murine tumor. They were shown to synthesize, store and release the appropriate neurotransmitters and to generate
action potentials following electrical stimulation. Fusion of the neuroblastoma clone N18TG-2 with the glioma cell line C6BU-1 has yielded the hybrid
NG108-15 (Amano et al., 1974) with enhanced electrical excitability and the
ability to form nicotinic cholinergic synapses when co-cultured with primary
or clonal myotubes (Nelson et al., 1976; Christian et al., 1977).

The synapses formed in co-cultures of NG108-15 cells and myotubes resemble those observed during early stages of skeletal muscle synaptogenesis in
vivo (Redfern, 1970; Dennis, 1975; Betz, 1976). Common features include
polyneuronal innervation, extrajunctional acetylcholine (ACh) sensitivity,

low acetylcholinesterase (AChE) activity and tetrodotoxin (TTX)-insensitive muscle action potentials. The spontaneous quantal discharges, in both systems, have a relatively low frequency, a slow time course and a skewed amplitude distribution (Diamond and Miledi, 1962).

In the present study, we examined some general properties of neuroblastoma/myotube co-cultures to determine their suitability as models for cholinergic synaptic transmission and neuromuscular development. To achieve this aim, we investigated the effects of external Ca^{2+}, osmotic strength, membrane potential and AChE activity on spontaneous miniature synaptic potentials (MSPs) in NG108-15/myotube synapses. The results indicate that MSP frequencies depend on Ca^{2+}, osmotic strength and nerve terminal depolarization. The synaptic potentials are, however, insensitive to variations in AChE levels.

MATERIALS AND METHODS

Culture Techniques

Neuroblastoma. Unless indicated otherwise, co-cultures were formed with the hybrid cell NG108-15 and primary rat myotubes. NG108-15 cells were grown in a humidified atmosphere of 10% CO_2/90% air in Dulbecco's modified Eagle's medium (DMEM, GIBCO) supplemented with 10% fetal bovine serum, 10^{-4} M hypoxanthine, 10^{-6} M aminopterin and 1.6×10^{-5} M thymidine. The neuroblastoma clone NS-26 was grown in DMEM and 10% fetal bovine serum.

Myotubes. Primary myotubes were obtained from hindlimb muscles of 1-3 day neonatal Wistar rats. Minced tissue fragments were incubated in 0.1% trypsin (Sigma) in Ca^{2+}-Mg^{2+}-free phosphate-buffered saline for 30 min and dissociated by trituration. The cell suspension was pelleted, resuspended in DMEM and preplated for 40-60 min to reduce the population of fibroblasts. The remaining suspension, enriched in myoblasts, was collected and passed through a Nitex 135 filter to remove large cellular aggregates. Myoblasts $(1-3 \times 10^5)$ were plated in 35 mm collagen-coated dishes and grown in DMEM with 10% fetal bovine serum and 10% heat-inactivated horse serum. Fusion of myoblasts to multinucleated myotubes was evident after 2 days. At this time, bovine serum was removed, and cells were fed with DMEM containing 10^{-5} M 5'-fluorodeoxyuridine and 10^{-4} M uridine to inhibit proliferation of fibroblasts and dividing myoblasts. The antimitotic agents were removed 2-3 days later. In some experiments clonal G8-1 myotubes were used (Christian et al.,

1977; Sugiyama, 1977; Adler et al., 1986). These were cultured essentially
as described above.

Co-culture. Dishes with 4-7 day myotubes were seeded with 2×10^5
NG108-15 cells and maintained in 90% DMEM, 10% horse serum, 10^{-4} M hypoxanthine, 1.6×10^{-5} M thymidine and 10^{-3} M dibutyryl cyclic adenosine monophosphate (dBcAMP). The latter was included to promote neuronal differentiation (Nirenberg et al., 1983).

Electrophysiology

For intracellular recordings, co-cultures were transferred to the heated
stage (37° C) of a Zeiss inverted microscope and superfused with a modified
Krebs-Ringer solution of the following composition (mM): NaCl, 145; KCl,
5.4; $CaCl_2$, 3.8; $MgCl_2$, 0.8; glucose, 25; choline, 0.075 and Hepes/NaOH, 10.
Cells were impaled with 3 M KCl-filled microelectrodes (10-30 megohms). ACh
potentials were elicited by iontophoretic application of agonist from high
resistance pipettes (150-200 megohms) filled with 2 M ACh. Single ACh channel currents were recorded by the improved patch-clamp technique (Hamill et
al., 1981). Data were low pass filtered at 1-5 kHz. Miniature endplate
currents were recorded from adult rat diaphragm muscle by a conventional two-
microelectrode voltage-clamp technique (Takeuchi and Takeuchi, 1959).

RESULTS AND DISCUSSION

Properties of Neuroblastoma/Myotube Synaptic Potentials

Synaptic transmission was investigated in the co-cultures by recording
from myotubes that appeared to be in contact with NG108-15 (or NS-26) neurites or soma. Functional innervation of myotubes was indicated by the presence of spontaneous MSPs. These MSPs resemble spontaneous miniature end-
plate potentials (MEPPs) of vertebrate skeletal muscle, and the available
evidence suggests that each results from the action of a single quantum of
ACh on postsynaptic nicotinic receptors (Del Castillo and Katz, 1954; Nelson
et al., 1976; Ceccarelli and Hurlbut, 1980). We have avoided designating the
myotube synaptic responses as MEPPs since junctional specializations characteristic of mature motor endplates are not generally observed on myotubes
(Nelson et al., 1978).

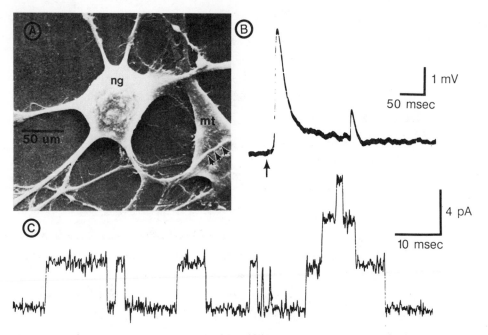

Fig. 1. Characteristics of NG108-15/myotube synapses. A. Scanning electron
micrograph of an NG108-15 cell (ng) in apparent synaptic contact with a myotube (mt) at the region indicated by arrowheads. B. ACh potential with a
spontaneous MSP on its decay phase. ACh was delivered by a brief iontophoretic pulse (6.6 nA, 0.3 msec) at the time indicated by the arrow.
C. Outside-out patch excised from a myotube perisynaptic region showing
single ACh channel currents. The patch pipette was filled with a high K^+
solution containing (mM): KCl, 140; $CaCl_2$, 0.55; EGTA, 1.1; $MgCl_2$, 2;
glucose, 25; Hepes/KOH, 10. The bath was maintained at 37° C and perfused
with physiological solution (see "Methods") containing 5×10^{-7} M ACh. The
membrane potential was -100 mV.

Fig. 1A shows a low power scanning electron micrograph of an NG108-15/
myotube co-culture incubated for 1 week in growth medium supplemented with
10^{-3} M dBcAMP. Treatment by dBcAMP caused somal enlargement, extensive process arborization, increased electrical excitability and enhanced secretory
activity. Cells thus treated showed a greater probability of forming functional synaptic connections than did untreated cells grown under otherwise
identical conditions (Higashida et al., 1978; Nirenberg et al., 1983). The
differentiation induced by dBcAMP appears to be exerted on the presynaptic
cell alone since no corresponding alterations have been observed on pure
myotube cultures.

The region of nerve-muscle contact is associated with high ACh sensitivity, as illustrated in Fig. 1B. The first potential was elicited with a
brief iontophoretic pulse delivered near a contacting neurite. The second
response is a spontaneous MSP with a comparable rise time. The ACh sensitivity at this junction was 2071 mV/nC. Sensitivities at other NG108-15/myo-
tube contacts ranged from 817 to 2469 mV/nC. Such high values are typical of
innervated regions of myotube and arise from neurally induced aggregation of
ACh receptors (Cohen and Fischbach, 1977). Postjunctional myotube ACh sensitivities are similar to those encountered at the adult neuromuscular junction
(Kuffler and Yoshikami, 1975; Land et al., 1977; Peper et al., 1982).

Synaptic responses at NG108-15/myotube junctions have a pharmacological
profile consistent with nicotinic receptors. Thus, ACh potentials, as well
as spontaneous and evoked synaptic potentials, are blocked by d-tubocurarine
and α-bungarotoxin (Christian et al., 1978), but not by low concentrations of
muscarinic antagonists such as atropine.

Nicotinic ACh channels responsible for the ACh potential and MSP have
been studied extensively since the introduction of the gigaohm seal patch-
clamp technique (Hamill et al., 1981). Fig. 1C shows a brief segment of data
from an outside-out membrane patch excised from a perisynaptic region.
Single channel currents were elicited by bathing the patch in physiological
solution containing 5×10^{-7} M ACh. Three superimposed openings are seen
near the end of the records, indicating that at least three ACh channels were
present in this patch. The channel open-time distributions were biphasic,
with a fast component of 0.16 msec and a slower component of 1.82 msec. The
former is likely to be an underestimate due to bandwidth limitations of the
recording system (Hamill et al., 1981). The slower time constant is within
the range reported by fluctuation analysis for myotube ACh channels (Rubin et
al., 1980). Values for single channel lifetimes did not depend on whether
measurements were made proximal to, or distal from, NG108-15 processes. This
differs from findings in adult muscle in which junctional and extrajunctional
receptors constitute separate populations with different open times (Peper et
al., 1982).

When NG108-15 cells are co-cultured with primary rat myotubes, under conditions similar to those used in this study, the majority of muscle fibers in
contact with hybrid neurites are found to generate MSPs (Nelson et al., 1976;
Higashida et al., 1978). A high efficiency of innervation has also been observed in NBr10A (N18TG-2 x BRL30-E)/myotube co-cultures (Higashida et al.,
1978). In contrast, non-hybrid neuroblastoma cell lines have generally been

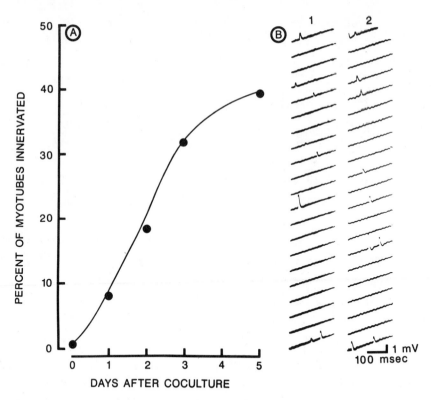

Fig. 2. Synapses between neuroblastoma clone NS-26 and primary rat myotubes. A. Percent of myotubes with functional synapses at various times after 1.3×10^5 NS-26 cells were seeded on a monolayer of myotubes. Co-cultures were maintained in 90% DMEM, 10% horse serum and 10^{-3} M dBcAMP. Myotubes selected for impalement were those in contact with NS-26 neurites or soma; 40% of such myotubes displayed MSPs 5 days after co-culture. B. Representative MSPs from NS-26/myotube pairs recorded 3 days (1) and 5 days (2) after co-culture. A small afterhyperpolarization is evident following the decay of some MSPs.

thought to innervate only a small fraction of the available postsynaptic target cells. A notable exception is the tetraploid neuroblastoma clone NS-26. Fig. 2A shows the percent of myotubes with MSPs after addition of a suspension of NS-26 cells. No synapses were detected within the first 2 hours of seeding; however, by day 1 nearly 10% of the myotubes were functionally innervated. The percent of innervated myotubes increased rapidly over the next 2 days and more gradually thereafter, reaching a maximum of 40% at 5 days. These levels were maintained for the subsequent 3 days but then declined as cultures deteriorated from overgrowth of NS-26 cells and atrophy

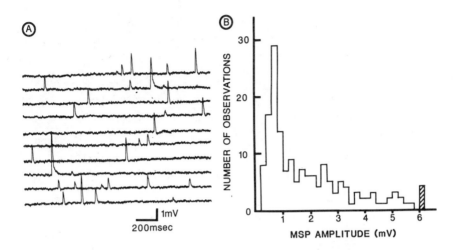

Fig. 3. A. Traces showing spontaneous MSPs from an NG108-15/myotube synapse. Note the marked variations in MSP amplitudes and their unusually high frequency. B. Histogram showing skewed distribution of MSP amplitudes. TTX (10^{-6} M) was added to inhibit spontaneous action potentials. The stippled bar denotes amplitudes $\geq$ 6 mV.

of myotubes. The MSPs from NS-26 cultures were qualitatively similar to those recorded from NG108-15 preparations (Fig. 2B).

MSPs display more variability in amplitude and frequency than do the corresponding MEPPs of adult skeletal muscle and are slower to rise and decay. Fig. 3A shows MSPs recorded from a myotube 4 days after seeding with NG108-15 cells and illustrates some of the salient characteristics of these synapses.

Amplitude

MSP amplitudes ranged from 0.2 to 23 mV (mean $\pm$ SEM = 1.78 $\pm$ 0.09 mV, n = 36 myotubes). A histogram of MSP amplitudes, from a representative synapse, is displayed in Fig. 3B. As indicated, the amplitude distribution is highly skewed, with the larger events ($\geq$ 6 mV) being nearly outside the limits encountered in a normal adult neuromuscular junction. The spread in the MSP amplitude is considerably greater than can be accounted for by variations in the size of the synaptic vesicles (Hubbard and Kwanbunbumpen, 1968; Whittaker et al., 1972; Nelson et al., 1978). Several factors may be responsible for the observed quantal distribution. The class of small MSPs ($\leq$ 1 mV) may originate at remote synapses and undergo spatial attenuation during passive spread to the recording electrode. A remote origin for small MSPs is unlikely, however, since their rise times did not exhibit a corresponding prolongation (Fig. 3A). The class of MSPs with large amplitudes may stem from action of multiquantal ACh packets due, perhaps, to spontaneous release of fused synaptic vesicles. Large MSPs are not likely to be responses elicited from spontaneous firing of the presynaptic membrane since TTX (10^{-6} M) was present during the recordings. Alternatively, the skewed distribution of MSP amplitudes may reflect differences in the diffusion paths of quantally-released ACh, secondary to the low postsynaptic AChE activity of these co-cultures (Rubin et al., 1980; Adler et al., 1986). This will be considered in a subsequent section.

Frequency

Although quantal frequencies comparable to those in adult muscle (1-3 sec^{-1}) are occasionally observed in co-culture (Hubbard et al., 1968a), MSP frequencies are more typically in the range 0.3-0.5 sec^{-1}, even for a synapse-competent cell line such as NG108-15. The lower rates of quantal secretion may stem from the paucity of synaptic vesicles in neuroblastoma-hybrid nerve terminals (Nelson et al., 1978). MSP frequencies were found to depend on temperature, Ca^{2+} concentration, membrane potential, osmotic strength, duration of dBcAMP treatment and hybrid cell density. The dependence of MSP frequency on nerve cell density results from the ability of myotubes to accept multiple innervation, with each functional terminal producing an approximately linear increment in the MSP frequency. Since attachment of NG108-15 cells to myotubes is somewhat random, multiple innervation can also account for part of the cell-to-cell variability in MSP frequency. Unlike developing muscles in vivo, myotubes retain multiple synaptic inputs during their lifespan in culture.

Effect of Ca^{2+}. Fig. 4 shows the influence of external Ca^{2+} on spontaneous release rates. Under control conditions, MSP frequencies averaged 16.7 min^{-1}. The quantal discharge rate fell below 4 min^{-1} following superfusion with a zero Ca^{2+} solution but returned to control levels within 3 min of restoration of external Ca^{2+}. In experiments in which zero Ca^{2+} was maintained for longer periods, MSPs were observed at approximately 10-30% of their control frequencies for up to 105 min. These results suggest that NG108-15 cells have both rapidly and slowly equilibrating pools of intracellular Ca^{2+}. Our findings that quantal release persists, albeit at reduced rates, in Ca^{2+}-free solutions is in agreement with the effects of Ca^{2+} deprivation in mammalian skeletal muscle (Hubbard et al., 1968a).

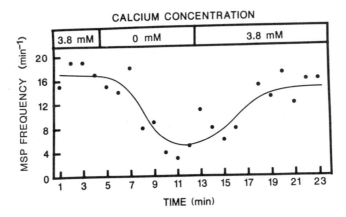

Fig. 4. Ca^{2+} sensitivity of NG108-15/myotube quantal secretion rates. Superfusion of co-cultures with a nominally Ca^{2+}-free solution (no chelating agents were added) led to a rapid, reversible decline in the MSP frequency. Solution changes are indicated by vertical bars.

Further evidence for the Ca^{2+}-dependence of MSP frequencies was obtained by use of the Ca^{2+} inhibitor YC-93 (2,6-dimethyl-4-(3-nitrophenyl)-1,4 dihydropyridine-3,5-dicarboxylic acid 3-[2-(N-benzyl-N-methyl-amino)] ethyl ester, 5-methyl ester HCl). Fig. 5A shows an NG108-15 Ca^{2+} spike recorded in physiological solution containing TTX to block Na^{+} entry. The Ca^{2+} spike was significantly inhibited by 5×10^{-6} M YC-93. Equivalent concentrations of D-600 or nifedipine were much less effective in blocking NG108-15 Ca^{2+} spikes (Atlas and Adler, 1981). Addition of YC-93 to co-cultures led to a concentration-dependent reduction in quantal release rates. Superfusion of 5×10^{-6} M YC-93 caused the MSP frequency to decline from 53.4 min^{-1} in control (Fig. 5B) to 28.2 min^{-1} (Fig. 5C) after equilibration with the dihydropyridine blocker. At this concentration YC-93 had little effect on the MSP amplitude or time course. Raising the YC-93 concentration to 10^{-5} M resulted in a more pronounced decrease in the MSP frequency such that it approached values obtained in Ca^{2+}-free solution.

Effect of osmotic strength. Increases in osmotic strength have been shown to enhance spontaneous transmitter release at vertebrate neuromuscular junctions by a process that requires neither Ca^{2+} entry nor depolarization

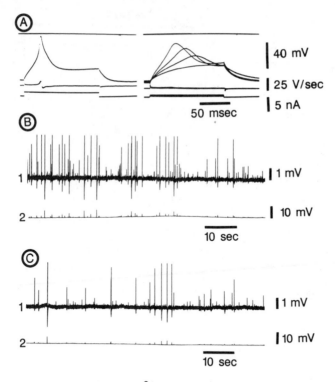

Fig. 5. Effect of the organic Ca^{2+}-inhibitor YC-93 on NG108-15 Ca^{2+} action potentials and MSPs. A. (left) Ca^{2+} spike elicited in physiological solution containing 10^{-6} M TTX to block regenerative Na^+ spike; (right) superimposed sweeps showing inhibition of the Ca^{2+} spike in another cell after addition of 5×10^{-6} M YC-93. The traces from top to bottom denote 0 mV, the action potential, its first derivative and the current pulse. B. Control MSPs recorded prior to addition of YC-93 with high gain AC (B1) and low gain DC (B2) coupling. C. MSPs from the same cell 13 min after addition of 5×10^{-6} M YC-93. (Some of the larger MSPs exceed the range of the high gain amplifier.)

(Furshpan, 1956; Hubbard et al., 1968b). MSP frequencies increased significantly when co-cultures were bathed in hypertonic Krebs-Ringer solution. For the synapse illustrated in Fig. 6, MSP frequencies were initially low

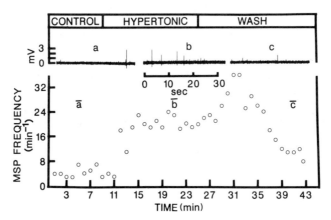

Fig. 6. Hypertonic sucrose increases MSP frequencies in NG108-15/myotube co-cultures. Superfusion with Krebs-Ringer containing 100 mM sucrose raised the osmolality from 323 to 411 mOsm/kg and led to a 5-fold increase in the MSP frequency. Solution changes are indicated by vertical bars. The inset shows records corresponding to the intervals denoted by short horizontal bars.

(4.9 min^{-1}), but increased by a factor of 5 in the presence of hypertonic sucrose. A secondary increase in frequency occurred during the early stages of washout, followed by restoration to near control levels with continued wash. Similar increases in MSP frequency were also observed in hypertonic Na^+ solutions. Other characteristics of synaptic responses were not altered by increases in osmotic strength.

Effect of membrane potential. At mature neuromuscular junctions, elevated extracellular K^+ concentrations produce a sustained increase in MEPP frequency (Liley, 1956). This increase has been attributed to an enhanced Ca^{2+} influx during K^+-induced depolarization of the nerve terminal. For NG108-15/myotube synapses, MSP frequencies increased following a rapid rise in external K^+ but showed an apparent decrease during slow bath perfusion of high K^+.

Fig. 7A shows MSPs prior to, during and following pressure ejection of Krebs-Ringer solution containing 29.5 mM K^+. Rapid elevation of K^+ caused a 30 mV depolarization and a transient, 10-fold increase in the MSP frequency.

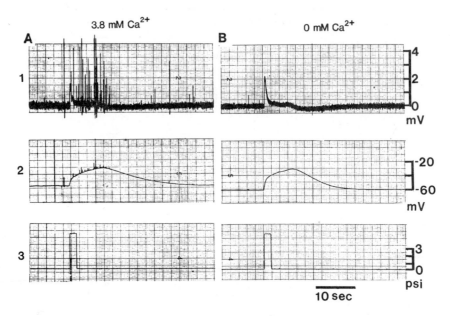

Fig. 7. Sudden elevation of extracellular K^+ by pressure ejection leads to a marked increase in MSP frequency in the presence (A) but not in the absence (B) of Ca^{2+}. The pressure pipette was filled with physiological solution containing 29.4 mM KCl (an excess of 24 mM). The solution was maintained isosmotic by appropriate reduction in NaCl. High K^+ was delivered by 5.5 psi pulses lasting 2 sec. Traces represent MSPs recorded with high gain AC (1) or low gain DC (2) coupling. Trace 3 denotes the pressure pulse.

The effect of high K^+ appears to be mediated by Ca^{2+} influx since no elevation of MSP frequency occurred in a nominally Ca^{2+}-free solution (Fig. 7B).

When high K^+ was delivered by slow bath perfusion, the MSPs underwent a reversible decrease in frequency (Fig. 8). The decrease was considered to arise from disappearance of small MSPs within the baseline noise due to postsynaptic depolarization and consequent reduction in the driving force. It is unlikely that the depolarization of the myotube could have masked an increase in the MSP frequency since an even larger depolarization occurred during pressure ejection of high K^+. In addition, a lower K^+ concentration (15.4 mM) also failed to produce an increase in the MSP frequency. The absence of an increase in spontaneous release rates with bath-applied high K^+ implies that the NG108-15 Ca^{2+} channels responsible for quantal transmitter release are inactivated with a maintained depolarization.

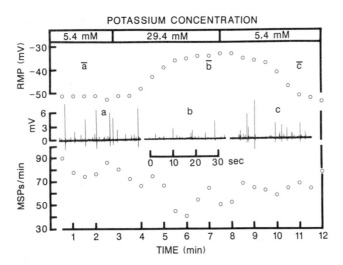

Fig. 8. Effect of gradual changes in external K^+ on quantal release. Slow bath perfusion (1.5 ml/min) of a high K^+ solution led to a gradual depolarization of the myotube (top) and an apparent decrease in MSP frequency. Solution changes are indicated by vertical bars. The middle traces show 40 sec segments corresponding to conditions denoted by horizontal bars.

Duration

At 37° C, MSPs recorded between 4-9 days of co-culture had rise times of 3.1 ± 0.04 msec and approximately exponential decays, with time constants of 6.9 ± 0.11 msec (n = 23 myotubes). The MSP time course is slow, relative to that of adult skeletal muscle, but is comparable to that observed in developing neuromuscular junctions (Diamond and Miledi, 1962). The slow MSP time course is due, in part, to the long passive time constant of the myotube (Christian et al., 1977). Other factors must also be responsible since, even under voltage-clamp, the decay time constant of the miniature synaptic current (MSC) is over 4 msec (Adler and Chang, 1985; Chang and Adler, 1985). In amphibian sympathetic neurons, long nicotinic synaptic current decays reflect correspondingly long open channel times (Schofield et al., 1985). However, this is not the case in the co-culture, since the mean open time for the nicotinic receptor-channel is only one third of the MSC decay time constant.

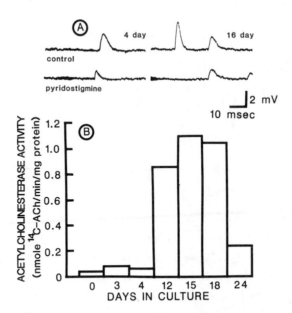

Fig. 9. Myotube AChE activities do not influence MSP lifetimes. A. MSPs under control conditions (upper) and after addition of 10^{-5} M pyridostigmine (lower) recorded from G8-1 myotubes 4 and 16 days after plating. Impalements were made within 2 hours of adding 1.7-1.9 x 10^6 NG108-15 cells per dish to G8-1 myotubes. The above NG108-15 density is much higher than that used elsewhere in the study (2 x 10^5 cells per dish) and was selected to permit rapid formation of synapses. B. Histogram showing G8-1 AChE activity with time in culture. The zero time point was obtained from stock cultures of myoblasts maintained in DMEM and 10% fetal bovine serum; cells were fed with DMEM and 10% horse serum from days 4 to 24. Between days 5 and 7, 5' fluoro-deoxyuridine and uridine were added to eliminate dividing myoblasts. To assay AChE activity the cells were washed twice with phosphate-buffered saline, detached from the substrate by use of 0.03% trypsin and homogenized in 1% Triton X-100. AChE activity was determined by the method of Siakotis et al. (1969). Protein was measured by the Coomassie Blue dye-binding assay (Bradford, 1976) using bovine serum albumen as a standard. Approximately 85% of the enzyme activity was true AChE; this is similar to the percentage of AChE in adult skeletal muscle.

An important factor underlying the slow MSP time course is the low AChE activity of the myotube. The influence of transmitter hydrolysis on MSP lifetimes was investigated in co-cultures of NG108-15 cells and G8-1 myotubes. The latter provided a more homogeneous population of myogenic cells for determination of AChE activity (Sugiyama, 1977). Synapses with G8-1 cells resembled, in most respects, those formed with primary myotubes. Notable exceptions were (1) the fraction of G8-1 myotubes innervated and the MSP frequencies were lower by 23 and 76% respectively and (2) the majority of G8-1 MSPs had hyperpolarizing tails (Christian et al., 1977; Adler et al., 1986), whereas only a small fraction of MSPs from primary myotubes had this component. The afterhyperpolarization was shown to be carried by K^+ ions and could be eliminated by holding the membrane potential between -70 and -80 mV (Adler et al., 1986).

A major problem in attempting to correlate MSP lifetime with AChE activity is the difficulty in measuring synaptic AChE levels in co-culture. This stems from the fact that both NG108-15 and G8-1 cells develop AChE activity, with the former accounting for the predominant fraction (Minna et al., 1972). To overcome this difficulty, AChE activities were determined on pure cultures of G8-1 myotubes. Synapses were formed rapidly by adding a high density suspension of NG108-15 cells, at various myotube ages, and MSPs were recorded for the first 2-4 hours of co-culture. Although innervation was sparse under these conditions (<1%), the brief contact with NG108-15 cells ensured that the G8-1 AChE levels did not change appreciably from possible induction by NG108-15 cells (Sanes et al., 1984).

The results of one such experiment are illustrated in Fig. 9. The traces show MSPs from 4 and 16 day G8-1 myotubes. The upper and lower records were obtained prior to and following exposure to the carbamate AChE inhibitor pyridostigmine (10^{-5} M). All recordings were performed within 2 hours of co-culture. Myotube AChE activities increased 20-fold between days 4 and 16, yet the MSP duration changed little over this period. Mean MSP decay time constants were 8.1 ± 0.67 msec (n = 6) for day 4 myotubes and 7.6 ± 0.39 msec (n = 8) for day 16 cultures. Addition of 10^{-5} M pyridostigmine, a concentration sufficient to block over 95% of muscle AChE activity, did not prolong the MSP decay in either 4 or 16 day cultures. Similar results were obtained in an earlier study in which NG108-15/G8-1 co-cultures were formed on day 8 and maintained for up to 6 weeks in vitro (Adler et al., 1986). These data suggest that synaptic AChE activity does not influence MSP lifetimes.

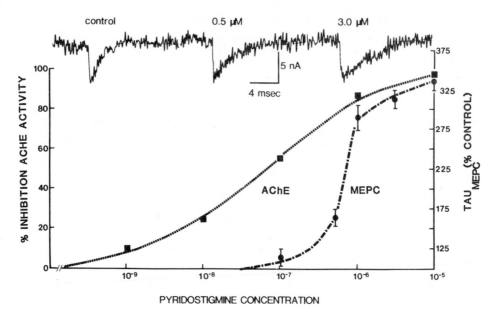

Fig. 10. Effect of pyridostigmine on AChE activity and MEPCs in adult rat diaphragm muscle. MEPCs were recorded at $24°$ C by a standard two-electrode voltage-clamp technique. The circles represent the mean $\pm$ SEM of MEPC decay time constant (TAU_{MEPC}) recorded at -70 mV. AChE activities (squares) were determined in triplicate on homogenized rat diaphragm tissue by the radiometric assay of Siakotis et al. (1969).

In contrast, synaptic events at the rat diaphragm endplate are highly sensitive to AChE activity. Fig. 10 illustrates the effects of pyrido-stigmine on AChE activity and miniature endplate current (MEPC) decay time constants. The inset shows the effects of pyridostigmine exposure on the MEPC. Prolongation of the MEPC decay was confined largely to pyridostigmine concentrations between 10^{-7} and 10^{-5} M. These drug concentrations broadened MEPC decays by 15 and 340%, respectively. The pyridostigmine-induced altera-tions were associated with decreases in AChE activities of 57% and 97%, res-pectively. Prolongation of the synaptic current decay was more pronounced during high frequency trains. Under these conditions, the decays became pro-gressively longer during the initial portion of the train. The MEPC ampli-tude increased slightly at concentrations below 3×10^{-6} M but was depressed with higher pyridostigmine concentrations. Only the inhibitory component of pyridostigmine, mediated by a direct action on the ACh receptor macromolecule (Pascuzzo et al., 1984), was evident on the MSP (Fig. 9).

At the vertebrate neuromuscular junction, ACh interacts with two macro-molecules, the ACh receptor and AChE. Interaction of ACh with its receptor initiates a sequence of events that begins with the opening of ion channels on the postjunctional membrane and culminates in muscle contraction. Interaction with AChE leads to rapid hydrolysis of ACh and cessation of transmitter action. Both macromolecules are under trophic control, as indicated by the disappearance of AChE and elaboration of extrajunctional ACh receptors following denervation (Dennis, 1975; Rubin et al., 1980; Peper et al., 1982). In NG108-15/myotube synapses, the same two macromolecules are present. However, while NG108-15 cells can induce postsynaptic receptor aggregation (Vogel et al., 1983), they apparently lack the ability to influence synaptic AChE levels. In the absence of neural induction, the increase in AChE activity that accompanies myogenesis is not sufficient to regulate the lifetime of quantally-released ACh (Fig. 9B). Possible reasons include low enzyme activity and incorrect synaptic localization (Adler et al., 1986). Thus, peak AChE levels in 15-18 day myotubes (Fig. 9) represent less than 10% of the activity associated with the adult neuromuscular junction.

Histochemical staining for AChE, using the method of Karnovsky and Roots (1964), indicates that the staining pattern is random and not well-correlated with synaptic contacts (Adler and Chang, unpublished observations). Sanes et al. (1984) have reported that myotubes grown in the presence of a soluble brain extract undergo increases in ACh receptor aggregation and AChE activity. Treated myotubes also exhibit primitive junctional folds and a well-developed synaptic basal lamina. The putative AChE-inducing components are apparently not expressed in adequate amounts in NG108-15 synapses. Other factors, such as sustained contractile activity and dibutyryl cyclic GMP, have been found to augment synaptic AChE levels in myotubes. These were shown by Rubin et al. (1980) to shorten the time constants of MSC decays to the limit imposed by the channel kinetics ($\leq$ 1.8 msec).

Myotubes in synaptic contact with NG108-15 cells did not undergo sustained contractions; instead they exhibited intermittent fasciculations. Consequently, AChE levels remained low leading to prolonged MSC durations. The ability of NG108-15 cells to increase receptor densities, but not AChE activities, suggests that these macromolecules are independently regulated.

In conclusion, neuroblastoma/myotube co-cultures possess a number of electrophysiological properties that are similar to both developing and mature vertebrate neuromuscular junctions. State-of-the-art techniques, such as patch-clamp recordings can be employed to obtain fundamental information on synaptic function at the molecular level. Thus, these co-cultures appear

to be useful model systems for studies of substances interacting at nicotinic
nerve-muscle synapses and for investigations of nervous system development.

ACKNOWLEDGMENTS

Portions of this work were performed in the Laboratory of Biochemical
Genetics, NHLBI, NIH under the expert guidance and direction of Dr. Marshall
Nirenberg. We also thank Drs. H. Higashida, N. Busis, F.-C. T. Chang and D.
Maxwell for their contributions to this study. YC-93 was a generous gift
from Dr. David J. Triggle.

The views, opinions, and/or findings contained in this report are those of
the author and should not be construed as an official Department of the Army
position, policy, or decision, unless so designated by other documentation.

REFERENCES

Adler, M. and Chang, F.-C. T., 1985, Role of acetylcholinesterase in
    cholinergic synaptic transmission, in: "Abstracts: Fifth Annual
    Chemical Defense Bioscience Review (USAMRDC)" p. 85.

Adler, M., Chang, F.-C. T., Maxwell, D., Mark, G., Glenn, J. F., and
    Foster, R. E., 1986 (in press), Effect of diisopropylfluorophosphate
    on synaptic transmission and acetylcholine sensitivity in neuro-
    blastoma-myotube co-culture, in: "Dynamics of Cholinergic Function"
    I. Hanin, ed., Plenum Press, New York.

Amano, T., Hamprecht, B., and Kemper, W., 1974, High activity of choline
    acetyltransferase induced in neuroblastoma x glia hybrid cells,
    Exp. Cell Res., 85:339.

Atlas, D. and Adler, M., 1981, α-Adrenergic antagonists as possible calcium
    channel inhibitors, Proc. Natl. Acad. Sci. USA, 78:1237.

Augusti-Tocco, G. and Sato, G., 1969, Establishment of functional clonal
    lines of neurons from mouse neuroblastoma, Proc. Natl. Acad. Sci.,
    64:311.

Betz, W., 1976, The formation of synapses between chick embryo skeletal
    muscle and ciliary ganglia grown in vitro, J. Physiol., 254:63.

Bradford, M. M., 1976, A rapid and sensitive method for the quantitation of
    microgram quantities of protein utilizing the principle of protein-dye
    binding, Anal. Biochem., 72:248.

Ceccarelli, B. and Hurlbut, W. P., 1980, Vesicle hypothesis of the release of quanta of acetylcholine, Phys. Rev., 60:396.

Chang, F.-C. T. and Adler, M., 1985, Acetylcholinesterase in clonal nicotinic synaptic transmission, Soc. Neurosci. Abstr., 11:304.

Christian, C. N., Nelson, P. G., Peacock, J., and Nirenberg, M., 1977, Synapse formation between two clonal lines, Science, 196:995.

Christian, C. N., Nelson, P. G., Bullock, P., Mullinax, D., and Nirenberg, M., 1978, Pharmacologic responses of cells of a neuroblastoma x glioma hybrid clone and modulation of synapses between hybrid cells and mouse myotubes, Brain Res., 147:261.

Cohen, S. A., and Fischbach, G. D., 1977, Clusters of acetylcholine receptors located at identified nerve muscle synapses in vitro, Dev. Biol., 59:24.

Del Castillo, J. and Katz, B., 1954, Quantal components of end-plate potential, J. Physiol., 124:560.

Dennis, M. J., 1975, Physiological properties of junctions between nerve and muscle developing during salamander limb regeneration, J. Physiol., 244:683.

Diamond, J. and Miledi, R., 1962, A study of foetal and new-born rat muscle fibers, J. Physiol., 162:393.

Furshpan, E. J., 1956, The effect of osmotic pressure changes on the spontaneous activity at motor nerve endings, J. Physiol., 134:689.

Hamill, O. P., Marty, A., Neher, E., Sakmann, B., and Sigworth, F. J., 1981, Improved patch-clamp techniques for high-resolution current recording from cells and cell-free membrane patches, Pflugers Arch., 391:85.

Higashida, H., Wilson, S. P., Adler, M., and Nirenberg, M., 1978, Synapse formation by neuroblastoma and hybrid cell lines, Soc. Neurosci. Abstr., 4:591.

Hubbard, J. I., Jones, S. F., and Landau, E. M., 1968a, On the mechanism by which calcium and magnesium affect the spontaneous release of transmitter from mammalian motor nerve terminals, J. Physiol., 194:355.

Hubbard, J. I., Jones, S. F., and Landau, E. M., 1968b, An examination of the effects of osmotic pressure changes upon transmitter release from mammalian motor nerve terminals, J. Physiol., 197:639.

Hubbard, J. I. and Kwanbunbumpen, S., 1968, Evidence for the vesicle hypothesis, J. Physiol., 194:407.

Karnovsky, M. and Roots, L., 1964, A "direct-coloring" thiocholine method for cholinesterases, J. Histochem. Cytochem., 12:219.

Kuffler, S. W. and Yoshikami, D., 1975, The distribution of acetylcholine sensitivity at the post-synaptic membrane of vertebrate skeletal twitch muscles: iontophoretic mapping in the micron range, J. Physiol., 244:703.

Land, B. R., Podleski, T. R., Salpeter, E. E., and Salpeter, M. M., 1977, Acetylcholine receptor distribution on myotubes in culture correlated to acetylcholine sensitivity, J. Physiol., 269:155.

Liley, A. W., 1956, An investigation of spontaneous activity at the neuro-muscular junction of the rat, J. Physiol., 132:650.

Minna, J., Glazer, D., and Nirenberg, M., 1972, Genetic dissection of neural properties using somatic cell hybrids, Nature New Biol., 235:225.

Nelson, P., Christian, C., and Nirenberg, M., 1976, Synapse formation between clonal neuroblastoma x glioma hybrid cells and striated muscle cells, Proc. Natl. Acad. Sci., 73:123.

Nelson, P. G., Christian, C. N., Daniels, M. P., Henkart, M.,Bullock, P., Mullinax, D., and Nirenberg, M., 1978, Formation of synapses between cells of a neuroblastoma x glioma hybrid clone and mouse myotubes, Brain Res., 147:245.

Nirenberg, M., Wilson, S., Higashida, H., Rotter, A., Krueger K., Busis, N., Ray, R., Kenimer, J. G., and Adler, M., 1983, Modulation of synapse formation by cyclic adenosine monophosphate, Science, 222:794.

Pascuzzo, G. J., Akaike, A., Maleque, M. A., Shaw, K.-P., Aronstam, R. S., Rickett, D. L., and Albuquerque, E. X., 1984, The nature of the inter-actions of pyridostigmine with the nicotinic acetylcholine receptor-ionic channel complex. I. Agonist, desensitizing and binding properties, Mol. Pharmacol., 25:92.

Peper, K., Bradley, R. J., and Dreyer, F., 1982, The acetylcholine receptor at the neuromuscular junction, Physiol. Rev., 62:1271.

Redfern, P. A., 1970, Neuromuscular transmission in new-born rats, J. Physiol., 208:701.

Rubin, L. L., Schuetze, S. M., Weill, C. L., and Fischbach, G. D., 1980, Regulation of acetylcholinesterase appearance at neuromuscular junc-tions in vitro, Nature, 283:264.

Sanes, J. R., Feldman, D. H., Cheney, J. M., and Lawrence, J. C., Jr., 1984, Brain extract induces synaptic characteristics in the basal lamina of cultured myotubes, J. Neurosci., 4:464.

Schofield, G. G., Weight, F. F., and Adler, M., 1985, Single acetylcholine channel currents in sympathetic neurons, Brain Res., 342:200.

Siakotis, A. N., Filbert, M., and Hester, R., 1969, A specific radioisotopic assay for acetylcholinesterase and pseudocholinesterase in brain and plasma, Biochem. Med., 3:1.

Sugiyama, H., 1977, Multiple forms of acetylcholinesterase in clonal muscle cells, FEBS Letters, 84:257.

Takeuchi, A. and Takeuchi, N., 1959, Active phase of frog's endplate potential, J. Neurophysiol., 22:395.

Vogel, Z. V. I., Christian, C. N., Vigny, M., Bauer, H. C., Sonderegger, P., and Daniels, M. P., 1983, Laminin induces acetyl-choline receptor aggregation on cultured myotubes and enhances the receptor aggregation activity of a neuronal factor, J. Neurosci., 3:1058

Whittaker, V. P., Essman, W. B., and Dowe, G. H. C., 1972, The isolation of pure cholinergic synaptic vesicles from the electric organs of elasmobranch fish of the family torpedinidae, Biochem. J., 128:833.

IDENTIFICATION OF A NEUROTROPHIC FACTOR FOR THE MAINTENANCE OF
ACETYLCHOLINESTERASE AND BUTYRYLCHOLINESTERASE IN THE PREGANGLIONICALLY
DENERVATED SUPERIOR CERVICAL GANGLION OF THE CAT

George B. Koelle

Department of Pharmacology, Medical School/G3
University of Pennsylvania
Philadelphia, PA 19104

Since this report forms part of a Festschrift volume for my old friend
Nicky Karczmar, I shall take the prerogative of putting it in the form of an
informal progress report. Supporting data will be found in the references
cited. One is denied this privilege in most publications.

Forty years ago Sawyer and Hollinshead (1) showed that preganglionic
denervation of the cat superior cervical ganglion (SCG) results within 3
days in a loss of 80% of its acetylcholinesterase (AChE; EC 3.1.1.7) and 30%
of its butyrylcholinesterase (BuChE; EC 3.1.1.8) contents. This was one of
the first phenomena that we investigated following the development, in
collaboration with Dr. Jonas S. Friedenwald, of the copper thiocholine
(CuThCh) histochemical method (2). It was found that in the normal cat SCG,
AChE is present in high concentrations throughout the neuropil and in the
somata of occasional (< 1%) ganglion cells, and in trace amounts in the
somata of the remainder. Butyrylcholinesterase activity was noted only in
the neuropil. Following denervation, AChE virtually disappeared from the
neuropil but remained unchanged in the ganglion cell somata; the concentration of BuChE in the neuropil fell. From these findings we concluded that
in the normal cat SCG, AChE is confined chiefly to the preganglionic fibers
and their terminals, and that BuChE is present only in the capsular glial
cells (3, 4). In order to account for the apparent presynaptic localization
of AChE and related pharmacological findings (5), a somewhat elaborate
working hypothesis was developed (6). Unfortunately, it attracted few
adherents.

The CuThCh method is unsatisfactory for electron microscopy (EM) for a
number of reasons. For this purpose we developed the bis-(thioacetoxy)
aurate (I) or Au $(TA)_2$ method (7). While the Au $(TA)_2$ method affords
excellent resolution of sites of enzyme activity, it is not highly specific
for AChE or BuChE; however, this limitation can be overcome by appropriate
controls. When the cat SCG was examined by EM with the Au $(TA)_2$ procedure,
the presynaptic localization of AChE was confirmed; however, it was found in
even higher concentrations at postsynaptic sites, along the full extent of
the dendritic and perikaryonal membranes of all ganglion cells. Butyrylcholinesterase was localized at only the latter, postsynaptic sites and
appeared in traces in the glial cells (8). Following denervation, in
confirmation of the earlier light microscopic findings, AChE disappeared
from both presynaptic and postsynaptic cell membranous sites, and the
concentration of BuChE at the latter fell (9). This raised the question of

why the integrity of the presynaptic fibers is essential for the maintenance of postsynaptic AChE, and the full component of postsynaptic BuChE. The most reasonable working hypothesis appeared to be that the preganglionic fibers release a neurotrophic factor (NF) that has this function. Its investigation is the subject of the present study (10-13).

In brief, aqueous extracts were prepared from the brain, spinal cord, and sciatic nerves of individual cats and infused via the right common carotid artery into test cats following bilateral preganglionic denervation of the SCG. In order to divert most of the infused extract to the SCG, which is supplied by the occipital and internal carotid arteries (14), the external carotid (EC) and lingual (L) arteries were ligated bilaterally. Exactly 48 hours following denervation, the SCG were excised, homogenized, and assayed for AChE, BuChE, and protein contents.

The ultimate controls consisted of cats that were treated as above and infused for 24 hours with 0.9% NaCl solution (Table 1, Group 5). Under these conditions, the AChE content of the SCG was reduced to approximately 55% of the normal value (Group 1).

Table 1. Control data

		Substrate hydrolyzed, nmol/mg of protein per min	
		AChE	BuChE
Group	Procedure	Mean ± S.E.M. (n)	Mean ± S.E.M. (n)
1	Normal cat SCG	449 ± 42 (8)	590 ± 61 (8)
2	SCG pregangionically denervated 48 hr previously	122 ± 5 (10)	349 ± 27 (10)
3	SCG denervated 48 hr previously; reanesthetized and EC and L arteries ligated 24 hr after denervation	177 ± 8 (12)	390 ± 22 (12)
4	SCG denervated 48 hr previously; continuous anesthesia until time of sacrifice; without EC and L arterial ligations	250 ± 23 (8)	444 ± 41 (8)
5	Same as group 4 excepting EC and L arteries ligated, and cat infused with 0.9% NaCl 24-48 hr post-denervation	254 ± 13 (6)	251 ± 33 (6)

Numbers of SCG in parentheses.

When the SCG were denervated and excised 48 hours later, with no intervening treatment, the AChE fell to 27% of normal (Group 2). Maintenance of continuous anesthesia alone, from the time of denervation to sacrifice (Group 4), resulted in the same fall as in the ligated, saline-infused cats. Temporary reanesthetization for arterial ligations caused an intermediate fall (Group 3). Thus, continuous anesthesia appears to be the critical factor for partially opposing the effect of denervation. In the foregoing control and subsequent test series, values for BuChE showed extreme, unexplainable variation.

In the initial test series, the SCG of cats infused for 24 hours with extract had a mean value for AChE (354 $\pm$ 35 nmol substrate hydrolyzed/mg protein/minute) that was significantly higher than that of the saline-infused controls (254 $\pm$ 13). When extracts were dialyzed overnight against a membrane with a molecular weight cut-off (MWCO) of 10,000, the retained portion was inactive, whereas the dialysate was active. Likewise, dialysates against membranes with MWCO's of 2,000 and 1,000 were highly active. When the latter were treated with carboxypeptidase A, type 1, activity was lost; the latter procedure included treatment of enzyme-treated and control aliquots at 80°C for 5 minutes. The NF therefore appeared to be a heat-stable peptide of low (< 1,000) molecular weight.

Negative results were obtained following infusion of extract for periods of 12 hours or less; with 24-hour infusions of similarly prepared extracts of skeletal muscle or liver; acetylcholine; and nerve growth factor (2.5 S and 7 S). Results were borderline following infusions of extracts of gut and cyclic AMP.

Of the many questions that remained to be answered regarding the NF, the first considered was its identification. It was obviously impossible to initiate this with the present assay procedure; a full week's work, including two all night stints, permits us to perform two assays. We therefore considered using an in-vitro organ culture procedure, several of which have been reported (e.g., 15-18), as a screening method. However, even this prospect seemed bleak in view of the saga of Schally and Guillemin. In the early 1950's Geoffrey Harris postulated that adenohypophyseal hormone-releasing factors are elaborated in the hypothalamus. Schally and Guillemin independently demonstrated the presence in the hypothalamus of an ACTH-releasing factor in 1957. They then set out, at first collaboratively then competitively, to identify it. Twenty-five years later they had both identified the thyrotropin-releasing factor and shared a Nobel Prize, but the ACTH-releasing factor remained elusive. To avoid such an impasse, we were looking for a hint, or a short-cut.

A real clue was provided by Laurie W. Haynes, then at the University of Birmingham. When Win and I visited there last summer, he showed us a manuscript still in press in which he and Margaret E. Smith had demonstrated that glycyl-1-glutamine (GlyGlu), the terminal dipeptide cleaved from beta-endorphin (19), markedly enhances conversion of the monomeric G_1 form of AChE to the G_4 and A_{12} forms in cultured preparations of denervated rat and chick muscle (20). This was precisely the effect we should have been seeking by a similar screening procedure.

Immediately following our return home we began testing GlyGlu (kindly provided by Dr. Haynes) by the cat in-vivo method. Initial results appeared inconsistent. Then as more data were accumulated a definite pattern emerged. The AChE of the right SCG of cats perfused with GlyGlu, 10^{-5} - 10^{-3} M, remained in the range of saline-perfused controls; however, the levels in the left SCG were significantly elevated. Since infusions were made into the right common carotid artery their contents arrived at the right SCG directly, but at the left SCG via a more circuitous route, chiefly through the anastomoses of the right and left internal carotid arteries. This suggested that a metabolite of GlyGlu functioned as a NF at the left SCG. Glycine and l-glutamine were found to be inactive. Glycyl-l-glutamic acid (GlyGA), which might be formed from GlyGlu by the action of glutaminase, was significantly active at concentrations of 10^{-6} and 10^{-5} M at both the right and left SCG; at 10^{-4} M, it was unexplainably inhibitory. (GlyGA showed no anti-ChE activity $\underline{in}$ $\underline{vitro}$ at 10^{-3} M).

Although GlyGA has been shown to be a NF for the maintenance of AChE and BuChE in the denervated cat SCG, several questions remain to be answered:

1. Is GlyGA the chief metabolite of GlyGlu, that is responsible for the latter's indirect neurotrophic effect? Or might GlyGA or GlyGlu act indirectly by releasing an endogenous NF?

2. Is GlyGA or GlyGlu the major NF present in (A) extracts of the central nervous system and its dialysates that maintains AChE and BuChE in denervated SCG, or (B) that is released by preganglionic fibers to maintain the enzymes at postsynaptic sites under physiological conditions?

3. Is the neurotrophic action of the identified compounds or from endogenous sources due to prevention or delay of degeneration of preganglionic fibers, or to maintenance of AChE and BuChE at postsynaptic sites (e.g., by regulating the conversion of the cytoplasmic G_1 forms to the membranous G_4 and A_{12} forms of the enzymes (21))?

4. Do GlyGlu, GlyGA, or related compounds affect other components of the cholinergic system, or of other systems?

We hope to report some of the answers by the time of Dr. Karczmar's eightieth birthday celebration.

ACKNOWLEDGEMENTS

I express my most appreciative thanks to my many collaborators in these studies: Dr. Winifred A. Koelle, Dr. Gerard A. Ruch, Dr. Richard Davis, Dr. Eiji Uchida, Ursula J. Sanville, Kathleen K. Rickard, Stephen J. Wall, James E. Williams, and Joseph M. Devlin.

This investigation was supported by Research Grant NS-00282 30-32 from the National Institute of Neurological and Communicative Disorders and Stroke, National Institutes of Health, and by contributions from the Barra Foundation, Inc., The Burroughs Wellcome Fund, the Foundation for Vascular-Hypertension Research (Philadelphia), and Whitehall Laboratories.

REFERENCES

1. C. H. Sawyer and W. H. Hollinshead, Cholinesterase in sympathetic fibers and ganglia, J. Neurophysiol. 8:137 (1945).
2. G. B. Koelle and J. S. Friedenwald, A histochemical method for localizing cholinesterase activity, Proc. Soc. Exp. Biol. Med. 70:617 (1949).
3. G. B. Koelle, The elimination of enzymatic diffusion artifacts in the histochemical localization of cholinesterases, and a survey of their cellular distributions, J. Pharmacol. Exp. Ther. 103:153 (1951).

4. W. A. Koelle and G. B. Koelle, The localization of external or functional acetylcholinesterase at the synapses of autonomic ganglia, J. Pharmacol. Exp. Ther. 126:1 (1959).

5. R. L. Volle and G. B. Koelle, The physiological role of acetylcholinesterase (AChE) in sympathetic ganglia, J. Pharmacol. Exp. Ther. 133:223 (1961).

6. G. B. Koelle, A new general concept of the neurohumoral functions of acetylcholine and acetylcholinesterase. J. Pharm. Pharmacol. 14:65 (1962).

7. G. B. Koelle, R. Davis, E. G. Smyrl, and A. V. Fine, Refinement of the bis-(thioacetoxy) aurate (I) method for the electron microscopic localization of acetylcholinesterase and nonspecific cholinesterase, J. Histochem. Cytochem. 22:252 (1974).

8. R. Davis and G. B. Koelle, Electron microscope localization of acetylcholinesterase and butyrylcholinesterase in the superior cervical ganglion of the cat I. Normal ganglion, J. Cell. Biol. 78:785 (1978).

9. R. Davis and G. B. Koelle, Electron microscope localization of acetylcholinesterase and butyrylcholinesterase in the superior cervical ganglion of the cat. II. Preganglionically denervated ganglion, J. Cell. Biol. 88:581 (1981).

10. G. B. Koelle and G. A. Ruch, Demonstration of a neurotrophic factor for the maintenance of acetylcholinesterase and butyrylcholinesterase in the preganglionically denervated superior cervical ganglion of the cat, Proc. Natl. Acad. Sci. USA 80:3106 (1983).

11. G. B. Koelle, G. A. Ruch, and E. Uchida, Effects of sodium pentobarbital anesthesia and neurotrophic factor on the maintenance of acetylcholinesterase and butyrylcholinesterase in the preganglionically denervated superior cervical ganglion of the cat, Proc. Natl. Acad. Sci. USA 80:6122 (1983).

12. G. B. Koelle, U. J. Sanville, K. K. Rickard, and J. E. Williams, Partial characterization of the neurotrophic factor for the maintenance of acetylcholinesterase and butyrylcholinesterase in the preganglionically denervated superior cervical ganglion of the cat in vivo, Proc. Natl. Acad. Sci. USA 81:6539 (1984).

13. G. B. Koelle, U. J. Sanville, and S. J. Wall, Glycyl-l-glutamine: a precursor, and glycyl-l-glutamic acid: a neurotrophic factor for maintenance of acetylcholinesterase and butyrylcholinesterase in the preganglionically denervated superior cervical ganglion of the cat in vivo, Proc. Natl. Acad. Sci. USA 82: In press (1985).

14. D. Chungcharoen, M. deB. Daly, and A. Schweitzer, The blood supply of the superior cervical sympathetic and the nodose ganglia in cats, dogs and rabbits, J. Physiol. (London) 118:528 (1952).

15. M. P. Rathbone, J. D. Vickers, and D. M. Logan, Neural regulation of cholinesterase in newt skeletal muscle II. The effects of denervation and of culture in vitro, J. Exp. Zool. 210:463 (1979).

16. B. Davey, L. H. Younkin, and S. G. Younkin, Neural control of skeletal muscle cholinesterase: A study using organ-cultured rat muscle, J. Physiol. (Lond.) 289:501 (1979).

17. T. L. Lentz, J. S. Addis, and J. Chester, Partial purification and characterization of a nerve trophic factor regulating muscle acetylcholinesterase activity, Exp. Neurol. 73:542 (1981).

18. T. H. Oh and G. J. Markelonis, Sciatin (transferrin) and other muscle trophic factors, in: "Growth and Maturation Factors, vol. 2," G. Guroff, ed., John Wiley and Sons, Inc., New York (1984).

19. D. C. Parish, D. G. Smyth, J. R. Normanton, and J. H. Wonstencroft, Glycyl glutamine, an inhibitory neuropeptide derived from beta-endorphin, Nature 306:267 (1983).

20. L. W. Haynes and M. E. Smith, Induction of endplate-specific acetylcholinesterase by beta-endorphin C-terminal dipeptide in rat and chick muscle cells, <u>Biochem</u>. <u>Soc</u>. <u>Trans</u>. 13:174 (1985).
21. J. Massoulie and S. Bon, The molecular forms of cholinesterase and acetylcholinesterase in vertebrates, <u>in</u>: "Annual Review of Neuroscience, Vol. 5," W. M. Cowan, ed., Annual Reviews Inc., Palo Alto, California (1982).

THE APPLICATION OF IMMUNOCHEMICAL TECHNIQUES TO THE STUDY OF CHOLINERGIC FUNCTION

Victor P Whittaker and Edilio Borroni

Abteilung Neurochemie
Max-Planck-Institut für biophysikalische Chemie
Postfach 2841, D-3400 Göttingen, FRG

THE ELECTROMOTOR SYSTEM OF THE ELECTRIC RAY

The electromotor system of the electric ray, *Torpedo marmorata*, is shown diagrammatically in Fig. 1a. The electrocytes of the electric organ develop embryologically from myotubes (Fig. 1b)[1,2]. Their ventral (under) surfaces are almost completely (80%) covered with synapses resembling – not unexpectedly – neuromuscular junctions; the transmitter is acetylcholine[3]. A single average-sized fish contains about 400 g of electric organ which in turn contains 500-1000 times more synaptic material per unit weight than muscle; thus electric organ is an ideal starting material for biochemical investigations of cholinergic function.

The cell bodies of the electromotor neurones are segregated in twin motor nuclei on the brain-stem of the fish just behind the cerebellum (Fig. 1a). The axons of these neurones run in eight large nerve trunks (four on each side) into the electric organs. Thus the cell bodies and axons of the electromotor neurones are also readily accessible and are being used in our group for various purposes including the identification, using recombinant DNA techniques, of the cholinergic portion of the genome[4], for the identification of trophic factors in development[5], and for axonal transport studies[6,7]. The embryological development of the system has been thoroughly described[1,2,8]

Means have been devised for isolating synaptic vesicles[9-12], detached, sealed portions of the network of presynaptic nerve terminals (synaptosomes)[13-15] and from the latter, presynaptic plasma membranes[16,17] The synaptic vesicles and plasma membranes have been used to raise antisera which, after suitable treatment, have found application in the development of new neuroanatomical methods and new techniques for investigating subcellular fractions. The general strategy is shown in Fig. 2.

It should be stressed at the outset that one cannot assume that antisera raised to subcellular organelles will be specific for these organelles; the mixture of antibodies they contain may be partly or wholly directed against highly antigenic contaminants rather than the main components of the subcellular fraction in question. Thus, to obtain an antiserum specific for a given organelle it is essential to remove by adsorption the unwanted antibodies and to demonstrate that the antigen(s)

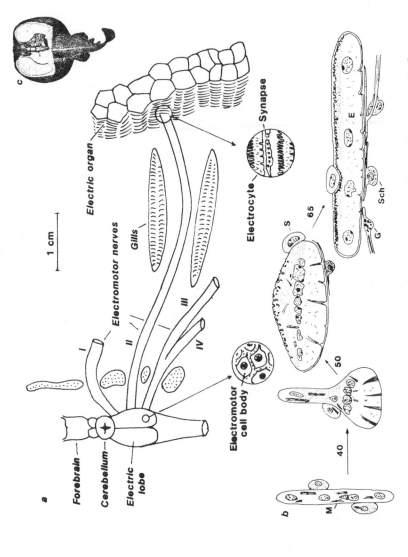

Fig. 1 Diagrams of (a) electromotor system of Torpedo marmorata, (b) development of electrocytes (E) from myo-tubes (M). Numbers are embryo lengths in mm. A population of satellite cells (S) fuses with the electrocytes, thereby increasing their size throughout life pari passu with the growth of the fish. G, growth cones; Sch, Schwann cells. (c) Drawing of whole fish showing location of brain stem and organ.

recognized by the adsorbed antiserum copurify with the organelle (Fig. 2).
In order to reduce the incidence of unwanted antibodies, organelles must
be as pure as possible; the usual criterion is purification to constant
composition.

It has been particularly difficult to satisfy these criteria with
synaptic vesicles since the only markers available until recently were
acetylcholine and vesicular ATP, both readily lost during purification.

However, an antiserum has recently been obtained which after analysis
and adsorption of unwanted antibodies recognizes a 200 kDa proteoglycan
(PG) which copurifies with synaptic vesicular acetylcholine and ATP in a
zonal density gradient[18,19] This antiserum detects a similar immunoreactive
substance in mammalian neuromuscular junctions[18] and retina[20].

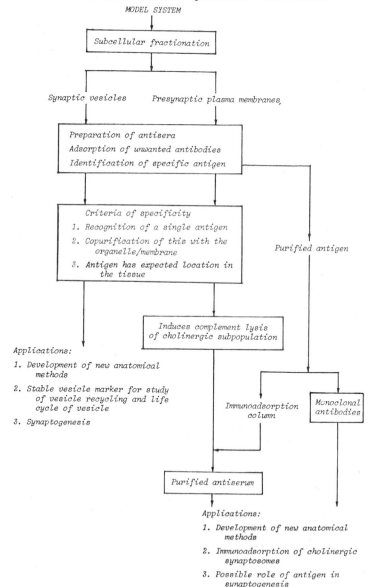

Fig. 2 Diagram illustrating the strategy of the research described in
this article.

With preparations of presynaptic plasma membranes similar problems arise[18,21] but it has proved possible to obtain a purified antiserum which recognizes several gangliosides mainly localized on the presynaptic plasma membranes of *Torpedo* electromotor nerve terminals[22,23] and two polysialogangliosides specific for cholinergic neurones in the mammalian central nervous system[23,24] The antiserum also specifically interacts with mammalian peripheral cholinergic neurones and nerve terminals, in ileum[21] retina[24] sympathetic ganglia[21] spinal cord[25] and muscle[21]

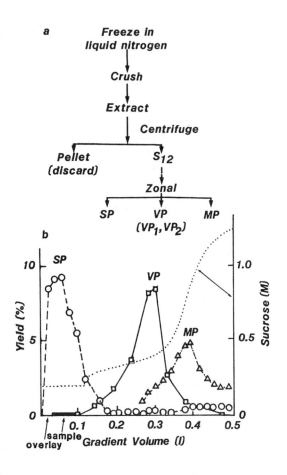

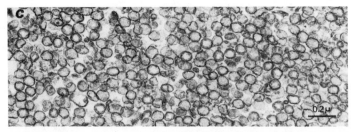

Fig. 3 *Summary of technique for isolating synaptic vesicles from electric organ. In (b) circles show protein, squares acetylcholine and triangles cholinesterase distribution in the zonal density gradient: SP, soluble protein peak; VP, vesicle peak; MP, membrane peak. (c) Shows vesicles isolated in VP.*

CHOLINERGIC SYNAPTIC-VESICLE-SPECIFIC PROTEOGLYCAN

Preparation of electromotor synaptic vesicles

The synaptic vesicles of electromotor nerve terminals may be isolated in bulk from electric organ by the technique summarized in Fig. 3[10,12] The advantages of this method are (a) deep-freezing of the tissue reduces adventitious stimulation and recycling or loss of vesicles (nevertheless careful handling of the tissue during excision from the fish is necessary), (b) unlike mammalian brain vesicles prepared from synaptosomes, electromotor vesicles are not exposed to hypoosmotic conditions, (c) use is made of the high resolving power and large capacity of the zonal rotor. As seen in Table 1, vesicles prepared by this method have an acetylcholine content of 6-7 nmol.(mg of protein)$^{-1}$ or 2-3.5 nmol.(mg of lipid)$^{-1}$ and cannot be significantly further purified by a second zonal run or chromatography on porous glass beads. This method can also be applied to perfused blocks of electric organ.

In a variant of this method[11], the vesicles and membrane fragments are first concentrated and partially freed from cytoplasmic proteins on a single step gradient before being separated in the zonal rotor. Such vesicles are of comparable purity (Table 1).

Table 1. Purification of synaptic vesicles from electromotor nerve terminals of *Torpedo marmorata*

Reference	Type of preparation[a]	Fraction designation	Acetylcholine content nmol/mg of protein[b]	nmol/mg of lipid[c]
9	SG	II	0.05	−
10	Z	VP	0.57±0.07(4)	−
12[d]	Z	vesicle peak	4.45±0.50(4)	2.76
	Z+G	vesicle peak	6.10±0.90(2)	3.57
11	SG+Z	vesicle peak	6.90±0.63(6)	1.99

[a]In col 2, SG = separation on a step gradient, Z = separation on a continuous density gradient in a zonal rotor, Z+G = separation in a zonal rotor followed by further purification on a column of porous glass beads, SG+Z = separation on a step gradient followed by density gradient separation in a zonal rotor. [d]Results taken from Tables I and II, ref 12.

[b]Means ± SEM (no of experiments in parentheses)

[c]Ratio of means

Vesicles prepared in this way were used as the source of vesicle antigens[18,19] At this stage the antiserum raised to the vesicles stained both the innervated, ventral, and non-innervated, dorsal surfaces of the electrocytes (Fig. 4a) (the highly polarized structure of the electric organ has provided a valuable tool for checking the localization of putative cholinergic-specific antigens).

The crude antiserum was analysed by immunoprecipitation of labelled vesicle proteins; it recognized two vesicle-specific protein constituents, a 34 kDa component, identified as the vesicular ATP translocase[26,27] and a

42 kDa component, identified as a special form of actin[28] but in addition, a number of other components which were not among those that copurify exclusively with vesicles but which are present as trace contaminants. Among these was acetylcholinesterase (molecular mass, 67 kDa).

Adsorption with liver membrane fragments and particle-free supernatant from electric organ homogenates resulted in an antiserum that stained only the ventral membrane (Fig. 4b). Adsorption of this antiserum with synaptic vesicles abolished the specific staining reaction (Fig. 4d) and the weak reaction of preimmune serum showed no dorsal/ventral selectivity (Fig. 4c).

The adsorbed serum (detected by means of a horse-radish peroxidase-conjugated second antibody technique) now failed to recognize any Coomassie-blue-positive proteins in immunoblots of vesicle proteins separated by gel electrophoresis, but was positive for a rather diffusely staining Alcian-blue-positive component of molecular mass ca. 200 kDa, identified as a PG (Fig. 5e). The disappearance of immunoreactivity towards the 34 kDa vesicle protein may have been brought about by adsorption onto liver mitochondrial fragments during the adsorption with liver membranes, since mitochondria contain a similar ATP translocase. A semi-quantitative analysis based on the densitometric scanning of the electrophoretically separated and immunostained 200 kDa PG showed that this copurified with electromotor synaptic vesicles (Fig. 5a). The analytical technique involved sedimentation of vesicles and/or other particulate material from the gradient, solubilization and polyacrylamide electrophoresis of the pellets in SDS buffer, immunoblotting and visualization of antigen by sequential reaction with antiserum, peroxidase-conjugated second antibody and diaminobenzene-H_2O_2.

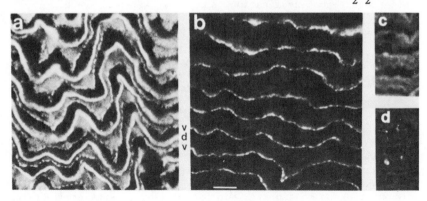

Fig. 4 Immunofluorescence of antisera to vesicles on 5-μm paraffin sections of Torpedo electric organ. (a) Unadsorbed antiserum; (b) adsorbed antiserum; (c) control serum; and (d) vesicle-adsorbed serum. Ventral (v) and dorsal (d) membranes are indicated. Scale bar = 10 μm.

Chemical work on the vesicular PG has shown that it consists of a protein backbone conjugated to a glycosaminoglycan[29] of the heparan sulphate type[30]. The antiserum does not recognize the glycosaminoglycan as such; the epitope must therefore involve the protein backbone.

Recent work on vesicular PG suggests that PGs of molecular mass considerably greater than 200 kDa occur in newly formed vesicles that have not yet taken up acetylcholine and ATP[31]. These are eliminated in the electrophoretic separation used in the immunoassay of the 200 kDa PG. Maturation of the vesicle may involve the formation of the 200 kDa PG from these higher molecular mass components.

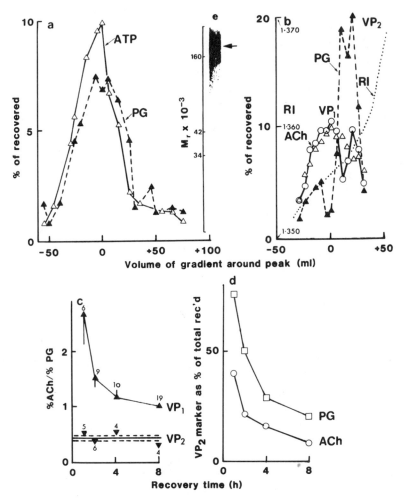

Fig. 5 (a) Copurification of proteoglycan (PG) with synaptic vesicles
from resting tissue (marker ATP). Correlation coefficient is +0.90.
(b) Vesicles from stimulated tissue after 1 h recovery. Note bimodal
distribution of acetylcholine (ACh), ATP (triangles) and PG with lower
ACh:PG ratios in VP_2 than in VP_1. (c,d) Recovery measured by (c) fall
in normalized ACh:PG ratio, (d) % of marker in VP_2. (e) Immune blot of
vesicle PG separated by SDS-PAGE. A single PG of M_r 200 000 is recognized (arrow).

Vesicle recycling

When synaptic vesicles are isolated from stimulated tissue, vesicular
acetylcholine is found to be bimodally distributed in the gradient[32,33] The
second vesicle peak consists of recycling vesicles which are only
partially loaded with acetylcholine and ATP. Several lines of evidence
identify this second population of isolated vesicles with a second
population of small vesicles detected by the statistical analysis of
vesicle profile diameters in electron micrographs of nerve terminals fixed
after similar periods of stimulation[34] The difference in diameter between
the two populations of isolated vesicles is the same as that between the
two populations seen *in situ*. If dextran particles are perfused through
the electric organ during stimulation, they enter the small vesicle

population, showing that these are vesicles that have undergone one or more cycles of exo- and endocytosis. After vesicle isolation, dextran-containing vesicles are confined to the second, denser (VP_2) vesicle peak. If an isotopically labelled acetylcholine precursor (acetate or choline) is perfused through the tissue, during or shortly after stimulation, labelled acetylcholine makes its appearance exclusively in the smaller, denser vesicle fraction; by contrast, labelled acetylcholine

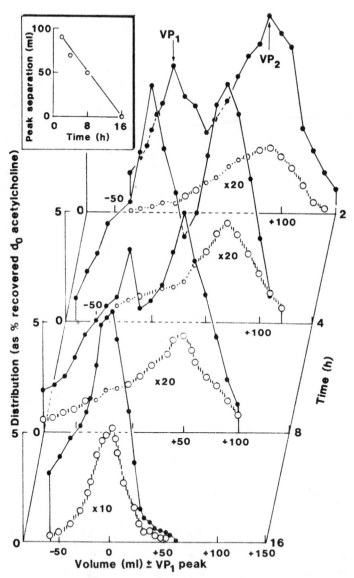

Fig. 6 Recovery by recycled vesicles (fraction VP_2) of the biophysical characteristics of reserve vesicles (fraction VP_1). The experimental technique was as in Fig. 5 a-c. Deuterated choline was perfused through the block of stimulated tissue for 0.5 h; the recycled vesicles were labelled by newly synthesized deuterated acetylcholine (o⁣—⁣o). After 16 h recovery was complete. Insert: progress of recovery measured as the separation of the VP_1 and VP_2 peaks.

is not significantly incorporated into vesicles in resting tissue. This is further grounds for identifying the small, dense vesicles as recycled vesicles since until vesicles have been unloaded they may be unable to take up newly synthesized transmitter from its site of synthesis in the cytoplasm.

During a period of rest following stimulation the small dense vesicles reacquire the biophysical properties of the 'reserve' population[33,35] This was clearly shown in experiments with perfused blocks of electric tissue one of which is presented in Fig. 6[36]

It will be seen that shortly after stimulation two fractions of vesicular acetylcholine could indeed be isolated and separated in the density gradient. Exposure for a short period to d_4 choline induced the formation of d_4 acetylcholine in the tissue; this was taken up mainly into the denser of the two vesicle peaks. As recovery continued, the density of the second peak became less until finally only one vesicle peak was present as in unstimulated tissue. However, unlike the corresponding peak for unstimulated tissue this peak now contained label, introduced when a proportion of these vesicles were recovering their acetylcholine content after recycling.

The change in the biophysical properties of the vesicles attendant on recycling has been accounted for by a loss of osmotically active water attendant on a reduced load of osmotically active acetylcholine and ATP[35] Water leaves the partially loaded vesicles in order to bring the osmolarity of the vesicle core into equilibrium with the cytoplasm. The recycling vesicles are thereby more easily able to resist a hypo-osmotic stress than the reserve vesicles, as has been demonstrated experimentally (Fig. 7)[37]

The availability of a stable vesicle marker which can be semiquantitatively assayed has enabled us to compare the acetylcholine content of the reserve and recycling vesicles directly by determining the ratio of acetylcholine to PG through the gradient[38] Figs. 8a-d and Fig. 5 b show that this ratio is considerably lower in the region of the gradient containing the recycling vesicles than in that containing the reserve vesicles[24,39] This is exactly what would be predicted from the relative osmotic fragilities of the two vesicle populations (Fig. 7).

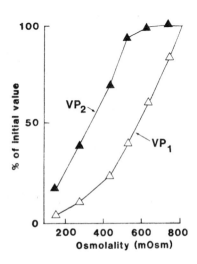

Fig. 7 Osmotic fragility of fractions
VP$_1$ and VP$_2$. Note lower osmotic pressure
required to bring about 50% lysis as
measured by loss of acetylcholine, thus
lower fragility of VP$_2$ vesicles compared
to VP$_1$.

Figs. 8a–d give the time course of recovery by the recycling vesicles of the biophysical properties of the reserve vesicles. As the two peaks merge, the ratio % acetylcholine ÷ % PG for the main peak must fall towards unity, the value for a single peak. On the other hand, the residual population of partially filled recycled vesicles will retain its initial value, though accounting for an ever smaller proportion of the total acetylcholine and PG[24] This is documented in Figs. 5c and d. One

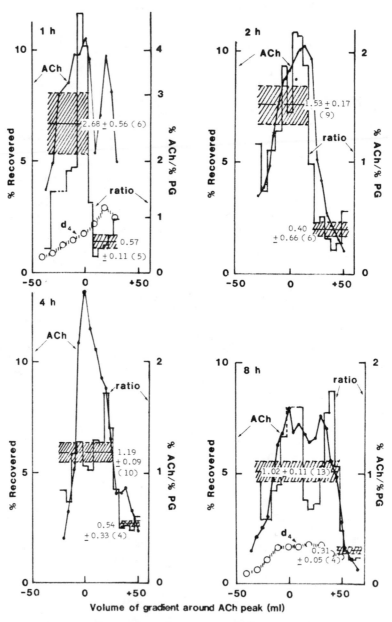

Fig. 8 Recovery, by recycled vesicles (identified at 1 h by their low ACh:PG ratio, high density and content of deuterated (d_4) ACh formed from d_4 choline perfused through the block during the first 0.5 h of recovery), of the biophysical characteristics of the reserve population. After 8 h recovery is almost complete, but the d_4 label originally intro- duced persists in the recovered vesicles. For abbreviations see Fig. 5.

hour after the stimulus given in the experiment shown in Fig. 8
(1800 pulses at 0.1 Hz) only 25% of the vesicles are in the reserve pool,
but these account for 60% of the acetylcholine remaining in the tissue.
After 8 h the reserve pool has risen to 80% of the total and accounts for
90% of the now greatly risen content of acetylcholine. After 16 h
recovery is complete (Fig. 8).

The life cycle of the synaptic vesicle

The availability of an antiserum recognizing a stable specific
vesicle component is permitting a study of the synthesis of vesicles in
the cell body, their axonal transport and their recycling in the terminal.
These methods are being supplemented by ^{35}S labelling of the
vesicle-specific PG. Fig. 9 illustrates some results obtained with
immunofluorescence histochemistry[40]. Fig. 9a shows what are presumed to be
fluorescent vesicles collecting in the axon-hillock region of an
electromotor neurone cell body waiting for axonal transport. Fig. 9b
shows the accumulation of fluorescent material in an electromotor axon
above a ligature. In both figures the vesicular PG has been rendered
accessible by the method of fixation. It is known that isolated vesicles
cannot be precipitated with anti PG antiserum unless they are first
disrupted, showing that the PG epitope is internal. In Fig. 9c and d,
frozen sections were used. Fig. 9c is a section through unstimulated

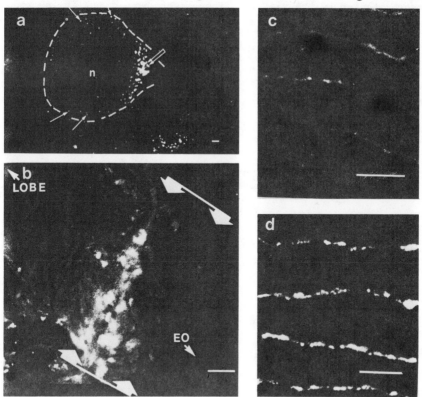

Fig. 9 *Immunofluorescence staining for vesicular proteoglycan.*
(a) Punctate staining of vesicles (arrows) in electromotor cell body and
accumulation (double arrows) of vesicles in axon hillock awaiting trans-
portation; the broken line is the outline of the cell obtained from phase
contrast. (b) Accumulation of vesicle-specific fluorescence in the axon
above a ligature. (c,d) Immunofluorescence of (c) resting, (d) stimulated
electromotor nerve terminals showing exteriorization of vesicle proteo-
glycan. Bars are 10 μm.

electric organ; fluorescence is low and diffuse. Fig. 9d, by contrast, is a section through stimulated electric organ. Strong fluorescence is now seen along the ventral surface of the organ. This demonstrates that vesicular PG becomes accessible to the antiserum during stimulus-induced vesicle exocytosis and transmitter release. When a period of recovery is allowed after stimulation and before freezing, sectioning and staining, the vesicular PG is reinternalized (not shown).

CHOLINERGIC PRESYNAPTIC PLASMA MEMBRANE-SPECIFIC ANTIGENS

Preparation of presynaptic plasma membranes

Presynaptic plasma membranes are prepared from synaptosomes by lysis and subsequent fractionation[16]. The various steps are summarized in Fig. 10. Synaptosome formation during the homogenization of electric organ was observed during our first attempts to prepare synaptic vesicles from the electromotor terminals[9], but it was a decade later before they were purified. The first synaptosomes[13,14] were rather small, but a technique of dispersion using stainless steel meshes of varying sizes produces larger ones[15,44-47]. Functionally there is little difference between the various preparations, where comparisons can be made. Recently, the presence of a membrane potential in metabolizing electromotor synaptosomes has been detected by the use of a fluorescent probe[48], but it is important to realise that a positive signal may be given by only a small proportion of the synaptosomes in the preparation; certainly bulk analyses do not show much of an ability to pump ions by these synaptosomes and it is likely that the majority are little more than inert sacs. This view is supported by the fact that the acetylcholine and choline acetyltransferase content of the synaptosomes per mg of protein is much lower than one would expect from intact preparations (Table 2) representing no more than a few percent of the tissue.

Table 2. Characteristics of large synaptosomes derived from electromotor nerve terminals of *Torpedo marmorata*

Preparation	Amount (units) per mg of protein			Intracellular potassium concentration (mM)
	Acetylcholine (nmol)	Choline acetyl-transferase (nmol/h)	High affinity choline uptake (pmol/min)	
Whole tissue	58[a]	452[b]	21[c]	116[d]
Synaptosomes				
expected[e]	1933	15065	700	116[d]
highest reported[f]	262[g]	680[g]	74[g]	28[h]
% intact (est.)	14	5	11	24

[abc]Calculated from data in (a) ref 41, (b) ref 42, (c) ref 43 assuming a protein content (ref 14, Table 2) of 16 mg/g.

[d]Assumed. [e]On assumption that terminals occupy 3% of tissue mass.

[f]For large synaptosomes prepared according to refs 15, 45 and 46.

[g]ref 46 (cf ref 44 and 45 which give 130, 450 and 23 respectively)

[h]ref 47.

For the purpose of preparing synaptosomal plasma membranes these deficiencies do not matter. The purified membranes contain a relatively limited number of proteins; one of 54 kDa has recently been tentatively identified as the choline transporter[17]. This component is functionally important in that it transfers the transmitter precursor choline into the nerve terminal at high rate and affinity in the presence of an inwardly-directed Na^+ gradient.

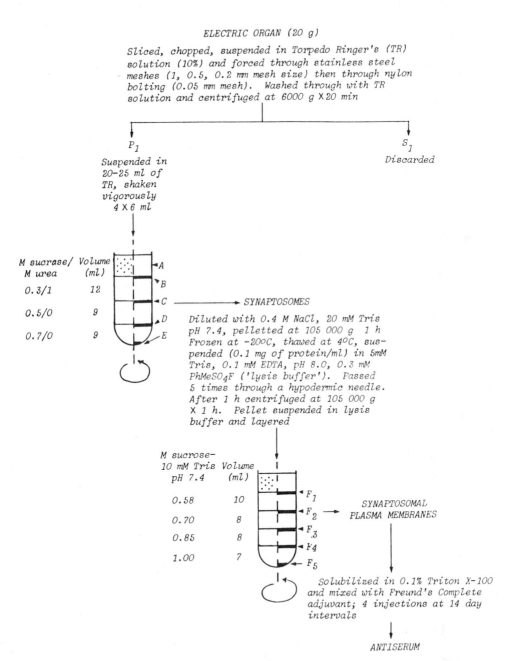

ELECTRIC ORGAN (20 g)

Sliced, chopped, suspended in Torpedo Ringer's (TR) solution (10%) and forced through stainless steel meshes (1, 0.5, 0.2 mm mesh size) then through nylon bolting (0.05 mm mesh). Washed through with TR solution and centrifuged at 6000 g × 20 min

P_1

Suspended in 20-25 ml of TR, shaken vigorously 4 × 6 ml

S_1

Discarded

M sucrase/ M urea	Volume (ml)	
0.3/1	12	A
		B
0.5/0	9	C
		D
0.7/0	9	E

SYNAPTOSOMES

Diluted with 0.4 M NaCl, 20 mM Tris pH 7.4, pelletted at 105 000 g 1 h Frozen at -20°C, thawed at 4°C, suspended (0.1 mg of protein/ml) in 5mM Tris, 0.1 mM EDTA, pH 8.0, 0.3 mM PhMeSO₄F ('lysis buffer'). Passed 5 times through a hypodermic needle. After 1 h centrifuged at 105 000 g × 1 h. Pellet suspended in lysis buffer and layered

M sucrose-10 mM Tris pH 7.4	Volume (ml)	
0.58	10	F_1
0.70	8	F_2
0.85	8	F_3
		F_4
1.00	7	F_5

SYNAPTOSOMAL PLASMA MEMBRANES

Solubilized in 0.1% Triton X-100 and mixed with Freund's Complete adjuvant; 4 injections at 14 day intervals

ANTISERUM

Fig. 10 Scheme showing the preparation of presynaptic plasma membranes from electromotor synaptosomes.

Injection of such preparations into sheep induces the formation of antibodies which specifically sensitize the cholinergic subpopulation of guinea-pig cortical synaptosomes to complement lysis (Fig. 11)[18,21,22] It will be recalled that such synaptosomes are sealed structures and have many properties in common with small cells[49-51] This selective complement lysis in the presence of the antiserum directed against electromotor synaptosomal plasma membrane implies the presence, on the cholinergic subpopulation of guinea-pig cortical synaptosomes, of an antigen resembling or identical to the *Torpedo* antigen which is specific for this subpopulation. The crude antiserum stained both the ventral and dorsal electrocyte membranes and recognized several proteins in Triton X-100 extracts of electric organ, but only two of these, of molecular masses 33 and 67 kDa, the latter identified as cholinesterase, copurified with the plasma membranes. Adsorption with a two-fold excess of membrane-bound cholinesterase removed the antibodies recognizing the 67 kDa protein and markedly attenuated the response to all other antigens except that of molecular mass 33. The adsorbed serum now selectively stained the ventral surface of the electrocytes.

In contrast to the results with electric organ extracts, the crude antiserum failed to precipitate any proteins from solubilized mammalian brain cortical synaptosomal membranes, showing that lysis of such synaptosomes was not due to components resembling any of the protein antigens present in *Torpedo*.

This led to an investigation of the lipids of mammalian cortical synaptosomes[22] Adsorption of the antiserum with *Torpedo* electric organ lipids greatly reduced its ability to sensitize mammalian cortical synaptosomes to complement lysis; the most effective class of lipids were the gangliosides. Consistent with this were the attenuation of the immunohistochemical response of tissue sections of electric organ and hippocampus caused by extracting them with chloroform-methanol (2:1 by volume) and the increase in the cytotoxicitiy of the antiserum resulting from adsorbing it onto a column of immobilized electric tissue ganglioside followed by elution[23,24]

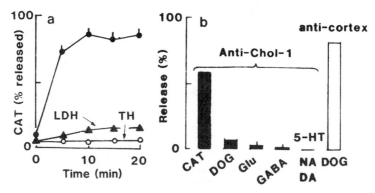

Fig. 11 (a) Selective complement-induced release of choline acetyl-transferase (CAT) from guinea-pig cortical synaptosomes sensitized with anti-Chol-1 antiserum. Lactate dehydrogenase (LDH) is partially released, tyrosine hydroxylase, a marker for catecholaminergic synaptosomes, not at all.[49] (b) Partial release of deoxyglucose (DOG), but no release of noncholinergic transmitters under same conditions as (a); over 80% release of DOG (white block) after sensitization with anti-cortex serum shows potential sensitivity of total population to complement lysis.[50] Synaptosomes were DOG-loaded beforehand.[51]

The purified antiserum recognizes several components in an immunoblot of electric tissue gangliosides separated by TLC (Fig. 12a) but only two in guinea-pig brain (Fig. 12b). Both are highly effective in blocking the lysis of cholinergic synaptosomes by complement after sensitizing with antiserum (Fig. 13). We refer to these as Chol-1 α and β. Chol-1β is enriched in a fraction enriched in polysialogangliosides (Fig. 12c). In extension of earlier work this antiserum identifies cholinergic neurones and nerve terminals in a wide variety of tissues; some examples are shown in Fig. 14.

Recently, monoclonal antibodies have been raised to gangliosides[52]. These have been screened by means of their ability to sensitize the mammalian brain cholinergic synaptosome subpopulation to complement lysis. One such antibody positive in the complement lysis test recognizes a third ganglioside, which we have named Chol-2. Histochemical work is now under way to see whether all cholinergic neurones respond similarly to the anti-Chol-1 and anti-Chol-2 antibodies or whether by differential staining one can recognize subclasses of cholinergic neurones.

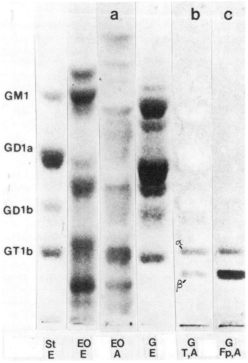

Fig. 12 Immunoblots of electric organ (EO) and guinea-pig cortical (G) gangliosides after TLC separation using affinity-purified anti-Chol-1 serum (A). E, Ehrlich reagent; St, standard ganglioside mixture; T, total gangliosides; Fp, fraction enriched in polysialogangliosides. Codes to left designate standard ganglioside classes.

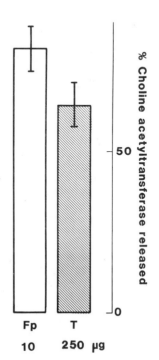

Fig. 13 Inhibition of complement lysis of cholinergic synaptosomes by total and polysialogangliosides.

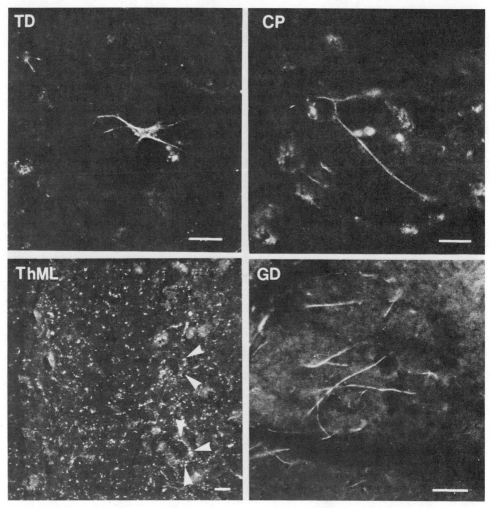

Fig. 14 Immunofluorescence histochemistry of rat cns neurones using affinity-purified anti-Chol-1 antiserum showing putative cholinergic neurones. TD, tractus diagonalis; CP, corpus putamen; ThML, thalamus nucleus medialis, pars lateralis; GD, gyrus dentatus. TD shows neurone cell body, CP, interneurone with cell body and axon, ThML, highly fluorescent nerve terminals on putative non-cholinergic cell bodies (arrows) and GD, axons. Bars are 1 μm.

Chol-1 appears to be highly concentrated in cholinergic nerve terminals, less so in cell bodies. This may make it possible to differentiate between cholinoceptive cells with numerous cholinergic synapses upon them, cholinergic cells with non-cholinergic innervation and cholinergic cells that are also cholinoceptive, a difficult task with present methods.

Other work, in collaboration with the group of Prof Tettamanti in Milan, involves the isolation of the pure gangliosides and their structural determination. In this way we hope to identify the structural features which make these gangliosides surface markers for cholinergic terminals.

An intriguing possibility that emerges from this work is that other transmitter-related surface antigens may exist for other transmitters. The monoclonal antibody technique utilizing synaptosomal plasma membranes combined with selective complement-induced lysis of synaptosomal subpopulations as a screening test may permit the identification of such transmitter-related surface antigens.

Isolation of cholinergic synaptosomes from brain

We conclude this account of cholinergic-specific antigens by mentioning their application in a new type of subcellular fractionation, utilizing immunoadsorption to antibody-coated cellulose[53].

In principle this method could be used to purify cholinergic vesicles, but the vesicle PG antigen as mentioned above is an internal not a surface antigen and intact vesicles are not sedimented by the anti-PG antiserum .

Recently, mammalian cortical cholinergic synaptosomes have been purified immunochemically, using an anti-Chol-1 antiserum and a column conjugated to a high-titre monoclonal second antibody[53]. As seen in Table 3, a relatively enriched fraction is obtained. In the future it may be possible to isolate other subpopulations of synaptosomes in this way using antibodies to other transmitter-related antigens.

It will be seen that the preparation of antisera which recognize one organelle or morphologically defined membrane have many uses once non-specific antibodies are removed. Among these are cell-biological investigations into the mechanism of synthesis, transport and utilization of the organelle in question, improved morphological methods to detect it in tissue sections and as the basis for immunoadsorption methods of purification.

Table 3. Isolation of cholinergic synaptosomes
by immunoadsorption[53]

Component	Activity in P_2 (u/min/mg of protein)[a]	Purification factor		Yield (%)
		found	expected[d]	
Cholinergic markers:				
choline acetyltransferase[b]	27.5 ± 3.3 (41)	18.9	160	9.5
acetylcholinesterase[c]	1.67 ± 0.14 (8)	14.1	160	7.1
Synaptosomal marker				
lactate dehydrogenase[c]	24.1 ± 2.3 (28)	1.5	10	0.8

[a]Units (b) pmol (c) nmol

[d]Calculation based on the assumption that: all lactate dehydrogenase in P_2 (synaptosomal-mitochondrial) fraction is synaptosomal; synaptosomes account for 10% of P_2 fraction; cholinergic synaptosomes account for 6% of all synaptosomes.[49,54]

REFERENCES

All references, except 3, 9, 10, 15, 41, 45, 46, 49, 51 and 54, are to publications of the Abteilung für Neurochemie, Max-Planck-Institut für biophysikalische Chemie, Göttingen. Quinquennial Reports (1973-78 and 1978-83) are of the work of the Abteilung and a limited number of reprints are available on request.

1. G.Q. Fox and G.P. Richardson, J. Comp. Neurol. **179**: 677 (1978)
2. G.Q. Fox and G.P. Richardson, J. Comp. Neurol. **185**: 293 (1979)
3. W. Feldberg and A. Fessard, J. Physiol. **101**: 200 (1942)
4. D. Schmid, Abstr. Colloquium on 'Biochemie des Nervensystems', Ges. f. biol. Chemie, Göttingen, Dec 1984
5. G.P. Richardson, B. Rinschen and G.Q. Fox, J. Comp. Neurol. **231**: 339 (1985)
6. L.P. Davies, V.P. Whittaker and H. Zimmermann, Exp. Brain Res. **30**: 493 (1977)
7. H. Stadler and M.-L. Kiene, Abstr. Colloquium on 'Biochemie des Nervensystems', Ges. f. biol. Chemie, Göttingen, Dec 1984
8. W.D. Krenz, T. Tashiro, K. Wächtler, V.P. Whittaker and V. Witzemann, Neuroscience **5**: 617 (1980)
9. M.N. Sheridan, V.P. Whittaker and M. Israël, Z. Zellforsch. **74**: 291 (1966)
10. V.P. Whittaker, W.B. Essman and G.H.C. Dowe, Biochem. J. **128**: 833 (1972)
11. T. Tashiro and H. Stadler, Eur. J. Biochem. **90**: 479 (1978)
12. K. Ohsawa, G.H.C. Dowe, S.J. Morris and V.P. Whittaker, Brain Res. **161**: 447 (1979)
13. M.J. Dowdall, G.Q. Fox, K. Wächtler, V.P. Whittaker and H. Zimmermann, Cold Spring Harbor Symp. quant. Biol. **40**: 65 (1975)
14. M.J. Dowdall and H. Zimmermann, Neuroscience **2**: 405 (1977)
15. M. Israël, R. Manaranche, P. Mastour-Franchon and N. Morel, Biochem. J. **160**: 113 (1976)
16. H. Stadler and T. Tashiro, Eur. J. Biochem. **101**: 171 (1979)
17. I. Ducis and V.P. Whittaker, Biochim. Biophys. Acta (in press)
18. J.H. Walker, R.T. Jones, J. Obrocki, G.P. Richardson and H. Stadler, Cell Tiss. Res. **223**: 101 (1982)
19. J.H. Walker, J. Obrocki and C.W. Zimmermann, J. Neurochem. **41**: 209 (1983)
20. N.N. Osborne, R. Beale, D. Nicholas, H. Stadler, J.H. Walker, R.T. Jones and V.P. Whittaker, Cell. Mol. Neurobiol. **2**: 157 (1982)
21. R.T. Jones, J.H. Walker, P.J. Richardson, G.Q. Fox and V.P. Whittaker, Cell Tiss. Res. **218**: 355 (1981)
22. P.J. Richardson, J.H. Walker, R.T. Jones and V.P. Whittaker, J. Neurochem. **38**: 1605 (1982)
23. P. Ferretti and E. Borroni, submitted for publication
24. V.P. Whittaker, E. Borroni, P. Ferretti and G.P. Richardson, in: 'Antibody Combining Sites: their Investigation and Exploitation in Subcellular Studies', E. Reid, ed., Plenum Press, New York (1985)
25. E. Borroni and J. Obrocki, unpublished results
26. D.A. Lee and V. Witzemann, Biochemistry **22**: 6123 (1983)
27. H. Stadler and E.M. Fenwick, Eur. J. Biochem. **136**: 377 (1983)
28. K. Zechel and H. Stadler, J. Neurochem. **39**: 788 (1982)
29. H. Stadler and V.P. Whittaker, Brain Res. **153**: 408 (1978)
30. H. Stadler and G.H.C. Dowe, EMBO J. **1**: 1381 (1982)
31. H. Stadler, Colloquium on 'Neurochemie', Ges. f. biol. Chemie, Mosbach, April 1985
32. H. Zimmermann and V.P. Whittaker, Nature, Lond., **267**: 633 (1977)
33. H. Zimmermann and C.R. Denston, Neuroscience **2**: 715 (1977)
34. H. Zimmermann and C.R. Denston, Neuroscience **2**: 695 (1977)

35. P.E. Giompres, H. Zimmermann and V.P. Whittaker, Neuroscience 6: 775 (1981)
36. V.P. Whittaker, G.H.C. Dowe and I.S. Roed, unpublished results
37. P.E. Giompres and V.P. Whittaker, Biochim. Biophys. Acta 770: 166 (1984)
38. V.P. Whittaker, Biochem. Soc. Trans. 12: 561 (1984)
39. V.P. Whittaker, G.H.C. Dowe, J.H. Walker and I.S. Roed, unpublished results
40. R.T. Jones, J.H. Walker, H. Stadler and V.P. Whittaker, Cell Tiss. Res. 223: 117 (1982)
41. H. Zimmermann and V.P. Whittaker, J. Neurochem. 22: 435 (1974)
42. R.R. Baker and M.J. Dowdall, Neurochem. Res. 1: 153 (1976)
43. M. Weiler, I.S. Roed and V.P. Whittaker, J. Neurochem. 38: 1187 (1982)
44. N. Morel, M. Israël, R. Manaranche and P. Mastour-Franchon, J. Cell Biol. 75: 43 (1977)
45. N. Morel, M. Israël, R. Manaranche and B. Lesbats, Prog. Brain Res. 49: 191 (1979)
46. H. Zimmermann, M.J. Dowdall and D.A. Lane, Neuroscience 4: 979 (1979)
47. P.J. Richardson and V.P. Whittaker, J. Neurochem. 36: 1536 (1981)
48. F.-M. Meunier, J. Physiol. 354: 121 (1984)
49. P.J. Richardson, J. Neurochem. 37: 358 (1981)
50. P.J. Richardson, J. Neurochem. 41: 640 (1983)
51. V.P. Whittaker, in: 'Handbook of Neurochemistry', A. Lajtha, ed., vol 7, pp 1-69, Plenum Press, New York (1984)
52. E. Borroni, unpublished results
53. P.J. Richardson, H. Siddle and J.P. Luzio, Biochem. J. 219: 643 (1984)
54. V.P. Whittaker, Prog. Brain Res. 45: 45 (1976)

BIOCHEMICAL STUDIES OF CHOLINERGIC SYSTEMS

THE EFFECT OF AH 5183 (2-(4-PHENYLPIPERIDINO)-CYCLOHEXANOL) ON ACETYLCHOLINE SYNTHESIS AND RELEASE IN THE ISOLATED GUINEA PIG ILEUM LONGITUDINAL MUSCLE/MYENTERIC PLEXUS PREPARATION

Donald J. Jenden, Margareth Roch, Ruth A. Booth,
Kathleen M. Rice, and Georgette M. Buga

Department of Pharmacology and Brain Research Institute
School of Medicine, Center for the Health Sciences
University of California, Los Angeles, CA 90024

INTRODUCTION

AH 5183 (2-(4-phenylpiperidino)-cyclohexanol) has been shown by Anderson et al. (1983) to be a potent inhibitor of the active transport of ACh into synaptic vesicles isolated from the electric organ of Torpedo. Toll and Howard (1980) and Melega and Howard (1984) reported that AH 5183 inhibited the loading of ACh into storage vesicles in PC 12 cells without affecting the vesicular storage of preformed ACh. They found no effect on choline uptake or ACh synthesis. Studies on synaptosomes and slices from rat and mouse brain (Otero et al., 1985; Carroll, 1985; Jope and Johnson, 1986) and perfused superior cervical ganglion of the cat (Collier et al., in press) have also shown an inhibition of evoked ACh release, with associated changes in Ch transport, ACh synthesis and levels. A recent electrophysiological study (Vyskocil, 1985) concluded that non-quantal leakage of ACh in mouse diaphragm was also inhibited by AH 5183.

We report here a study of the effect of AH 5183 on isolated strips of longitudinal muscle and attached myenteric plexus from the guinea pig ileum. This preparation has been extensively employed in studies of ACh release and is well suited to an analysis of the other component processes in ACh turnover (Kilbinger, 1982). The results show that while resting ACh release is unchanged by AH 5183, electrically induced release is markedly inhibited; tissue levels increase and synthesis is slowed.

METHODS

The procedure used to measure ACh and Ch release from guinea pig ileum was similar to that employed by Kilbinger (1982). Male English short-hair guinea pigs weighing 300-450 gm were stunned and decapitated. Strips of ileum 4 cm in length were removed, beginning 8-12 cm from the ileocecal junction. A total of 8 strips was used in most experiments. The strips were cleaned and dissected free of mesentery. The longitudinal muscle layer with the attached myenteric plexus was teased free and mounted on platinum electrodes 12 mm apart supported in a polyacrylate holder. Details of the holder and constant current stimulating circuit are being published separately. The holders with attached muscle strips were placed in 3 ml baths containing modified Tyrode solution of the following composition, and saturated with 95% O_2 and 5% CO_2: NaCl: 137 mM; KCl: 2.7 mM; $CaCl_2$: 1.8 mM; $MgSO_4$: 1.0 mM; NaH_2PO_4: 0.4 mM; $NaHCO_3$: 11.9 mM, glucose: 5.6 mM; EDTA: 10 µM; physostigmine, 30 µM and atropine, 1 µM. One hour was allowed for equilibration, during which the bath fluid was changed every 15 min. Thereafter, AH 5183 (1 µM) was added to some preparations, while others served as controls. $[^2H_4]$-Ch was added to some preparations to estimate the kinetics of Ch uptake and utilization. The preparations were stimulated at 3 Hz (1 msec, 11 V cm^{-1}) as indicated in the text. The polarity of the stimuli alternated with successive pulses to prevent polarization. The bath fluid was changed every 10 min and analyzed for ACh and Ch by GCMS, using $[^2H_9]$-ACh and $[^2H_9]$-Ch as internal standards, as we have described previously (Jenden et al., 1973; Freeman et al., 1975). The tissue was analyzed at the end of the experiment. Tissue concentrations are expressed as nmol gm^{-1} wet weight, and release rates as nmol gm^{-1} min^{-1}. The statistical significance of comparisons between tissues was estimated by Student's t test. Exact probabilities were calculated by series summation using a Hewlett Packard 41 CX calculator.

RESULTS

Figure 1 shows the results of an experiment in which guinea pig longitudinal muscle/myenteric plexus preparations were incubated without stimulation for one hour, followed by stimulation at 3 Hz for one hour. Every 10 min the bath fluid was removed for analysis and replaced. At the end of the second hour the tissues were analyzed for choline and acetylcholine. AH 5183 (1 µM) had no significant effect on resting ACh release at any time during the first hour (Table 1). Stimulation at 3 Hz caused a substantial ($\sim$ 30-fold) increase in the rate of ACh release in the control preparations; this declined by 58% during the 1 hour period of stimulation. A dramatic inhibition of ACh release by AH 5183 was immediately apparent after stimulation began (by 55%; t_6 = 6.853; P = 4.8 x 10^{-4}) and increased during the second hour to 61%. Choline release was also unaffected during the resting phase of the experiment, and declined by about 25% in both control and AH 5183-treated preparations. Stimulation caused an abrupt decrease in choline release (by 31 and 32% in control and experimental preparations respectively), and a further decline throughout the 1 hour period of stimulation. This decline was significantly less in the AH 5183-treated preparations (37%) than in the controls (60%; t_6 = 3.323; P = 1.6 x 10^{-2}).

Table 1. Average ACh release rates during a 1 hr period of rest followed by 1 hr of stimulation at 3 Hz in control tissues and tissues treated with AH 5183 (1 µM) starting at the beginning of the 1 hr rest period. Data are presented as mean ± standard error of 4 replicates.

	Control	AH 5183	t_6	P
Resting	0.066±0.006	0.062±0.003	0.531	6.1 x 10^{-1}
Stimulated	2.17 ±0.12	0.89 ±0.03	10.206	5.2 x 10^{-5}

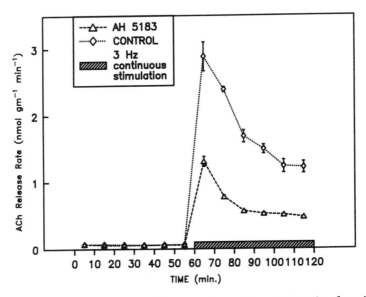

Figure 1. ACh release rates from strips of guinea pig longitudinal muscle/myenteric plexus. Tissues were resting from 0-60 min and were stimulated at 3 Hz from 60-120 min. ◇ Control. △ AH 5183 (1 μM). Bars indicate standard errors of 4 replicates.

Tissue levels of ACh at the end of the experiment were more than doubled in the preparations treated with AH 5183 (94.0 compared with 46.2 nmol gm^{-1}; t_6 = 26.509; P = 1.9 x 10^{-7}). The sum of ACh released and remaining in the tissue was less in the AH 5183-treated preparations (139.3 ± 0.6) than in controls (159.4 ± 3.5; t_6 = 5.650; P = 1.3 x 10^{-3}), suggesting that AH 5183 had a net inhibitory effect on ACh synthesis. Tissue choline levels were significantly higher in the preparations treated with AH 5183 (20.10 ± 0.88 compared to 14.84 ± 0.63 nmol gm^{-1}; t_6 = 4.883; P = 2.8 x 10^{-3}); the sum of choline released and remaining in the tissue (137.9 ± 4.6 nmol gm^{-1}) was also larger than in the control preparations, but the difference was not significant (114.42 ± 9.6 nmol gm; t_6 = 2.202; P = 7.0 x 10^{-2}).

These results were confirmed and extended in a second experiment, depicted in Fig. 2, in which similar preparations were stimulated continuously for 2 hr, during which the bath fluid was changed for analysis every 10 min. As before, tissue levels were measured at the end of the experiment. Again, ACh release declined slowly but progressively during constant stimulation at 3Hz. At every time point ACh release was less in the presence of AH 5183 than in control preparations, the ratio varying from 29% at 20-30 min to 50% at 110-120 min. In every case the difference was highly significant

(P $<10^{-3}$). Choline release was greater in the presence of AH 5183 in 10 of the 12 periods. Tissue levels of ACh were again higher in the presence of AH 5183 (116.5 ± 5.3 compared to 42.2 ± 1.95); the difference was highly significant (t_6 = 13.109, P = 1.2 x 10^{-5}). In preparations treated with AH 5183, but not in controls, ACh levels were significantly higher (t_6 = 4.190; P = 5.7 x 10^{-3}) after 2 hr of stimulation than in the first experiment. As in the previous experiment, the sum of the ACh released and remaining in the tissue was greater in control preparations (248.2 ± 12.5 nmol gm^{-1}) than in those treated with AH 5183 (203.1 ± 4.4 nmol gm^{-1}; t_6 = 3.407; P = 1.4 x 10^{-2}), confirming that AH 5183 inhibits ACh synthesis.

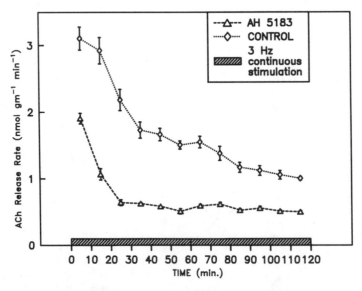

Figure 2. ACh release rates from strips of guinea pig longitudinal muscle/myenteric plexus, stimulated at 3 Hz throughout the 2 hr period. ◇ Control. △ AH 5183 (1 μM). Bars indicate standard errors of 4 replicates.

Table 2. ACh and Ch release rates at the beginning and end of a 2 hr period of continuous stimulation at 3 Hz and tissue levels at the end of the 2 hr period, with and without $[^2H_4]$-Ch (5 µM) in the bath fluid. No AH 5183 was added. Data are presented as mean ± standard error.

Medium $[^2H_4]$-Ch (µM)		n	Release Rate nmol gm^{-1} min^{-1}		Tissue nmol gm^{-1}
			0-10 min	110-120 min	
0	ACh	4	3.11±0.17	1.01±0.03	42.23±1.95
	Ch	4	0.92±0.08	0.53±0.14	18.10±3.51
5	$[^2H_4]$-ACh	10	0.24±0.04	1.13±0.06	27.87±2.55
	Total ACh	10	2.90±0.08	2.26±0.12	91.54±4.40
	$[^2H_4]$-Ch	10	-	-	3.83±0.41
	$[^2H_0]$-Ch	10	1.20±0.13	0.27±0.04	25.62±3.58
	Total Ch	10	-	-	29.45±3.48

A third experiment was carried out in the presence of $[^2H_4]$-choline (5 µM) to assess the effect of AH 5183 on the kinetics of Ch uptake and acetylation as well as on ACh release. In control preparations (Table 2), ACh release was better maintained in the presence of 5 µM choline than in its absence. The decline in release (from 2.90 to 2.26 nmol gm^{-1} min^{-1}) is significantly less than in the absence of added choline (t_{10} = 7.047; P = 3.5 x 10^{-5}). Of the ACh released in the final epoch, 48.7 ± 3.1% was derived from the added $[^2H_4]$-Ch. Tissue levels of ACh were also better maintained in the presence of supplemental Ch (t_{12} = 6.832; P = 1.8 x 10^{-5}). Of the tissue ACh 29.9 ± 2.5% was derived from $[^2H_4-]$Ch. Tissue levels of Ch were as expected higher than when the medium contained no Ch; the difference is suggestive but not significant (t_{12} = 1.889; P = 8.3 x 10^{-2}). 14.7 ± 2.1% of the tissue Ch was labelled.

The major effects of AH 5183 observed in the first two experiments were also seen in the third (Table 3). ACh release was progressively inhibited during exposure to the drug, reaching a plateau of 26.6 ± 2.8% of control at the end of 2 hrs. The release of $[^2H_4]$-Ch was increased from a control rate of 268 ± 39 pmol gm^{-1} min^{-1} to 711 ± 8 pmol gm^{-1} min^{-1} (t_{12} = 39.659; P < 10^{-9}). Tissue levels of ACh (176.5 ± 2.3 nmol gm^{-1}) were significantly increased compared to control (91.5 ± 4.4 nmol gm^{-1}; t_{12} = 17.539; P = 1.5 x 10^{-9}), but Ch levels were not significantly affected. The sum of the ACh released and remaining in the tissue (264.5 ± 3.7 nmol gm^{-1}) was significantly less than in control strips (426.9 ± 15.7 nmol gm^{-1}; t_{12} = 6.346; P = 3.7 x 10^{-5}) indicating that ACh synthesis was reduced by AH 5183. If tissue levels in the strips treated with AH 5183 were initially the same as those in control preparations and remained constant throughout the experiment, the inhibition of synthesis was 26.2%.

Table 3. ACh and Ch release rates at the beginning and end of a 2 hr period of continuous stimulation at 3 Hz and tissue levels at the end of the 2 hr period, with and without $[^2H_4]$-Ch (5 μM) in the bath fluid. All tissues were exposed to AH 5183 (1 μM) throughout the experiment. Data are presented as mean ± standard error.

Medium [Ch] (μM)		n	Release Rate (nmol gm^{-1} min^{-1})		Tissue (nmol gm^{-1})
			0-10 min	110-120 min	
0	ACh	4	1.90±0.08	0.50±0.02	116.51±5.32
	Ch	4	0.98±0.04	0.41±0.02	23.51±1.64
	$[^2H_4]$-ACh	4	0.03±0.00	0.28±0.03	73.22±3.61
	Total ACh	4	1.82±0.05	0.63±0.06	176.49±2.31
5	$[^2H_4]$-Ch	4	–	–	8.90±0.06
	$[^2H_0]$-Ch	4	1.34±0.11	0.71±0.01	27.61±3.08
	Total Ch	4	–	–	36.52±3.13

In addition to these conclusions, the rate of incorporation of $[^2H_4]$-Ch provides additional information about the effect of AH 5183 on the dynamics of ACh metabolism. The total uptake of $[^2H_4]$-Ch, as indicated by the sum of tissue $[^2H_4]$-Ch and tissue $[^2H_4]$-ACh at the end of the experiment and $[^2H_4]$-ACh release during the experiment, was 149.0 ± 12.8 nmol gm^{-1}, or 1.242 ± 0.107 nmol gm^{-1} min^{-1}, in the control tissues compared to 103.4 ± 5.4 nmol gm^{-1}, or 0.862 ± 0.045 nmol gm^{-1} min^{-1} in strips treated with AH 5183. This inhibition of $[^2H_4]$-Ch uptake (30.6%) is not quite significant (t_{12} = 2.166; P = 5.1 x 10^{-2}). The percentage of this $[^2H_4]$-Ch which was acetylated was much greater in control strips than in those treated with AH 5183 (97.44 ± 0.151 and 91.41 ± 0.142 respectively), but neither of these figures take into account the incorporation of $[^2H_4]$-Ch into the phospholipid pathway. The total synthesis of $[^2H_4]$-ACh during the 2 hr experiment (sum of release and tissue levels) was 94.5 ± 4.8 and 145.2 ± 12.6 nmol gm^{-1} for AH 5183-treated and control preparations respectively. This inhibition of 34.9% is significant (t_{12} = 2.453; P = 3.0 x 10^{-2}). However, it is not an absolute estimate of ACh synthesis, since the mole ratio of $[^2H_4]$-Ch in the nerve terminals is not known. The mole ratio of $[^2H_4]$-Ch in the tissue at the end of the experiment is larger in the strips treated with AH 5183 (24.84 ± 2.29%) than in controls (14.73 ± 2.06%), but this is evidently not an accurate reflection of the mole ratio in the pool of Ch available for synthesis, because the mole ratio of $[^2H_4]$-ACh in the tissue at the end of the experiment was considerably larger (29.9 ± 2.5% and 41.5 ± 2.4% for control and experimental respectively), and the mole ratio of label in released ACh was still larger (48.8 ± 3.1% and 43.6 ± 2.1% respectively).

In control preparations the rate of release of $[^2H_0]$-Ch from the tissue decreased progressively throughout the period of stimulation (from 1.204 ± 0.100 to 0.268 ± 0.036 nmol gm^{-1} min^{-1}). In the presence of AH 5183 the initial rate of release was not significantly different $(1.338 \pm 0.107$ nmol gm^{-1} $min^{-1})$ but it decreased much less during the 2 hr of stimulation (to 0.711 ± 0.008 nmol gm^{-1} min^{-1}). The difference in the final efflux rate was highly significant $(t_{12} = 7.489; P = 7.3 \times 10^{-6})$. It was evidently not caused by a difference in the concentration gradient, since tissue levels of $[^2H]$-Ch were not significantly affected by AH 5183 $(t_{12} = 0.328; P = 7.5 \times 10^{-1})$. It appears likely that the faster loss of $[^2H]$-Ch in the presence of AH 5183 is due to the capture of a smaller proportion of $[^2H_0]$-Ch for synthesis of ACh, since the evidence presented above indicates that the total rate of ACh synthesis is slower in the presence of the inhibitor.

DISCUSSION

The data presented clearly indicate that AH 5183 (1 μM) inhibits the release of ACh evoked in the guinea pig myenteric plexus by electrical stimulation, while resting release was not significantly affected. Similar results have been reported by Collier et al. (in press) in the cat superior cervical ganglion. AH 5183 has also been reported to inhibit ACh release induced by potassium depolarization of rat cortical minces (Jope and Johnson, 1986), mouse forebrain minces (Carroll, 1985) and rat cortical synaptosomes (Otero, 1985), and by Ba^{++} in PC 12 cells (Melega and Howard, 1984). Resting release has generally been found to be unaltered by AH 5183, but Vyskocil (1985) has reported that the mouse diaphragm end plate region is hyperpolarized by AH 5183, and interpreted this as an inhibition of non-quantal leakage. A selective inhibition of evoked release by an established inhibitor of vesicular ACh transport (Anderson et al., 1983) must be considered strong evidence for a vesicular role in evoked release, but Vyskocil (1985) has pointed out that exocytosis of vesicles might be expected to leave the ACh transporter in the plasma membrane where it could also favor leakage of cytoplasmic ACh. Thus AH 5183 might also inhibit spontaneous release from a cytosolic compartment.

Evidence has been presented in this report that ACh synthesis and Ch uptake are also inhibited by AH 5183. It seems likely that these effects are secondary to the inhibition of ACh release, although a direct effect of AH 5183 on high affinity Ch transport cannot be ruled out (Jope and Johnson, 1986). Inhibition of synthesis is in any event not sufficient to prevent a rise in ACh levels, as others have also observed (Jope and Johnson, 1986; Collier et al., in press). This increase is greater after 2 hr of stimulation than after 1 hr, and did not occur in resting preparations (data not shown). We conclude that stimulation has a direct effect on ACh synthesis when ACh release is inhibited by AH 5183, and in a subsequent paper data will be presented to show that this increase is mediated by increased influx of Ca^{++}.

Like most isolated preparations, the guinea pig longitudinal muscle/myenteric plexus preparation releases Ch, presumably as a result of phospholipid degradation. This Ch can be utilized for ACh synthesis, since there was an abrupt fall in the rate of Ch release in experiment 1 at the onset of stimulation. This utilization of endogenous Ch is presumably the reason why the tissue levels and net efflux of Ch tend to be greater in preparations treated with AH 5183, in which less Ch is taken up for ACh synthesis.

Despite the endogenous supply of Ch, ACh metabolism in the myenteric plexus is better maintained in the presence of an exogenous source. A similar dependence on exogenous Ch was reported many years ago for the superior cervical ganglion of the cat (Birks and MacIntosh, 1961). During sustained stimulation (2 hr), ACh release declined much less when 5 μM Ch was present in the bathing fluid (Table 2), and tissue ACh levels at the end of the experiment were significantly greater when 5 μM Ch was present, both in the presence of AH 5183 (Table 3) and in control prepartions (Table 2). Not unexpectedly, tissue Ch levels were also higher when exogenous Ch was provided (Tables 2 and 3); the difference (11.35 and 11.01 nmol gm^{-1} in control and AH 5183-treated preparations respectively) was greater than the concentration of Ch provided in the bathing fluid (5 nmol ml^{-1}). This must indicate that most of the Ch is intracellular, where it could be retained electrochemically by the membrane potential.

When $[^2H_4]$-Ch was added to the medium $[^2H_4]$-ACh progressively replaced $[^2H_0]$-ACh in the released transmitter, whether or not AH 5183 was present. Under all conditions and in all preparations, the mole ratio of $[^2H_4]$-label was greater in the released ACh than in the tissue ACh, where it was in turn greater than in the tissue Ch. This familiar pattern of apparently selective release of the most recently synthesized transmitter is consistent with the existence of a small, rapidly turning over pool of transmitter or vesicles, but is more generally attributable to heterogeneity in the preparation (Weiler et al., 1981), which undeniably exists in this preparation because of diffusion gradients of both Ch and ACh. Caution should therefore be exercised in interpreting this phenomenon in a more specific way.

ACKNOWLEDGMENTS

These authors are grateful to Dr. Stanley M. Parsons for a gift of AH 5183 and to Dr. Brian Collier for permission to quote data in press. This research was supported by MH 17691. We gratefully acknowledge the valuable editorial assistance of Ms. Nelly Canaan.

REFERENCES

Anderson, D.C., King, S.C., and Parsons, S.M., 1983, Pharmacological characterization of the acetylcholine transport system in purified Torpedo electric organ synaptic vesicles, Mol. Pharmacol., 24:48.

Birks, R.I., and MacIntosh, F.C., 1961, Acetylcholine metabolism of a sympathetic ganglion, Canad. J. Biochem. Physiol., 39:787.

Carroll, P.T., 1985, The effect of the acetylcholine transport blocker 2-(4-phenylpiperidino)cyclohexanol (AH5183) on the subcellular storage and release of acetylcholine in mouse brain, Brain Res., 358:200.

Collier, B., Welner, S.A., Ricny, J., and Araujo, D.M., Acetylcholine synthesis and release by a sympathetic ganglion in the presence of 2-(4-phenylpiperidino) cyclohexanol (AH5183), J. Neurochem., In press.

Freeman, J.J., Choi, R.L., and Jenden, D.J., 1975, Plasma choline: its turnover and exchange with brain choline, J. Neurochem., 24:729.

Jenden, D.J., Roch, M,, and Booth, R.A., 1973, Simultaneous measurement of endogenous and deuterium-labelled tracer variants of choline and acetylcholine in subpicomole quantities by gas chromatography/mass spectrometry, Anal. Biochem., 55:438.

Jope, R.S., and Johnson, G.V.W., 1986, Quinacrine and 2-(4-phenylpiperidino)cyclohexanol (AH5183) inhibit acetylcholine release and synthesis in rat brain slices, Mol. Pharmacol., 29:45.

Kilbinger, H., 1982, The myenteric plexus-longitudinal muscle preparation, in: "Progress in Cholinergic Biology: Model Cholinergic Synapses", I. Hanin and A.M. Goldberg, ed., Raven Press, New York, p. 137.

Melega, W.P., and Howard, B.D., 1984, Biochemical evidence that vesicles are the source of the acetylcholine released from stimulated PC12 cells, Proc. Natl. Acad. Sci. USA, 81:6535.

Otero, D.H., Wilbekin, F., and Meyer, E.M., 1985, Effects of 4-(2-hydroxyethyl)-1-piperazine-ethanesulfonic acid (AH5183) on rat cortical synaptosome choline uptake, acetylcholine storage and release, Brain Res., 359:208.

Toll, L., and Howard, B.D., 1980, Evidence that an ATPase and a protonmotive force function in the transport of acetylcholine into storage vesicles, J. Biol. Chem., 255:1787.

Vyskocil, F., 1985, Inhibition of non-quantal acetylcholine leakage by 2(4-phenylpiperidine)cyclohexanol in the mouse diaphragm, Neurosci. Lett., 59:277.

Weiler, M.H., Gundersen, C.B., and Jenden, D.J., 1981, Choline uptake and acetylcholine synthesis in synaptosomes: investigations using two different labeled variants of choline, J. Neurochem., 36:1802.

BRAIN ACETYLCHOLINE - A VIEW FROM THE CEREBROSPINAL FLUID

Ezio Giacobini, Robert Becker, Rodger Elble, Thomas Mattio,
Michael McIlhany and G. Scarsella

Departments of Pharmacology, Internal Medicine (Division
of Neurology), Psychiatry and Surgery (Division of
Neurosurgery), Southern Illinois University
School of Medicine, Springfield, IL 62708 and
Department of Cell Biology, University of Rome
Rome, Italy

INTRODUCTION

Is acetylcholine (ACh) metabolism in brain reflected by changes in
the cerebrospinal fluid (CSF)?   Are there specific changes in enzyme
activities associated with ACh synthesis and hydrolysis, levels of the
precursor (choline) and the neurotransmitter, which can be related to
physiological and pathological conditions of the central cholinergic
nervous system? This question has become more acute as several authors
have reported a selective impairment of the cholinergic system with a
marked decrease of cholineacetyltransferase (ChAc) and acetylcholinesterase (AChE) activity in several cortical and subcortical areas of the brain
of patients affected by presenile (AD) and senile dementia of Alzheimer
type (SDAT) (Davies, 1979; Perry et al., 1977; Rossor et al., 1982;
Whitehouse et al., 1981). We have recently reported (Giacobini et al.,
1985) changes in choline (Ch), AChE and ChAc activity in the CSF of a
group of SDAT patients showing characteristic symptoms of dementia of
different grades of severity, as compared to the CSF of healthy
age-matched controls. In this review, we shall examine and discuss our
recent results and some data found in the literature which might answer,
although not completely, the question posed by the title of this paper.

ORIGIN OF ACETYLCHOLINESTERASE IN CEREBRAL SPINAL FLUID (CSF)

The soluble AChE which is localized in the cell bodies of cholinergic
as well as non-cholinergic neurons (Giacobini, 1959) is transported to the
periphery as a mobile fraction by axoplasmic flow at a relatively rapid
rate (Lubinska and Niemerko, 1971; Fig. 1).   Acetylcholinesterase is
present in peripheral nerve endings of cholinergic neurons (Giacobini,
1959) where it represents 20% of the total neuronal activity as compared
to 70% for the cell body and 10% for the axon (Giacobini et al., 1979).
Acetylcholinesterase decreases in response to denervation and its levels
are regulated by trans-synaptic effects (Giacobini et al., 1979).   Its
activity has also been demonstrated in extracellular fluids such as plasma
and CSF of several species including man (Augustinsson, 1963; Plattner and

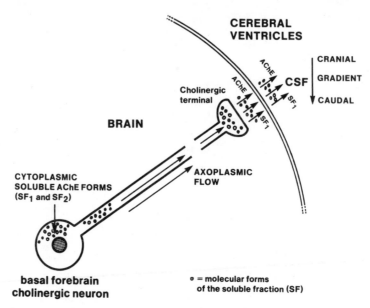

FIGURE 1: Secretory hypothesis of AChE in dog CSF (Bareggi and Giacobini, 1978; Scarsella et al, 1979).

Table I
Acetylcholinesterase Activity in CSF and Plasma of the Dog

	Total ChE Activity (μmole ACh hydrol/ml/hr)	AChE Activity (μmole ACh hydrol/ml/hr)	Protein (mg/ml)	AChE specific Activity (μmole ACh hydrol/hr/mg protein
Plasma	42.3 + 1.4 (3)	9.3 + 0.2 (3)	53.8 + 2 (3)	0.17 + 0.009 (3)
CSF				
Ventricular	1.32 + 0.1 (4)	1.2 + 0.2 (4)*	0.55 + 0.1 (4)*	2.18 + 0.2 (4)*
Cisternal	4.84 + 0.4 (6)	4.4 + 0.3 (6)*	0.68 + 0.2 (6)*	6.5 + 2.5 (6)*
CSF/Plasma ratio				
Ventricular	0.03	0.13	0.01	16
Cisternal	0.11	0.47	0.013	81

All values are mean $\pm$ S.E.M. Numbers in parenthesis indicate number of samples. Statistical significance of CSF values are relative to the corresponding plasma value. * $p < 0.1$ (modified from Bareggi and Giacobini, 1978)

Hintner, 1930). Plasma AChE activity in dog is significantly higher than in either ventricular or cisternal CSF (Table I). However, since protein levels in plasma are about 100-fold higher than that in CSF, the specific activity of AChE is lower in plasma than in CSF (Bareggi and Giacobini, 1978 and Table I). Acetylcholinesterase activity in plasma represents only 22% of total cholinesterase activity while in canine ventricular and cisternal CSF it is about 80%. Scarsella et al. (1979) compared the activity of AChE and butyrylcholinesterase (BuChE) in the cisternal CSF, plasma and brain of beagle dogs and described the characteristics of the molecular forms of both enzymes. Based on their distribution and similarities it was concluded that the single soluble form (SF) of AChE present in the CSF corresponds to the slower of the two forms (SF_1 and SF_2) found in the soluble fraction from brain tissue (Fig. 2) and, therefore,

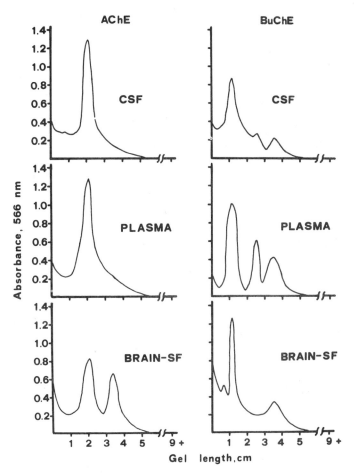

FIGURE 2: Pattern of AChE and BuChE molecular forms in dog CSF, plasma and brain (mod. from Scarsella et al., 1979)

it could be expected to be present in the CSF as a result of leakage or secretion from the nervous tissue (Fig. 1). A combined origin from blood plasma and brain tissue appears to be probable for the BuChE of the CSF. Additional evidence for the neuronal origin of AChE in CSF is the significant increase in AChE specific activity seen by Bareggi and Giacobini (1978) in the CSF following the administration of chlorpromazine (10 mg/kg i.v.), a drug which increases ACh turnover and ACh output. Taking these results together, we proposed (Bareggi and Giacobini, 1978) that in the dog, AChE activity present in CSF is mostly of cerebral origin and may reflect changes in neuronal AChE activity. This hypothesis is supported by the results of several investigators. Release of AChE was demonstrated by Chubb and Smith (1975) in the perfusate from the ox adrenal gland, by Chubb et al. (1974, 1976) in the rabbit CSF following peripheral nerve stimulation and by Gisiger and Vigny (1977) in perfusate from stimulated sympathetic ganglia. As for the origin of the single form of AChE found in blood plasma (Fig. 2) it appears most likely that its source is the CSF while a combined origin from both blood plasma and brain tissue (soluble fraction) appears to be probable for the BuChE of the CSF. Our results have also demonstrated a craniocaudal (i.e., ventricular vs. cisternal) gradient of AChE activity (Table I). The gradient reflects the different locations of the sites of AChE outflow from the brain into CSF (Fig. 1), mostly in the lateral and the fourth ventricles, in addition, AChE is secreted from CSF to blood mostly in the subarachnoidal spaces. We suggest that there is a continuous, rather slow rate of exit of AChE into the CSF resulting in an accumulation of the soluble enzyme form along the ventricular system (Fig. 1). The demonstration of such a gradient for AChE in canine CSF is in agreement with our hypothesis of a cerebral origin of AChE. In this case, CSF on its way from the lateral ventricles to subarachnoidal spaces would receive a continuous input of AChE from brain tissue.

The most widely accepted classifications of AChE molecular forms is presently based on both solubility characteristics and sedimentation velocities of the enzyme (Massoulié and Bon, 1982). This classification comprises two groups: globular forms as monomeric (G_1), dimeric (G_2)

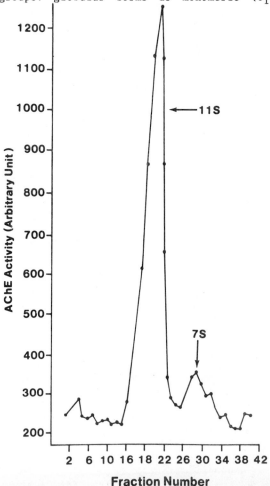

FIGURE 3: Pattern of molecular forms of AChE of human CSF of a normal subject. Observe the two different forms (11S and 7S).

or tetrameric (G_4) structures, and asymmetric forms with various configurations and catalytic subunits. In the human brain, using density gradient centrifugation, three molecular forms have been distinguished in both normal and SDAT post-mortem samples of neocortex (Atack et al., 1983). While the levels of the light and heavy forms were unaltered, there was a selective and extensive loss (73%) of the intermediate tetrameric globular G_4 form (Atack et al., 1983) in SDAT.

The molecular forms of AChE are being investigated in our laboratory in the human CSF by means of electrophoretic analysis and density gradient microsedimentation. Recent findings from our laboratory show that two molecular forms of AChE (11S and 7S) (Fig. 3) are detected in the CSF of normal human subjects, which represent the globular, tetramer and dimer forms, respectively. These forms are the same which are found in human brain (Massoulié and Bon, 1982). Preliminary findings also indicate that the 11S molecular form may be decreased in the Alzheimer patients. This particular form could represent the isozymic component secreted or leaked out from the nervous tissue under specific pathological conditions such as Alzheimer disease.

In conclusion, according to our present hypothesis, under conditions of cholinergic hyperactivity, following the action of drugs acting upon the CNS such as chlorpromazine (Bareggi and Giacobini, 1978) or amphetamines (Greenfield and Shaw, 1982), a particular AChE molecular form could be released by the CNS and accumulated in the CSF. These CSF changes in AChE activity could be used to monitor central cholinergic activity. Under particular pathological conditions, such as in Alzheimer, specific losses of cholinergic neurons and synapses could be reflected, within a certain period of the disease, by measurable changes of specific molecular forms of AChE in the CSF (Figs. 1 and 3).

THE EFFECT OF ACETYLCHOLINESTERASE INHIBITION ON ACETYLCHOLINESTERASE ACTIVITY IN CSF AND PLASMA

Little data are available on the effect of ChE inhibitors on human CSF (Thal et al., 1983) and none are available on CSF in animals. In order to further explore the validity of our hypothesis and to study the relation between peripheral and central effects of reversible cholinesterase (ChE) inhibitors, we monitored the levels of AChE activity (ChE activity was inhibited by 10^{-5}M iso-OMPA) following intravenous (i.v.) and intracerebral ventricular (i.c.v.) administration of various doses of a reversible ChE inhibitor, physostigmine (Phy) which has ready access to the CNS. In a second group of experiments (Giacobini et al., to be published), we related the changes in ChE activity of plasma and CSF to changes in these enzyme activities and ACh levels of various brain regions as well as to concentrations of Phy. The doses used in our experiments were 10, 20, 40, 80 and 120 μg for the i.c.v. administration and 250, 500 and 1000 μg for the i.v. administration. Six adult male beagle dogs (8.5-10.5 kg b.w.) were implanted with Rickham® nylon reservoirs which communicated with the respective lateral ventricle through a silastic catheter. The position of the catheter as well as the conditions of the ventricules were verified at autopsy. Both mono- and bilateral implant of reservoirs were used, so that the CSF could be sampled from, or the drug injected into, the contralateral ventricle, in the awake, non-anesthetized dog. The time of the drug infusion was 90 sec. The infusion was followed by a 1 cc 90 sec wash with saline. The animals were trained so that no visible stress was apparent before or during perfusion or sampling. Symptoms of peripheral or central cholinergic hyperactivity and behavior were recorded and rated according to an arbitrary scale. Each experiment lasted 24 hrs during which AChE activity was monitored both in plasma and CSF at fixed intervals in at least three dogs for each concentration.

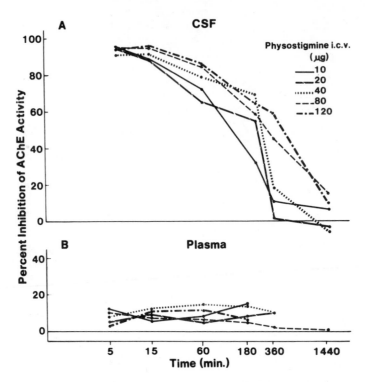

FIGURE 4: Changes in AChE activity in CSF and plasma following i.c.v. administration of various doses of physostigmine.

The different effects of the two routes of administration (i.c.v. and i.v.) of various doses of Phy on AChE activity in CSF and plasma are shown in Figs. 4,5. In the CSF, with the i.c.v. route, over 90% AChE inhibition was reached in 5 min at all dosages (Fig. 4A). With the lowest dose (10 µg), 50% inhibition was present in the CSF at 90 min, while with the highest dose (120 µg) the same inhibition was still present at 360 min. At 1440 min (24 hr) AChE inhibition was less than 20% at all doses. A dose/AChE inhibition relationship was present at most time points, however, it was most evident at the later ones such as at 360 and 1440 min (24 hr). With i.c.v. administration, the inhibitory effect of Phy on AChE activity in plasma was minimal as compared to CSF (Fig. 4B). Using this route, AChE inhibition was never higher than 15% at any time and at any Phy dosage. With i.v. administration, approximately 60% AChE inhibition (mean 57%) was present in plasma at 5 min at all dosages (Fig. 5A). Fifty percent inhibition was still present at 8 min with the two lower doses (250 and 500 µg) and at 25 min with the highest dose (1000 µg). At 24 hr (1440 min), AChE inhibition in plasma was less than 5% at all doses. No significant AChE inhibition was seen in CSF at any time and any dosage with i.v. administration (Fig. 5B). On the contrary, at 180 min, AChE activity was increased by 58, 48 and 36% with 1000, 500 and 250 µg Phy, respectively. At 24 hr, AChE activity reached normal levels at all doses. Three dogs administered the highest doses by the i.c.v. route (120 µg), showed symptoms of both central and peripheral hyperactivity such as: hypersalivation, laryngospasm, bronchospasm, generalized tremor and hind-leg rigidity (Table II). The symptoms appeared generally 5 min after the injection and lasted 15-20 min. One dog (injected i.c.v.) developed a generalized seizure which was promptly blocked by 1.5 mg atropine i.v. Three other dogs (injected i.c.v or i.v.) showed only mild hypersalivation, mild bronchospasm, fasciculations and tremor (Table II).

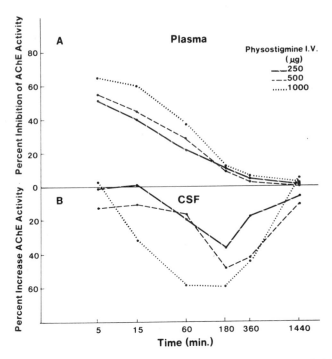

FIGURE 5: Changes in AChE activity in CSF and plasma following i.v. administration of various doses of physostigmine.

The sharp differences in AChE inhibition shown by the two routes of administration demonstrate that the i.c.v. route is very effective in inhibiting AChE activity in CSF with a minimal effect on activity in plasma. On the other hand, intravenous administration, even at the high dosage of 1000 µg (corresponding to about 100 µg/kg b.w.) does not inhibit significantly AChE in CSF. On the contrary, a progressive increase of enzyme activity is seen in CSF. The increase in AChE activity seen by us is similar in magnitude and time pattern to the increase in cortical ACh release seen by Bartolini et al. (1973) in cats at the same dose of Phy (100 µg/kg) and with the same route of administration (i.v.). This ACh increase was antagonized by a dose of 1 mg/kg i.v. of scopolamine administered 30 min before Phy. This effect of Phy was explained by the authors as a result of increased ACh available at subcortical receptors producing an evoked stimulation of the ascending cholinergic pathways.

The increased AChE activity measured by us in the CSF may be related to an increased secretion of AChE from the CSN caused by a low-dose presynaptic facilitation of ACh release by Phy. There is considerable evidence that cholinergic terminals both in the central (Marchi et al., 1983; Consolo et al., 1984) and in the peripheral (Kilbinger, 1984a,b; Mattio et al., 1984) nervous system are endowed with inhibitory muscarinic receptors whose activation by various agonists causes a reduction of ACh release evoked by electrical stimulation or high potassium. The inhibition of such receptors by antagonists (eg. atropine) or by low doses of agonists could produce the opposite effect, that is increase the release of both ACh and AChE from the terminals and subsequently increase the latter in the CSF. High concentrations (1 µM) of Phy depresses the output of ACh from peripheral terminals either by a direct effect on the ACh presynaptic muscarinic receptor or through a secondary effect via high concentrations of ACh in the synaptic cleft (Bourdois and Mitchell, 1974).

TABLE II: Symptoms of Cholinergic Hyperactivity
Following Administration of Physostigmine

Degree of Severity	Characteristic Symptoms	intracerebral ventricular		intravenous	
		Dose* (μg)	# Dogs*** Showing Symptoms	Dose** (μg)	# Dogs*** Showing Symptoms
I	Mild salivation	80	1/3	500	1/3
	Fasciculations	40	1/4		
	Mild hyperventilation				
II	Mod. salivation,	80	1/3	1,000	4/4
	restlessness	40	1/4		
	Mild bronchospasm,	20	1/4		
	defecation				
	Fasciculations, tremor				
III	Pronounced salivation,	120	3/4	--	--
	miosis				
	Bronchospasm, laryngospasm				
	Myoclonus, tremor				
	Muscular weakness				
	Stereotypism				
IV	Severe bronchospasm and	120	1/4	--	--
	laryngospasm	40	1/4		
	Tonic-clonic seizure				
	Atropine admin. required				

* 10 μg produced no symptoms
** 250 μg produced no symptoms
*** Ratio of number of dogs showing symptoms to number of dogs tested

High concentrations of Phy also inhibit Ch uptake in the rat iris (Mattio et al., 1985). On the contrary, low concentrations of Phy in CNS such as those reached by i.v. doses in the range of 100 μg/kg (Hallak and Giacobini, 1985) might inhibit the autoreceptor-mediated inhibition of ACh release and consequently increase AChE secretion. Dose-dependent effects of opposite sign (excitatory vs. inhibitory) on receptors are known. An example is the action of drugs acting on presynaptic dopamine autoreceptors (Grigoriadis and Seeman, 1984). Peripheral nerve stimulation has been seen to produce AChE release in CSF (Chubb et al., 1974), therefore, a second possibility to explain the increased AChE activity in CSF would be the stimulation of peripheral cholinergic synapses by Phy.

Finally, large rises in AChE activity in CSF could be attributed to rapid fluid expulsion within the ventricular system, resulting from a sudden brain edema or from sudden expansion of the cerebral vascular bed. This phenomenon could be due to a sudden vasodilation or from rises in the ventricular pressure as a result of an opening of the blood-brain barrier. Similar possibilities have been discussed for several noncholinergic drugs by Vogt et al. (1984). It is known that in rats, Phy injected intraventricularly or systemically can cause a pressor response, probably via central muscarinic cholinoceptors (Brezenoff, 1973). The ability of Phy to increase the cerebral blood flow following electrical stimulation of peripheral nerves and the close association between ACh release and blood flow in the cerebral cortex would support the idea that endogenously released ACh may play a role in controlling cerebral blood flow (cf.

Lee, 1985).   This view, however, is not generally accepted (cf. Lee, 1985).

Further considerations in comparing the two routes of administration are of clinical interest.   First, not only has i.v. administration been proven by our experiments to be much less effective in inhibiting AChE activity in CSF than the i.c.v. route, but the duration of AChE inhibition was shown to be much more long-lasting with the latter.   Secondly, symptoms of peripheral cholinergic hyperactivity seem to be less severe with i.c.v. than with i.v. administration, while the opposite is true for central symptoms.   All of these observations may have important clinical implications for the treatment of Alzheimer patients (Table II).   In therapy, a prolonged high AChE inhibitory effect (<50% for 6 hrs) resulting in high steady levels of ACh in the CNS could be obtained only by the intraventricular administration.   Since at best only short-lasting effects on AChE activity can be reached by the i.v. route, this could explain the short-lasting therapeutic effect of Phy on memory and cognitive function in Alzheimer (Table II).   In a final analysis, the presence of side effects and the development of tolerance to the therapeutic effect of the drug will be determinant in choosing one or the other route of administration.

CHOLINERGIC MARKERS IN HUMAN CSF

The CSF represents the most direct physiological compartment accessible to diagnostic evaluation of the CNS in the living patient or animal. However, as the CNS is effectively isolated from other organs, this compartmentalization not only provides protection to neural function but also makes it more difficult to evaluate the significance of its extracellular environment.

The cerebrospinal fluid represents a potential source of metabolic products, neurotransmitters, precursors and metabolites derived from the brain and related to CNS dysfunction and neuropsychiatric disorders. Lumbar CSF has been mainly used to study psychiatric (psychoses or depression) and neurological illnesses (Parkinson, Huntington).   A major attempt has been done to link biogenic amine metabolites found in the CSF to particular behavioral disturbances, mainly schizophrenia and various forms of depression.   This has given a great impulse to the field and produced a series of interesting results.   At the same time, several methodological questions have arisen from such studies, mainly related to the origin of the substances identified in the CSF and their relationship to neuronal metabolism and function.

In addition, problems such as size and selection of the control group, the "normal" range of the substances to be analyzed and their chemical identification (chromatographic, electrophoretic or mass-spectrometric) have also been under discussion.

It is generally accepted that CSF proteins can originate from cells found in the CSF, cells in the central nervous system (glial cells, neurons) or from the choroid plexus. The relative contribution of each of these three sources is not known. The problem becomes even more difficult when measurable enzyme activity related to neurotransmitter synthesis and metabolism is found in the CSF.

We have been specifically interested in the process of aging of the nervous system as it relates to synaptic function and more recently to pathological aspects of senescence and have been trying to identify specific molecular markers of neuronal aging.

TABLE III: COMPARISON OF PHYSOSTIGMINE TREATMENTS OF ALZHEIMER

Author/Year	Single Dose Nr. of Patients ( )	Daily Dose	Duration	Effect on Memory
	Normal Aged (64-82 yrs)			
Davis et al., 1978	1 mg (i.v./60 min) (19)	1 mg	2 days	+
Drachman & Sahakian, 1980	.80 mg (s.c.) (13)	.80 mg	acute	+
Drachman et al., 1982	.5 mg (i.v.) (16)	.5 mg	5 weeks	0
	Amnestic Syndromes			
Laurent et al., 1981	1 mg (s.c.) (23)	1 mg	acute	++
	* Oral Administration			
Peters & Levin, 1982	1.5-9 mg (oral) (3)	9 mg	3-18 mo	+++
Thal & Fuld, 1983	.5-1.0 mg x 6 (oral) (8)	3-16 mg	2 days	+++
Thal et al., 1983	.5 mg (oral/2 hrs) (12)	3 mg-upward max. 16 mg	--	+
Wettstein, 1983	1-2 mg (oral) (8)	3-10 mg	2-6 weeks	0
Levin & Peters, 1983	.5-1.5 mg (oral) (3)	1.5 mg	3-11 mo	++
Jotkowitz, 1983	1.25-2.5 mg (oral) (10)	10-15 mg	10 mo	0
Muramoto et al., 1984	.3-.8 mg (i.v.) 1-3 mg (oral or s.c.) (6)	.3-.8 mg	acute	+++
	* s.c. Administration			
Smith & Swash, 1979	1mg (s.c.) (1)	1 mg	acute	(0)
	* i.v. Administration			
Peters & Levin, 1979	.005-.015 mg (i.v.) (3)	.015 mg	acute	+++
Davis et al., 1979	.125-5 mg (i.v.) (2)	-	acute	+++
Christie et al., 1981	.25-1 mg (i.v./30 min) (11)	--	acute	+++
Ashford et al., 1981	.5 mg (i.v./30 min) (6)	.5 mg	acute	(0)
Davis & Mohs, 1982	.125-.50 mg (i.v./30 min)(10)	--	acute	+++
Sullivan et al., 1982	.25-.5 mg (i.v.) (18)	--	acute	+++

* Alzheimer's patients

Our longitudinal studies on animals (Giacobini, 1982; Giacobini et al., 1984) have shown that the cholinergic terminal is selectively vulnerable to the process of aging and that presynaptic mechanisms are more affected than postsynaptic ones (Giacobini, 1982). In particular, two membrane-related mechanisms are affected by age. First, an early failure in the uptake mechanism (V_{max}) for Ch occurs which is followed by a decrease in ACh. Second, the senescent cholinergic synapse releases, under experimental conditions, significantly less ACh than the adult one (Giacobini et al., 1984). These biochemical data correlate well with the EM morphometric data which demonstrate that two important features for neurotransmitter storage and release, total vesicular volume and appositional membrane, are decreased (Giacobini et al., 1984). These results, obtained in the normal aging animal support the hypothesis that cholinergic transmission is an age-dependent phenomenon which declines in conjunction with increasing age (Giacobini, 1983). Whether such "normal" age-dependent modifications of cholinergic function are also related to pathological processes such as in senile dementia remain to be demonstrated.

The marked reduction in synaptosomal high affinity Ch transport recently found in SDAT patients by Rylett et al. (1983) could be indicative of degenerative process in cholinergic nerve terminal boutons resulting from an overall decrease in the number of carrier sites per nerve terminal as demonstrated in our experiments in aging animals (Giacobini, 1982, 1983).

In order to determine the degree of involvement of cholinergic structures in SDAT patients, we assayed AChE activity in the CSF of SDAT patients showing various grades of severity of dementia and in healthy age-matched control subjects. Diagnostic categories were established as described by Hughes et al. (1982). In addition, in order to correlate our

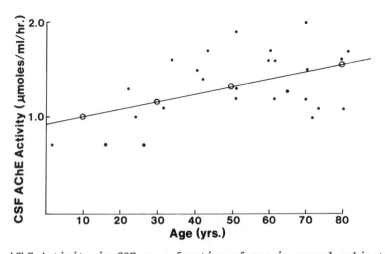

FIGURE 6: AChE Activity in CSF as a function of age in normal subjects.

biochemical data to the progression of the disease, the CSF was re-examined at intervals of 3 and 6 months in the same patient and the biochemical parameters were correlated to the severity of dementia. In six healthy subjects, AChE activity was measured in five consecutive 2 ml samples of the same spinal tap. The variation between the first ml and the tenth ml were not higher than 12%. As determined by specific inhibitors (iso-OMPA and BW), 95% of ChE activity in CSF was found to be AChE activity. When the CSF was re-examined in the same patient following a period of only one month, the levels of AChE were found to be highly reproducible (less than 6% difference).

Acetylcholinesterase activity in CSF is shown as a function of age in 26 normal control subjects (age range from 3 to 83) in Fig. 6. The figure shows a tendency for the average AChE activity to increase with age. Over the 80 year span, the average AChE activity increases in CSF by a factor of 25. This result confirms the finding of Tune et al. (1985).

The data found in the literature for AChE activity are mainly based on relatively small groups of controls and patients and often no relationship has been established with the grade of severity of the diagnoses and/or with the progression of the disease.

As shown in Fig. 7C, the mean AChE activity in CSF does not differ between normal age-matched controls (n=16) and early and/or less severe dementia patients (Group I, n=16). A clear decrease is seen only if the more severe groups of dementia (Group III, n=3) patients are compared with controls. With regard to ChAc activity (Fig. 7A), an apparent increase in enzyme activity is seen between normal age matched controls and SDAT patients (Groups I, n=5, II, n=3 and III, n=1 together). Choline (Fig. 7B) by contrast shows a decrease (p < .01) when normal controls (n=15) are compared with Groups I (n=14); II (n=8) and III (n=3) diagnostic categories. These results from our laboratory indicate that changes in all three CSF parameters studied may occur in SDAT patients. However, it is necessary to extend our study to a larger number of patients and controls to draw any definitive conclusions. On the other hand, when a larger interval (6 months) between CSF analysis was used, indicative changes in one direction, an increase for Ch and a decrease for ChAc and AChE were seen. These changes seen in Ch and ChAc after a 6 month follow-up may be indicative of the progression of the disease.

Choline acetyltransferase was first detected in human CSF by Johnson and Domino in 1971. These authors found CSF levels in healthy college students to be in the range of 11 nmoles ACh/ml/hr which is somewhat higher than our own values, which might be due to the age factor (college students versus elderly). No significant difference was seen in their study between normal young subjects and SD dementia patients. Choline acetyltransferase activity was also found at low levels in human serum and erythrocytes. There was a relationship for both ChAc and AChE activities between CSF and cortex and CSF and caudate suggesting a common source for these enzymes. Choline acetyltransferase activity was also detected in CSF by Rimon et al. (1973). More recently, Haber and Grossman (1983) reported ChAc activity values of the order of 480 nmoles/hr in patients with minimal pathology. These values are much higher than previously described. Aquilonius and Eckernas (1975) investigated the specificity of the assay procedure in relation to the origin of the ChAc activity found in the CSF. Their conclusion was that whenever ChAc activity is determined in CSF, special care should be taken to eliminate possible errors due to non-enzymatically catalyzed formation of ACh. The presence of low molecular weight compounds responsible for the non-enzymatic ACh formation was suggested by these authors.

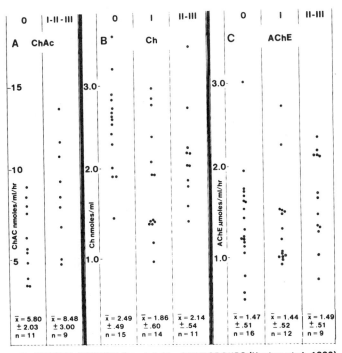

FIGURE 7: AChE and ChAc Activity as well as Ch levels in CSF of healthy age-matched controls and SDAT patients.

DeKosky et al. (1985) found that CSF which was treated to denature ChAc still produces ACh and CSF filtrates of < 10,000 m.w. retain ACh-synthesizing activity. The same authors claim to have isolated an endogenous ChAc inhibitor from bovine brain, raising the question of such a compound suppressing ChAc activity in the CSF. It is, therefore, possible that synthesis of ACh in CSF could be partially non-enzymatically catalyzed or mediated by low molecular weight compounds which have not yet been identified.

Haber and Grossman (1983) found ACh and Ch levels in the lumbar CSF of patients with minimal pathology to be of the order of 187 and 1745 pmoles/ml, respectively, by using a radiometric method. Ventricular and cisternal levels were twice as high and the CSF collected from cerebral convexities showed ACh levels as high as 1350 pmoles/ml. The age of the patients is not reported in this study and no data are available on SDAT patients. Davis et al. (1982) and Johns et al. (1985) reported ACh and Ch levels of the order of 42 pmoles/ml and 3260 pmoles/ml, respectively, in SDAT patients, aged 53-80. Both ACh and Ch were measured by GC-MS. There was an inverse correlation between memory impairment measured as MIT scores expressing severity of dementia and ACh levels. Patients with greater memory impairment tended to have a lower CSF ACh. There was no significant correlation between severity of dementia and level of other neurotransmitter metabolites (5-HIAA, HVA and MHPG) measured in the same CSF. There was a trend for higher Ch levels to be associated with greater severity of dementia, however, the ratio of Ch/ACh was inversely correlated to MIT dementia scores.

Measurable ACh levels found by us in the CSF were in the range of 100 to 800 pmoles/ml. By using new approaches, we are presently attempting to conclusively determine whether the ACh we have measured in the CSF of both normals and SDAT patients is of CNS origin.

ACKNOWLEDGEMENTS

Supported in part by funds for pilot project from S.I.U. School of Medicine; E.F. Pearson Foundation and S.I.U. Alzheimer Research Fund. The authors gratefully acknowledge the technical skills of Virginia Hoban and Diana Smith for typing the manuscript.

REFERENCES

Aquilonius, S.-M. and Eckernas, S.-Å, 1975, Choline acetyltransferase in human cerebrospinal fluid: non-enzymatically and enzymatically catalyzed acetylcholine synthesis, J. Neurochem., 27:317-318.

Ashford, J.W., Soldinger, S., Schaeffer, J., Cochran, L. and Jarvik, L., 1981, Physostigmine and its effect on six patients with dementia, Amer. J. Psychiatry, 138:829-830.

Atack, J.R., Perry, E.K., Bonham, J.R., Perry, R.H., Tomlinson, B.E., Blessed, G. and Fairbairn, A., 1983, Molecular forms of acetylcholinesterase in senile dementia of Alzheimer type: selective loss of the intermediate (10S) form, Neurosci. Letters, 40:199-204.

Augustinsson, K.B., 1963, Classification and comparative enzymology of the cholinesterases and methods for their determination, Handb. Exp. Pharmakol., 15:89-128.

Bareggi, S.R. and Giacobini, E., 1978, Acetylcholinesterase activity in ventricular and cisternal CSF of dogs, J. Neurosci. Res., 3:335-339.

Bartolini, A., Bartolini, R. and Domino, E.F., 1973, Effects of physostigmine on brain acetylcholine content and release, Neuropharmacology, 12:15-25.

Bourdois, P.S. and Mitchell, J.F., 1974, The output per stimulus of acetylcholine from cerebral cortical slices in the presence or absence of cholinesterase inhibition, Br. J. Pharmac., 52:509-517.

Brezenoff, H.E., 1973, Centrally induced pressor responses to intravenous and intraventricular physostigmine evoked via different pathways, Eur. J. Pharmac., 23:290-292.

Christie, J.E., Shering, A., Ferguson, J. and Glen, A.I.M., 1981, Physostigmine and arecoline: effects of intravenous infusions in Alzheimer presenile dementia, Brit. J. Psychiatry, 138:46-50.

Chubb, I.W. and Smith, A.D., 1975, Isoenzymes of soluble and membrane-bound acetylcholinesterase in bovine splachnic nerve and adrenal medulla, Proc. R. Soc. Lond. (Biol.), 191:245-261.

Chubb, I.W., Goodman, S. and Smith, A.D., 1974, Increased concentration of an isoenzyme of acetylcholinesterase in rabbit cerebrospinal fluid after peripheral stimulation, J. Physiol. (Lond.), 242:118-120P.

Chubb, I.W., Goodman, S. and Smith, A.D., 1976, Is acetylcholinesterase secreted from central neurons into the cerebrospinal fluid? Neuroscience, 1:57-62.

Consolo, S., Wang, J-X., Fusi, R., Vinci, R., Forloni, G. and Ladinsky, H., 1984, In vitro and in vivo evidence for the existence of presynaptic muscarinic cholinergic receptors in the rat hippocampus, Brain Res., 309(:147-151.

Davies, P., 1979, Neurotransmitter-related enzymes in senile dementia of the Alzheimer type, Brain Res., 171:319-327.

Davis, K.L. and Mohs, R.C., 1982, Enhancement of memory processes in Alzheimer's disease with multiple-dose intravenous physostimgine, Am. J. Psychiatry, 139:1421-1424.

Davis, K.L., Mohs, R.C., Tinklenberg, J.R., Pfefferbaum, A., Hollister, L.E. and Kopell, B.S., 1978, Physostigmine: improvement of long-term memory processes in normal subjects, Science, 201:272-274.

Davis, K.L., Mohs, R.L. and Tinklenberg, J.R., 1979, Enhancement of memory by physostigmine, New Eng. J. Med., 301:946.

Davis, K.L., Hsieh, J.Y-K., Levy, M.I., Horvath, T.B., Davis, B.M. and Mohs, R.C., 1982, Cerebrospinal fluid acetylcholine, choline and senile dementia of the Alzheimer type, Psychopharm. Bull., 18:193-195.

DeKosky, S.T., Hackney, C. and Scheff, S.W., 1985, Acetylcholine (ACh) synthesis and endogenous choline acetyltransferase (CAT) inhibitory activity in human CSF, Neurology, 35(Suppl 1):258.

Drachman, D.A., Glosser, G., Fleming, P. and Longenecker, G., 1982, Memory decline in the aged: treatment with lecithin and physostigmine, Neurology, 32:944-950.

Drachman, D.A. and Sahakian, B.J., 1980, Memory and cognitive function in the elderly, A preliminary trial of physostigmine, Arch. Neurol., 37:674-675.

Giacobini, E., 1959, The distribution and localization of cholinesterases in nerve cells, Acta Physiol. Scand., 45(Suppl 156):1-45.

Giacobini, E., 1982, in: "Aging of the Brain: Molecular and Cellular Mechanisms of Aging", Raven Press, New York, pp. 271-284.

Giacobini, E., 1983, in: "Aging of the Brain", Raven Press, New York, pp. 197-210.

Giacobini, E., Pilar, G., Suszkiw, J. and Uchimura, H., 1979, Normal distribution and denervation changes of neurotransmitter related enzymes in cholinergic neurones, J. Physiol., 286:233-253.

Giacobini, E., Mussini, I. and Mattio, T., 1984, Aging of cholinergic synapses in the avian iris, In: "Developmental Neuroscience: Physiological and Pharmacological Control of Nervous System Development", F. Caciagli, E. Giacobini and R. Paoletti, ed., Elsevier, pp. 89-93.

Giacobini, E., Becker, R., Elble, R., Mattio, T. and McIlhany, 1985, Acetylcholine metabolism in brain. Is it reflected by CSF changes? in: "OHOLO Biological Conference", A. Fisher, Ed., Plenum Press.

Gisiger, V. and Vigny, M., 1977, A specific form of acetylcholinesterase is secreted by rat sympathetic ganglia, FEBS Lett., 84:253-256.

Greenfield, S.A. and Shaw, S.G., 1982, Release of acetylcholinesterase and aminopeptidase in vivo following infusion of amphetamine into the substantia nigra, Neuroscience, 7:2883-2893.

Grigoriadis, D. and Seeman, P., 1984, The dopamine/neuroleptic receptor, Can. J. Neurolog. Sci., 11:108-113.

Haber, B. and Grossman, R.G., 1983, Acetylcholine metabolism in intracranial and lumbar cerebrospinal fluid and in blood, in: "Neurobiology of Cerebrospinal Fluid", H. Wood, Ed., Plenum Press.

Hallak, M.E. and Giacobini, E., 1985, Effects of physostigmine on cholinesterase activity, choline and acetylcholine levels in rat brain, J. Neurochem., Suppl. 44:S105A.

Hughes, C.P., Berg, L., Danziger, W.L., Coben, L.A. and Martin, R.L., 1982, A new clinical scale for the staging of dementia, Brit. J. Psychiatry, 140:566-572.

Johns, C.A., Haroutunian, V., Greenwald, B.S., Mohs, R.C., Davis, B.M., Kanof, P., Horvath, T.B. and Davis, K.L., 1985, Development of cholinergic drugs for the treatment of Alzheimer's disease, Drug. Dev. Res., 5:77-96.

Johnson, S. and Domino, E.F., 1971, Cholinergic enzymatic activity of cerebrospinal fluid of patients with various neurologic diseases, Clin. Chim. Acta, 35:421-428.

Jotkowitz, S., 1983, Lack of clinical efficacy of chronic oral physostigmine in Alzheimer's disease, Ann. Neurol., 14:690-691.

Kilbinger, H., 1984a, Facilitation and inhibition by muscarinic agonists of acetylcholine release from guinea pig myenteric neurons: mediation through different types of neuronal muscarinic receptors, Trends in Pharmacol. Sci., Suppl:49-52.

Kilbinger, H., 1984b, Presynaptic muscarinic receptors modulating acetyl-
choline release, Trends in Pharmacol. Sci., 55:103-105.
Laurent, B., Hibert-Kuntzler, O., Chazot, G., Michel, D. and Schott, B.,
1981, Effets de la physostigmine sur les syndromes amnesiques, Rev.
Neurol., 137:649-660.
Lee, T.J-F., 1985, Cholinergic mechanisms in the cerebral circulation, in:
"Trends in Autonomic Pharmacology, Vol. 13", S. Kalsner, Ed., Urban &
Schwarzenberg, Baltimore-Munich.
Levin, H.S. and Peters, B.H., 1983, Long-term administration of oral
physostigmine and lecithin improve memory in Alzheimer's disease,
Notes and Letters, p. 210, 1983.
Lubinska, L. and Niemerko, S., 1971, Velocity and intensity of bidirec-
tional migration of acetylcholinesterase in transected nerves, Brain
Res., 27:329-342.
Marchi, M., Paudice, P., Caviglia, A. and Raiteri, M., 1983, Is acetyl-
choline release from striatal nerve endings regulated by muscarinic
autoreceptors? Eur. J. Pharmacol., 91:63-68.
Massoulié, J. and Bon, S., 1982, The molecular forms of cholinesterase
and acetylcholinesterase in vertebrates, Ann. Rev. Neurosci.,
5:57-106.
Mattio, T.G., Richardson, J.S. and Giacobini, E., 1984, Effects of DFP on
iridic metabolism and release of acetylcholine and on pupillary
function in the rat, Neuropharmacology, 23:1207-1214.
Mattio, T.G., Richardson, J.S. and Giacobini, E., 1985, Acute effects of
cholinesterase inhibitors on uptake of choline in the rat iris,
Neuropharmacology, 24:325-328.
Muramoto, O., Sugishita, M. and Ando, K., 1984, Cholinergic system and
constructional praxis: a further study of physostigmine in
Alzheimer's disease, J. Neurol. Neurosurg. Psych., 47:485-491.
Perry, E., Perry, R., Blessed, G. and Tomlinson, B., 1977, Necropsy
evidence of central cholinergic deficits in senile dementia, Lancet,
1:189.
Peters, B.H. and Levin, H.S., 1979, Effects of physostigmine and lecithin
on memory in Alzheimer's disease, Ann. Neurol., 6:219-221.
Peters, B.H. and Levin, H.S., 1982, Chronic oral physostigmine and
lecithin administration in memory disorders of aging, in: "Aging -
Alzheimer's Disease: A Report of Progress", S. Corkin, K.L. Davis,
J.H. Growdon, E. Usdin and R.J. Wurtman, eds., pp. 421-426, Raven
Press, New York.
Plattner, F. and Hintner, H., 1930, Die spaltung von acetylcholin durch
organextrakte and koperflussigkeiten, Pflug Arch. Ges. Physiol.,
225:19-25.
Rimon, R., Puhakka, P., Venolainen, E. and Mandel, A.J., 1973, Psychiatria
Fennica, 265-267.
Rossor, M.N., Garrett, N.J., Johnson, A.L., Mountjoy, C.Q., Roth, M. and
Iversen, L.L., 1982, A post-mortem study of the cholinergic and GABA
systems in senile dementia, Brain, 105:313-330.
Rylett, R.J., Ball, M.J. and Calhoun, E.H., 1983, Evidence for high
affinity choline transport in synaptosomes prepared from hippocampus
and neocortex of patients with Alzheimer's disease, Brain Res.,
289:169-175.
Scarsella, G., Toschi, G., Bareggi, S.R. and Giacobini, E., 1979, Molecu-
lar forms of cholinestereases in cerebrospinal fluid, blood plasma,
and brain tissue of the beagle dog, J. Neurosci. Res., 4:19-24.
Smith, C.M. and Swash, M., 1979, Physostigmine in Alzheimer's disease,
Lancet, 1:42.
Sullivan, E.V., Shedlack, K.J., Corkin, S. and Growdon, J.H., 1982,
Physostigmine and lecithin in Alzheimer's disease, in: "Aging -
Alzheimer's Disease: A Report of Progress", S. Corkin, K.L. Davis,
J.H. Growdon, E. Usdin and R.J. Wurthman, eds., pp. 361-367, Raven
Press, New York.

Thal, L.J. and Fuld, P.A., 1983, Memory enhancement with oral physo-
    stigmine in Alzheimer's disease, New Eng. J. Med., 308:720.
Thal, L.J., Fuld, P.A., Masur, D.M. and Sharpless, N.S., 1983, Oral physo-
    stigmine and lecithin improve memory in Alzheimer disease, Ann.
    Neurol., 13:491-496.
Thal, L.J., Masur, D.M., Fuld, P.A., Sharpless, N.S. and Davies, P., 1983,
    Memory improvement with oral physostigmine and lecithin in
    Alzheimer's disease, in: "Banbury Report 15", Cold Spring
    Laboratory.
Tune, L., Gucker, S., Folstin, M., Oshida, L. and Coyle, J.R., 1985,
    Cerebrospinal fluid acetylcholinesterase in senile dementia of the
    Alzheimer type, Ann. Neurol., 17:46-48.
Vogt, M., Smith, A.D. and Fuenmayor, L.D., 1984, Factors influencing the
    cholinesterases of cerebrospinal fluid in the anaesthetized cat,
    Science, 12:979-995.
Wettstein, A., 1983, No effect from double-blind trial of physostigmine
    and lecithin in Alzheimer disease, Ann. Neurol., 13:210-212.
Whitehouse, P.J., Price, D.L., Clark, A.W., Coyle, J.T. and DeLong, M.R.,
    1981, Alzheimer disease: evidence for selective loss of cholinergic
    neurons in the nucleus basalis, Ann. Neurol., 10:122-126.

ACETYLCHOLINESTERASE ACTIVITY IN USE AND DISUSE OF MUSCLE

Wolf-D. Dettbarn, Gary T. Patterson, and
Ramesh C. Gupta and Karl E. Misulis

Pharmacology Department and
The Jerry Lewis Neuromuscular Research Center
Vanderbilt University
Nashville, Tennessee

INTRODUCTION

Intact neural innervation is necessary for the maintenance of normal skeletal muscle structure and function and in the control of acetylcholinesterase activity. Features of innervation that may contribute to this influence include nerve and muscle electrical activity, neurotrophic substances transported through the axon, acetylcholine, and perhaps mechanical factors involved in muscle action (Ranish et al., 1981).

Acetylcholinesterase (AChE) is present in both skeletal muscle and motoneurons, though its chief physiological role is as a part of the post-synaptic membrane and basal lamina at the motor end plate where it hydrolyzes acetylcholine (Brzin et al., 1980). While most muscle AChE is synthesized in the muscle fiber, some may be released into the synaptic clefts from the innervating axon terminal. This latter amount, however, is insufficient to account for the turnover of muscle AChE, especially during reinnervation (Wooten and Chang, 1980; Dettbarn, 1981). Therefore, it would appear that synthesis of AChE is initiated by innervating nerve fibers, while the potential to synthesize AChE is an endogenously programmed event in both fast and slow muscle.

Previous studies have shown that with denervation there is a large decrease in total muscle AChE activity (Guth et al., 1964; Crone and Freeman, 1972; Dettbarn, 1981). This is to a greater extent than can be accounted for by muscle fiber atrophy. With reinnervation there is restoration of previous enzyme activity, but the patterns of change are different in fast non-postural muscle, such as the extensor digitorum longus (EDL) and in slow postural muscle, such as the soleus (Dettbarn, 1981). The EDL exhibits a gradual recovery of AChE activity towards control. In contrast, the soleus has a large overshoot in AChE activity well above that of control. This occurs at a time when innervation is just being established, and is prevented if reinnervation does not occur. We have previously demonstrated that this overshoot was not due to initial preferential innervation of the soleus by axons destined for fast fibers (Misulis and Dettbarn, 1985).

Therefore, some feature of early reinnervation must cause this change.

In this study we have examined the influence of neural input on AChE of slow and fast rat skeletal muscle. To investigate this role of neural influence, disuse of the hindlimb was produced by lesions at three levels of the neuraxis: 1) sciatic nerve crush resulting in denervation with subsequent reinnervation, 2) spinal cord section with resultant paraplegia, and 3) hypokinesia, imparted by hindlimb suspension leaving ambulation to the forelimbs. The first lesion is of the lower motoneuron, the second is of the upper motoneuron leaving the segmental motor system intact, and the third is disuse without a structural lesion to the neuraxis. For adequate evaluation of the influence of these treatments, the changes in AChE were correlated with muscle electrical activity for each model of disuse. Further delineation of changes in AChE were achieved by analysis of individual molecular forms of the enzyme (Groswald and Dettbarn, 1983a,b; Brimijoin, 1983).

MATERIALS AND METHODS

Adult Sprague-Dawley rats weighing 160-180 grams were used throughout this study. Animals were maintained with 12 hr light/dark cycles with ad libitum access to food and water. All surgical procedures were performed under aseptic conditions.

Denervation

The animals were anesthetized with ether and the sciatic nerve of one hindlimb exposed in the upper thigh, near the sciatic notch. The nerve was crushed over a 2 mm segment by means of modified mosquito forceps. This resulted in interruption of all axons through the crush site, but allowed for faster and more directed reinnervation, by maintaining the intact connective tissue sheath. The skin was closed with sterile stainless steel wound clips.

Spinal cord section

Animals were anesthetized with ether and their mid-thoracic spinal cords exposed via a dorsal laminectomy. The spinal cord was sectioned by a scalpel with care taken to not damage the anterior spinal artery. The posterior circulation was sacrificed. The protection of the anterior spinal artery resulted in better preservation of blood flow to the distal cord, thus diminishing the likelihood of infarction of the spinal segments of concern in this study (distal to L3). The skin was closed with wound clips without closure of the muscle layers.

Hypokinesia

Hypokinesia was accomplished by suspension of the hindlimbs of the animal off the floor of the cage, such that stance and gait were performed solely by the forelimbs. This involved a modification of the technique of Morey-Holton (Morey, 1979; Musacchia and Deavers, 1980). The unanesthetized animals were placed in restrainer cages, their tails cleaned and prepared with isopropyl alcohol and Benzoin (Lilly), and a swivel clip attached to the base of the tail by means of Durapore tape (3M). For freedom of movement around the cage the clip traveled along a runner on the top of the cage. Using this technique there was no breakdown of tissue and animals continued to gain weight at the same rate as their age-matched controls.

Muscle electrical activity

Electromyography (EMG) was performed on both the soleus and EDL by two methods to assess the muscle electrical activity imparted by neural innervation in each of the preparations. The first involved recording EMG's from the soleus and EDL while the animals were in their normal caged state for evaluation of baseline muscle electrical activity. Electrodes were 0.003" enamelled nichrome wire with approximately 100 square microns exposed on the recording surface. These were inserted percutaneously via a 25 gauge hypodermic needle which was subsequently withdrawn leaving two recording electrodes in the muscle. The animals were un-anesthetized in restraint cages and tolerated the procedure well. The animals were then returned to their usual cages and the electrodes attached via light-weight shielded cables to the electrophysiological apparatus. This consisted of Grass P-15 preamplifiers, Tektronix oscilloscopes, and an Ampex tape recorder. Muscle fiber electrical activity was monitored over a 30 minute period and the relative frequency and patterns of discharge observed. Evaluations were made both at rest and with ambulation. Long term quantification was not performed for this study.

The second procedure involved recording of EDL and soleus EMG in sodium pentobarbital (Nembutal) anesthetized experimental and control animals in response to direct electrical stimulation of the sciatic nerve. The purpose of this portion of the study was to evaluate the security of neuromuscular transmission especially in spinal and hypokinetic animals, but also in denervated animals. This was performed using extra-fine coaxial needle electrodes for unit analysis, and an un-insulated monopolar reference electrode along the long axis of the muscle for recording a compound potential from the muscle. Supra-maximal stimulation of the distal end of the cut sciatic nerve or of a dissected fascicle was provided by a Grass S88 stimulator. The EMG response to varying rates of stimulation was recorded.

Acetylcholinesterase assays

At intervals of one week, four animals from each treatment group, including controls, were sacrificed and the soleus and extensor digitorum longus (EDL) muscles removed for biochemical analysis. Total muscle acetylcholinesterase (AChE) activity was assayed by determining the hydrolysis of acetylthiocholine colorimetrically after pre-incubation with 0.1 mM iso-OMPA, a specific inhibitor of Butyro-cholinesterase (Ellman et al., 1961). AChE was expressed as micromoles of acetylthiocholine hydrolyzed/hr/gram tissue wet weight. Statistical evaluation was by an ANOVA blocked for treatment group and weeks.

Individual molecular forms of AChE were separated by velocity sedimentation on 5-20% linear sucrose density gradients, as described by Groswald and Dettbarn, (1983a,b), and were quantitated by the radiometric assay of Johnson and Russell (1975). Proteins with sedimentation constants, alkaline phosphatase (6.1S), catalase (11.1S), and beta-galactosidase (16S), were added to the gradients for determination of the sedimentation values of the AChE molecular forms, as previously described (Groswald and Dettbarn, 1983a,b).

RESULTS

All animals tolerated the surgical and restraint procedures well with no significant morbidity and mortality. Denervation, spinal cord section, and hypokinesia resulted in no significant difference in body weight as compared to age-matched controls.

Quantification of muscle activity

Four animals in each treatment group were assayed for muscle electrical activity. Real time analysis of motor unit discharge characteristics was performed during rest and during encouraged ambulation. Control animals at rest exhibited minimal spontaneous activity in the EDL with limited activity in the soleus. Denervation resulted in the expected fibrillations and positive sharp waves at 2 weeks after operation in both muscles, with there being little motor unit activity. Spinal cord section resulted in spontaneous activity in the EDL that was not observed in controls. The soleus had some spontaneous activity that did not qualitatively differ from control animals. In hypokinetic animals the soleus and the EDL were virtually silent. Hypokinesia and spinal cord section produced no electrical signs of denervation.

With denervation the phasic activation was of a much lesser degree than age-matched controls, at 2 weeks. Spinal animals had no voluntary activation, but did have some phasic activity of both the soleus and EDL associated with spasticity. Hypokinetic animals had little or no phasic activation associated with ambulation within the suspension apparatus. This adaptation occurred within 3 days in all animals, when the hindlimb muscles were found to be virtually quiescent during all phases of rest and activity.

Direct electrical stimulation of the sciatic nerve produced normal muscle action potentials in soleus and EDL of spinal and hypokinetic animals in response to both single and repetitive stimuli. In contrast, with denervation at 2 weeks the rate of rise of the muscle action potentials was prolonged, the number of active fibers greatly reduced, and the response rapidly fatiguing at rates above 10/sec. This indicated a stage of early reinnervation.

Total acetylcholinesterase activity

AChE activity in both the soleus and EDL decreased following nerve crush (Table 1). Within 3 weeks after sciatic nerve crush, when reinnervation was occurring, there was an increase in soleus AChE activity to over 176.6% of control. Following this increase, the soleus AChE activity gradually decreased towards normal level over the following 2 weeks (not shown). The EDL exhibited only a gradual recovery of AChE activity to its normal level and was still only 50% of control values after 3 weeks.

Spinal cord section produced an increase in the AChE activity of the soleus within 1 week. Two weeks after spinal cord section the AChE activity of the soleus was 75% greater than control values. After 3 weeks, the AChE activity of the soleus was found to be decreasing towards the control value. The EDL exhibited declining AChE activity from 1 to 3 weeks after spinal cord section. Three weeks after spinal cord section EDL AChE activity was about 60% that of control values.

Table 1. Total Acetylcholinesterase (AChE) Activities
Expressed as a Percent of Control Values[a]

Total AChE (percent control)

EDL

Weeks	Nerve Crush	Spinal	Hypokinetic
1	28.2$\pm$ 7.0[b]	79.5+7.0[b]	125.9+6.5
2	22.2$\pm$10.2[b]	70.8$\pm$6.8[b]	95.3+6.0
3	49.6$\pm$ 5.8[b]	56.8$\pm$5.6[b]	78.1$\pm$9.2

Soleus

Weeks	Nerve Crush	Spinal	Hypokinetic
1	54.5+12.0[b]	123.0+13.2[b]	140.6+17.5[b]
2	50.3$\pm$11.0[b]	175.5$\pm$24.9[b]	228.9$\pm$27.0[b]
3	176.6$\pm$ 5.3[b]	129.0$\pm$ 9.0[b]	187.1$\pm$32.7[b]

[a] Values are the mean $\pm$ standard deviation for 4 to 8 animals
compared to aged-matched controls. Control values for EDL
AChE activity ranged from 95 to 110 uM/hr/gram tissue wet
weight and for the soleus AChE activity from 50 to 65
uM/hr/gram tissue wet weight.
[b] $p < 0.05$ when compared to aged-matched controls.

Hypokinesia resulted in a significant increase in soleus AChE activity
similar to that seen with spinal cord section. After two weeks of
hypokinesia, the AChE activity of the soleus was more than twice that
of controls. The AChE activity of the EDL was less affected by
hypokinesia and the changes found were not statistically significant.

Activity of acetylcholinesterase molecular forms

Three weeks after nerve crush, when the total AChE activity showed
a marked increase over control in the soleus, the increase was most
marked in the activity of the 4S form and to a lesser extent in the 16S
form. The 10S and 12S forms lagged behind the other forms. In the EDL
there was slow recovery of all molecular forms but the 16S recovered
first followed by the 4S. The 10S lagged significantly behind the
other forms.

After 2 weeks of spinal cord section there were no changes in the
relative proportions of the individual molecular forms in either the
soleus or EDL. However, in the soleus after 2 weeks of hypokinesia
there was an increase in the activity of all molecular forms. No
change in the relative proportions of the individual forms was found
with this concurrent increase in total activity (Figure 1). The
profile of the activity of the molecular forms of the EDL was the same
as control.

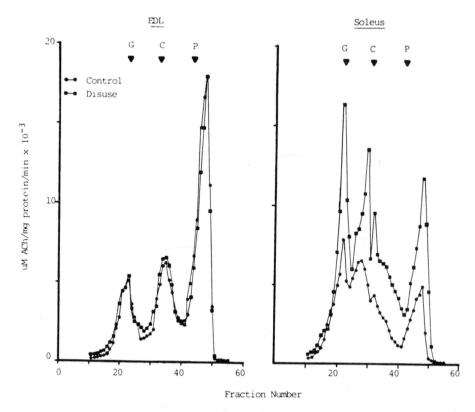

Figure 1.

Velocity sedimentation profiles of AChE molecular forms from
extensor digitorum longus (EDL) and soleus muscle after 2
weeks of hypokinetic suspension. Arrows represent fraction
location of protein standards G = B-galactosidase (16,0S);
C = catalase (11.1S); and, P = alkaline phosphatase (6.1S).

DISCUSSION

     All of the treatments employed in this study resulted in the lack
of use of the hindlimbs in stance and gait, and thus are models of
"disuse". However, they are associated with very different patterns of
muscle activation.

     Denervation abolished neurally imparted action potentials, although
it did result in increased irritability of the muscle fiber membrane,
manifested on EMG as fibrillations and positive sharp waves. The large
increase in soleus AChE activity was associated with early
reinnervation, and this overshoot was previously shown to be specific
to the soleus muscle and not due to initial fast fiber innervation
(Misulis and Dettbarn, 1985). The overshoot was also shown to be
dependent on reinnervation and to not occur if the sciatic nerve was
resected. At this same time, when there are few functionally
transmitting neuromuscular junctions, there is a shift in histochemical

fiber type profile towards an increased proportion of type 2 (fast) fibers. Thus, this transformation occurred without the benefit of substantial neural electrical input and with the limb not yet being used successfully for ambulation. This suggests that in the absence of neural innervation the soleus reverts to a faster, and perhaps more primitive state (Rubenstein and Kelley, 1978). The conversion to more type 2 (fast) fibers could be responsible for the overshoot in AChE, since fast muscles have a higher intrinsic AChE activity. The pattern of molecular forms remained the same, however, arguing against a shift from slow fiber AChE characteristics to that of a fast fiber. The other two models of disuse were designed to evaluate the relative importance of activity and features of neural innervation independent of activity, such as neurotrophic substances.

Both spinal cord section and hypokinesia resulted in disuse of the hindlimbs. Spinal cord section resulted in no obvious change in motor unit activity of the soleus while hypokinesia was associated with a substantial decrease in fiber activation. In spite of this difference, both produced marked changes in AChE activity as well as fiber type profile, such that the soleus fiber composition more resembled a fast muscle. In soleus the changes in AChE activity were comparable to those seen with early reinnervation after denervation. Thus, the overshoot appears to be a common feature of disuse, relatively independently of neural electrical activity. The fact that the AChE activity decreased so markedly with early denervation indicates that innervation is required for muscle AChE synthesis, although its level is regulated at least in part by use. Weightbearing activity may play a role in this since it was this factor that all three models of disuse had in common.

In the EDL, there was little change in AChE activity with any of these treatments. This distinct difference in response compared to the soleus is undoubtedly due to several factors. First, the EDL is not normally tonically active in sustained stance. Therefore, the removal of load was not a major perturbation with either of these models, as it was in the soleus. Secondly, the EDL is already composed predominantly of type 2 fibers, so any trend towards a faster character with higher AChE activity would be more difficult to elucidate.

The quantitatively less impressive yet still significant effects of spinal cord section and hypokinesia on the EDL were, therefore, most likely due to the quantity of imparted neural activity. The activity with spinal cord section was not greatly different from that of controls. There was a mild increase in resting activity, but phasic activation also intermittently occurred secondary to spasticity. Thus, if there was any quantitative change, there was an increase in total muscle fiber activation. This may have been responsible for the mild decrease in AChE activity. Hypokinesia, on the other hand, produced a pronounced decrease in activation, chiefly through a reduction in phasic ambulatory activation which could have produced a transient elevation.

In summary, the predominantly slow soleus and the predominantly fast EDL both depend on intact neural innervation and activity for the maintenance of normal AChE activity. AChE activity of the soleus, which normally subserves a postural role in stance and gait, increases towards the level of a faster muscle, not only when the muscle is denervated, but also when its role in posture is removed, relatively independently of quantity of activity. Perhaps the mechanical effects of sustained load, as in stance, are important for maintaining enzyme activity in soleus. In contrast, AChE activity of the EDL, which is most active in gait, and does not support a tonic load, is more dependent upon the quantity and pattern of neural activation for maintenance of normal muscle structure and function.

ACKNOWLEDGEMENTS

This study was supported by NASA Grants #NAGW-469 and #NAG 2-301. The authors acknowledge the technical assistance of Renee Martens and Carolyn Petrone, and the secretarial assistance of Barbara Page.

REFERENCES

Brimijoin S., 1983, Molecular forms of acetylcholinesterase in brain, nerve and muscle: nature, localization and dynamics, Prog. in Neurobiol. 21:291-322,.

Brzin, M., Sketelj, J., Grubic, Z., Kiauta, T., 1980, Cholinesterases of neuromuscular junction, Neurochem. Intl., 2:149-159.

Crone H. D., Freeman S. E., 1972, The acetylcholinesterase activity of the denervated rat diaphragm, J. Neurochem. 19:1207-1208.

Dettbarn W-D., 1981, A distinct difference between slow and fast muscle in acetylcholinesterase recovery after reinnervation in the rat, Exp. Neurol. 74:33-50.

Ellman G. L., Courtney U. D., Andres Jr., V., Featherstone R.M., 1961, A new and rapid colorimetric determination of AChE activity, Biochem. Pharmacol. 7:88-95.

Groswald D. E., Dettbarn W-D., 1983a, Nerve crush induced changes in molecular forms of AChE in soleus and EDL, Exp. Neurol. 79:519-531.

Groswald D. E., Dettbarn W-D., 1983b, Characterization of acetylcholinesterase molecular forms in slow and fast muscle of rat, Neurochem. Res. 8:935- 995.

Guth L., Albers R. W., Brown W. C., 1964, Quantitative changes in cholinesterase activity of denervated muscle fibers and soleplates, Exp. Neurol. 10:236-250.

Johnson C. D., Russell R, L., 1975, A rapid, simple radiometric assay for cholinesterase, suitable for multiple determinations, Anal. Biochem. 64:229-238.

Misulis K. E., Dettbarn W-D., Is fast fiber innervation responsible for increased AChE activity in reinnervating soleus muscle?, Exp. Neurol., 1985, (in press).

Morey E. R., 1979, Spaceflight and bone turnover: correlation with a new rat model of weightlessness, Bio. Science 29:168-179.

Musacchia X. J., Deavers D. R., 1980, A new rat model for studies of hypokinesia and antiorthostasis, Physiologist 23 (suppl):s91-s92.

Rubinstein N. A., Kelly A. M., 1978, Myogenic and neurogenic contributions to the development of fast and slow twitch muscles in rat, Dev. Biol. 62:473-485.

Wooten G. F., Chang C-H., 1980, Transport and turnover of acetylcholinesterase and choline acetyltransferase in rat sciatic nerve and skeletal muscle, J. Neurochem. 34:359-366.

PROTEIN PHOSPHORYLATION AND PHOSPHOLIPID METABOLISM IN THE

SUPERIOR CERVICAL GANGLION

Robert L. Perlman, Anne L. Cahill, and Joel Horwitz

Department of Physiology and Biophysics
University of Illinois College of Medicine at Chicago
Box 6998
Chicago, IL 60680

Our laboratory has been interested in the mechanisms by which
neuronal activity regulates neuronal metabolism. Specifically, we have
been studying the mechanisms by which neuronal activity regulates tyrosine hydroxylase (tyrosine 3-monooxygenase, EC 1.14.16.2) activity and
catecholamine synthesis in the superior cervical ganglion (SCG). The
SCG is a prototypical sympathetic ganglion. The noradrenergic principal
neurons in this ganglion innervate the pineal gland, the salivary
glands, the thyroid gland, smooth muscles of the iris, and blood vessels
in the head and neck. These neurons are innervated by preganglionic
sympathetic nerves whose cell bodies lie in the intermediolateral
column of the spinal cord and which release acetylcholine (ACh) as their
classical neurotransmitter. The principal ganglionic neurons contain
both nicotinic and muscarinic cholinergic receptors. Stimulation of the
nicotinic receptors produces a rapid depolarization that is due to a
generalized increase in the permeability of the neurons to cations.
Nicotinic stimulation typically leads to the generation of action potentials in the neurons. Stimulation of the muscarinic receptors produces
a slower depolarization that is due at least in part to the inhibition
of K^+ efflux from the cells. These neurons also contain voltage-sensitive Ca^{2+} channels; depolarization activates these channels and thereby
causes an additional influx of Ca^{2+} into the cells. Finally, the preganglionic neurons contain a variety of peptides in addition to ACh; the
physiological effects of these peptides have not yet been determined.

The SCG of the rat weighs about 1 mg. It can easily be removed
from the animal and incubated in vitro. The ganglion can be isolated
together with short lengths of preganglionic and postganglionic nerves,
so that it is possible to stimulate the ganglion via the preganglionic
cervical sympathetic trunk and to monitor synaptic transmission by
electrical recording from the postganglionic internal carotid nerve.
Since the ganglion is a paired structure, it is convenient to stimulate
one member of the pair and to use the other member as a non-stimulated
control (McAfee, 1982).

In our initial experiments, carried out in collaboration with Nancy
Ip and Richard Zigmond at Harvard Medical School, we studied the effects
of cholinergic agonists and of preganglionic stimulation on tyrosine
hydroxylase activity in the SCG. We measured tyrosine hydroxylase acti-

vity in intact ganglia by monitoring the accumulation of dopa in ganglia
that were incubated with brocresine, an inhibitor of dopa decarboxylase.
We measured dopa accumulation by high-performance liquid chromatography
with electrochemical detection. Ganglia incubated under control conditions produced dopa at a rate of approximately 100 pmol/ganglion/hour.
Incubation of the ganglia with nicotinic or muscarinic cholinergic
agonists increased the rate of dopa accumulation (Ip et al., 1982b).
Nicotinic agonists typically produced a 4- to 5-fold increase in dopa
accumulation, whereas muscarinic agonists caused about a 2-fold increase
in dopa production. The action of nicotinic agonists was dependent upon
extracellular Ca^{2+} and was inhibited by nicotinic antagonists such as
hexamethonium. In contrast, the action of muscarinic agonists was not
dependent upon extracellular Ca^{2+} and was specifically inhibited by low
concentrations (2-10 µM) of atropine. Nicotinic and muscarinic agonists
appeared to produce additive increases in dopa accumulation. These
results were consistent with the idea that nicotinic and muscarinic
agonists increase tyrosine hydroxylase activity in the SCG by distinct
mechanisms.

Electrical stimulation of the preganglionic cervical sympathetic
trunk (10 Hz, 30 min) produced a 4- to 6-fold increase in dopa accumulation (Ip et al., 1983). This increase was partially inhibited by
hexamethonium but was not affected by atropine. Thus, although exogenous muscarinic agonists can increase dopa synthesis in the SCG, the
activation of muscarinic receptors does not appear to play a major
role in the response of the ganglion to preganglionic stimulation. In
the presence of both hexamethonium and atropine, preganglionic stimulation still caused a 2- to 4-fold increase in dopa accumulation.
These studies suggested that the effect of preganglionic stimulation
on tyrosine hydroxylase activity was due in part to the release of ACh
from preganglionic nerve terminals and in part to the release of an
as-yet-unidentified noncholinergic transmitter. The SCG contains
vasoactive intestinal peptide (VIP)-like immunoreactivity (Hokfelt et
al., 1977) and VIP can also increase tyrosine hydroxylase activity in
the ganglion (Ip et al., 1982a); the putative noncholinergic transmitter may be VIP or a related peptide.

Tyrosine hydroxylase activity is thought to be regulated by phosphorylation and dephosphorylation reactions. To understand the mechanisms by which preganglionic stimulation and cholinergic agonists increase tyrosine hydroxylase activity in the SCG, we have studied the
effects of a variety of agents that are thought to regulate the activities of specific protein kinases (Horwitz and Perlman, 1984a; Cahill
et al., 1985). The following substances were found to increase dopa
synthesis: 8-bromo cAMP and agents that raise the content of cAMP in
the ganglion, including VIP and related peptides, and forskolin;
phorbol 12,13-dibutyrate; depolarizing agents, including veratridine
and elevated K^+; and the Ca^{2+} ionophore, ionomycin. Since all of
these agents increased dopa synthesis in decentralized ganglia, their
effects appeared to be due at least in part to a direct action on the
principal neurons in the ganglion. The actions of 8-bromo cAMP and of
agents that raise ganglionic cAMP levels are presumably mediated by a
cAMP-dependent protein kinase. Since protein kinase C appears to be
the cellular receptor for phorbol esters (Neidel et al., 1983), it is
likely that the effect of phorbol dibutyrate involves the activation
of protein kinase C. Finally, the effects of depolarizing agents and
of ionomycin are dependent upon extracellular Ca^{2+} and are presumably
due to a Ca^{2+}-dependent process, possibly the activation of a
Ca^{2+}/calmodulin-dependent protein kinase. Preganglionic stimulation
and cholinergic agonists may increase tyrosine hydroxylase activity by
a combination of these mechanisms.

We have also measured tyrosine hydroxylase activity in homogenates of the SCG (Horwitz and Perlman, 1984b). In these experiments, we have again assessed tyrosine hydroxylase activity by measuring dopa production by high-performance liquid chromatography. The agents that increased dopa synthesis in the intact ganglion all produced a stable increase in tyrosine hydroxylase activity that could be measured in ganglionic homogenates. This increase in tyrosine hydroxylase activity was manifest kinetically by a shift in the pH optimum of enzyme activity and by a decrease in the $K_m$app of the enzyme for its pterin cofactor. Thus, the increase in dopa synthesis produced by these agents in the intact ganglion appears to be due at least in part to the activation of tyrosine hydroxylase.

More recently, we have studied the phosphorylation of tyrosine hydroxylase in the SCG (Cahill and Perlman, 1984a, 1984b; Cahill et al., 1985). In these experiments, we have incubated ganglia with $^{32}P_i$, stimulated the ganglia, and then isolated tyrosine hydroxylase by immunoprecipitation followed by SDS-polyacrylamide gel electrophoresis. (The anti-tyrosine hydroxylase antiserum used in these experiments was generously provided by Norman Weiner and A. William Tank of the University of Colorado School of Medicine.) We localized the ^{32}P-labeled tyrosine hydroxylase by autoradiography and quantitated the incorporation of $^{32}P_i$ into tyrosine hydroxylase by densitometry of the autoradiograms or by liquid scintillation counting of the tyrosine hydroxylase bands in the gels. All of the stimuli that increased dopa synthesis in the SCG also increased the incorporation of $^{32}P_i$ into tyrosine hydroxylase in the ganglion. Of greatest interest was the observation that preganglionic stimulation increased the labeling of tyrosine hydroxylase. The effect of preganglionic stimulation on tyrosine hydroxylase labeling, like its effect on dopa synthesis, appeared to be due in part to a nicotinic mechanism and in part to a noncholinergic mechanism. The effect of preganglionic stimulation on the labeling of tyrosine hydroxylase was reversible. Moreover, preganglionic stimulation did not cause a generalized increase in the incorporation of $^{32}P_i$ into all ganglionic phosphoproteins. Therefore, the increased incorporation of $^{32}P_i$ into tyrosine hydroxylase appeared to represent a real increase in the phosphorylation of the enzyme and not merely an increase in the specific activity of the enzyme-bound phosphate. The increases in dopa synthesis produced by electrical and chemical stimulation of the SCG are presumably due, at least in part, to increases in the phosphorylation of the tyrosine hydroxylase.

We have also studied the effects of various agonists on the pattern of protein phosphorylation in the SCG. In these experiments, we have incubated ganglia with $^{32}P_i$, stimulated the ganglia, separated the ganglionic phosphoproteins by two-dimensional gel electrophoresis, and observed the patterns of protein phosphorylation by autoradiography of the gels. With these methods, we could visualize approximately 40 distinct phosphoproteins in the ganglion. Tyrosine hydroxylase was identified as a doublet of two closely-moving radioactive spots. The most heavily labeled phosphoprotein in the ganglion was an acidic protein with an Mr of approximately 83,000. This protein is apparently identical to the "87k" synaptosomal protein described by Wu et al., (1982). Treatment of the ganglion with agents that raise cAMP levels, with phorbol dibutyrate, or with depolarizing agents increased the incorporation of $^{32}P_i$ into distinct but overlapping groups of ganglionic phosphoproteins. While all of these agents increased the labeling of tyrosine hydroxylase, only phorbol dibutyrate increased the incorporation of $^{32}P_i$ into the 83,000 Mr protein. These results are consistent with the idea that tyrosine hydroxylase may be a substrate for several different protein kinases in the ganglion, whereas the 83,000 Mr protein is a specific substrate for protein kinase C.

We have also studied protein kinase activities in homogenates of the SCG. Using exogenous histone as a substrate, we could detect cAMP-dependent protein kinase, Ca^{2+}/calmodulin-dependent protein kinase, and protein kinase C activities in ganglionic homogenates. Protein kinase C activity in crude homogenates was not dependent upon exogenous phospholipids, but exhibited a strong phospholipid dependence after the enzyme had been partially purified by ion-exchange chromatography. We have also begun to characterize the endogenous substrates for the various protein kinases in the ganglion. These experiments have shown that tyrosine hydroxylase can be phosphorylated by all three protein kinases in ganglionic homogenates and that the 83,000 Mr protein can be phosphorylated by protein kinase C. The study of protein phosphorylation in ganglionic homogenates supports our conclusions about protein phosphorylation in the intact ganglion.

Muscarine not only increases the phosphorylation of tyrosine hydroxylase in the SCG, but also increases the metabolism of inositol-containing phospholipids in the ganglion (Hokin, 1965). The hydrolysis of inositol-containing phospholipids may lead to the accumulation of diacylglycerol, which can activate protein kinase C, and to the accumulation of inositol 1,4,5-trisphosphate (Ins-P_3), which can release Ca^{2+} from intracellular stores and thereby activate Ca^{2+}/calmodulin-dependent enzymes. To understand the mechanisms by which muscarine regulates ganglionic functions, we have studied phospholipid metabolism in the SCG (Horwitz et al., 1984, 1985). We have used several methods to study the metabolism of inositol-containing phospholipids in the ganglion. In some experiments, we have measured the incorporation of $^{32}P_i$ into phospholipids. In other experiments, we have incubated ganglia with [^{3}H]inositol ([^{3}H]Ins) to label the ganglionic phospholipids and have then measured the release of [^{3}H]inositol phosphates from these lipids. The [^{3}H]inositol phosphates were separated by ion-exchange chromatography or by high-voltage electrophoresis. These experiments were carried out in the presence of Li^+, which inhibits inositol 1-phosphatase and thereby allows the accumulation of inositol 1-phosphate (Ins-P). Muscarinic agonists increased the incorporation $^{32}P_i$ into ganglionic phospholipids and also increased the accumulation of [^{3}H]inositol phosphates in labeled ganglia. These effects occurred without a detectable lag, were independent of extracellular Ca^{2+}, and were blocked by atropine. Muscarine was more effective than bethanechol in stimulating phospholipid metabolism and in increasing dopa synthesis in the ganglion. These results are consistent with the idea that the stimulation of phospholipid metabolism may play a role in the mechanism by which muscarinic agonists increase tyrosine hydroxylase activity. In addition, these results support the concept that the activation of muscarinic receptors leads to an increase in the activity of a phospholipase C that hydrolyzes inositol-containing phospholipids to yield inositol phosphates and diacylglycerol. The identity of the substrates(s) for this receptor-linked phospholipase C is still unclear. Studies in other tissues have led to the concept that the receptor-coupled phospholipase C preferentially hydrolyzes phosphatidylinositol (PtdIns)-P and PtdIns-P_2. The hydrolysis of these phospholipids should result in the formation of Ins-P_2 and Ins-P_3, respectively. To date, however, we have not observed a significant accumulation of [^{3}H]Ins-P_2 or of [^{3}H]Ins-P_3 in muscarine-treated ganglia, but have only found an increase in the accumulation of [^{3}H]Ins-P. We have also not observed a consistent decrease in any of the labeled inositol-containing phospholipids in muscarine-treated ganglia. The receptor-coupled phospholipase C in the SCG may hydrolyze PtdIns instead of or in addition to the other inositol-containing phospholipids. Alternately, the ganglion may contain phosphatases that rapidly convert Ins-P_2 and Ins-P_3 to Ins-P.

In collaboration with Donald McAfee and Clark Briggs of the City of Hope Medical Center, we have studied the effects of preganglionic stimulation on the metabolism of inositol-containing phospholipids in the SCG (Briggs et al., 1985). Stimulation of the preganglionic cervical sympathetic trunk increased the accumulation of [^{3}H]Ins-P in [^{3}H]Ins-labeled ganglia. Experiments with cholinergic antagonists suggested that this effect was mediated in part by the stimulation of muscarinic receptors and in part by the stimulation of nicotinic receptors. It is interesting that preganglionic stimulation increased phospholipid metabolism by a muscarinic mechanism but did not appear to cause a muscarinic receptor-mediated increase in the phosphorylation of tyrosine hydroxylase. Exogenous muscarinic agonists caused a much greater increase in [^{3}H]Ins-P accumulation than did preganglionic stimulation; the increase in phospholipid metabolism produced by preganglionic stimulation may not have been sufficient to cause a measurable increase in tyrosine hydroxylase phosphorylation. It is also interesting that, although exogenous nicotinic agonists had little effect on ganglionic phospholipid metabolism, preganglionic stimulation appeared to increase the accumulation of [^{3}H]Ins-P by a nicotinic mechanism. Exogenous nicotinic agonists cause a profound desensitization of the nicotinic receptor; this desensitization may prevent these agonists from causing a significant increase in phospholipid metabolism. On the other hand, the idea that preganglionic stimulation increases phospholipid metabolism by a nicotinic mechanism is based solely on the observation that this effect was blocked in part by hexamethonium. Although hexamethonium is thought to be a specific nicotinic antagonist, it is conceivable that this drug inhibited [^{3}H]Ins-P accumulation by a mechanism that was unrelated to the blockade of nicotinic receptors. Finally, the apparent nicotinic stimulation of [^{3}H]Ins-P accumulation does not necessarily indicate that the nicotinic receptor is directly coupled to a phospholipase C; nicotinic stimulation may lead to the release of some substance that in turn activates phospholipase C. The SCG has been reported to contain a protein with vasopressin-like immunoreactivity (Hanley et al., 1984). Moreover, vasopressin increases the hydrolysis of inositol-containing phospholipids in the ganglion (Bone et al., 1984). However, a vasopressin receptor antagonist that blocked the effect of exogenous vasopressin did not inhibit the effect of preganglionic stimulation on [^{3}H]Ins-P accumulation. Therefore, this endogenous vasopressin-like protein does not appear to play a role in the mechanism by which preganglionic stimulation increases the hydrolysis of inositol-containing phospholipids.

We have also studied phospholipase C activity in homogenates of the SCG. In these experiments, we incubated ganglia with [^{3}H]Ins, homogenized the ganglia, and then measured the hydrolysis of [^{3}H]inositol-labeled phospholipids and the production of [^{3}H]inositol phosphates in these homogenates. The ganglion contained a phospholipase C activity that was dependent on Ca^{2+} and that hydrolyzed [^{3}H]PtdIns-P and [^{3}H]PtdIns-P_2 more actively than [^{3}H]PtdIns. This phospholipase C may be the enzyme that is activated in response to muscarine, vasopressin, or preganglionic stimulation. However, we have not observed an effect of muscarine or of vasopressin on phospholipase C activity in vitro. The mechanism by which stimulation of the muscarinic and vasopressin receptors leads to the activation of phospholipase C remains to be determined.

In our studies of phospholipid metabolism in the SCG, we have measured the accumulation of inositol phosphates that results from the action of phospholipase C. The other product of phospholipase C activity is diacylglycerol, which is thought to be the endogenous regulator of protein kinase C activity in eukaryotic cells. Therefore, agents that stimulate the hydrolysis of inositol-containing phospholipids might be expected to increase the activity of protein kinase C in their target cells. We have taken advantage of the fact that the 83,000 Mr protein is a specific substrate for protein kinase C to monitor the activity of this enzyme in th SCG. Muscarine, vasopressin, and bacterial phospholipase C (B. cereus) increased phosphorylation of this protein; accordingly, all of these agents appear to increase the activity of protein kinase C in the ganglion. We have not observed a consistent effect of preganglionic stimulation on the labeling of the 83,000 Mr protein. Thus although exogenous muscarinic agonists appear to activate protein kinase C in the SCG, there is as yet no evidence that ACh released by preganglionic stimulation can activate this enzyme. Again, this may reflect the fact that exogenous muscarinic agonists cause greater increases in phospholipid metabolism than does preganglionic stimulation.

The observation that phorbol dibutyrate increased the phosphorylation of tyrosine hydroxylase suggested that the activation of protein kinase C might lead to the phosphorylation of tyrosine hydroxylase. Bacterial phospholipase C also increased the phosphorylation and the activity of tyrosine hydroxylase in the ganglion. In contrast, vasopressin had no effect on the phosphorylation of tyrosine hydroxylase or on dopa synthesis. It is possible that vasopressin increases phospholipid metabolism and therefore activates protein kinase C in a cellular or subcellular compartment that does not contain significant amounts of tyrosine hydroxylase. We have recently carried out experiments with Conwell Anderson of the Department of Anatomy at the University of Illinois College of Medicine to localize the effects of muscarine and of vasopressin on ganglionic phospholipid metabolism. These experiments were based on the observation that agents that increased the hydrolysis of inositol-containing phospholipids also increased the incorporation of [^{3}H]Ins into these lipids. To study the sites of action of muscarine and of vasopressin, we incubated ganglia with [^{3}H]Ins in the presence of these agents and then localized the labeled phospholipids in the ganglion by autoradiography. Muscarine appeared to increase the incorporation of [^{3}H]Ins into phospholipids in the cell bodies of the principal ganglionic neurons, whereas vasopressin increased phospholipid labeling primarily in the neuropil. These experiments support the idea that muscarine and vasopressin stimulate the metabolism of different pools of phospholipids, but they have not yet clarified the relationships between phospholipid metabolism, protein kinase C activity, and the phosphorylation of tyrosine hydroxylase in the ganglion.

Table 1 summarizes the mechanisms by which preganglionic stimulation may regulate tyrosine hydroxylase activity in the SCG. The effects of preganglionic stimulation appear to be due in part to the release of ACh and in part to the release of a noncholinergic transmitter, which may be VIP or a related peptide. ACh, in turn, may interact with nicotinic and with muscarinic receptors. The effects of ACh and of the noncholinergic transmitter appear to be mediated by the activation of specific protein kinases. Nicotinic stimulation is accompanied by an increase in the influx of Ca^{2+} into the ganglion (Volle et al., 1981). Thus, it is likely that nicotinic stimulation

TABLE 1. MECHANISMS BY WHICH PREGANGLIONIC STIMULATION MAY REGULATE TYROSINE HYDROXYLASE ACTIVITY IN THE SUPERIOR CERVICAL GANGLION

Transmitter	Receptor	Effector	Intracellular Mediator	Protein Kinase
Acetylcholine	Nicotinic	Ion channel	Ca^{2+}	Ca^{2+}/calmodulin-dependent
	Muscarinic	Phospholipase C	Diacylglycerol	Protein kinase C
Peptide	Peptidergic	Adenylate cyclase	cAMP	cAMP-dependent

leads to a rise in intracellular Ca^{2+} and to the activation of Ca^{2+}/calmodulin-dependent enzymes, including Ca^{2+}/calmodulin-dependent protein kinases. Muscarinic stimulation results in the activation of phospholipase C and in the hydrolysis of inositol-containing phospholipids. By this mechanism, preganglionic stimulation may increase the accumulation of diacylglycerol and activate protein kinase C in the ganglion. Finally, preganglionic stimulation increases the content of cAMP in the ganglion, and presumably thereby the activity of the cAMP-dependent protein kinase, by a noncholinergic mechanism (Briggs et al., 1982; Volle et al., 1982). All three of these protein kinases appear to phosphorylate tyrosine hydroxylase and increase the rate of catecholamine synthesis in the ganglion. These kinases may regulate other ganglionic functions by phosphorylating other proteins. Future experiments will be required to identify the other substrates for these protein kinases, to determine the effects of phosphorylation on the functions of these proteins, and to elucidate the roles of these various pathways in mediating the effects of preganglionic stimulation on the functions of the ganglion.

ACKNOWLEDGEMENTS

This research was supported in part by research grant HL29025 from the National Institutes of Health and by a grant from the Earl M. Bane Charitable Trust. J. H. was the recipient of NRSA HL06701 from the National Institutes of Health.

REFERENCES

Bone, E. A., Fretten, P., Palmer, S., Kirk C. J., and Michell, R. H., 1984, Rapid accumulation of inositol phosphates in isolated rat superior cervical sympathetic ganglia exposed to V_1-vasopressin and muscarinic cholinergic stimuli, Biochem. J., 221:803-811.

Briggs, C. A. Whiting, G. J., Ariano, M. A., and McAfee, D. A., 1982, Cyclic nucleotide metabolism in the sympathetic ganglion, Cell Molec. Neurobiol., 2:129-141.

Briggs, C. A., Horwitz, J., McAfee, D. A., Tsymbalov, S., and Perlman, R. L., 1985, Effects of neuronal activity on inositol phospholipid metabolism in the rat autonomic nervous system, J. Neurochem., 44:731-739.

Cahill, A. L., and Perlman, R. L., 1984a, Phosphorylation of tyrosine hydroxylase in the superior cervical ganglion, Biochem. Biophys. Acta, 805:217-226.

Cahill, A. L., and Perlman, R. L., 1984b, Electrical stimulation increases phosphorylation of tyrosine hydroxylase in superior cervical ganglion of rat, Proc. Natl. Acad. Sci. USA, 81:7243-7247.

Cahill, A. L., Horwitz, J., and Perlman, R. L., 1985, Low-Na^+ medium increases the activity and the phosphorylation of tyrosine hydroxylase in the superior cervical ganglion of the rat, J. Neurochem., 44:680-685.

Hanley, M. R., Benton, H. P., Lightman, S. L., Todd, K., Bone, B. A., Fretten, P., Palmer, S., Kirk, C. J., and Michell, R. H., 1984, A

vasopressin-like peptide in the mammalian sympathetic nervous
system, Nature, 309:258-261.

Hokfelt, T., Elfvin, L.-G., Schultzberg, M., Fuke, K., Said, S. I.,
Mutt, V., and Goldstein, M., 1977, Immunohistochemical evidence of
vasoactive intestinal polypeptide-containing neurons and nerve
fibers in sympathetic ganglia, Neuroscience, 2:885-896.

Hokin, L. E., 1965, Autoradiographic localization of the acetylcholine-
stimulated synthesis of phosphatidylinositol in the superior
cervical ganglion, Proc. Natl. Acad. Sci., 53:1369-1376.

Horwitz, J., and Perlman, R. L., 1984a, Stimulation of DOPA synthesis
in the superior cervical ganglion by veratridine, J. Neurochem.,
42:384-389.

Horwitz, J., and Perlman R. L., 1984b, Activation of tyrosine
hydroxylase in the superior cervical ganglion by nicotinic and
muscarinic agonists, J. Neurochem., 43:546-552.

Horwitz, J., Tsymbalov, S., and Perlman, R. L., 1984, Muscarine
increases tyrosine 3-monooxygenase activity and phospholipid metabolism in the superior cervical ganglion of the rat, J. Pharmacol.
Exp. Ther., 229:577-582.

Horwitz, J., Tsymbalov, S., and Perlman, R. L., 1985, Muscarine
stimulates the hydrolysis of inositol-containing phospholipids in
the superior cervical ganglion, J. Pharmacol. Exp. Ther., 233:235-
241.

Ip, N. Y., Ho, C. K., and Zigmond, R. E. 1982a, Secretin and vasoactive
intestinal peptide acutely increase tyrosine 3-monooxygenase in the
rat superior cervical ganglion, Proc. Natl. Acad. Sci. USA,
79:7566-7569.

Ip, N. Y., Perlman, R. L., and Zigmond, R. E., 1982b, Both nicotinic
and muscarinic agonists acutely increase tyrosine 3-monooxygenase
activity in the superior cervical ganglion, J. Pharmacol. Exp.
Ther., 223:280-283.

Ip, N. Y., Perlman, R. L., and Zigmond, R. E., 1983, Acute transsynaptic
regulation of tyrosine 3-monooxygenase activity in the rat superior
cervical ganglion: Evidence for both cholinergic and noncholinergic
mechanisms, Proc. Natl. Acad. Sci., USA, 80:2081-2085.

McAfee, D. A., 1982, Superior cervical ganglion: Physiological
considerations, in: "Progress in Cholinergic Biology: Model
Cholinergic Synapses," I. Hanin and A. M. Goldberg, eds., Raven
Press, New York.

Neidel, J. E., Kuhn, L. J., and Vandenbark, G. R., 1983, Phorbol
diester receptor copurifies with protein kinase C, Proc. Natl.
Acad. Sci., USA, 80:36-40.

Volle, R. L., Quenzer, L. F., Patterson, B. A., Alkadhi, K. A., and
Henderson, E. G., 1981, Cyclic guanosine 3':5'-monophosphate
accumulation and ^{45}Ca-uptake by rat superior cervical
ganglia during preganglionic stimulation, J. Pharmacol.
Exp. Ther., 219:338-343.

Volle, R. L., Quenzer, L. G., and Patterson, B. A., 1982, The regulation of cyclic nucleotides in a sympathetic ganglion, <u>J. Autonomic Nervous System</u>, 6:65-72.

Wu, W. C.-S., Walaas, S. I., Nairn, A. C., and Greengard, P., 1982, Calcium/phospholipid regulates phosphorylation of a M_r "87k" substrate protein in brain synaptosomes, <u>Proc. Natl. Acad. Sci. USA</u>, 79:5249-5253.

AF64A: A USEFUL TOOL IN CHOLINERGIC RESEARCH

Israel Hanin

University of Pittsburgh School of Medicine
Western Psychiatric Institute and Clinic
3811 O'Hara Street
Pittsburgh, Pennsylvania 15213

INTRODUCTION

AF64A (ethylcholine aziridinium) has generated considerable interest following the demonstration by Fisher and colleagues, in 1980 (1, 2), that it can induce a persistent central cholinergic hypofunction in vivo. A variety of studies have since been conducted using this compound, in several laboratories, employing a wide array of applications. Neurochemical, electrophysiological, biochemical, morphological and behavioral studies have been completed to date. Data obtained are beginning to provide information regarding the possible mode of action of AF64A, and its selectivity vis-a-vis the cholinergic system in vivo. Findings reported from these studies (excluding the behavioral observations) will be surveyed in this chapter, and our current understanding of the mode of action of AF64A will be discussed in light of these findings.

NEUROCHEMICAL OBSERVATIONS

Major emphasis has been placed in the neurochemical studies, on the evaluation of the selectivity of action of AF64A vis-a-vis the cholinergic system. Treatment of animals with AF64A in vivo has been shown to result in a significant inhibition of a variety of markers of cholinergic activity. These include the high affinity choline uptake (HAChT) system (the rate limiting step in the synthesis of acetylcholine), activity of the enzymes choline acetyltransferase (ChAT) and acetylcholinesterase (AChE), levels of acetylcholine (ACh), and potassium-stimulated release of ACh from perfused hippocampal slices (3-7). This effect has occurred primarily in the hippocampus following intracerebroventricular (icv) administration of the toxin (7), or within the region of administration, when the substance has been injected into a specific brain area (5, 8). The effect is first observed within 24-48 hours after administration, and reaches a plateau by seven days (9). The attenuation of cholinergic function subsequently is long-lasting, and has been found to persist for up to one year following treatment with AF64A (10; Leventer et al., unpublished observation).

If AF64A is a selective cholinotoxin, then, by definition, its effect should be targeted primarily to the cholinergic system. If other neurotransmitter systems are perturbed, then, accordingly this effect should be secondary to the initial perturbation by AF64A of cholinergic neurons. Several studies consequently have been conducted, in which concurrent analysis was made of cholinergic as well as other neurotransmitter parameters in the same animal, following AF64A administration in vivo. A brief summary of findings reported to date from these particular studies follows.

In our laboratories we have administered AF64A to rats at several different sites, and have observed cholinergic selectivity of action of AF64A. Thus, stereotaxically administered intrahippocampal (2 nmol; 5 days) AF64A significantly reduced hippocampal ACh levels, HAChT, and ChAT activity (5). In addition, this treatment also markedly reduced acetylcholinesterase (AChE) staining in the hippocampus 20 hours following DFP administration (11). In the same tissues, however, there was no effect at all on norepinephrine (NE) levels or serotonin (5HT) uptake.

Sandberg and coinvestigators (8) have observed similar effects following stereotaxic administration of AF64A (2-26 nmol; up to 90 days post-treatment) directly into the striatum of rats. In a dose-response study they established that doses of up to 8 nmol of AF64A caused a significant decrease in striatal ChAT activity, ACh levels and HAChT, with minimal effects on the activities of glutamate decarboxylase (GAD) activity, GABA levels and uptake, tyrosine hydroxylase (TH) activity, and dopamine (DA) levels and uptake. Interestingly, these authors also noted nonspecific, dose related decreases of GAD and TH activities, when doses of AF64A used exceeded 16 nmol. The selective inhibition of ChAT activity persisted for at least three months, which was the time span of this study.

Following intracerebroventricular (icv) administration of AF64A to rats, Walsh et al. (10) have also demonstrated selectivity of action of AF64A towards the cholinergic system. At 120 days post dosing with either 7.5 or 15 nmol AF64A, bilaterally, significant reductions were observed in hippocampal ACh levels, as well as in cortical ACh levels after the higher dose of AF64A. Levels of choline, as well as concentrations of NE, DA, 5HT, and the metabolites DOPAC, HVA and 5-HIAA, respectively, were not affected in the same tissues following AF64A treatment. Also, histochemical analysis revealed no damage due to the treatment of AF64A on hippocampus, fimbria-fornix, septum, or caudate nucleus.

Jarrard and coinvestigators (12) have injected either 3 or 6 nmol of AF64A, bilaterally, into rats, icv. After 7 days neurochemical analyses revealed large depletions of ACh in hippocampus and in striatum, with no concurrent depletions of either NE or DA. Histological evaluation of the animals' brains indicated, however, damage to the fornix-fimbria region. The authors concluded on this basis, that the effects of AF64A are possibly due to some nonspecific action of the toxin. This difference in histochemical evidence between the present data and those of Walsh and his coinvestigators has yet to be resolved.

AF64A has also been administered directly into the substantia nigra of rats (13). A dose of 3 nmol AF64A was administered unilaterally by stereotaxic injection. Two weeks after surgery striatal DA levels were found to be depleted by 50%, and extensive damage was found at the site of injection of AF64A. Concurrent analysis of cholinergic markers was not conducted in these studies. The implication in these studies nevertheless was that AF64A produces nonspecific lesions in the brain.

Villani and coworkers (14) also found that AF64A, when administered into the interpeduncular nucleus at doses ranging from 1 to 30 nmoles, will significantly reduce ChAT activity in the interpeduncular nucleus as well as in the hippocampus. However, while only the cholinergic system was affected by such treatment in the hippocampus, within 24 hours after injection of AF64A even 1 nmol of AF64A caused a reduction of GAD activity and of high affinity uptake of GABA in synaptosomes obtained from the interpeduncular nucleus.

Arbogast and Kozlowski, on the other hand, have shown selective cholinotoxicity following administration of AF64A (0.02 and 0.2 nmol, unilaterally) by stereotaxic injection, at two sites along the rostrocaudal axis of the nucleus basalis of Meynert in rats (15). ChAT activity was reduced significantly in the ipsilateral cortex, with no concurrent effect on cortical levels of DA or 5HT. Very little necrosis/nonspecific damage was evident, and a substantial loss of AChE histochemical staining activity was observed at the site of AF64A injection. These findings would indicate a selectivity of action of AF64A for cholinergic components in the nucleus basalis area, at the low doses used in these studies.

All of these above findings, while at first glance possibly contradictory, do not necessarily negate one another. They do imply, however, that different brain areas are differentially sensitive to AF64A-induced toxicity. Thus, it is extremely important that a dose response toxicity analysis be conducted whenever the toxin is applied for the first time in a new brain area, and that the dose to be used be titrated carefully. Otherwise, it is not unexpected that, at high enough doses, nonspecific damage due to AF64A will be incurred.

We cannot ignore, however, the findings mentioned above, in which AF64A has also been reported to alter steady state levels of other neurotransmitters besides ACh. As stated above, even assuming that the primary effect of AF64A is at the cholinergic nerve terminal, it is conceivable that other neurotransmitter systems may be affected secondarily to the initial perturbation by AF64A of cholinergic neurons. Studies by Potter and coinvestigators imply that might, in fact, be the case (16, 17). They have demonstrated that within 4 days after icv adminis- tration of AF64A (10 nmol, unilaterally, icv) to rats, adrenergic, dopaminergic and serotonergic neurons also appeared to be perturbed in an inhibitory manner. These effects were transient, in that NE, DA, and 5HT levels reached a nadir at 4 days, but had returned to normal by 7 days following AF64A treatment. Serotonergic neurons appeared, moreover, to be more responsive to the toxin than were the catecholaminergic neurons. When AF64A was administered bilaterally, icv, at a dose of 5 nmol per side, only 5HT levels were reduced within 4 days, and had returned to normal by 7 days post-treatment. Levels of DA and NE were not affected in all brain regions tested, under these experimental circumstances. A time and dose related study of this phenomenon should provide important information regarding the interactive effect of cholinergic and other aminergic systems in the brain in vivo.

ELECTROPHYSIOLOGICAL OBSERVATIONS

Electrophysiological approaches also have been employed in the study of the mode of action of AF64A in vivo.

The work by Mantione and coinvestigators, in cats (18), was designed to evaluate the site of action of AF64A at the cholinergic nerve terminal. The effect of AF64A was studied in the periphery in the intact, anesthetized cat, at the level of the superior cervical ganglion, the neuromuscular junction of the tongue, and the nictitating membrane. In the superior

cervical ganglion, postganglionic action potentials following preganglionic stimulation were reduced in amplitude after each AF64A injection
(1 mg, intraarterially administered into the common carotid artery).
The effect was cumulative, and resulted (within about 1 hour) in a
complete loss of cholinergic transmission. This irreversible consequence
of AF64A administration lasted for the course of the experiment (12-18
hours). Contractions of the neuromuscular junction produced by preganglionic stimulation were also almost completely abolished. However,
postganglionic stimulation, or administration of tetraethylammonium (a
ganglionic stimulant), ACh or NE (which would be expected to act postsynaptically, at the level of the ganglion, or directly on the smooth muscle
of the nictitating membrane, respectively), elicited normal contractions
of the neuromuscular junction. Throughout the experiment, there was a
progressive depression of transmission at the neuromuscular junction of
the tongue, which was most pronounced at higher frequencies of motor
nerve stimulation, implying progressive depletion of the ACh available
for release. Thus, in these studies AF64A produced a long lasting
cholinergic hypofunction without compromising adrenergic transmission.
Moreover, the results indicated that the site of action of AF64A is at
the presynaptic site on the cholinergic nerve terminal.

McArdle and coinvestigators have recently completed some preliminary
studies on the effect of in vivo AF64A administration to mice ($2XLD_{50}$,
i.p., 30 min) on subsequent secretion of ACh from the isolated soleus
nerve-muscle preparation (19). Spontaneous (mepp) and stimulus evoked
(epps, 1 Hz) endplate potentials were monitored, at 22°C, in the crushed
muscle preparation. A significant reduction was observed in mepp
frequency (sec^{-1}; controls: $0.70^{\pm}0.02$, treated: $0.20^{\pm}0.02$); mean quantal
content ($mean^{\pm}SEM$; controls: $35.2^{\pm}0.98$, treated: $6.11^{\pm}0.9$), and mean
binomial probability of quantal release ($mean^{\pm}SEM$; controls: $0.93^{\pm}0.02$,
treated: $0.36^{\pm}0.06$). These attenuative effects of AF64A were similar
to those induced in the presence of elevated extracellular Mg^{++}, and
were partially restored by treatment of the preparation with 5-6uM 3,4
diaminopyridine. McArdle et al. have suggested, based on these studies,
that AF64A has an immediate action on the mechanism of quantal release
of ACh which is partially antagonized by blockade of K^{+} channels at the
motor nerve terminal.

Yet another electrophysiological approach to the study of the
effects of in vivo AF64A administration has been conducted by Lehr et
al. (20). These investigators have studied the effects of icv administration of AF64A (20 nmol; 3 months) on cortical EEG and neck EMG for
sleep studies; as well as on spontaneous unit activity, population
spikes, frequency potentiation, and responses to microiontophoretic
application of ACh in dorsal hippocampal cells of urethane anesthetized
rats. AF64A treatment had no effect on responses due to the microiontophoretic application of ACh, on spontaneous unit activity, on population
spikes evoked by stimulation of Schaffer collaterals, or on frequency
potentiation. AF64A treated animals did, however, show a sleep profile
similar to that of old rats (age >30 months) but different from that
seen in controls. This was evident in a shorter sleep time, a longer
REM latency, and a higher proportion of slow-wave sleep in the AF64A
treated rats, than that seen in young control animals. Based on these
observations the authors concluded that the AF64A treated rat should
serve as a good model in Alzheimer's disease research.

BIOCHEMICAL OBSERVATIONS

A number of biochemical studies have been conducted, primarily in
vitro, in an attempt to evaluate the mechanism of action of AF64A at a

more molecular level. Primary emphasis to date has been placed on the evaluation of its mechanism of action on the HAChT system.

Thus, Rylett and Colhoun (21) reported, using rat forebrain synaptosomes in vitro, that a number of choline mustard analogs, including the ethylcholine mustard, will selectively inhibit the HAChT system. Choline transport was not restored following several washes of the synaptosomes treated with the monomethyl aziridinium analog of choline. However, a reversible inhibition was obtained following treatment of the synaptosomes with the monoethyl-aziridinium analog of choline. These investigators concluded that these mustard analogs competitively alkylate the high affinity transporter of choline, and that some of these aziridinium compounds (but not AF64A) will inhibit HAChT in an irreversible manner.

We have also studied the effect of AF64A on HAChT in vitro. In our hands, the inhibition of HAChT by AF64A differs in different brain regions (22). Hippocampal as well as striatal synaptosomes obtained from rat brain were preincubated with AF64A, then washed successively, and tested for extent of HAChT activity at 1.5 uM choline. The inhibition of HAChT in hippocampal synaptosomes was of a mixed noncompetitive type, whereas striatal HAChT was competitively inhibited by AF64A. These data were interpreted as indicating that the HAChT system may exist in at least two different forms in the brain, which may also be brain area-specific. One system (in hippocampus) interacts noncompetitively with AF64A and can become irreversibly inactivated by the compound; another form (in striatum) interacts competitively with AF64A, and is reversible in nature.

Curti and Marchbanks (23) have investigated the kinetics of irreversible inhibition by AF64A of choline transport in guinea pig cortical synaptosomes. They have demonstrated that choline influx as well as choline efflux is inhibited by the neurotoxin. This inhibition of HAChT is reversible in the presence of choline or hemicholinium-3, which apparently compete with AF64A for the active transport site. Moreover, at low concentrations of AF64A (5-500 uM), the rate of HAChT inhibition appears to be that of a first order reaction with the choline carrier. At high (>2mM) AF64A concentrations, however, these investigators claim that the rate of inhibition of choline transport is controlled by translocation of the choline carrier to an outward-facing conformation.

Other components of the cholinergic nerve terminal have also been investigated vis-a-vis the effect of AF64A treatment on their integrity and function.

ChAT activity is significantly reduced following administration of AF64A in vivo (4-9, 15). This presumably is secondary to the effect of AF64A treatment on HAChT, ultimately resulting in destruction of cholinergic neurons, since ChAT is quite resistent to inhibition by AF64A in vitro. We measured the IC_{50} for inhibition of ChAT in vitro in rat hippocampal synaptosomes and found it to be $5.1X10^{-3}M$ (for comparison, the IC_{50} for HAChT was $3.0X10^{-6}M$). Similarly, Barlow and Marchbanks (24) found that exposure to 50 uM AF64A had no effect on ChAT activity in mouse cortex synaptosomes, and that as much as 500 uM AF64A was required to inhibit ChAT activity by 40%. We also did discover that AF64A can be acetylated by ChAT (apparent $K_m = 5.1$ mM) in the presence of a cholinesterase inhibitor (eserine) to form a possible false transmitter (25). This phenomenon may be an important consideration in understanding the mechanism of the neurotoxic action of AF64A.

AChE (5) and choline kinase activity (24) in intact rat and mouse brain synaptosomes, respectively, were essentially not affected by AF64A. However, AF64A was found to be an extremely potent inhibitor of a number of choline-recognized enzymes, when they were prepared and tested in partially purified form. Thus, choline dehydrogenase, extracted from washed acetone powder of liver mitochondria was readily inhibited with an IC_{50} of 6uM (24). This inhibition was prevented by incubation with choline, but once it occurred, it was essentially irreversible. Similarly, commercially available partially purified choline kinase, ChAT and AChE were inhibited by 88%, 87%, and 60%, respectively, in the presence of 100 uM AF64A (30 min at 37°C). Other enzymes which do not use choline as a natural substrate, including lactate dehydrogenase, chymotrypsinogen, carboxypeptidase A and alcohol dehydrogenase were minimally affected under the identical conditions (26). Moreover, key phospholipids extracted from cell cultures of the cholinergic neuroblastoma x glioma hybrid cell line NG-108-15 were decreased following 24 hours of continuous exposure of the cells to 50 uM AF64A. Phosphatidylcholine, phosphatidylethanolamine and phosphatidylserine concentrations were decreased by 35, 30 and 22% respectively. Addition of choline (500 uM) to the medium both enhanced cell survival and reduced the attenuating effect of AF64A on phospholipid concentrations (26).

The difference in effects induced by AF64A in vivo and in vitro shown above clearly has to be explored further. The data do however provide encouraging results vis-a-vis the possible mode of action of AF64A at the molecular level, with particular inclination for activity targeted toward the cholinergic system.

The site of binding of AF64A at the level of the nerve terminal has also been studied. Our in vivo studies indicated that tritiated quinuclidynyl benzilate (QNB) binding was not altered in various brain regions following icv and intrahippocampal administration of AF64A to mice and rats, respectively (4, 5). A more extensive drug binding study of the effect of icv administration of AF64A (3nmol per side, 7 and 21 days) showed that such treatment had no effect at all in cortex, hippocampus or striatum, on high affinity binding of [3H](-)QNB (a classical muscarinic antagonist), [3H]pirenzepine (a selective antagonist of the putative M_1 muscarinic receptor subclass), and [3H](+)cis- methyl-dioxolane (a potent muscarinic agonist). A 59-65% reduction in high affinity binding of [3H]hemicholinium-3 (a putative radioligand for sodium-dependent HAChT sites on cholinergic nerve terminals) was however found in the hippocampus of these AF64A treated rats, indicating that the effect of the neurotoxin most probably is presynaptic, with minimal influences upon muscarinic cholinergic receptor populations (27).

MORPHOLOGICAL OBSERVATIONS

Extensive morphological studies of the effects of AF64A administration in vivo have only been conducted during the past 2-3 years. These studies were prompted by several earlier reports in the literature claiming that the action of AF64A is not selective for cholinergic nerve terminals alone, and that its administration to experimental animals results in nonspecific damage to nerve terminals at, and around the site of its administration (12-14, 28). All of the studies which will be described below were conducted in parallel with biochemical analyses of the cholinergic system. In each case, clear biochemical evidence for cholinergic hypofunction was observed, concurrent with the reported morphological findings.

Kasa and his coinvestigators have conducted an extensive dose dependent light and electron microscopic analysis of the effects of

126

AF64A administration in vivo (29, 30). These studies focussed on the
effect of icv and intrastriatal administration of AF64A to rats. These
investigators observed a definite dose-dependent effect of the compound. Five nmol of AF64A, icv, produced selective cholinotoxic effects
in the brain. Axons were selectively degenerated in the cingular
cortex, fimbria, hippocampus, habenula, septum, striatum, and in fibers
arising from the nucleus basalis of Meynert - all these sites are
cholinergic in nature. It is intriguing to note, that the degenerated
axon terminals always were of the type that contained spherical vesicles;
axon terminals having ovoid or dense core vesicles were not altered by
the above treatments. Higher icv concentrations of AF64A (> 10 nmol),
on the other hand, produced nonspecific degeneration. Neuronal perikarya
were found to be affected at the higher doses of AF64A, in the CA2 and
CA3 fields of the hippocampus, and in the temporal and frontal cortex.
Moreover, necrosis was quite evident around the lateral ventricles, in
animals treated with 10 nmol AF64A or more.

The authors concluded, based on these observations, that at doses
below 5 nmol, icv administered AF64A exerts its specific toxic effects
primarily on cholinergic axons and axon terminals. At higher concentrations, however, nonspecific lesions of non-cholinergic cell bodies will
occur in different brain regions.

Similar observations and conclusions have been obtained by Gaal
and her coinvestigators, following the unilateral icv administration of
10 or 40 nmols of AF64A in rats (31).

Eight nmol AF64A, when injected intrastriatally, exerted a necrotic
effect near the injection site, and caused some distinct degeneration
of axons in the treated striatum and in the ipsilateral frontal cortex.
A similar effect was found with 0.5 nmol AF64A, except that the necrotic
region was very small and no degeneration was found in the cortex.

McGurk and Butcher have recently studied the neuropathologic
consequences of unilateral, stereotaxic AF64A infusion into the striatum
and the nucleus basalis of Meynert in rats (32). They have reported
nonselective tissue necrosis in both regions following 0.5 nmol of the
neurotoxin. More selective effects were observed in the range of
0.1-0.5 nmol, although, in their hands this was paralelled with only
minimal cholinergic deficits.

In a similar vein, Kozlowski and Arbogast have conducted some
parallel histochemical and biochemical studies on the effect of AF64A
injection directly into the nucleus basalis of Meynert in rats (33).
Using 0.02 and 0.05 nmol of AF64A they have been able to observe reduction
of ChAT activities in the central cortex of the injected hemisphere,
concurrent with clear cut loss of both diffuse staining for AChE and
loss of Nissl stained darkly labelled cell bodies at the site of the
injection. No apparent nonspecific tissue necrosis was observed with
these low doses of AF64A.

Thus, morphologic results obtained to date favor the concept of a
cholinotoxic effect of AF64A, although several reports have claimed a
nonspecific effect of action of this substance. Some of the discrepancies
may be attributable to differences in site of drug administration as
well as in the doses which were used. The source and purity of the
injected product may also be a critical factor in the observed results
(A. Fisher, unpublished observation). Clearly, attempts must be made
to resolve the differences reported in this area of investigation as
well.

DISCUSSION AND CONCLUSIONS

In this chapter an attempt has been made to survey and to present, in a cohesive manner, all information currently available, regarding the mode of action of AF64A in vivo.

Emphasis has been placed on the effects of the compound at the level of the nerve terminal; behavioral consequences of AF64A administration have not been described, since this information was not relevant to the topic of the present chapter. It should be mentioned, however, that AF64A administration results in distinct deficiencies in memory and learning in rats (10, 12). Hence we have suggested that the AF64A treated animal may also serve as a useful animal model of Alzheimer's Disease (6).

Although the exact mechanism of action of AF64A at the nerve terminal is still not determined definitively, we have access to enough information to allow us to render a working hypothesis in this regard.

Based upon all the information described above, it would appear that the immediate and primary effect of AF64A following its administration in vivo, is to interact in an irreversible manner with the HAChT system at the presynaptic site of cholinergic nerve terminals. This results in an inhibition of the rate limiting step for ACh synthesis, and a consequent reduction in ACh levels.

While AF64A does not readily cross the blood-brain barrier, some of it may in fact eventually be transported across the membrane into the nerve terminal (23). There, it could conceivably interact with a number of choline related enzymes and substrates, and serve to reduce their function or activity. This effect would be secondary to the initial effect on HAChT, but it could be significant, depending on the accessibility of the target enzymes or substrates, as well as the concentration of AF64A. Possible candidates for such interaction would include: ChAT, AChE, choline dehydrogenase, choline kinase, as well as phosphatidylcholine, phosphatidylethanolamine and phosphatidylserine. The interaction with phospholipid substrates could of course also occur on the outside of the nerve terminal and, in fact, could involve terminals of neurons that are not necessarily cholinergic in nature. AF64A accumulating on the inside of the nerve terminal could conceivably also inhibit quantal ACh release via K^+ channels at the nerve terminal.

The extent and relevance of this interaction of AF64A with the various enzymes listed is, however, not entirely clear at present. This is especially so in view of the fact that the inhibitory effect of AF64A on the above enzymes occurred with the partially purified preparation, but was not evident in the intact tissue when it was incubated with AF64A. It seems more appropriate to suggest at this time, therefore, that the loss in ChAT and AChE activity, and in ACh levels and release, all result from actual destruction of cholinergic nerve terminals in vivo. This destruction presumably is initiated via the mechanism of irreversible inhibition of the HAChT system, and possibly combined with some, as yet not clarified interaction with phospholipids comprising the presynaptic nerve terminal membrane.

This destructive effect on cholinergic nerve terminals is not evident at terminals pertaining to catecholaminergic, serotonergic or GABAergic neurons and thus can be considered to be selective for the cholinergic system. Some nonspecific destruction may admittedly occur following administration of high doses of AF64A, and hence some reduction of levels of transmitters other than ACh have been reported following

128

treatment with such concentrations. However, if the dose of AF64A is carefully titrated for the particular brain region studied, one will obtain selective cholinergic hypofunction in vivo. This destruction of cholinergic nerve terminals occurs within 48 hours following AF64A administration, reaches a maximal effect within 5-7 days, and has been shown to last for as long as a year following treatment with AF64A.

As more investigators become interested in using AF64A in their investigations, we will gain additional information regarding its mode of action, and its potential as a useful tool in cholinergic research.

Acknowledgements

This work encompasses results obtained in a number of laboratories. It includes also the cumulative effort of several valuable colleagues, listed in the bibliography, without whose collaboration these studies would not have been completed. Major portions of this report were supported by NIMH Grant #34893.

REFERENCES

1. A. Fisher and I. Hanin, Minireview. Choline analogs as potential tools in developing selective animal models of cholinergic hypofunction, Life Sci. 27:1615 (1980).
2. A. Fisher, C.R. Mantione, D.J. Abraham, and I. Hanin, Ethylcholine mustard aziridinium (AF64A): A potential irreversible cholinergic neurotoxin in vivo, Fed. Proc. 39:411 (1980).
3. C.R. Mantione, A. Fisher, and I. Hanin, The AF64A-treated mouse: Possible model for central cholinergic hypofunction, Science 213:579 (1981).
4. A. Fisher, C.R. Mantione, D.J. Abraham, and I. Hanin, Long-term central cholinergic hypofunction induced in mice by ethyl- choline aziridinium ion (AF64A) in vivo, J. Pharmacol. Exp. Therap. 222:140 (1982).
5. C.R. Mantione, M.J. Zigmond, A. Fisher, and I. Hanin, Selective presynaptic cholinergic neurotoxicity following intrahippocampal AF64A injection in rats, J. Neurochem. 41:251 (1983).
6. I. Hanin, W.C. DeGroat, C.R. Mantione, J.T. Coyle, and A. Fisher, Chemically-induced cholinotoxicity in vivo: Studies utilizing ethylcholine aziridinium ion (AF64A), in: Banbury Report 15: Biological Aspects of Alzheimer's Disease, R. Katzman, ed., Cold Spring Harbor Laboratory (1983).
7. S. Leventer, D. McKeag, M. Clancy, E. Wulfert, and I. Hanin, Intra- cerebroventricular administration of ethylcholine mustard aziridinium (AF64A) reduces release of acetylcholine (ACh) from rat hippocampal slices, Neuropharmacology, In Press (1985).
8. K. Sandberg, I. Hanin, A. Fisher, and J.T. Coyle, Selective cholinergic neurotoxin: AF64A's effects in rat striatum, Brain Research 293:49 (1984).
9. S. Leventer, D. McKeag, D. VanLear, E. Wulfert, and I. Hanin, AF64A (ethylcholine mustard aziridinium) in vivo: time course of cholinotoxicity, Fed. Proc. 44:896 (1985).
10. T.J. Walsh, H.A. Tilson, D.L. DeHaven, R.B. Mailman, A. Fisher, and I. Hanin, AF64A, a cholinergic neurotoxin, selectively depletes acetylcholine in hippocampus and cortex, and produces long-term passive avoidance and radial-arm maze deficits in the rat, Brain Research 321:91 (1984).
11. D.S. Arst, T.W. Berger, A. Fisher, and I. Hanin, AF64A reduces acetylcholinesterase (AChE) staining, and uncovers AChE-positive cell bodies in rat hippocampus in vivo, Fed Proc. 42:657 (1983).

12. L.E. Jarrard, G.J. Kant, J.L. Meyerhoff, and A. Levy, Behavioral and neurochemical effects of intraventricular AF64A administration in rats, Pharmacol. Biochem. Behav.21:273 (1984).

13. A. Levy, G.J. Kant, J.L. Meyerhoff, and L.E. Jarrard, Noncholinergic neurotoxic effects of AF64A in the substantia nigra, Brain Research 305:169 (1984).

14. L. Villani, A. Contestabile, A. Poli, P. Migani, and F. Fonnum, Neurotoxic effects of the presumed cholinergic toxin AF64A, Neurosci. Lett.Suppl. 18 :S228 (1984).

15. R.E. Arbogast, and M.R. Kozlowski, Reduction of cortical choline acetyltransferase (CAT) activity following injections of ethylcholine mustard aziridinium ion (AF64A) into the nucleus basalis of Meynert (NBM), Soc. Neurosci. Abst. 10:1185 (1984).

16. P.E. Potter, L.G. Harsing, Jr., I. Kakucska, Gy. Gaal, E.S. Vizi, A. Fisher, and I. Hanin, Effects of AF64A on hippocampal and monoaminergic systems in vivo, Fed. Proc. 44:897 (1985).

17. P.E. Potter, L.G. Harsing, Jr., I. Zimanyi, I. Kakucska, Gy. Gaal, A. Fisher, I. Hanin, and E.S. Vizi, Use of HPLC in characterizing the effects of AF64A, a potential cholinergic neurotoxin, in Proceedings of the 4th Annual Eastern European Symposium on Liquid Chromatography, H. Kalasz and L.S. Ettre, eds, Elsevier, Holland (1985).

18. C.R. Mantione, W.C. DeGroat, A. Fisher, and I. Hanin, Selective inhibition of peripheral cholinergic transmission in the cat produced by AF64A, J. Pharmacol. Exp. Therap. 225:616 (1983).

19. J.J. McArdle, T.M. Argentieri, D. Gargano, I. Hanin, and A. Fisher, Acute effects of the cholinergic neurotoxin AF64A on the secretion of acetylcholine, The Pharmacologist 27: (1985).

20. E. Lehr, F.J. Kuhn and D.H. Hinzen, AF64A neurotoxicity: Behavioral and electrophysiological alterations in rats, Soc. Neurosci. Abstr. 10:775 (1984).

21. B.J. Rylett and E.H. Colhoun, Kinetic data on the inhibition of high-affinity choline transport into rat forebrain synaptosomes by choline-like compounds and nitrogen mustard analogues, J. Neurochem. 34:713 (1980).

22. C.R. Mantione, A.Fisher, and I. Hanin, Biochemical heterogeneity of high affinity choline transport (HAChT) systems demonstrated in mouse brain using ethylcholine mustard aziridinium (AF64A), Trans. Am. Soc. Neurochem. 12:219 (1981).

23. D. Curti and R.M. Marchbanks, Kinetics of irreversible inhibition of choline transport in synaptosomes by ethylcholine mustard aziridinium, J. Membrane Biol. 82:259 (1984).

24. P. Barlow and R.M. Marchbanks, Effect of ethylcholine mustard on choline dehydrogenase and other enzymes of choline metabolism, J. Neurochem. 43:1568 (1984).

25. C.R. Mantione, A. Fisher, and I. Hanin, Possible mechanisms involved in the presynaptic cholinotoxicity due to ethylcholine aziridinium (AF64A) in vivo, Life Sci. 35:33 (1984).

26. K. Sandberg, R.L. Schnaar, M. McKinney, I. Hanin, A. Fisher, and J.T. Coyle, AF64A: An active site directed irreversible inhibitor of choline acetyltransferase, J. Neurochem. 44:439 (1985).

27. T.W. Vickroy, S.M. Leventer, M. Watson, W.R. Roeske, I. Hanin, and H.I. Yamamura, Selective reduction of central cholinergic parameters following ethylcholine mustard aziridinium ion (AF64A) administration, The Pharmacologist 27: (1985).

28. J.W. Asante, A.J. Cross, J.F.W. Deakin, J.A. Johnson, and H.R. Slater, Evaluation of ethylcholine mustard aziridinium ion (ECMA) as a specific neurotoxin of brain cholinergic neurons, Brit. J. Pharmacol. 573P (1983).

29. P. Kasa and I. Hanin, Light and electron microscopic investigation of the selective cholinotoxicity of AF64A (ethylcholine mustard aziridinium) in the rat CNS, Fed. Proc. 44:896 (1985).

30. P. Kasa, Z. Farkas, P. Szerdahelyi, Z. Rakonczay, A. Fisher, and I. Hanin, Effect of cholinotoxin (AF64A) in the central nervous system: Morphological and biochemical studies, in: Regulation of Transmitter Function: Basic and Clinical Aspects, E.S. Vizi and K. Magyar, eds, Akademiai Kiado, Budapest (1984).

31. Gy. Gaal, P.E. Potter, L.G. Harsing, Jr., I. Kakucska, A. Fisher, I. Hanin, and E.S. Vizi, Histological changes caused by AF64A in rat hippocampus, in: Regulation of Transmitter Function: Basic and Clinical Aspects, E.S. Vizi and K. Magyar, eds, Akademiai Kiado, Budapest (1984).

32. S.R. McGurk and L.L. Butcher, Neuropathology following intracerebral infusion of ethylcholine mustard aziridinium (AF64A), Fed. Proc. 44:897 (1985).

33. M.R. Kozlowski and R.E. Arbogast, Histochemical and biochemical effects of the injection of AF64A into the nucleus basalis of Meynert: Relevance to animal models of senile dementia of the Alzheimer type, in: Dynamics of Cholinergic Function, I. Hanin, ed., Plenum Press, New York (1985).

A PHARMACOLOGICAL STUDY OF ACETYLCHOLINE SYNTHESIS STORAGE AND RELEASE

B. Collier, J. Říčný and S.A. Welner

Department of Pharmacology
McGill University
Montreal, Quebec

INTRODUCTION

The effect of drugs on physiological processes has long been a fruitful way to obtain important information about the neurobiology of acetylcholine (ACh). It seems particularly appropriate to present such an attempt as a contribution to this symposium in recognition of the survival for so many years of Alexander G. Karczmar as the Chairman of his Department of Pharmacology.

The drug that is the object of our attention in this study is 2-(4-phenylpiperidino) cyclohexanol, which is now known to block the uptake of ACh by synaptic vesicles. It is usually considered that ACh is synthesized in the cytosol of cholinergic nerve terminals and that the newly synthesized ACh is translocated into synaptic vesicles from which it can be released. Thus, it might reasonably be expected that a drug that blocks this sequestration process would have somewhat interesting consequences to ACh turnover, and it was the purpose of this present study to explore such.

This drug was synthesized first in the research laboratories of Allen and Hanbury (now a member of the Glaxo group); hence its identification as AH5183. Dr. Mervyn Peel provided me with a little of its early history: it was isolated as a product of a reaction of N-nitroso-4-phenylpiperidine with cyclohexene using an actinic lamp, an undertaking prompted by their interest in photochemistry, not so much in pharmacology, and certainly not in the pharmacology of cholinergic nerve terminals. The compound is prepared most easily by reacting 4-phenylpiperidine with cyclohexene oxide, which is the way used by the Allen and Hanbury chemists to confirm the structure as:

This was also the reaction used by Dr. Tak-Hang Chan (McGill University, Dept. Chemistry) to prepare our supply of AH 5183 that supplemented a sample provided by Dr. S. Parsons (University of California, Santa Barbara).

The initial observations on the pharmacological activity of the

AH5183 were made at the Allen and Hanbury laboratories by Dr. R.T. Brittain. The toxicity test in mice showed death resulted from skeletal muscle paralysis; in chicks, the compound provoked a flaccid paralysis, so Brittain et al (1969) compared the AH5183 to tubocurarine in standard nerve-muscle preparations. The drug produced a junctional block, but with characteristics that differed from that induced by tubocurarine. They suggested AH5183 to have presynaptic depressant activity, and supported the idea by a test on guinea-pig ileum preparation: AH5183 depressed responses to co-axial stimulation without blocking responses to exogenously added ACh.

Marshall (1970 a,b) explored the neuromuscular blocking activity of AH5183 in more detail, showing the pharmacological properties were consistent with an effect of the compound to block ACh release indirectly, but by an action distinct from that of hemicholinium. He suggested the AH5183 did not act to inhibit choline uptake by the nerve terminal, but blocked ACh uptake by synaptic vesicles. This idea was tested directly by Anderson et al. (1983) with a preparation of synaptic vesicles isolated from Torpedo; such isolated synaptic vesicles possess an ACh uptake mechanism and this was inhibited potently by AH5183. This confirmed Marshall's suggestion and was compatible with the result of Toll and Howard (1980) showing that AH5183 reduced the amount of newly synthesized ACh recovered from a granule fraction prepared from PC12 cells that had been exposed to radioactive choline.

The objective of our work was to test the effects of AH5183 on neurochemical measures of ACh turnover in mammalian nervous tissue.

EFFECT OF AH5183 ON ACH RELEASE IN SYMPATHETIC GANGLION

For these experiments, we perfused superior cervical ganglia of the cat with medium containing physostigmine and measured the amount of ACh released at rest and during preganglionic nerve stimulation. The drug had no effect on spontaneous ACh release collected from ganglia. When stimulation was at 5Hz for 10 min, the AH5183 (10^{-5} M) reduced the amount of ACh collected by some 50%; increasing drug concentration 4-fold did not further suppress ACh release (Table 1).

Table 1. Effect of AH5183 on ACh Released from Superior Cervical Ganglia at Rest and During Preganglionic Stimulation (5Hz)

	Spontaneous Release (pmoles/10 min)	Evoked Release (pmoles/10 min)
Control	40 ± 7	457 ± 39
AH5183 (10^{-5} M)	52 ± 11	228 ± 19
AH5183 (4.10^{-5} M)	41 ± 10	220 ± 16

The effect of AH5183 to block ACh release was not the result of a direct effect on ACh release and was not associated with an effect on Ca influx during depolarization. The first point is evident from the result above that increased drug concentration did not have increased effect. It is also evident from the results of experiments that measured ACh release during short periods of preganglionic nerve stimulation: during 1-2 min stimulation at 5Hz, ACh release in presence of AH5183 was 102±7%

that in its absence. Thus, in ganglia exposed to the drug during preganglionic activity, initial ACh release is normal, but release subsequently declines. This pattern of effect is not characteristic of a Ca^{++}-influx blocking compound and tests of the effect of AH5183 on stimulation-induced increase of ^{45}Ca accumulation in ganglia were negative. Preganglionic stimulation increased the influx of ^{45}Ca as shown before (e.g. Blaustein, 1971; Lamarca and Collier, 1983), and this parameter was not affected by AH5183 (up to $4.10^{-5}M$).

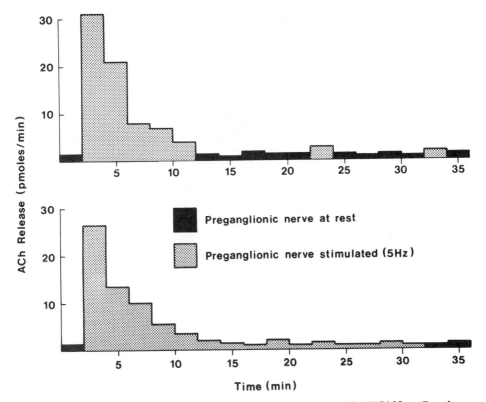

Fig. 1   The release of ACh from ganglia perfused with AH5183. In the upper experiment, the preganglionic nerve was stimulated (5Hz) for 10 min; then the ganglion was at rest and evoked release was tested every 10 min. In the lower experiment, preganglionic stimulation (5Hz) was for 30 min.

The time-course of the effect of AH5183 on ACh release during preganglionic nerve stimulation is shown in Fig. 1 which shows the results of 2 experiments. In one, stimulation was continuous and in the other it was interrupted. In both cases, evoked release after 10-15 min was fully suppressed in the presence of AH5183, and periods of rest did not result in partial recovery. The size of the pool of ACh releasable in AH5183's presence was calculated from this sort of an experiment: it was 189 pmoles (average of 18 tests), or 13% of the ganglion's total store of ACh; its size was the same whatever the frequency of preganglionic nerve stimulation used to evoke its release.

This store of ACh releasable in the presence of AH5183 presumably represents that part of the transmitter store that pre-exists in synaptic vesicles available to the release mechanism. It is substantially (Fig. 2) less than the 85% of stored transmitter available to be released from ganglia when ACh synthesis is blocked by hemicholinium (Birks and

MacIntosh, 1961; Matthews, 1966; Collier, 1973). It is often considered that the transmitter store in cholinergic nerve terminals exists in two pools, one being more available for release than the other, which replenishes the releasable pool by a process of mobilization (see MacIntosh and Collier, 1976). It seems that the AH5183 blocks the process of mobilization, allowing the release of only the pool of ACh readily available for release.

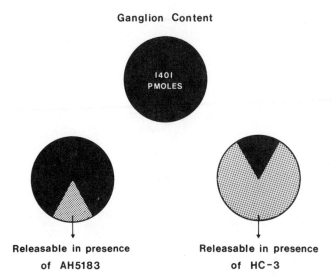

Ganglion Content

1401 PMOLES

Releasable in presence of AH5183

Releasable in presence of HC-3

Fig. 2   Schematic representation of the proportion of ganglionic ACh store releasable by preganglionic stimulation in presence of AH5183 or of hemicholinium (HC-3).

This concept of two ACh pools is illustrated by Fig. 3. The idea is presented as if two populations of synaptic vesicles exist and as if ACh can move from one to the other, rather than the more-often expressed view that vesicles from the reserve population can move to become active vesicles. The idea that two populations of vesicles might exist is well supported by the literature (see Zimmermann, 1979) and it is reasonable to presume that the metabolically more active vesicles identified by Dr. V.P. Whittaker and his colleagues might represent those that discharge their ACh during stimulation in AH5183's presence. The idea that ACh should move out of reserve into active vesicles is less well written about, but supportable by some good evidence (Elmqvist and Quastel, 1965; Large and Rang, 1978). This notion of intervesicular movement of ACh is prescribed because the only known effect of AH5183 is to block ACh uptake into synaptic vesicles; it remains possible that the drug, in addition, interacts with whatever mechanism might be responsible for synaptic vesicle mobility within the nerve terminal.

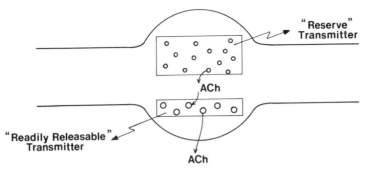

Fig. 3 Schematic representation of two ACh stores in a preganglionic
nerve terminal and the postulated relationship between the two.

REVERSABILITY OF EFFECT OF AH5183

    The effect of AH5183 on ACh release from ganglia was reversible:
during perfusion with drug-free medium, evoked ACh release returns toward
control values (Table 2).

Table 2. Reversal by Washing of Depressant Effect of
AH5183 on ACh Release from Ganglia

	ACh Release (pmoles/min)
Release before exposure to AH5183	50
Release after 15 min stimulation in presence of AH5183	2
Release after 20 min wash	6
Release after 40 min wash	18
Release after 60 min wash	30
Release after 80 min wash	41
Release after 120 min wash	60

    The source of ACh that becomes available for release during the
recovery from AH5183 could be from new synthesis to replenish that
depleted from the releasable pool, or it could be by mobilization from
that not releasable in AH5183's presence. Both processes seem to occur.
We tested this point by exposing ganglia to [^{3}H]choline during the
development of the AH5183-induced block to label the residual ACh, and to
[^{14}C]choline during wash-out of AH5183 to label the pool of ACh depleted
in the presence of AH5183. Test of isotope ratio of ACh released during
recovery showed it to be similar to that of ACh in tissue; thus both
synthesis and mobilization contribute to replenishment under the
conditions of this experiment and neither seems to be preferred over the
other.

ACH RELEASE AND SUBCELLULAR DISTRIBUTION IN BRAIN

The main objective of these experiments was to obtain information about the effect of AH5183 on the ACh content of subcellular fractions prepared from tissue stimulated to release ACh. The drug clearly depressed ACh release from slices of rat striatum stimulated by K^+: about half-maximum suppression of evoked ACh release was apparent with 70nM AH5183.

The amount of ACh in a cytoplasmic fraction prepared from lysed synaptosomes from tissue incubated in presence of AH5183 and stimulated by K^+ was greater than the amount of ACh in this fraction prepared from tissue stimulated in the absence of the drug. Conversely, the ACh content of the pellet prepared from lysed synaptosomes was reduced when this was prepared from tissue stimulated in presence of AH5183. And when these pellets were subject to density gradient centrifugation, the ACh content of the fraction containing monodispersed synaptic vesicles was severely depleted by exposure of tissue to AH5183; there was not measurable depletion of fractions denser than synaptic vesicle fraction.

Thus, these experiments have shown stimulation in presence of AH5183 to be associated with vesicular, but not cytoplasmic ACh depletion, and it seems reasonable to suppose that the block of ACh release is a consequence of the loss of vesicular ACh. The idea that cytoplasmic ACh is the origin of releasable transmitter (e.g. Israël et al., 1979; Tauc, 1982) seems not to hold under the conditions of the present experiments, a conclusion similar to that reached by Melega and Howard (1984) on the basis of their studies on the effect of AH5183 in ACh storage in PC12 cells.

The idea expressed earlier in this article about two populations of synaptic vesicles with different susceptibility to depletion in the presence of AH5183 is compatible with the subcellular fractionation results described above, if the denser gradient fractions whose ACh was not depleted in the presence of AH5183 contain much of the reserve ACh. It is not altogether clear what is the nature of the bound ACh in these denser fractions, although there is evidence suggesting that they contain a part of rapidly turning-over ACh (Barker et al, 1972), an idea the opposite to the present one that reserve ACh is contained therein.

ACH SYNTHESIS

The consequence of AH5183 to transmitter synthesis was measured in sympathetic ganglion. The initial test of this that we made was of AH5183's effect on the uptake and acetylation of a choline analogue. This experiment provides information about the delivery of precursor as well as the generation of product. We used diethylhomocholine, an analogue that is taken up by the choline transport mechanism, some of what is taken up is acetylated, but the acetyldiethylhomocholine is not releasable (Welner and Collier, 1984). The AH5183 did not alter either choline analogue uptake or its acetylation, suggesting that the drug has no effect on the process of transmitter synthesis. This result was somewhat unexpected, because the AH5183 clearly decreases ACh release and most drugs that decrease ACh release have the consequence to decrease ACh synthesis, the two processes normally being coupled.

The mechanism by which ACh release triggers an increase in ACh synthesis is not known; the evidence well reviewed by Tuček (1984) tends to the conclusion that the ACh synthetic reaction approaches equilibrium at rest and is disturbed toward product formation as the result of ACh

release. This idea implies (Fig. 4) that activation of transmitter
synthesis is triggered by the uptake of cytoplasmic ACh into synaptic
vesicles, because synthesis occurs in the cytoplasm and release occurs
from vesicles. The prediction from this hypothesis would be that AH5183,
by blockade of ACh uptake by vesicles, would block stimulation-induced
increase in ACh synthesis.

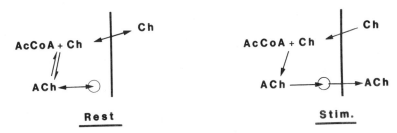

Fig. 4.   Scheme to illustrate the idea that ACh synthesis is at
          equilibrium during rest and displaced toward ACh production as
          the result of ACh release during stimulation (stim.)

        Thus, we estimated the effect of AH5183 on ACh synthesis by
measuring ACh release and ACh content of ganglia and subtracting from the
sum of these two measures, the estimate of initial ACh content provided
by measure of ACh in the ganglion contralateral to the test one. During
30 min of preganglionic nerve stimulation, AH5183 did not alter the ACh
synthesis (Table 3).

Table 3.   ACh Synthesis in Presence or Absence of
           AH5183

		ACh (pmoles)	
		Control	AH5183
a)	Release	1401	344
b)	Final Content	2436	3528
	a + b	3837	3872
c)	Initial Content	1323	1378
d)	Synthesis (a+b)-c	2514	2494

        It appears, therefore, that ACh synthesis can be dissociated from
ACh release by the use of AH5183 and that something other than mass
action regulates transmitter synthesis.

The activation of ACh synthesis during stimulation in the presence of AH5183 was confirmed by experiments which measured [3H]ACh formed from [3H] choline (Table 4). Preganglionic stimulation (5Hz) increased [3H] ACh synthesis and this increase was similar whether AH5183 was present or not.

Table 4. Synthesis of [3H]ACh from [3H]choline by Ganglia in Presence or Absence of AH5183

	[3H]ACh (10^3 dpm)
Resting Ganglia	40.0 ± 11.1
Stimulated Ganglia – AH5183	160.5 ± 8.2
Stimulated Ganglia + AH5183	172.6 ± 24.3

The ACh that is synthesized during blockade of release by AH5183 mixes well with pre-existing ACh stores and becomes releasable upon wash-out of AH5183. This is shown by Fig. 5. In this experiment, the ganglion was exposed to [3H]choline during stimulation in the presence of AH5183; then drug and [3H]choline were washed out with choline-free medium to discourage synthesis, and release of ACh was tested by preganglionic stimulation. Clearly, both [3H] and ACh were released; the evoked release of [3H] was mostly [3H]ACh, and its specific activity (94 dpm/pmole) was similar to that measured in tissue (99 dpm/pmole).

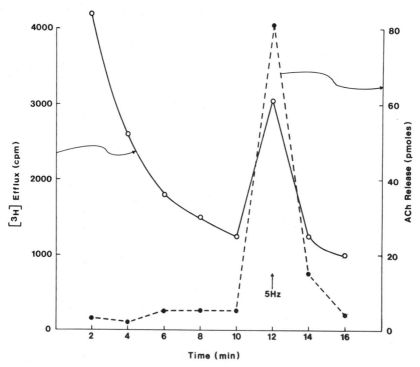

Fig. 5. An experiment that shows the availability for release of ACh synthesized during exposure to AH5183. The ganglion was perfused first with AH5183 and [3H]choline during preganglionic nerve stimulation (5Hz for 30 min). Then, at rest, it was perfused with choline- and AH5183-free medium and after 30 min wash, the preganglionic nerve was again stimulated.

The consequence of increased ACh synthesis when ACh release is reduced by AH5183 is evident from the Table 3: tissue ACh increases. This increase in tissue ACh shown in the above experiments was apparent in the presence of inhibitor of cholinesterase, necessary to preserve released ACh. But it is not necessary to inhibit esterase to increase tissue ACh during stimulation in the presence of AH5183 (Table 5).

Table 5. Effect of Preganglionic Stimulation on ACh Content of Ganglia Perfused with AH5183

Medium	ACh Content (pmoles)	
	Test	Control
Normal	2561	1581
Ca-free	1875	1584
4-aminopyridine	3210	1600
↑Mg	2028	1502
↓Ca	2148	1591
↑Mg + ↓Ca	1669	1653

The Table 5 also includes test of the effects of procedures that alter Ca influx during stimulation on the increase of ACh content measured in AH5183-treated ganglia. It is evident that procedures that lower Ca influx lessen the magnitude of the phenomenon, and that 4-aminopyridine, which increases Ca influx (Thesleff, 1980), increases the phenomenon. Thus, it seems possible that changed intracellular Ca during activity is involved in ACh synthesis activation.

SUMMARY

The objective of the experiments summarized was to use the drug AH5183 to tell something about the processes of ACh release, storage and synthesis. The results support the notion that synaptic vesicles contain releasable transmitter, they identify the readily releasable fraction of transmitter as being some 13% of the total store, and they suggest that some mechanism other than mass action regulates ACh synthesis.

ACKNOWLEDGEMENTS

The author's work is supported by the Medical Research Council of Canada. They are grateful to Drs. Peel, Chan and Parsons for their help in providing the AH5183, and to Maureen Levore for preparing this camera-ready copy.

REFERENCES

Anderson, D.C., King, S.C., and Parsons, S.M., 1983, Pharmacological characterization of the acetylcholine transport system in purified Torpedo electric organ synaptic vesicles, Mol. Pharmacol. 24:48-54.

Barker, L.A., Dowdall, M.J., and Whittaker, V.P., 1972, Choline metabolism in the cerebral cortex of guinea pig, Biochem. J. 130: 1063-1080.

Birks, R.I., and MacIntosh, F.C., 1961, Acetylcholine metabolism of a sympathetic ganglion, Can. J. Biochem. Physiol. 39:787-827.

Blaustein, M.P., 1971, Preganglionic stimulation increases calcium uptake by sympathetic ganglia, Science, 172:391-393.

Brittain, R.T., Levy, G.P., and Tyers, M.B., 1969, The neuromuscular blocking action of 2-(4-phenylpiperidino)cyclohexanol (AH5183), Eur. J. Pharmacol., 8:93-99.

Collier, B., 1973, The accumulation of hemicholinium by tissues that transport choline, Can. J. Physiol. Pharmacol. 51:491-495.

Elmqvist, D., and Quastel, D.M.J., 1965, Presynaptic action of hemicholinium at the neuromuscular junction, J. Physiol. (Lond.), 177:463-482.

Israël, M., Dunant, Y., and Manaranche, R., 1979, The present status of the vesicular hypothesis, Prog. Neurobiol., 13:237-275.

Lamarca, M.V., and Collier, B., 1983, Effects of 4-aminopyridine on the cat superior cervical ganglion, J. Pharmacol. Exp. Therap., 226:249-257.

Large, W.A., and Rang, H.P., 1978, Variability of transmitter quanta released during incorporation of a false transmitter into cholinergic nerve terminals, J. Physiol. (Lond.), 285:25-34.

MacIntosh, F.C., and Collier, B., 1976, Neurochemistry of cholinergic terminals, pp. 99-228, in: "Neuromuscular Junction," E. Zaimis, ed., Springer-Verlag, Berlin.

Marshall, I.G., 1970a, Studies on the blocking action of 2-(4-phenyl piperidino)cyclohexanol (AH5183), Br. J. Pharmacol., 38:503-516.

Marshall, I.G., 1970b, A comparison between the blocking actions of 2-(4-phenylpiperidino)cyclohexanol (AH5183) and its N-methyl quaternary analogue (AH5954), Br. J. Pharmacol., 40:68-77.

Matthews, E.K., 1966, The presynaptic effects of quaternary ammonium compounds on the acetylcholine metabolism of a sympathetic ganglion, Br. J. Pharmacol., 26:552-566.

Melega, W.P., and Howard, B.D., 1984, Biochemical evidence that vesicles are the source of the acetylcholine released from stimulated PC12 cells, Proc. Nat'l Acad. Sci. USA, 81:6535-6538.

Tauc, L., 1982, Nonvesicular release of neurotransmitter. Physiol. Rev., 62:857-893.

Thesleff, L., 1980, Aminopyridine and synaptic transmission, <u>Neuroscience</u> 5:1413-1419.

Toll, L., and Howard, B.D., 1980, Evidence that an ATPase and a protonmotive force function in the transport of acetylcholine into storage vesicles, <u>J. Biol. Chem.</u> 255:1787-1789.

Tuček, S., 1984, Problems in the organization and control of acetylcholine synthesis in brain neurons, <u>Prog. Biophys. Molec. Biol.</u>, 44:1-46.

Welner, S.A., and Collier, B., 1984, Uptake, metabolism, and releasability of ethyl analogues of homocholine by rat brain, <u>J. Neurochem.</u>, 43:1143-1151.

Zimmermann, H., 1979, Vesicle recycling and transmitter release, <u>Neuroscience</u>, 4:1773-1804.

REGULATION OF CHOLINE PHOSPHORYLATION IN RAT STRIATUM

R.R. Reinhardt and L. Wecker

Department of Pharmacology, Louisiana State University

Medical Center, New Orleans, Louisiana 70112, USA

INTRODUCTION

In cholinergic nerve terminals, choline is an important precursor molecule for the synthesis of both acetylcholine (ACh) and phosphorylcholine (PCh) through reactions catalyzed by choline acetyltransferase (CAT) and choline kinase (CK), respectively. While studies have indicated that CAT exists in both soluble and membrane associated forms which may subserve different primary functions in the nerve terminal (Smith and Carroll, 1980; Benishin and Carroll, 1983), little similar information has been available for CK. This enzyme catalyzes the first and possibly rate-limiting step (Infante, 1977) in the cytidine pathway (Kennedy and Weiss, 1956) which is the major pathway for the incorporation of choline into phosphatidylcholine in brain (Ansell and Spanner, 1968). Since choline serves as a substrate for both CAT and CK, it might be expected that the nerve terminal has regulatory mechanisms to channel choline through the pathway that requires the precursor most at any given instant. Indeed, an association between the acetylation and phosphorylation pathways has been suggested (Ansell and Spanner, 1970; Collier, 1970). Therefore, to further our understanding of the utilization of choline by the cholinergic neuron, we studied the properties of CK and the modulation of choline phosphorylation by endogenous agents.

Choline Kinase

Early studies suggested that CK activity was localized exclusively to the cytosol of nerve endings in brain (Spanner and Ansell, 1978; 1979). However, there was some evidence for membrane associated activity in brain (McCaman and Cook, 1966; Upreti et al., 1976), as well as in the anaerobic protozoon Entodinium caudatum (Bygrave and Dawson, 1976). Furthermore, it had been suggested that in this latter preparation, CK played a key role in the high affinity transport of choline. Since Massarelli and Wong (1981) suggested that CK activity may be coupled to the transport of choline in neuronal membranes, we investigated the subcellular distribution of CK activity in rat striatum (Reinhardt and Wecker, 1983).

CK activity in the supernatant isolated from hypoosmotically shocked crude mitochondrial (P_2) or synaptosomal (B) preparations was 4.16 and 2.13 umoles/g initial wet weight/hr, respectively. When the particulate fractions from these preparations were assayed, they were essentially devoid of enzyme activity. In addition, incubation of the membrane fractions with NaCl (up to 1.5 M) did not lead to measurable CK activity. However, when membranes were dissolved in 2% Triton X-100, significant enzyme activity was apparent (1.40 and 0.77 umoles/g initial wet weight/hr for membrane fractions from the P_2 and B preparations, respectively). The addition of Triton X-100 to the soluble fractions did not significantly alter enzyme activity. When enzyme activity in the membrane and soluble fractions was compared to the activity present in the unfractionated preparation treated with detergent, 26% of the total activity was attributed to the particulate fraction and 72% to the soluble portion. The distribution of enzyme activity in a P_2 preparation is shown in Figure 1. A subcellular profile of CK activity in rat striatum (each fraction treated with Triton X-100) indicated that of the total enzyme activity in a tissue homogenate (16.3 umoles/g initial wet weight/hr), 33% was associated with the P_2 fraction, 18% with the B fraction, and 6% with the microsomal fraction. The remaining activity (62%) was localized to the cytosolic (S_3) fraction.

To determine whether any differences existed between enzyme activities associated with the two fractions, the optimal ionic requirements for ATP and Mg^{2+} were determined. Under the conditions of our assay, the optimal ATP concentration was 1.5 mM for both soluble and membrane associated activity and the optimum Mg^{2+} concentration was

146

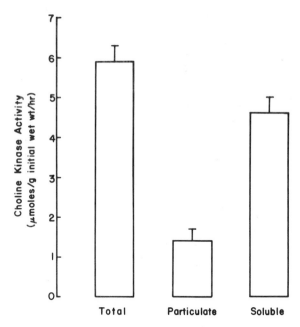

Fig. 1. Distribution of choline kinase activity in a P_2 preparation from rat striatum. For measurements of total enzyme activity, Triton X-100 (final concentration 2%, v/v) was added to the P_2 pellet following resuspension. For soluble and particulate activities, detergent was added following hypoosmotic rupture and centrifugation of P_2. Choline kinase activity was determined by incubating samples with (^{14}C)choline for 1 hour at 37°C. Values are the means of 12 observations and bars are standard errors.

between 20 and 50 mM. Hence, the enzymes were indistinguishable on the basis of ionic requirements.

Kinetic experiments were performed to determine whether a difference existed between particulate and soluble CK and to determine the kinetic mechanism for striatal CK. No kinetic differences were detected between the cytoplasmic and particulate forms (Reinhardt et al., 1984). However, it should be noted that the activity of CK was measured in a solubilized membrane fraction, not in an intact membrane preparation. Interpretation of initial velocity, product inhibition, and substrate inhibition data indicated a rapid equilibrium addition of MgATP prior to Mg^{2+}, but a random addition of choline and MgATP. On the basis of kinetic data, it appears that a single CK exists.

Table 1. Choline Kinase Activity in Soluble and Particulate Fractions of a P_2 Preparation from Different Brain Regions

Fraction	Striatum	Hippocampus	Frontal Cortex	Cerebellum
	CK activity (umoles/h/mg protein)			
Total P_2	0.59 ± 0.03	0.72 ± 0.03	0.59 ± 0.04	0.62 ± 0.03
Soluble	0.51 ± 0.02	0.63 ± 0.02	0.51 ± 0.02	0.56 ± 0.02
Particulate	.072 ± .002	.080 ± .002	.075 ± .002	.055 ± .002

For measurements of total enzyme activity, Triton X-100 (final concentration 2%, v/v) was added to the P_2 pellet following resuspension. For soluble and particulate activities, detergent was added following hypoosmotic rupture and centrifugation of P_2. Enzyme activity was determined by incubating samples with (^{14}C)choline for 1 hour at 37°C. Each value is the mean ± the SEM of 6 observations.

To determine whether particulate enzyme activity was specifically associated with cholinergic neurons, we investigated the distribution of soluble and particulate CK activity in P_2 fractions from different brain regions. Total CK activity was highest in the hippocampus, but all brain areas studied, including the cerebellum, had relatively comparable enzyme activities (Table 1). Further comparisons indicated that the Michaelis-Menten constants for both choline and MgATP (for both forms of CK) were the same in both striatum and cerebellum. Hence, data suggested that there was no unique distribution or kinetic constant of membrane bound CK in a cholinergic versus noncholinergic region. Further studies to determine whether membrane bound CK was specific for cholinergic neurons included experiments in which the cholinergic septal-hippocampal pathway of rats was destroyed. Lesions of the medial septal area resulted in large decreases in ACh levels, in the activity of both soluble and membrane bound CAT, and in the rate of high affinity choline uptake in the hippocampus. However, there was no change in the rate of low affinity choline transport or in the activity of either form of CK, suggesting that CK was not specifically associated with cholinergic neurons.

Since membrane bound CK activity could only be assayed by disruption of membranes, we attempted to determine the function of this form of CK in unsolubilized preparations using reconstituted synaptosomes.

Synaptosomes were osmotically shocked to remove soluble CK and were refilled with MgATP and Mg^{2+}. In this manner, upon choline uptake, all of the substrates for CK would be present. The rate of choline uptake into this preparation was reduced to 25% of control and no appreciable synthesis of PCh could be measured. Perhaps disruption of the synaptosomes during osmotic shock altered the membrane characteristics such that membrane bound CK could no longer effectively metabolize its substrates.

Although the function of membrane associated CK could not be determined in brain synaptosomes, results from studies in other preparations have suggested a relationship between enzyme activity and the high affinity transport of choline (Bygrave and Dawson, 1976; Yavin, 1976; Massarelli and Wong, 1981; Meyer et al., 1982). Perhaps the membrane associated enzyme converts choline to PCh as choline is transported through the membrane, similar to the mechanism postulated for the transport of choline and its acetylation to ACh (Barker and Mittag, 1975). Under conditions of high neuronal activity, it is likely that choline transported into the nerve terminal will be used predominantly to support ACh synthesis (Kuhar and Murrin, 1978). When neuronal activity is low, however, transported choline may be used mainly for phospholipid synthesis. Hence, CK might play an important role in regulating the metabolism of choline as it is transported into the nerve terminal. This would suggest that CK may control the supply of a pool of choline for the synthesis of ACh. This idea is supported by studies indicating that the concentrations of ACh and choline in brain following the administration of choline may be modulated by CK activity (Millington and Wurtman, 1982). Indeed, studies have suggested that exogenous choline is converted to a bound form prior to its use for the synthesis of ACh (Schmidt and Wecker, 1981).

Modulation of Choline Phosphorylation

Although much evidence suggests that cholinergic activity and the synthesis of ACh can be modulated by numerous endogenous substances, the possible regulation of choline phosphorylation has not been investigated. It is well documented that adenosine decreases the release of ACh from rat brain slices (Harms et al., 1979; Pedata et al., 1983) and adenosine analogues decrease ACh turnover in brain (Murray et al., 1982; Haubrich et al., 1981; Jackisch et al., 1984). To determine whether the synthesis of PCh is subject to endogenous modulation and to further elucidate a possible relationship between choline acetylation and phosphorylation, we studied the effects of adenosine on the level of newly synthesized (^{3}H)PCh subsequent to (^{3}H)choline transport into synaptosomes. Incubation of synaptosomes with various concentrations of adenosine indicated a concentration-dependent decrease in the levels of (^{3}H)PCh with a significant effect at a concentration of 0.1 mM (Figure 2A). Since studies have indicated that adenosine may be a Ca^{2+} antagonist and its inhibitory effects can be attenuated by increasing extracellular Ca^{2+} (Daly, 1982; Stone, 1981; Dowdle and Maske, 1980), we determined the effects of Ca^{2+} on the levels of (^{3}H)PCh and on the adenosine-induced decrease. Increasing the extracellular Ca^{2+} concentration above 1 mM resulted in a significant decrease in (^{3}H)PCh levels (Figure 2B). In addition, when the concentration of Ca^{2+} was increased in the presence of adenosine (0.25 mM), the effects of adenosine were masked. Since the effects of adenosine and Ca^{2+} were not additive, it is likely that these agents share a common pathway or mechanism to decrease the level of newly synthesized PCh.

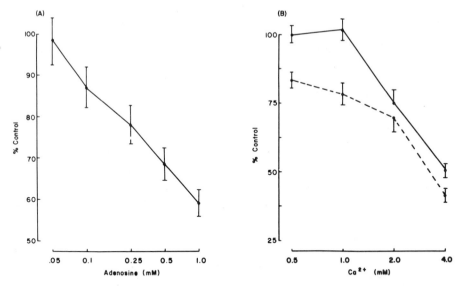

Fig. 2. Effects of Adenosine and Ca^{2+} on the levels of newly synthesized PCh in rat striatal synaptosomes. Synaptosomes were incubated for 10 min at 37°C with choline (25 uM) and the levels of (^{3}H)PCh subsequent to (^{3}H)choline uptake were determined. (A) The concentration of adenosine in the incubation medium was varied. (B) The concentration of Ca^{2+} in the incubation medium was varied alone (●——●) or in the presence of 0.25 mM adenosine (●----●). Values are the means of 9 determinations and bars represent standard errors. The control mean value was 19.3 pmoles (^{3}H)PCh/mg protein.

To determine the mechanism mediating the adenosine-induced decrease in (^{3}H)PCh levels, we investigated the effects of adenosine analogues known to interact at different sites at the nerve terminal. Three adenosine receptors have been described, viz., A_1 which has a high affinity (nanomolar) for adenosine, A_2 which has a lower affinity (micromolar) for adenosine and is coupled to adenylate cyclase in a stimulatory manner, and P which is an intracellular site on adenylate cyclase that is inhibitory (for review see Daly, 1982). The A_1 site need not be considered because nanomolar concentrations of adenosine had no effect on (^{3}H)PCh levels. The possibility that A_2 receptor activation was responsible for the depression of (^{3}H)PCh levels was tested using 2',5'-dideoxyadenosine, an analogue that is inactive at this site (Daly, 1982). 2',5'-dideoxyadenosine (0.25 mM) decreased the level of newly synthesized PCh by 35% (Figure 3), suggesting that the effect of

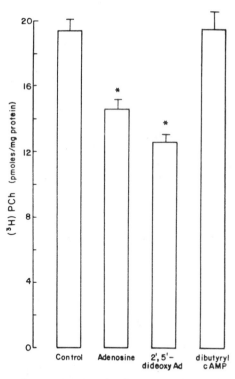

Fig. 3. Effect of Adenosine, 2',5'-Dideoxyadenosine, and Dibutyryl-cAMP on levels of newly synthesized PCh in rat striatal synaptosomes. Synaptosomes were incubated for 10 min at 37°C with choline (25 uM) and 0.25 mM concentrations of each compound. The levels of (^{3}H)PCh subsequent to (^{3}H)choline uptake were determined. Values are the means of 9 observations and bars represent standard errors. *Significantly different from control values (p < 0.05) as determined by Dunnett's test.

adenosine was not mediated by A_2 receptor stimulation. To confirm this finding, synaptosomes were incubated with dibutyryl-cAMP. This stable analogue, which readily crosses membranes and is resistant to hydrolysis by phosphodiesterase, had no effect on (^{3}H)PCh levels, even when the concentration was raised to 1 mM (Figure 3). Similar results were obtained with dibutyryl-cGMP. Hence, data indicated that an extracellular site of action of adenosine was not responsible for its effect to decrease the level of newly synthesized PCh.

The possibility that the effect of adenosine involved actions at the intracellular P site was investigated using L-N^6-(phenylisopropyl)-adenosine and 2-chloroadenosine, analogues that are inactive at this site (Daly, 1982). These compounds (0.25 mM) significantly decreased the levels of (^{3}H)PCh to the same extent as adenosine (Figure 4). Thus, data were not consistent with an action at this intracellular site. However,

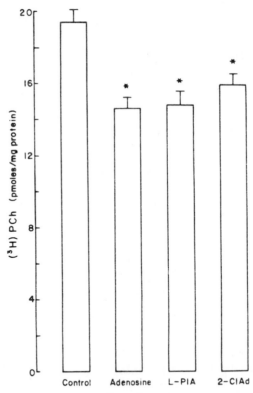

Fig. 4. Effect of Adenosine, L-N^6-(phenylisopropyl)-adenosine (L-PIA), and 2-chloroadenosine (2-ClAd) on levels of newly synthesized PCh in rat striatal synaptosomes. Synaptosomes were incubated for 10 min at 37°C with choline (25 uM) and 0.25 mM concentrations of each compound. The levels of (^{3}H)PCh subsequent to (^{3}H)choline uptake were determined. Values are the means of 9 observations and bars represent standard errors. *Significantly different from control values (p < 0.05) as determined by Dunnett's test.

it was possible that another intraterminal site was involved. The adenosine uptake inhibitors dipyridamole and papaverine could not be used to confirm this hypothesis because these compounds inhibited choline uptake and decreased (^{3}H)PCh levels by an unknown mechanism.

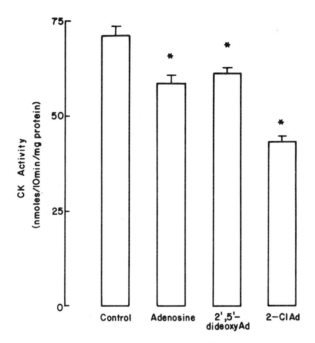

Fig. 5. Effect of Adenosine, 2',5'-Dideoxyadenosine, and 2-Chloroadenosine (2-ClAd) on CK activity. Rat striatal synaptosomes were incubated for 10 min at 37°C in buffer containing 0.5 mM (^{14}C)choline and 0.25 mM concentrations of each compound. Values are the means of 6 observations and bars represent standard errors. *Significantly different from control values ($p < 0.05$) as determined by Dunnett's test.

If adenosine was not working through one of its proposed receptor mediated mechanisms, then it was possible that adenosine had an effect on the enzyme mediating the phosphorylation of choline. To test this possibility, we studied the effects of adenosine and its derivatives on CK activity. Adenosine and its analogues inhibited the activity of choline kinase with the following order of potency: 2-chloroadenosine > adenosine = 2',5'-dideoxyadenosine (Figure 5). Kinetic experiments were performed to characterize the inhibition of CK by adenosine and its analogues. When the velocity of the reaction was measured using various concentrations of choline, several concentrations of inhibitor, a single concentration of MgATP, and a saturating concentration of Mg^{2+}, all the inhibitors were shown to be noncompetitive versus choline. When the velocity of the reaction was measured using various concentrations of

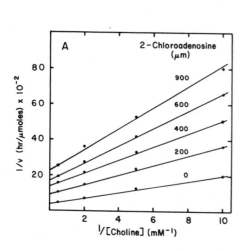
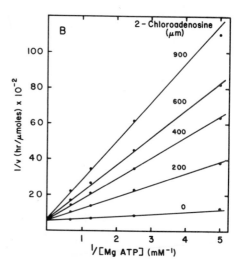

Fig. 6. Dead-end inhihibtion of CK activity by 2-chloroadenosine. Enzyme activity was measured in the particulate fraction of rat striatal synaptosomes. A, the concentrations of choline were 0.1, 0.2, 0.5, and 2 mM with concentrations of 2-chloroadenosine as shown and a single concentration of MgATP (0.8 mM) and Mg^{2+} (28 mM uncomplexed). B, the concentrations of MgATP were 0.2, 0.4, 0.8, and 1.5 mM with concentrations of 2-chloroadenosine as shown and a single concentration of choline (0.5 mM) and Mg^{2+} (28 mM uncomplexed).

MgATP, several concentrations of inhibitor, a single concentration of choline, and a saturating concentration of Mg^{2+}, all the inhibitors were shown to be competitive versus MgATP. The inhibition plots for 2-chloroadenosine are shown in Figure 6. Hence, data indicated that the effect of adenosine to decrease the levels of newly synthesized $(^{3}H)PCh$ was due to inhibition of CK activity. It is interesting to note that adenosine also inhibits cAMP dependent protein kinase from bovine skeletal muscle, another MgATP requiring enzyme (Cook et al., 1982). Varying the Ca^{2+} concentration from 0.1 to 2 mM did not alter CK activity.

CONCLUSION

CK, the enzyme that catalyzes the phosphorylation of choline, has been demonstrated to be present in both the soluble and membrane fractions isolated from rat brain synaptosomes. Membrane associated enzyme activity represents approximately 1/4 of the total activity present in the synaptosome and the membrane and soluble forms of the enzyme are indistinguishable on the basis of their ionic requirements, kinetic constants, and distribution in various brain regions.

We have shown that the level of newly synthesized (^{3}H)PCh subsequent to the transport of (^{3}H)choline into synaptosomes is decreased by both Ca^{2+} and adenosine. The effect of adenosine is not mediated by an interaction at an adenosine receptor, but rather appears to be due to inhibition of CK activity. The inhibitory effect of adenosine on choline phosphorylation may indicate a modulatory role for adenosine in rat striatum to provide more choline to support the synthesis of ACh. This would suggest a unique role for adenosine in the striatum for it has been shown that adenosine and its analogues inhibit ACh release and turnover in the hippocampus and cortex, but not in the striatum (Haubrich et al., 1981; Murray et al., 1982; Jackisch et al., 1984). Hence, data suggests that choline availability for the synthesis of ACh in rat striatum may be influenced by endogenous modulators of CK activity.

ACKNOWLEDGEMENTS

These studies were supported by a grant from the National Institute of Mental Health, DHHS #MH-33443.

REFERENCES

Ansell, G.B. and Spanner, S. (1968) The metabolism of (Me-^{14}C) choline in the brain of the rat in vivo, Biochem. J., 110:201-206.

Ansell, G.B. and Spanner, S. (1970) The origin and turnover of choline in the brain, in: "Drugs and Cholinergic Mechanisms in the CNS," E. Heilbronn and A. Winter, eds., Forsvarets Forskningsanstalt, Stockholm, Sweden, pp.143-159.

Barker, L.A. and Mittag, T.W. (1975) Comparative studies of substrates and inhibitors of choline transport and choline acetyltransferase, J. Pharmacol. Exp. Ther., 192:86-94.

Benishin, C.G. and Carroll, P.T. (1983) Multiple forms of choline-O-acetyltransferase in mouse and rat brain: Solubilization and characterization, J. Neurochem., 41:1030-1039.

Bygrave, F.L. and Dawson, R.M.C. (1976) Phosphatidylcholine biosynthesis and choline transport in the anaerobic protozoon Entodinium caudatum, Biochem. J., 160:481-490.

Collier, B. (1970) Biosynthesis of acetylcholine in vitro and in vivo, in: "Drugs and Cholinergic Mechanisms in the CNS," E. Heilbronn and A. Winter, eds., Forsvarets Forskningsanstalt, Stockholm, Sweden, pp. 163-172.

Cook, P.F., Neville, M.E.,Jr., Vrana, K.E., Hartl, T. and Roskoski,R., Jr., (1982) Adenosine cyclic 3',5'-monophosphate dependent protein kinase: Kinetic mechanism for the bovine skeletal muscle catalytic subunit, Biochem., 21:5794-5799.

Daly, J.W. (1982) Adenosine receptors: Targets for future drugs, J. Med. Chem., 25:197-207.

Dowdle, E.B. and Maske, R. (1980) The effects of calcium concentration on the inhibition of cholinergic neurotransmission in the myenteric plexus of guinea-pig ileum by adenine nucleotides, Brit. J. Pharmacol., 71:245-252.

Harms, H.H., Wardeh, G. and Mulder, A.H. (1979) Effects of adenosine on depolarization-induced release of various radiolabelled neurotransmitters from slices of rat corpus striatum, Neuropharmacol., 18:577-580.

Haubrich, D.R., Williams, M., Yarbrough, G.G. and Wood, P.L. (1981) 2-Chloroadenosine inhibits brain acetylcholine turnover in vivo, Can. J. Physiol. Pharmacol., 59:1196-1198.

Infante, J.P. (1977) Rate-limiting steps in the cytidine pathway for the synthesis of phosphatidylcholine and phosphatidylethanolamine, Biochem. J., 167:847-849.

Jackisch, R., Strittmatter, H., Kasakov, L. and Hertting, G. (1984) Endogenous adenosine as a modulator of hippocampal acetylcholine release. Naunyn-Schmiedeberg's Arch. Pharmacol., 327:319-325.

Kennedy, E.P. and Weiss, S.B. (1956) The function of cytidine coenzymes in the biosynthesis of phospholipids, J. Biol. Chem., 222:193-214.

Kuhar, M.J. and Murrin, L.C. (1978) Sodium-dependent high affinity choline uptake, J. Neurochem., 30:15-21.

Massarelli, R. and Wong, T.Y. (1981) Choline uptake in nerve cultures and in synaptosomal preparation is regulated by the endogenous pool of choline, in: Cholinergic Mechanisms. Pepeu, G. and Ladinsky, H., eds., Vol. 25, Plenum Press, New York, pp. 511-520.

McCaman, R.E. and Cook, K. (1966) Intermediary metabolism of phospholipids in brain tissue. III. Phosphocholine-glyceride transferase, J. Biol. Chem., 241:3390-3394.

Meyer, E.M., Jr., Engel, D.A. and Cooper, J.R. (1982) Acetylation and phosphorylation of choline following high or low affinity uptake by rat cortical synaptosomes, Neurochem. Res., 7:749-759.

Millington, W.R. and Wurtman, R.J. (1982) Choline administration elevates brain phosphorylcholine concentrations, J. Neurochem., 38: 1748-1752.

Murray, T.F., Blaker, W.D., Cheney, D.L. and Costa, E. (1982) Inhibition of acetylcholine turnover rate in rat hippocampus and cortex by intraventricular injection of adenosine analogs, J. Pharmacol. Exp. Ther., 222:550-554.

Pedata, F., Antonelli, T., Lambertini, L., Beani, L. and Pepeu, G. (1983) Effect of adenosine, adenosine triphosphate, adenosine deaminase, dipyridamole and aminophylline on acetylcholine release from electrically-stimulated brain slices, Neuropharmacol., 22:609-614.

Reinhardt, R.R. and Wecker, L. (1983) Evidence for membrane-associated choline kinase activity in rat striatum, J. Neurochem., 41:623-629.

Reinhardt, R.R., Wecker, L. and Cook, P.F. (1984) Kinetic mechanism of choline kinase from rat striata, J. Biol. Chem., 259:7446-7452.

Schmidt, D.E. and Wecker, L. (1981) CNS effects of choline administration: Evidence for temporal dependence, Neuropharmacol., 20:535-539.

Smith, C.P. and Carroll, P.T. (1980) A comparison of solubilized and membrane-bound forms of choline-O-acetyltransferase (EC 2.3.1.6) in mouse brain nerve endings, Brain Research, 185:363-371.

Spanner, S. and Ansell, G.B. (1978) Choline and ethanolamine kinase activity in the cytoplasm of nerve endings from rat forebrain, Adv. Exp. Med. Biol., 101:237-245.

Spanner, S. and Ansell, G.B. (1979) Choline kinase and ethanolamine kinase activity in the cytosol of nerve endings from rat forebrain, Biochem. J., 178:753-760.

Stone, T.W. (1981) Physiological roles for adenosine and adenosine 5'-triphosphate in the nervous system, Neurosci., 6:523-555.

Upreti, R.K., Sanwal, G.G. and Krishnan, P.S. (1976) Likely individuality of the enzymes catalyzing the phosphorylation of choline and ethanolamine, Arch. Biochem. Biophys., 174:658-665.

Yavin, E. (1976) Regulation of phospholipid metabolism in differentiating cells from rat brain cerebral hemispheres in culture: Patterns of acetylcholine, phosphocholine and choline phosphoglycerides labeling from (methyl-^{14}C)choline, J. Biol. Chem., 25:1392-1397.

THE MECHANISMS OF ACTION OF NOREPINEPHRINE AND ACETYLCHOLINE ON THE HEART: ROLE OF PROTEIN PHOSPHORYLATION

H. Criss Hartzell

Department of Anatomy and Cell Biology

Emory University School of Medicine, Atlanta, GA. 30322

INTRODUCTION

The heart does not beat with the same frequency or force all the time: the heartbeat is constantly regulated by various neurotransmitters and hormones. In particular, norepinephrine (NE) released from the sympathetic nervous system causes an increase in the frequency and force of contraction, whereas acetylcholine (ACh) has the opposite effects. During the past decade, our understanding of the mechanisms by which neurotransmitters produce their effects on heart has increased significantly, but at the same time it has become clear that these mechanisms are extremely complicated. The effects of NE and ACh are mediated through a variety of different effector systems including several kinds of ionic channels in the plasma membrane, the sarcoplasmic reticulum, and the contractile apparatus. The purpose of this review is to summarize how these various systems interact to regulate cardiac contraction.

Fig. 1 illustrates the effects of β-adrenergic and cholinergic agonists on contraction of the frog heart. In this experiment, a frog heart was attached to a force transducer and the heart was perfused with Ringer solution. At the first arrow, 1µM ISO was added to the perfusion solution and the force of contraction approximately doubled. At the second arrow, 1µM carbamylcholine (CCh) was added to the ISO-containing solution and the contraction declined to control levels. In addition to changing the amplitude of the contraction, ISO and CCh also altered the kinetics of the contraction (Fig. 1B). In the presence of ISO, the contraction was much more rapid than it was in the presence of CCh. In the absence of both transmitters, the waveform of the contraction was intermediate between that in ISO and in CCh.

It appears that the effects of ISO and CCh on the peak amplitude and the timecourse of the contraction are mediated by different mechanisms, because the two effects can be separated in time under certain circumstances. In Fig. 2 (left), 1 µM ISO was added to the perfusion at the arrow. The peak contractile force increased about two-fold. Coincident with the increase in peak force, the decay-time of the contraction, which is arbitrarily defined as the time it takes for the contraction to decline from the peak amplitude to 25% of the peak amplitude, increased. In contrast, when 1 µM CCh was added to the perfusion medium in the presence of 1µM ISO (Fig. 2,right), the amplitude of the contraction declined much more rapidly than the decay-time increased. Although the peak amplitude of

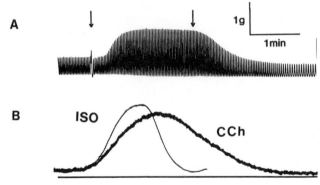

Fig. 1. Effects of isoproterenol and carbamylcholine on contraction of frog heart (<u>Xenopus laevis</u>). The heart was perfused with Ringer solution and connected to a force transducer. A. At the first arrow, 1 μM ISO was added to the perfusion medium. At the second arrow,1 μM CCh was added to the ISO-containing Ringer solution. B. Twitch tensions shown at a faster chart speed to illustrate the difference in timecourse of the contractions. The trace labelled ISO was taken ≈1 min after adding ISO. The trace labelled CCh was taken from the same heart 6 min after adding CCh. Hartzell, 1984; reprinted with permission of Rockefeller Univ. Press.

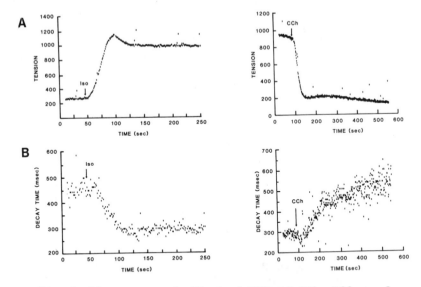

Fig. 2. Time course of effect of ISO and CCh. Effect of ISO (left) and CCh (right) on peak systolic tension (A) and decay time (B). Left panel: a spontaneously beating heart was perfused with Ringer solution for 1 hour without drugs and then 1 μM ISO was added at the arrow. Right panel: 0.5 μM CCh was added to the ISO-containing solution 3 min after beginning perfusion with ISO. Hartzell,1984; reprinted with permission of Rockefeller Univ. Press.

the contraction decreased within 60 sec to a new level, the decay-time gradually increased over several hundred seconds.

MOLECULAR MECHANISMS OF NE AND ACh ACTION

It now seems clear that at least some of the effects of NE on cardiac contraction are mediated by cAMP-dependent phosphorylation of a variety of substrate proteins. This hypothesis is supported by several lines of evidence. β-agonists stimulate adenylate cyclase both in intact cardiac cells and in sarcolemmal membranes and increase cAMP levels and cAMP-dependent protein kinase activity in cardiac cells (see reviews by Tsien, 1977; Drummond & Severson, 1979; Reuter, 1983). The effects of β-agonists can be mimicked by external application of membrane-permeable analogs of cAMP and by phosphodiesterase inhibitors. Application of cAMP also increases tension in cut-end trabeculae (Tsien & Weingart, 1976) and in skinned fibers (Fabiato & Fabiato, 1978; Winegrad, 1984). A variety of substrate proteins become phosphorylated in intact cells in response to β-agonists. These include ionic channels, phospholamban (a protein in the sarcoplasmic reticulum that regulates Ca-uptake by the sarcoplasmic reticulum), and several proteins in the contractile apparatus.

The mechanisms by which ACh regulates contraction are less well understood than the mechanisms of NE action. ACh has the ability to inhibit adenylate cyclase activity and thus reduce cAMP levels (Murad et al., 1962; Watanabe & Besch, 1975; Watanabe et al., 1978; Brown, 1979; Jakobs et al., 1979; Biegon & Pappano, 1980; Flitney & Singh, 1981; Pappano et al., 1982; Watanabe et al., 1984). However, dissociation between cAMP levels and the effects of ACh have been demonstrated in a variety of studies (Löffelholz & Pappano, 1985; Watanabe et al., 1984). For example, ACh can produce negative inotropic effects without reducing cAMP levels in guinea pig or rat ventricle (Watanabe & Besch; 1975; Keeley et al., 1976) and ACh can inhibit Ca-dependent action potentials without affecting cAMP levels in embryonic chick ventricle (Biegon & Pappano; 1980). Furthermore, ACh is able to produce inhibitory physiological effects even when cAMP levels are elevated "irreversibly" with cholera toxin, exogenous lipophilic derivatives of cAMP, or phosphodiesterase inhibitors (Biegon et al., 1980; Pappano et al., 1982; Hartzell & Titus, 1982). Thus, it has been suggested that ACh may not only inhibit adenylate cyclase but may also stimulate a protein phosphatase or inhibit a protein kinase (Hartzell & Titus, 1982; Watanabe et al., 1984; Winegrad, 1984; Löffelholz & Pappano, 1985). However, no direct or compelling evidence exists at present to support this view (Ingebretsen, 1980).

The finding that cAMP levels do not correlate well with contractile force has lead to a search for other second messenger systems for ACh. Two second messenger systems in particular have received attention: cGMP and phospholipids. cGMP levels increase in response to ACh (Gardner & Allen, 1976; 1977; George et al., 1973). Contractile force correlates extremely well with the ratio between cAMP and cGMP (Goldberg et al., 1975; Flitney & Singh, 1981). Furthermore, application of 8-bromo cGMP (Nawrath, 1977) or cGMP-containing liposomes (Bkaily & Sperelakis, 1985) to cardiac cells mimics some of the effects of ACh. However, other investigators have suggested that cGMP is not a second messenger for ACh. Brooker (1977) and Linden & Brooker (1979) have argued that cGMP levels do not correlate at all well with contractile force. Furthermore, a light-activated cGMP derivative produced no effect in frog atrium (Nargeot et al., 1983) and, unlike ACh, cGMP injected into cells first shortened and then prolonged the action potential (Trautwein et al., 1982). Since specific proteins phosphorylated by cGMP-dependent protein kinase in response to ACh have not been identified, the role of cGMP in mediating the response to ACh remains unclear.

ACh also stimulates the turnover of phospholipids in cardiac muscle (Quist, 1982; Brown & Brown, 1984; Masters et al., 1985). This results in the production of inositol trisphosphate, which is involved in calcium mobilization in other cell types, and diacylglycerol, which activates protein kinase-C (see reviews by Nishizuka, 1984; Berridge & Irvine, 1984),but there is no direct evidence that either inositol trisphosphate or diacylglycerol are involved in mediating the effects of ACh.

REGULATION OF CONTRACTILE FORCE

Ca-influx

In principle, the amplitude of the contraction is determined by the concentration of intracellular calcium and by the sensitivity of the contractile apparatus to Ca. In the frog heart, virtually all of the Ca which activates the contractile apparatus enters the cell from the extracellular space through sarcolemmal Ca channels (Morad et al., 1983). In mammalian heart, additional Ca is released from the sarcoplasmic reticulum. In both amphibian and mammalian species, however, the amplitude of the contraction correlates well with the amplitude of the slow inward calcium current (I_{Ca}) (Trautwein et al., 1975; Ouedraogo et al., 1982).

It is well established that β-adrenergic stimulation increases I_{Ca} in both mammalian (Reuter, 1974; Reuter & Scholz; 1977; Pappano & Carmeliet, 1979; Kass & Wiegers, 1982; Noma et al., 1980) and amphibian myocardium (Vassort et al., 1969; Brown et al., 1975; Morad et al., 1981). Although the effect of ACh alone on basal I_{Ca} may depend upon experimental conditions and the preparation, ACh is able to decrease I_{Ca} which has been elevated by catecholamines in both ventricular and atrial muscle (Inui & Imamura, 1977; Prokopczuk et al., 1973; Giles & Noble, 1976; Ikemoto & Goto, 1977; Ten Eick et al., 1977; Garnier et al., 1978; Nargeot & Garnier, 1982; Hino & Ochi, 1980; Josephson & Sperelakis, 1982; Inoue et al.,1983; Fischmeister & Hartzell, 1986).

Although ACh decreases I_{Ca} in atrial tissue, it is unclear whether this is a direct effect of ACh. In atrium, ACh can increase a time-dependent K conductance in addition to decreasing I_{Ca} (Prokopczuk et al., 1973; Giles & Noble, 1976; Ikemoto & Goto, 1977; Ten Eick et al., 1977; Garnier et al., 1978; Nargeot & Garnier, 1982). Recently, Iijima et al., (1985) have suggested that the apparent effect of ACh on I_{Ca} in mammalian atrium (in the absence of exogenous catecholamines) is due to an artifact caused by contamination of I_{Ca} by the time-dependent ACh-activated K current. It is clear, however, that the effect of ACh on catecholamine-stimulated I_{Ca} in both atrium and ventricle of amphibians is a direct effect, because I_{Ca} is decreased by ACh in cells in which K currents have been blocked by intracellular and extracellular Cs (Fischmeister & Hartzell, 1986; and unpublished).

The increase in I_{Ca} produced by NE has been shown to be due to an increase in the probability of opening of the Ca channel and also the number of calcium channels available for activation by voltage (Bean et al., 1984; Cachelin et al., 1983; Brum et al., 1984; Kamayama et al., 1985). The conductance of the channel, however, does not seem to be affected by NE. The effects of ACh on Ca channel kinetics have not yet been thoroughly examined.

Another mechanism that regulates Ca influx is the period of time over which Ca channels are activated. This is determined by the kinetics of Ca channel inactivation as well as the duration of the action potential, which depends upon the K currents which repolarize the membrane. Fischmeister & Hartzell (1986) have recently shown that inactivation of I_{Ca} is unaffected and the kinetics of I_{Ca} reactivation are affected less than 20% by ACh and isoproterenol. In most species, ACh increases K conductance in both atrium and ventricle and thus produces a shortening of the action potential (but see Inoue et al, 1985).

Role of cAMP in regulating ICa

From several lines of evidence, it is now well established that the effects of β-agonists on I_{Ca} are mediated by cAMP-dependent protein phosphorylation. I_{Ca} is increased by external application of cAMP, its analogues or phosphodiesterase inhibitors (Tsien et al., 1972; Tsien, 1973; Reuter, 1974; Morad et al., 1981; Cachelin et al., 1983) and by intracellular application of cAMP or cAMP-dependent protein kinase (Tsein, 1973; Tsien & Weingart, 1976; Vogel & Sperelakis, 1981; Trautwein et al., 1982; Osterrieder et al., 1982; Brum et al., 1983; Brum et al., 1984; Kamayama et al., 1985; Fischmeister & Hartzell, 1986). It has been suggested that cAMP dependent protein kinase activates calcium channels by phosphorylation of either the Ca channel itself or a protein that regulates the Ca channel (Rinaldi et al., 1981; Rinaldi et al., 1982; Manalan & Jones, 1982; Flockerzi et al., 1983; Horne et al., 1984).

It appears that the effects of ACh on I_{Ca} can be completely explained by an inhibitory effect of ACh on adenylate cyclase activity because ACh is incapable of reducing I_{Ca} elevated by intracellularly applied cAMP (Fischmeister & Hartzell, 1986) even though it has been reported that other effects of cAMP can be reduced by ACh (Hartzell & Titus, 1982; Löffelholz & Pappano, 1985; Watanabe et al., 1984).

Sarcoplasmic Reticulum

Although the effects of NE and ACh on contractile force in amphibians can be explained by their effects on membrane currents, in mammals these neurotransmitters also produce effects on Ca release and storage by the sarcoplasmic reticulum. In frog heart, the majority of the Ca which is responsible for activation of the contractile apparatus originates from the extracellular space and enters through the sarcolemma. In mammal, however, additional calcium is released from the sarcoplasmic reticulum and NE increases the amount of calcium released from these intracellular stores. The reason for this increased release is not fully understood, although it is known that NE causes an increased uptake of Ca into the SR as the result of cAMP-dependent phosphorylation of phospholamban. Phospholamban, which is phosphorylated in vivo in response to β-adrenergic stimulation (Kranias & Solaro, 1982; Lindemann et al., 1983, 1985) and in vitro by cAMP-dependent protein kinase (Kirchberger et al., 1972; Wray et al., 1973; LaRaia & Morkin, 1974; Tada et al., 1975), regulates Ca uptake by the sarcoplasmic reticulum (Kirchberger et al., 1974; Katz et al., 1975; Schwartz et al., 1976; Wray & Gray, 1977; Katz, 1979). Thus, NE increases the store of Ca in the SR and this may be directly related to the amount of Ca released.

Contractile Proteins

Although the idea that ACh and NE may regulate contractile force by producing effects on contractile proteins has received considerable attention (Stull, 1980; Winegrad, 1984), at present phosphorylation of contractile proteins seem to be related to the kinetics of the contraction and not to contractile force itself.

KINETICS OF THE CONTRACTION

Relaxation of the heart is mediated by several different processes. First, influx of Ca is terminated by repolarization of the membrane and by inactivation of Ca channels. Intracellular Ca concentration is then reduced (1) by sequestration of Ca by the sarcoplasmic reticulum and (2) by Ca extrusion into the extracellular space by sodium-calcium exchange and by ATP-dependent Ca pumping. As intracellular Ca declines, Ca dissociates from troponin and the interaction between actin and myosin is terminated and the muscle relaxes. As noted above, NE and ACh produce very marked effects on the kinetics of the contraction: the contraction is faster in the presence of NE. This "relaxant effect" of NE is related to several different effects of NE.

As discussed above, NE stimulates phosphorylation of phospholamban in the sarcoplasmic reticulum. This causes an increase in the affinity and the turnover of the Ca pump in the sarcoplasmic reticulum in mammalian muscle and results in a more rapid uptake of calcium after a contraction. In amphibian muscle, where the sarcoplasmic reticulum is not well developed, however, it seems unlikely that increased pumping by the sarcoplasmic reticulum plays an important role in relaxation.

NE also produces in a change in the sensitivity of the contractile apparatus to Ca which seems to be related to troponin phosphorylation. Troponin-I is phosphorylated in vivo in response to β-adrenergic stimulation (England, 1975, 1976, 1977; Solaro et al., 1976; Stull, 1980) and in vitro by cAMP dependent protein kinase (Reddy et al., 1973; Cole & Perry, 1975; Ray & England, 1976; Stull & Buss, 1977; Blumenthal et al., 1978). Troponin-I phosphorylation is likely to be involved in regulating the calcium sensitivity of the contractile apparatus because the affinity of troponin-C for calcium is decreased and rate of dissociation of Ca from troponin-C is increased when troponin-I is phosphorylated (Ray & England, 1976; Reddy & Wyborny, 1976; Bailin, 1979; Holroyde et al., 1979; McClellan & Winegrad, 1980; Mope et al., 1980; Herzig et al., 1981; Stull, 1980; Robertson et al. 1982). This decreased sensitivity of the contractile apparatus for Ca is thought to be involved in mediating the increased relaxation produced by β-adrenergic stimulation.

Recently, it has been found that C-protein, which is a component of the myosin thick filament (Offer, 1972; Offer et al., 1973), is phosphorylated in a cAMP-dependent manner in cardiac muscle exposed to β-adrenergic agonists (Jeacocke & England, 1980; Hartzell & Titus, 1982; England, 1983; Hartzell 1984). C-protein purified from cardiac muscle is phosphorylated at 3 - 5 sites by purified cAMP-dependent protein kinase (Hartzell & Glass, 1984; Lim & Walsh, 1985). Although the function of C-protein remains obscure, we have shown that the level of C-protein phosphorylation correlates with the rate at which cardiac muscle relaxes after a twitch (Hartzell, 1984). We have proposed that C-protein is involved in regulating twitch relaxation in cardiac muscle by modulating actin-myosin interaction.

The remainder of this review will summarize our data suggesting that C-protein, in addition to the calcium channel, phospholamban, and troponin, may play a role in regulating cardiac contraction.

PHOSPHORYLATION AND DEPHOSPHORYLATION OF C-PROTEIN

In our initial experiments, we simply asked the question: "what proteins are reversibly phosphorylated in frog heart in response to β-adrenergic agonists and acetylcholine?" Hearts were perfused with ^{32}P, rinsed, and then perfused with solution containing ISO, ACh, or a combination of the two. After various periods of time, the hearts were frozen by clamping them with clamps cooled with liquid nitrogen. The frozen hearts were homogenized in a buffer that inhibited protein kinase and protein phosphatase activity and the radioactive proteins were identified by SDS-polyacrylamide gel electrophoresis and quantitative autoradiography. In addition, since changes in ^{32}P incorporation into proteins could also be caused by changes in specific activity of the ATP pool, we measured the specific activity of the cellular ATP pools and corrected the radioactivity of the proteins for the specific activity of the ATP pool.

Fig. 3 shows the results of a typical experiment. We found that ISO stimulated ^{32}P incorporation into a protein with a molecular weight of 165,000, whereas ACh decreased the ^{32}P incorporation that was stimulated by ISO. The 165,000 dalton protein was identified as C-protein by immunological criteria. Antibodies prepared against the 165,000 protein from frog heart cross-reacted with purified C-protein from rabbit heart and stained the "C-protein" region of the sarcomere (Hartzell & Titus, 1982).

Although relatively little is known about cardiac muscle C-protein, C-protein from skeletal muscle has been studied extensively by Moos & colleagues. C-protein is a component of the thick filament of striated muscles (Offer et al., 1973; Yamamoto & Moos, 1983) and is located in the middle third of each half of the A-band (Craig & Offer, 1976; Dennis et al., 1984; Offer, 1972; Pepe & Drucker, 1975; Rome et al., 1973). It has been suggested that C-protein may regulate thick filament assembly and length (Koretz et al., 1982; Squire, 1981), participate in thick filament structure (Offer et al., 1973; Pepe & Drucker, 1975), or regulate cross-bridge movement during contraction. In addition, C-protein has a number of properties that suggest it might play a role in regulation of contractile activity. C-protein binds to both actin (Moos et al., 1978) and myosin (Moos et al., 1975; Starr & Offer, 1978) and can affect the ability of actin to activate myosin ATPase (Moos & Feng, 1980; Moos et al., 1978, Offer et al., 1973; Yamamoto & Moos, 1983). It has been suggested that the physiological mechanism of C-protein action may involve a calcium-regulated binding of C-protein to thin filaments, because C-protein binding to the sarcomere occurs only in the presence of micromolar concentrations of calcium (Moos, 1981).

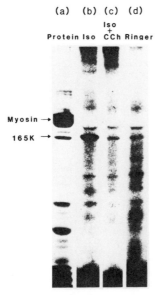

Fig. 3. Effects of ISO and CCh on ^{32}P incorporation into intact frog atria. (a). Coomassie-blue stained gel. (b) to (d). Autoradiograms of SDS gels. Intact atria were incubated in Ringer solution containing 100 μCi/ml ^{32}P for 3 hrs, rinsed, and exposed to 10 μM ISO for 5 min (b), 10 μM ISO for 5 min followed by 10 μM ISO and 10 μM CCh for 15 min (c) or Ringer solution for 5 min (d). Reprinted from Hartzell & Titus (1982).

Our first hypothesis was that the phosphorylation of C-protein was related to the peak force of the contraction. However, several experiments demonstrated that this hypothesis was not correct (Fig. 4). Although ^{32}P incorporation into C-protein occurred very rapidly and paralleled the timecourse of increase in tension in response to ISO, the dephosphorylation was much slower than the decrease in tension in response

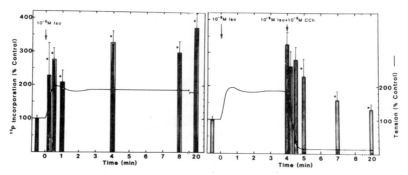

Fig. 4. Timecourse of effects of ISO and CCh on tension and ^{32}P incorporation into C-protein. Left panel: atria were preincubated in ^{32}P and exposed to 10 μM ISO for the times shown. Right panel: 10 μM CCh was added after 4 min exposure to ISO. Stippled bars are relative ^{32}P incorporation into C-protein expressed as a percentage of ^{32}P incorporation in Ringer solution. Solid line is tension measured from a typical atrium. Error bars are ± 1 standard error. Reprinted from Hartzell & Titus (1982).

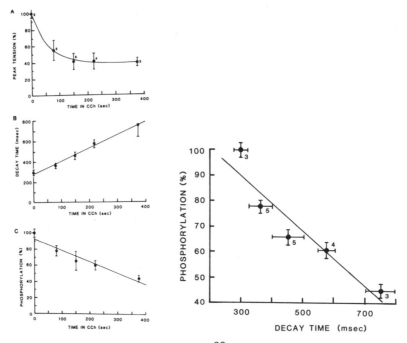

Fig. 5. Correlation between ^{32}P incorporation into C-protein and decay time. Frog ventricles were perfused with ^{32}P, rinsed, and exposed to 1 μM ISO for 4 min. At zero-time, 0.5 μM CCh was added to the perfusion medium. A. Peak systolic tension as a percentage of the peak tension in 1 μM ISO. B. Decay time. C. ^{32}P incorporation into C-protein as a percentage of the incorporation after 4 min exposure to ISO alone. The right portion of the figure shows the correlation between decay time and ^{32}P incorporation into C-protein. Hartzell, 1984; reprinted with permission of Rockefeller Univ. Press.

to CCh. However, we found that the timecourse of dephosphorylation of C-protein paralleled the slowing of relaxation produced by CCh (Fig. 5). The correlation between decay time and ^{32}P incorporation into C-protein was very good.

From many experiments of this type we proposed the working hypothesis that C-protein phosphorylation is involved in regulation of relaxation of the cardiac contraction. One can think of several different mechanisms by which this could occur. One possibility is that phosphorylated C-protein could inhibit actin-myosin interaction at the end of a contraction and thus speed relaxation, while dephosphorylated C-protein would be inactive. The opposite possibility is that dephosphorylated C-protein slows down relaxation and that phosphorylated C-protein is inactive. Regardless of the exact mechanism, our hypothesis predicted that C-protein should have an effect on actin-activated myosin ATPase and that phosphorylated and dephosphorylated states of C-protein should act differently.

In order to test this prediction, we set about to purify C-protein from cardiac muscle and to determine its effect on reconstituted actin-myosin systems. For these experiments (Hartzell & Glass, 1985; Hartzell, in press) we have used chicken heart C-protein.

C-protein purified from detergent-washed cardiac myofibrils was found to be a protein of molecular weight 155,000 composed of a single polypeptide. Hydrodynamic measurements and electron microscopy have shown that the protein is an asymmetric molecule with the predominant form being V-shaped with each arm of the V being about 20 nm in length (Fig. 6) (Hartzell & Sale, 1985).

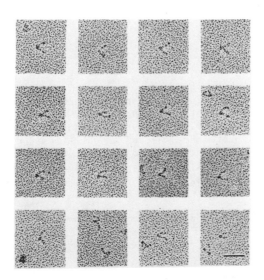

Fig. 6. Selected C-protein particles viewed by rotary shadowing of purified cardiac C-protein. Calibration: 50 nm. Hartzell & Sale, 1986; reprinted with permission of Rockefeller Univ. Press.

PHOSPHORYLATION OF PURIFIED C-PROTEIN

We first wanted to characterize C-protein phosphorylation by purified protein kinases and determine the number of phosphorylation sites. Purified C-protein contained an average of 0.2 mole of phosphate per mole

of C-protein (Hartzell & Glass, 1985). Up to 2.5 moles of phosphate were
incorporated into C-protein by purified catalytic subunit of cAMP-
dependent protein kinase (Hartzell & Glass, 1985; Fig. 7). This suggested
that C-protein contained 3 phosphorylation sites. In order to examine
further the number of phosphorylation sites, we digested C-protein with
trypsin or chymotrypsin and subjected the digests to peptide mapping by
high pressure liquid chromatography. Although we generally found more than
3 phosphopeptides (Fig. 8), the results were consistent with 3 to 5 sites
being phosphorylated by cAMP-dependent protein kinase. C-protein was also
phosphorylated by a calcium-calmodulin dependent protein kinase and cGMP
dependent protein kinase. The sites phosphorylated by these kinases seemed
to be the same as those phosphorylated by cAMP-dependent protein kinase,
since phosphorylation by the different protein kinases was not additive.

C-protein was an excellent substrate for cAMP-dependent protein
kinase. The kinetic constants for C-protein phosphorylation by cAMP-
dependent protein kinase are shown in Fig. 9. The K_m of 4 µM was well
within the physiological concentration of C-protein in the cell and the
V_{max} of 19 µmol/min/mg was one of the highest velocities that has been
reported for a substrate of cAMP-dependent protein kinase.

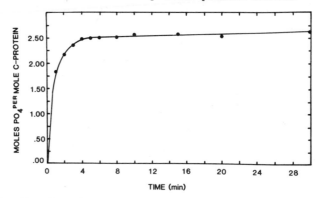

Fig. 7. Stoichiometry of phosphorylation of C-protein
by cAMP-dependent protein kinase. C-protein (13.4 µM)
was incubated with catalytic subunit (2 µg/ml) at
30°C. Aliquots were removed at the times indicated and
the amount of incorporated phosphate was determined by
a phosphocellulose paper assay. Reprinted from
Hartzell & Glass (1984).

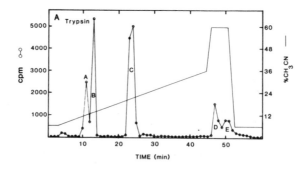

Fig. 8. Peptide mapping of C-protein. ^{32}P-labelled C-
protein was digested with trypsin and the
phosphopeptides analyzed by high pressure liquid
chromatography. Reprinted from Hartzell & Glass
(1984).

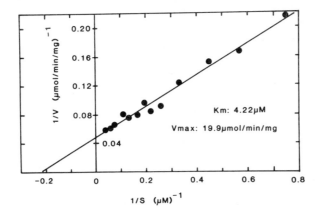

Fig. 9. Kinetics of phosphorylation of C-protein by catalytic subunit of cAMP-dependent protein kinase. C-protein (1.9 to 52 μM) was incubated with 0.12 μg/ml catalytic subunit and ^{32}P-ATP for 1 min. Reprinted from Hartzell & Glass (1984).

EFFECTS OF C-PROTEIN ON MYOSIN ATPase

Having purified C-protein in the unphosphorylated (0.2 mol phosphate per mol C-protein) and phosphorylated (2.5 to 2.9 mol/mol) forms, we were then able to examine the effects of C-protein on myosin ATPase activities. We purified myosin and actin from chicken heart by standard methods. The proteins were homogeneous by SDS-polyacrylamide gel electrophoresis (Fig. 10).

At the low ionic strengths which are necessary for activation of myosin ATPase by actin, myosin precipitates. The formation of these

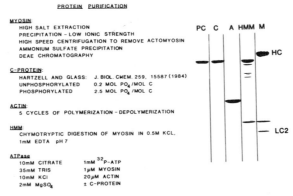

Fig. 10. Purification of proteins for ATPase experiments. Left panel: summary of protein purification procedures used. Right panel: SDS-polyacrylamide gels of purified proteins. PC: phosphorylated C-protein. C: unphosphorylated C-protein. A: actin. M: myosin. HMM: heavy meromyosin. HC: myosin heavy chain. LC2: myosin light chain.

aggregates complicates the determination of kinetic constants. This problem is often circumvented by use of proteolytic subfragments of myosin (i.e., heavy meromyosin or subfragment-1). However, we did not want to use myosin subfragments because we did not know to which region of myosin C-protein might bind. For this reason, we chose to measure ATPase activity of myosin minifilaments (Reisler et al., 1980). Minifilaments are myosin filaments composed of ∿18 myosin molecules, which do not precipitate upon addition of actin and are much more suitable for kinetic studies.

Minifilaments in the absence of actin had a very low ATPase activity and C-protein had no effect on this ATPase activity. In the presence of actin, the ATPase activity was increased 20 - 100 fold. C-protein stimulated this actin-activated ATPase activity several-fold. The maximum effect of C-protein was observed with equimolar ratios of C-protein and myosin (Fig. 11). Phosphorylated C-protein also stimulated ATPase activity but to a lesser extent than unphosphorylated C-protein (Hartzell, 1985).

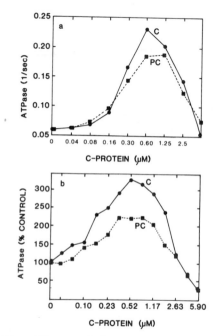

Fig. 11. The effect of C-protein on actin-activated myosin ATPase activity of myosin minifilaments. Minifilaments were pre-incubated with unphosphorylated (circles) or phosphorylated (squares) C-protein at 4°C. The ATPase reaction was initiated by addition of ATP and actin. [Actin] = 5 μM; [Myosin] = 0.85 μM. ATPase activity in the absence of actin was subtracted from the activity in the presence of actin to give the myosin. (b). Another experiment. ATPase activity is expressed as % activity in absence of C-protein. Reprinted from Hartzell (1985).

In order to gain insight into the mechanism by which C-protein stimulated the actin-activated ATPase activities of myosin filaments, ATPase activity was measured as a function of actin concentration in the presence and absence of 1 μM C-protein (Fig. 12). The solid lines are the best fit lines to the data using the Michaelis-Menten equation. The effect of C-protein was to increase the V_{max} of the ATPase reaction to 250% of control and to increase the affinity of myosin for actin 44%. The differences between the kinetic parameters in the presence and absence of C-protein were statistically significant at 1%.

These kinetic data demonstrated that C-protein increased the velocity of the actin-activated ATPase and the affinity of actin for myosin. Since the myosin was in a filamentous form, it seemed possible that C-protein altered the structure of the myosin filaments and increased the number of myosin heads available for interaction with actin. In order to test this possibility, the effect of C-protein on acto-HMM ATPase activity was examined. I reasoned that if C - protein produced its effects on actin-

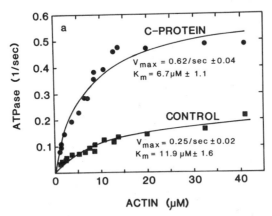

Fig. 12. Kinetic parameters of actin-activated ATPase. Actin-activated minifilament ATPase was measured in the absence (squares) or the presence (circles) of 1 μM unphosphorylated C-protein. [Myosin] = 1.17 μM. Reprinted from Hartzell (1985).

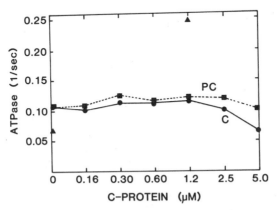

Fig. 13. Effect of C-protein on actin-activated ATPase of HMM. ATPase activity was measured as a function of unphosphorylated (circles) and phosphorylated (squares) C-protein. [Actin] = 5 μM, [myosin] = 1.12 μM. In the same experiment, the ATPase activity of minifilaments was also measured (triangles). Reprinted from Hartzell (1985).

activated myosin ATPase activity by producing changes in filament structure, C-protein would not affect the actin-activated ATPase activity of soluble, non-filamentous HMM. In these experiments, the ATPase assays were performed in buffer of exactly the same composition as used for the minifilament ATPase assays. The actin-activated HMM ATPase activity in the absence of C-protein was only slightly higher than that of the same concentration of minifilaments in the absence of C-protein in the same experiment. C-protein, whether in the phosphorylated or dephosphorylated forms, however, had no effect on ATPase activity, except at high concentrations of C-protein where an inhibition was noted (Fig. 13).

These data were consistent with the hypothesis that the stimulatory effect of C-protein either required myosin in a filamentous form or required a portion of the light meromyosin segment of the myosin molecule in order to exert its effect. There was also another interesting possibility. The HMM that we used for our experiments contained myosin light chain-2 that was partly degraded. The possibility that C-protein action on myosin ATPase activity requires light chain-2 has been suggested by Margossian & Slayter (1985).

LIGHT SCATTERING

To examine the effect of C-protein on the structure of myosin filaments, we examined the absorbance at 350 nm of minifilaments in the presence and absence of C-protein. The data below are consistent with the suggestion that C-protein produces a structural change in myosin filaments that results in a change in actin-myosin interaction.

Minifilaments alone had a very low A_{350}, usually less than 0.05 (Fig. 14). 1 µM C-protein by itself had an A_{350} of <0.01. Addition of increasing amounts of C-protein to minifilaments caused abrupt, but small, increases

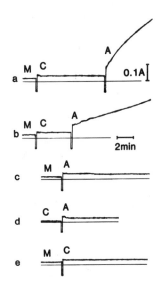

Fig. 14. Effect of C-protein on actin and myosin light-scattering. Light scattering was measured by absorbance (A) at 350 nm. M: myosin, A: actin, C: C-protein, PC: phosphorylated C-protein. Reprinted from Hartzell (1985).

in light scattering. The increase in light scattering was distinctly greater than the sum of the light scattering of the individual components. C-protein had no effect on light scattering of actin solutions.

Addition of actin to minifilaments in the absence of C-protein caused an abrupt increase in light scattering that was very close to the sum of the light scattering of the separate actin and minifilament solutions (Fig. 14c). The level of light scattering of the acto-minifilaments was stable and there was no precipitation of the actomyosin as long as ATP was present (for at least 10 min) (Fig. 14c). When actin was added to minifilaments that had been pre-incubated in the presence of unphosphorylated C-protein, however, a different result was obtained. Even in the presence of 1 mM ATP, light scattering increased with time after addition of actin (Fig. 14b). The increase in light scattering was accompanied by visible turbidity in the cuvette and, after 10 minutes, formation of an actomyosin precipitate.

The rate of increase in light scattering was dependent upon the time of preincubation of the minifilaments with C-protein. The rate of light scattering increase was distinctly slower if C-protein was incubated with minifilaments for only 4 min, rather than 8 min, before addition of actin (Fig. 14 a & b).

The rate of increase in light scattering produced by unphosphorylated C-protein was greater than the rate produced by phosphorylated C-protein (Fig. 15). Regardless whether the minifilaments were preincubated with C-protein for 2 min (Fig. 15, a & b) or >8 min (not shown), the increase in light scattering was less with phosphorylated C-protein than with unphosphorylated C-protein. These results suggested that C-protein was stimulating the formation of aggregates of actin and myosin and that unphosphorylated C-protein was more effective than phosphorylated C-protein in producing this aggregation.

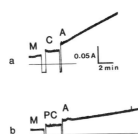

Fig. 15. The effect of phosphorylated and unphosphorylated C-protein on light scattering of minifilaments. Reprinted from Hartzell (1985).

ROLE OF C-PROTEIN IN REGULATING CARDIAC CONTRACTION

The biochemical experiments with C-protein are difficult to relate directly to the experiments with intact cells. However, it seems clear that C-protein is phosphorylated reversibly in intact cells in response to neural transmitters and that C-protein has effects on the interaction between actin and myosin. How the effect of C-protein on actin-myosin interaction is translated into changes in relaxation is unclear. There are several testable hypotheses that can be offered, however. Our data suggest that when C-protein is unphosphorylated, it stimulates the interaction of actin and myosin more than when C-protein is phosphorylated. This increased interaction could be responsible for the slowed relaxation of the heart when the heart is exposed to ACh. Alternatively, the increased interaction of actin and myosin could be secondary to other structural changes that are caused by C-protein and that these structural changes would be responsible for mediating cardiac relaxation.

SUMMARY

From this brief review, it should be obvious that regulation of the heartbeat by neurotransmitters is an extremely complicated process that involves the interaction between membrane conductances, calcium buffering systems, and the contractile apparatus. At the present time, it appears that changes in the sarcolemmal calcium current are largely responsible for changes in contractile force, whereas changes in calcium sequestration and phosphorylation of proteins in the contractile apparatus are responsible for changes in the time course of the contraction.

ACKNOWLEDGEMENTS

I would like to thank all my colleagues at Emory University and at the University of Paris, Orsay, for their stimulating conversations and for providing many of the ideas in this review. In particular, I thank the colleagues who have collaborated with me on these studies: Mark Simmons, Tony Creazzo, Rodolphe Fischmeister, David Glass, Winfield Sale, Louisa Titus, and Edward King, and Winifred Scherer for help with the manuscript.

REFERENCES

Bailin, G. (1979). Am J. Physiol. 236, C41-C46.
Bean, B.P., Nowycky, M.C. & Tsien, R.W. (1984). Nature 307, 371-375.
Berridge, M. & Irvine, R. (1984). Nature 312, 315-321.
Biegon, R.L., Epstein, P.M. & Pappano, A.J. (1980). J. Pharmac. Exp. Ther. 215, 348-356.
Biegon, R.L. & Pappano, A.J. (1980). Circ. Res. 46, 353-362.
Bkaily, G. & Sperelakis, N. (1985). Am. J. Physiol. 248, H745-H749.
Blumenthal, D.K., Stull, J.T. & Gill, G.N. (1978). J. Biol. Chem. 253, 334-336.
Brooker, G. (1977). J. Cyclic Nucleotide Res. 3, 407-413.
Brown, J.H. & Brown, S.L. (1984). J. Biol. Chem. 259, 3777-3781.
Brown, H.F., McNaughton, P.A., Noble, D. & Noble, S. (1975). Phil. Trans. R. Soc. B270, 527-537.
Brown, J.H. (1979). J. Cyclic Nucleotide Res. 5, 423-433.
Brum, G., Flockerzi, V., Hofmann, F., Osterrieder, W. & Trautwein, W. (1983). Pflügers Arch. 398, 147-154.
Brum, G., Osterrieder, W. & Trautwein, W. (1984). Pflügers Arch. 401, 111-118.
Cachelin, A.B., de Peyer, J.E., Kokubun, S. & Reuter, H. (1983). Nature 304, 462-464.

Cole, H.A. & Perry, S.V. (1975). Biochem. J. 149, 525-533.

Craig, R. & Offer, G. (1976). Proc. R. Soc. Lond.B 192, 451-461.

Dennis, J.E., Shimizu, T., Reinach, F.C. & Fischman, D.A. (1984). J. Cell Biol. 98, 1514-1522.

Drummond, G.I. & Severson, D.L. (1979). Circ. Res. 44, 145-153.

England, P.J. (1975). FEBS Lett. 50, 57-60.

England, P.J. (1976). Biochem. J. 160, 295-304.

England, P.J. (1977). Biochem. J. 168, 307-310.

England, P.J. (1983). Phil. Trans. R. Soc. Lond. B 302, 83-90.

Fabiato, A. & Fabiato, F. (1978). Ann. N.Y. Acad. Sci. 307, 491-522.

Flockerzi, V., Mewes, R., Ruth, P. & Hofman, F. (1983). Eur. J. Biochem. 135, 131-142.

Flitney, F.W. & Singh, J. (1981). J. Mol. Cell. Cardiol. 13, 963-979.

Gardner, R.M. & Allen, D.O. (1976). J. Pharmac. Exp. Ther. 198, 412-419.

Gardner, R.M. & Allen, D.O. (1977). J. Pharmac. Exp. Ther. 202, 346-353.

Garnier, D., Nargeot, J., Ojeda, C. & Rougier, O. (1978). J. Physiol. 274, 381-396.

George, W.J., Wilkerson, R.D. & Kadowitz, P.J. (1973). J. Pharmac. Exp. Ther. 184, 228-235.

Giles, W. & Noble, S. (1976). J. Physiol. 261, 103-123.

Goldberg, N.C., Haddox, M.R., Nicol, S.E., Glass, D.B., Sandford, C.H., Kuehl, F.A. & Estensen, R. (1975). Adv. Cyclic Nucleotide Res. 5, 307-330.

Hartzell, H.C. & Titus, L. (1982). J. Biol. Chem. 257, 2111-2120.

Hartzell, H.C. (1984). J. Gen. Physiol. 83, 563-588.

Hartzell,H.C. & Glass,D.B. (1984). J. Biol. Chem. 259, 15587-15596.

Hartzell, H.C. & Sale, W.S. (1985). J. Cell Biol. 100, 208-215.

Hartzell, H.C. (1985). J. Mol. Biol. 185, 185-195.

Hartzell, H.C. & Fischmeister, R. (1986). J. Physiol. in press.

Herzig, J.W., Kohler, G., Pfizer, G., Ruegg, J.C. & Wolfe, G. (1981). Pflügers Archiv. 391, 208-212.

Hino, N. & Ochi, R. (1980). J. Physiol. 307, 183-197.

Holroyde, M.J., Howe, E. & Solaro, R.J. (1979). Biochim. Biophys. Acta 586, 63-69.

Horne, P., Triggle, D.J. & Venter, J.C. (1984). Biochim. Biophys. Res. Commun. 121, 890-898.

Iijima, T., Irisawa, H. & Kameyama, M. (1985). J. Physiol. 359, 485-501.

Ikemoto, Y. & Goto, M. (1977). J. Mol. Cell. Cardiol. 9, 313-326.

Ingebretsen, C.G. (1980). J. Cyclic Nucleotide Res. 6, 121-132.

Inoue, D., Hachisu, M. & Pappano, A.J. (1983). Circ. Res. 53, 158-167.

Inui, J. & Imamura, H. (1977). Naunyn-Schmiedeberg's Arch. Pharmacol. 299, 1-7.

Jakobs, K.H., Aktories, K. & Schultz, G. (1979). Naunyn-Schmiedeberg's Arch. Pharmacol. 310, 113-119.

Jeacocke, S.A. & England, P.J. (1980). FEBS Lett. 122, 129-132.

Josephson, I. & Sperelakis, N. (1982). J. Gen. Physiol. 79, 69-86.

Kamayama, M., Hoffman, F. & Trautwein, W. (1985). Pflügers Archiv. 405, 285-293.

Kass, R.A. & Wiegers, S.E. (1982). J. Physiol. 322, 541-558.

Katz, A.M., Tada, M. & Kirchberger, M.A. (1975). Adv. Cyclic Nucleotide Res. 5, 453-472.

Katz, A.M. (1979). Adv. Cyclic Nucleotide Res. 11, 303-343.

Keeley, S.L., Lincoln, T.M. & Corbin, J.D. (1978). Am. J. Physiol. 234, H432-H438.

Kirchberger, M.A., Tada, M., Repke, D.I. & Katz, A.M. (1972). J. Mol. Cell. Cardiol. 4, 673-680.

Kirchberger, M.A., Tada, M. & Katz, A.M. (1974). J. Biol. Chem. 249, 6166-6173.

Koretz, J.F. (1979). Biophys. J. 27, 433-446.

Kranias, E.G. & Solaro, R.J. (1982). Nature, Lond. 298, 182-184.

LaRaia, P.J. & Morkin, E. (1974). Circ. Res. 35, 298-306.

Lim, M.S. & Walsh, M.P. (1985). Biophys. J. 47, 471a.

Lindemann, J.P., Jones, L.R., Hathaway, D.R., Henry, B.G. & Watanabe, A.M. (1983). J. Biol. Chem. 258, 464-471.

Lindemann, J.P. & Watanabe, A.M. (1985). J. Biol. Chem. 260, 4516- 4525.

Linden, J. & Brooker, G. (1979). Biochem. Pharmacol. 28, 3351-3360.

Löffelholz, K. & Pappano, A.J. (1985). Pharmacol. Rev. 37, 1-24.

Manalan, A.S. & Jones, L.R. (1982). J. Biol. Chem. 257, 10052-10062.

Margossian, S.S. & Slayter, H.S. (1985). Biophys. J. 47, 309a.

Masters, S.B., Martin, M.W., Harden, T.K. & Brown, J.H. (1985). Biochem. J. 227, in press.

McClellan, G.B. & Winegrad, S. (1980). J. Gen. Physiol. 75, 283-295.

Moos, C., Offer, G., Starr, R. & Bennett, P. (1975). J. Mol. Biol. 97, 1-9.

Moos, C., Mason, C.M., Besterman, J.M., Feng, I.M., & Dubin, J.H. (1978). J. Mol. Biol. 124, 571-586.

Moos, C. & Feng, I.M. (1980). Biochim. Biophys. Acta 632, 141-149.

Moos, C. (1981). J. Cell Biol. 90, 25-31.

Mope, L., McClellan, G.B. & Winegrad, S. (1980). J. Gen. Physiol. 75, 271-282.

Morad, M., Sander, C. & Weiss, J. (1981). J. Physiol. 311, 585-604.

Morad, M., Goldman, Y.E. & Trentham, D.R. (1983). Nature 304, 635-638.

Murad, F., Chi, Y.M., Rall, T.W. & Sutherland, E. (1962). J. Biol. Chem. 237, 1233-1238.

Nargeot, J. & Garnier, D. (1982). J. Pharmacol. (Paris). 13, 431-445.

Nargeot, J., Nerbonne, J.M., Engels, J. & Lester, H. (1983). Proc. Natl. Acad. Sci. USA. 80, 2395-2399.

Nawrath, H. (1977). Nature 267, 72-74.

Nilius, B., Hess, P., Lansman, J.B. & Tsien, R.W. (1985). Nature 316, 443-446.

Nishizuka, Y. (1984). Nature 308, 693-698.

Noma, A. Kotake, H. & Irisawa, H. (1980). Pflügers Archiv. 388, 1-9.

Offer, G. (1972). Cold Spring Harb. Symp. Quant. Biol. 37, 87-95.

Offer, G., Moos, C. & Starr, R. (1973). J. Mol. Biol. 6, 653-675.

Osterrieder, W.G., Brum, G., Hesheler, J., Trautwein, W., Flockerzi, V. & Hofmann, F. (1982). Nature (Lond.) 298, 576-578.

Ouedraogo, C.O., Garnier, D., Nargeot, J. & Pourrias, B. (1982). J. Mol. Cell. Cardiol. 14, 111-121.

Pappano, A.J. & Carmeliet, E.E. (1979). Pflügers Archiv. 382, 17-26.

Pappano, A.J., Hartigan, P.M. & Coutu, M.D. (1982). Am. J. Physiol. 342, H434-H441.

Pepe, F.A. & Drucker, B. (1975). J. Mol. Biol. 99, 609-617.

Prokopczuk, A., Lewartowski, B. & Czarnecka, M. (1973). Pflügers Archiv. 339, 305-316.

Quist, E.E. (1982). Biochem. Pharmacol. 31, 3130-3133.

Ray, K.P. & England, P.J. (1976). FEBS Lett. 70, 11-16.

Reddy, Y.S., Ballard, D., Giri, N.Y. & Schwartz, A. (1973). J. Mol. Cell. Cardiol. 5, 461-471.

Reddy, Y.S. & Wyborny, L.E. (1976). Biochim. Biopyhs. Res. Comm. 73, 703-709.

Reisler, E., Smith, C. & Seegan, G. (1980). J. Mol. Biol. 143, 129-145.

Reuter, H. (1974). J. Physiol. 242, 429-451.

Reuter, H. (1983). Nature 301, 569-574.

Reuter, H. & Scholz, H. (1977). J. Physiol. 264, 49-62.

Rinaldi, M., LePeuch, C.J. & Demaille, J.G. (1981). FEBS Lett. 129, 277-281.

Rinaldi, M., Capony, J.P. & Demaille, J.G. (1982). J. Mol. Cell. Cardiol. 14, 279-289.

Robertson, S.P., Johnson, J.D., Holroyde, M.J., Kranias, E.G., Potter, J.D. & Solaro, R.J. (1982). J. Biol. Chem. 257, 260-263.

Rome, E., Offer, G. & Pepe, F. (1973). Nature New Biol. 244, 152-154.

Schwartz, A., Entman, M.L., Kaniike, K., Lane, L.K., VanWinkle, W.B. & Bornet, E.P. (1976). Biochim. Biophys. Acta 426, 57-72.

Solaro, R.J., Moir, A.J.G. & Perry, S.V. (1976). Nature, 262, 615-616.

Squire, J. (1981). The Structural Basis of Muscular Contraction, Plenum Press, New York

Starr, R. & Offer, G. (1978). Biochemistry 171, 813-816.

Stull, J.T. & Buss, J.E. (1977). J. Biol. Chem. 252, 851-857.

Stull, J.T. (1980). Adv. Cyclic Nucleotide Res. 13, 39-93.

Tada, M., Kirchberger, M.A. & Katz, A.M. (1975). J. Biol. Chem. 250, 2650-2647.

Ten Eick, R., Nawrath, H., McDonald, T.F. & Trautwein, W. (1976). Pflügers Archiv. 361, 207-213.

Trautwein, W., McDonald, T.F. & Tripathi, O. (1975). Pflügers Archiv. 354, 55-74.

Trautwein, W., Taniguchi, J. & Noma, A. (1982). Pflügers Archiv. 392, 307-314.

Tsien, R.W., Giles, W.R. & Greengard, P. (1972). Nature New Biol. 240, 181-183.

Tsien, R.W. (1973). Nature New Biol. 245, 120-122.

Tsien, R.W. (1977). Adv. Cyclic Nucleotide Res. 8, 363-420.

Tsien, R.W. & Weingart, R. (1976). J. Physiol. 260, 117-141.

Vassort, G., Rougier, O., Garnier, D., Sauviat, M.P., Coraboeuf, E. & Gargouil, Y.M. (1969). Pflügers Archiv. 309, 70-81.

Vogel, S. and Sperelakis, N. (1981). J. Mol. Cell Cardiol. 13, 51-64.

Watanabe, A.M. & Besch, H.R. (1975). Circ. Res. 37, 309-317.

Watanabe, A.M., Lindemann, J.P. & Fleming, J.W. (1984). Fed. Proc. 43, 2618-2623.

Watanabe, A.M., McConnaughey, M.M., Strawbridge, R.A., Fleming, J.W., Jones, L.R. & Besch, H.R. (1978). J. Biol. Chem. 253, 4833-4836.

Winegrad, S. (1984). Circ. Res. 55, 565-574.

Wray, H.L., Gray, R.R. & Olsson, R.A. (1973). J. Biol. Chem. 248, 1496-1498.

Wray, H.L. & Gray, R.R. (1977). Biochim. Biophys. Acta 461, 441-459.

Yamamoto, K. & Moos, C. (1983) J. Biol. Chem. 258, 8395-8401.

PRESYNAPTIC MODULATION OF CORTICAL ACETYLCHOLINE RELEASE: INFLUENCE OF AGE AND ADENOSINE

F.Pedata, L.Giovannelli, M.G.Giovannini and G.Pepeu

Department of Pharmacology, University of Florence

Viale G.B. Morgagni 65, 50134 Florence, Italy

INTRODUCTION

Histochemical and neurochemical investigations demonstrate that the mammalian cerebral cortex contains a diffuse cholinergic network formed prevalently by nerve endings whose somata are located in the basal forebrain nuclei (Mesulam et al., 1983; Wainer et al.,1984). Minor contributions to the cortical cholinergic network are due to a direct projection from the large choline acetyltransferase (ChAT) immunoreactive cells in the pontomesencephalon (Mesulam et al.,1983) and, in the rat, by interneurons scattered throughout all cellular layers in all cortices which contain approximately 30% of total ChAT (Levey et al.,1984; McGeer et al.,1984).

The release of acetylcholine (ACh) from the cortical cholinergic nerve endings is influenced by physiological conditions and by a large number of drugs as demonstrated by both in vivo (Pepeu,1973) and in vitro (Vizi,1979) studies.

The stimulation of subcortical regions in vivo (Pepeu, 1983; Szerb,1967) demonstrates that a relationship exists between the amount of ACh release and the activity of the neurons ascending to the cortex. However, measuring ACh release from the cerebral cortex in vivo makes it impossible to distinguish between events and drugs which influence the release by acting on the neuronal somata and those which act on the nerve endings through presynaptic mechanisms.

Cortical slices and synaptosomes are therefore useful tools for investigating the presynaptic mechanisms regulating ACh release.

ACh release from the cortical slices is influenced by age and modulated by autoreceptors (Hadhazy and Szerb,1976) and heteroreceptors including alpha receptors (Beani et al.,1979) as well as by purinergic receptors (Pedata et al.,1983). It has been shown that ACh release taken from 24 month old rats is approximately 50% smaller than in 3 month old rats.

Similar results were obtained in K^+-depolarized slices from aged mouse whole brain (Gibson and Peterson,1981).

In the present study we investigated whether a decrease in ACh output from the electrically stimulated cortical slices can be also seen in 15 month old rats.

Adenosine modulates neurotransmitter release from central and peripheral nerve endings (Stone,1981) by acting on specific purinergic receptors (Daly,1982). The effect of adenosine on ACh release is decreased in senescent rats (Pedata et al.,1983). This decrease could be related to the disappearance of a low affinity subpopulation of A_1 receptors, as observed by Corradetti et al. (1984) in the old rat brain. In order to better understand the influence of age on the purinergic receptors modulating ACh release, the effect of adenosine and caffeine on ACh release from cortical slices was investigated in 22-24 month old rats.

MATERIALS AND METHODS

Animals

The experiments were carried out in 3, 15 and 22-24 month old male Wistar rats obtained from Charles River, Italia. The rats were killed by decapitation and the right and left parietal cortices were rapidly dissected.

Preparation and electrical stimulation of brain slices

The cortices were plunged into cold Krebs solution with the following composition (mM): NaCl 118.5, KCl 4.7, $CaCl_2$ 2.5, $MgSO_4$ 1.2, KH_2PO_4 1.2, glucose 10, $NaHCO_3$ 25, choline 0.02. The slices were prepared and superfused according to the procedure previously described by Pedata et al. (1983) in Perspex superfusion chambers of 0.9 ml volume with Krebs solution gassed with 95% O_2 and 5% CO_2, containing physostigmine sulphate, at the rate of 0.5 ml/min at 37°C.

After 20 min equilibration, the experimental design was the following: 5 min rest; 5 min stimulation at rates of 1, 2 and 5 Hz with rectangular pulses of alternating polarity, using a current strength of 30 mA/cm^2 and a pulse duration of 5 msec; 10 min rest to allow the washout of all ACh released by electrical stimulation.

The actual net extra release of ACh caused by electrical stimulation was estimated by subtracting the amount of release expected during 15 min rest (calculated by multiplying by 3 the amount released during the 5 min rest preceeding each stimulation period), from the total amount of ACh found in the 15 min of stimulation and washout. In Ca-free Krebs solution no extra release was detectable.

Acetylcholine assay

ACh content of the superfusate samples was quantified on the isolated guinea pig ileum perfused with Tyrode solution (Pedata et al.,1983). The identity of ACh as the active substance was routinely checked by adding atropine or by alkaline hydrolysis of the samples. ACh release was expressed as ng/g of wet tissue/min of superfusion $\pm$ S.E.

Drugs

Freshly prepared solutions of the following drugs were used: acetylcholine (Sigma), atropine sulphate and physostigmine sulphate (BDH), tetrodotoxin (Biochemia), morphine sulphate (Carlo Erba), caffeine (Sigma), adenosine (Calbiochem).

RESULTS

Fig. 1 shows the ACh release from cortical slices taken from 3 and 15 month old rats. The release in the 15 month old rats was markedly lower than in the 3 month old rats at 1, 2 and 5 Hz stimulation frequency. No difference was seen at 0.2 Hz. When Ca^{++} concentration in the superfusing Krebs solution was increased from 2.5 to 5 mM the release in the 15 month old rats was significantly greater than in slices taken from rats of the same age but superfused with normal Krebs solution.

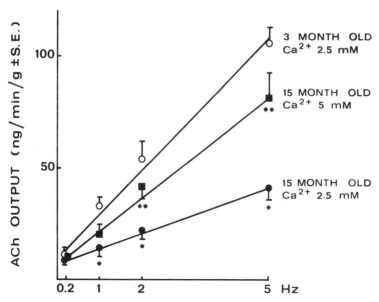

Fig. 1 - Acetylcholine output from electrically stimulated cortical slices. Each point is the mean of 5-6 experiments. Vertical bars = standard error of the mean. Statistically significant difference with $p < 0.01$:*from 3 month old rats; **from 15 month old rats, 5 mM Ca^{++}.

Fig. 2 shows the effect of adenosine on ACh release from cortical slices from adult and aged rats. The stimulation frequency was 5 Hz. It can be seen that the concentration of 30 μM adenosine resulting in a 50% decrease of ACh release in the 3 month old rats had no effect in the aged animals.

In the latter, a 10 fold adenosine concentration was necessary to obtain a similar decrease in ACh output.

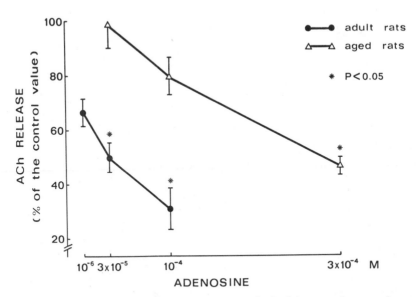

Fig. 2 - Effect of adenosine on acetylcholine release from electrically stimulated cortical slices from adult and aged rats.Stimulation frequency was 5 Hz.Each point is the mean of 5-8 experiments. Vertical bars = standard error of the mean. *Statistically significant difference from controls.

Table 1 summarizes the effect of caffeine at 50 and 500 μM concentrations on ACh release from cortical slices taken from 3 and 24 month old rats. The table demonstrates that ACh release from 24 month old rats was 47% and 42% less than that from the 3 month old rats at 1 and 5 Hz stimulation frequency, respectively. The superfusion with 50 uM of caffeine in slices taken from 3 month old rats brought about an increase in ACh release of 127% at 0.2, 75% at 1, and 50% at 5 Hz stimulation frequency, respectively. On the contrary, 50 uM concentration of caffeine had no effect on ACh release from slices taken from 24 month old rats. Finally, caffeine in 3 month old rats at the concentration of 500 μM brought about a 50% decrease in ACh release at 0.2, a 50% at 1 and a 46% at 5 Hz stimulation frequency, respectively. In the 24 month old rats, however, 500 μM of caffeine exerted no significant effect on ACh release from the stimulated slices and a 47% increase from the unstimulated slices.

TABLE 1

Effect of caffeine on acetylcholine release (ng/g/min±S.E.) from electrically-stimulated cortical slices from young and old rats.

AGE Months	DOSE uM	STIMULATION FREQUENCY (Hz)			
		0	0.2	1	5
3	0	6.5+0.3	9.7+2.2	34.8+5.7	90.8+ 5.2
24	0	5.5+0.5	8.8+0.8	18.5+2.3*	53.1+ 8.7*
3	50	6.5+0.4	22.1+2.9*	61.2+2.9*	136.4+ 9.1*
24	50	6.4+0.9	7.8+0.3	18.1+2.8	55.2+10.3
3	500	5.8+0.4	4.2+0.7*	17.7+3.2*	49.1+ 6.0*
24	500	8.1+1.0*	6.7+0.7	19.4+3.7	72.2+11.8

Each value is the mean $\pm$ S.E. of 6-9 rats. *Statistically significant difference from 3 months, no caffeine: P< 0.01.

DISCUSSION

The present experiments confirm previous results (Pedata et al.,1983) that ACh release from electrically-stimulated cortical slices is much smaller in 24 month old than in 3 month old rats. However, a decrease in ACh output of the same size was also found in 15 month old rats indicating that the age-dependent impairment of ACh output begins at an earlier stage in the rat life.

The decrease in ACh release in the 15 month old rats was partially corrected by increasing Ca^{++} concentration in the superfusing Krebs solution. The increase in Ca^{++} concentration also enhances ACh release from unstimulated (Mantovani et al.,1981) and stimulated (unpublished results) slices taken from 3 month old rats. However, the finding that raising Ca^{++} concentration increases ACh release in aging rats indicates that age does not impair markedly ACh synthesis. On the other hand, the decrease in ACh release observed in aging animals cannot be explained by a comparable decrease in choline acetyltransferase which, if occurring, is generally small (Bartus et al.,1982). Furthemore, in the cerebral cortex steady state ACh levels do not change with age (Meek et al.,1977). Age does not significantly decrease "K^{+}-stimulated" ACh synthesis in slices of rat cortex and hippocampus (Sherman et al.,1981), human cortex (Sims et al., 1981) or whole brain slices in the mouse (Gibson and Peterson,1981). It is therefore possible that the release mechanism might be directly altered by aging.

A marked decrease in Ca^{++} uptake into synaptosomes prepared from the brain of old rats has been demonstrated (Peterson and Gibson,1983; Pepeu et al.,in press). This finding and the present observation that Ca^{++} restores ACh release in aging rats suggest that a reduced Ca^{++} availability could be responsible for the decrease of the stimulus-evoked ACh release observed in the aging rats.

The inhibitory effect of adenosine on ACh release from electrically-stimulated cortical slices is strongly reduced in 24 month old rats as previously shown (Pedata et al.,1983). Moreover, the dose-dependent stimulatory and inhibitory effects of caffeine on ACh release are also abolished in senescent rats.

It has been demonstrated that aging affects brain adenosine receptors. In rat cerebral cortex and hippocampus aging is associated with the disappearance of low affinity binding sites (Corradetti et al.,1984). In the whole brain of 12 month old rats an apparent decrease in affinity of adenosine receptors has been reported by Virus et al. (1983).

It is difficult to understand the mechanism and the functional meaning of the changes in adenosine receptors and adenosine and methylxanthine actions in aging rats. The possibility that they may depend on age-related changes in adenosine metabolism needs to be explored. Questions may be raised as to whether peripheral actions of adenosine are also affected by aging.

In conclusion, from the results reported here it appears, however, that in evaluating the age-related impairment of brain cholinergic mechanism, which is believed to be responsible for geriatric memory dysfunctions (Bartus et al.,1982), alterations in the presynaptic release mechanism and its regulation should be taken into account. Drugs aimed at correcting these alterations can be envisaged (Pedata et al., 1985; Peterson and Gibson,1983).

Acknowledgments
This work was supported by grant n° CT 83.02771.56 target project "Preventive Medicine and Rehabilitation", subproject Aging Mechanisms, and also by a grant from the University of Florence. The old rats were a generous gift of the Italian Study Group for Brain Aging.

REFERENCES

Bartus,R.T., Dean,R.L., Beer,B. and Lippa,A.S., 1982, The cholinergic hypothesis of geriatric memory dysfunction. Science, 217: 408.
Beani,L., Bianchi,C., Giacomelli,A. and Tamberi,F., 1978, Noradrenaline inhibition of acetylcholine release from guinea-pig brain. Eur.J.Pharmacol.,48: 179.

Corradetti,R., Kiedrowski,L., Nordström,O and Pepeu,G., 1984, Disappearance of low affinity adenosine binding sites in aging rat cerebral cortex and hippocampus. Neurosci.Lett., 49: 143.

Daly,J.W., 1982, Adenosine receptors: targets for future drugs. J. Med. Chem., 25: 197.

Gibson,G.E. and Peterson,C., 1981, Aging decreases oxidative metabolism and the release and synthesis of acetylcholine. J.Neurochem., 37: 978.

Hadhazy,P. and Szerb,J.C., 1976, The effect of cholinergic drugs on ^{3}H-acetylcholine release from slices of rat hippocampus, striatum and cortex. Brain Res., 123: 311.

Levey,A.I., Wainer,B.H., Rye,D.B., Mufson,E.J. and Mesulam, M.M., 1984, Choline acetyltransferase-immunoreactive neurons intrinsic to rodent cortex and distinction from acetylcholinesterase-positive neurons. Neuroscience, 13: 341.

Mantovani,P. and Pepeu,G., 1981, Interactions between ionophores, Mg^{2+} and Ca^{2+} on acetylcholine formation and release in brain slices. Pharmacol.Res.Commun., 13: 175.

McGeer,P.L., McGeer,E.G. and Peng,J.H., 1981, Choline acetyltransferase: purification and immuno istochemical localization. Life Sci., 34: 2319.

Meek,J.L., Bertilsson,L., Cheney,D.L., Zsilla,G. and Costa,E., 1977, Aging-induced changes in acetylcholine and serotonin content of discrete brain nuclei. J.Gerontol., 32: 129.

Mesulam, M.M., Mufson,E.J., Wainer,B.H. and Levey,A.I., 1983, Central cholinergic pathway in the rat: an overview based on an alternative nomenclature (Ch1 - Ch6). Neurosci., 10:1185.

Pedata,F., Antonelli,T., Lambertini,L., Beani,L. and Pepeu,G., 1983, Effect of adenosine, adenosine triphosphate, adenosine deaminase, dipyridamole and aminophylline on acetylcholine release from electrically-stimulated brain slices. Neuropharmacol., 22: 609.

Pedata,F., Slavikova,J., Kotas,A. and Pepeu,G., 1983, Acetylcholine release from rat cortical slices during postnatal development and aging. Neurobiol. Aging, 4: 31.

Pedata,F., Giovannelli,L., Giovannini, M.G. and Pepeu,G., 1985, Effect of phosphatidylserine on cortical acetylcholine (ACh) release in adult and senescent rats. Abstracts Meeting on: Phospholipids in the Nervous System: Biochemical and Molecular Pharmacology. Mantova, p.42.

Pepeu,G., 1973, The release of acetylcholine from the brain: an approach to the study of the central cholinergic mechanisms. Progr. Neurobiol., 2: 257.

Pepeu,G., 1983, Brain acetylcholine: an inventory of our knowledge on the 50th anniversary of its discovery. Trends Pharmacol.Sci., 4: 416.

Pepeu,G., Giovannelli,L., Giovannini,M.G. and Pedata,F., Effect of phosphatidylserine on cortical acetylcholine release and calcium uptake in adult and aging rats. in:"Phospholipids in the nervous system" L.A.Horrock,G.Toffano and L.Freyz eds,Fidia Research Series,Liviana Press,Padova, in press.

Peterson,C. and Gibson,G.E., 1983, Aging and 3,4-diamino-pyridine alter synaptosomal calcium uptake. J.Biol.Chem., 258: 11482.

Sherman,K.A., Kuster,J.E., Dean,R.L., Bartus,R.T. and Friedman,E., 1981, Presynaptic cholinergic mechanisms in brain of aged rats with memory impairments. Neurobiol.Aging, 2: 99.

Sims,N.R., Bowen,D.M. and Davison,A.N., 1981, ^{14}C acetylcholine synthesis and ^{14}C carbon dioxide production from U - [14]C glucose by tissue prisms from human neocortex. Biochem.J., 196: 867.

Stone,T.W., 1981, Physiological roles for adenosine and adenosine 5'-triphosphate in the nervous system. Neurosci., 6:523.

Szerb,J.C., 1967, Cortical acetylcholine release and electroencephalographic arousal. J.Physiol., 192: 329.

Virus,R.M., Baglajewski,T. and Radulovacki,M., 1983, Adenosine receptor binding in whole brains from young and old rats. Abstracts Soc.Neurosci., 9: 1202.

Vizi,E.S., 1979, Presynaptic modulation of neurochemical transmission. Progr.Neurobiol., 12: 181.

Wainer,B.H., Levey,A.I., Mufson,E.J. and Mesulam,M.M., 1984, Cholinergic system in mammalian brain identified with antibodies against choline acetyltransferase. Neurochem.Int., 6: 163.

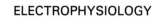

ELECTROPHYSIOLOGY

THE STORY OF THE RENSHAW CELL

John C. Eccles

Max-Planck-Institut fur Biophysikalische Chemie
Göttingen

The story begins in many apparently unrelated findings. The axon collaterals of neurons had been described by neuroanatomists from the 1890's on. Then neurophysiologists speculated about the function of motor axon collaterals. In particular Renshaw (1941) depicted motor axon collaterals ending either on motoneurons or adjacent interneurons. Meanwhile there had grown up a literature on the inhibitory action of antidromic impulses in motor axons, the time course being precisely investigated by Renshaw (1941) and by Lloyd (1946). In a later investigation Renshaw (1946) discovered that interneurons in the ventral horn gave an extraordinary high frequency discharge (over 1000/sec) in response to an antidromic volley. Renshaw tentatively suggested that such interneurons could be involved in the antidromic inhibition. I met him in February, 1946 at the Rockefeller Institute. He was an exciting personality who inexplicably left for Portland soon after and there died from a fulminating polio. Strangely enough his story seemed to be dying with him. One knew of these extraordinary interneurons, but suspected that in some way injury by the penetrating microelectrode might be involved.

And so the story remained for many years. My move to Canberra from Dunedin interrupted my experimentation for over a year, but in March, 1953, Paul Fatt and I started experiments in the temporary Canberra laboratory.

Our plan was to study further the IPSP's generated by afferent inputs from muscle. To our chagrin dorsal roots were blocked, but the ventral roots still functioned. So perforce we had to investigate the central effects of antidromic volleys in motor axons. To our delight we discovered the interneuronal responses just as Renshaw had described them. We recognized that the dorsal root blockage was due to a defective medicinal paraffin contaminated by volatile hydrocarbons. The deeply lying ventral roots were apparently unaffected. So by an accident we were driven to work on the absolutely unique Renshaw cells, as we felicitiously named them. Meanwhile Dr. Koketsu had joined us and together we three embarked on one of the most satisfactory investigations of my life.

In the first stage we studied the Renshaw cell responses to antidromic volleys from a variety of muscles. There was convergence onto one cell from the axon collaterals of motoneurons supplying many muscles, with a wide range of gradation of effect. Always there was an initial response of very short latency (0.6 - 1.0 msec) followed by a repetitive discharge

at an initial frequency up to 1500/sec with the strongest excitations and
with a rapid decline to fade out in 50 - 100 msec at the longest (Fig. 1B).
This time course of the Renshaw cell responses fitted them precisely for
the role of inhibitory interneurons responsible for the antidromic inhibition that had orginally been described by Renshaw (1941). Correspondingly
we recorded intracellularly the antidromically evoked IPSP's which were
exactly in accord with the earlier studies on reflex inhibition (Fig. 1C,
D, E, F). A new neuronal system had been discovered (Fig. 1A). Antidromic
impulses in collaterals of a motor axon converged onto and excited many
Renshaw cells and their axons in turn converged on to many motoneurons to
produce the antidromically evoked inhibition.

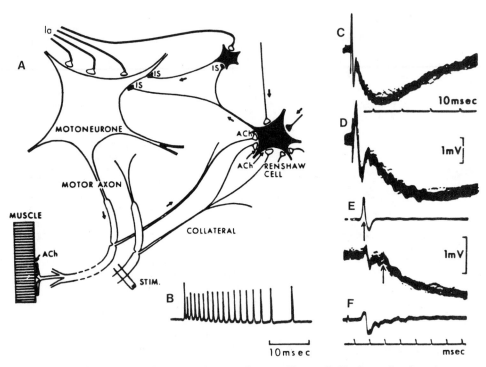

Fig. 1   Feed back inhibition via Renshaw cells. Full description in text.
IS signifies inhibitory synapses and ACh excitatory synapses operating with acetylcholine as transmitter. (J. C. Eccles, P. Fatt,
and K. Koketsu, J. Physiol., 126:524 (1954)).

Even more interesting were the results of our pharmacological investigation. We were mindful of Dale's Principle that would require the axon
collaterals of motoneurons to act by the same transmitter as the peripheral axonal synapses on muscle, namely ACh at both sites. But our first
experiments were disappointing. D-tubocurarine that so effectively
blocked the periperal cholinergic synapses of motoneurons had almost no
action on the synaptic excitation of Renshaw cells by the axon collater-

als; and atropine was similarly ineffective. The anticholinesterase, prostigmine, that was so effective peripherally failed to cause the expected prolongation of the Renshaw cell discharge. We suspected that these pharmacological failures were due to the inability of substances with a particular molecular configuration to cross the blood-brain barrier. It was encouraging to find that the anticholinesterase eserine very effectively prolonged the responses of Renshaw cells so that a single antidromic volley could evoke a Renshaw cell repetitive discharge for over a second. Two other anticholinesterases, tetraethylpyrophosphate (TEPP) and NU 2126 (Roche) were equally effective. However, for some days we were frustrated by the failure of d-tubocurarine. Then I remembered that I had two glass-sealed tubes of curare substitutes β-erythroidine and dihydro-β-erythroidine. I got them originally in Sydney many years before, then took them to New Zealand where they lay unopened in a drawer. Just before leaving for Canberra I had noticed them and packed them for transport. During an unsuccessful curare experiment it all came back to me and Paul Fatt instantly opened them and made up the solution for injection. We chose a rather large dose - 1 mg/Kg as I remember. The Renshaw cell discharge so dramatically disappeared that we thought we had lost the cell, but on close inspection there were still the first two spikes that are so resistant to depression. It turned out that 0.1 mg/Kg was quite satisfactory for dihydro-β-erythroidine.

Conclusive evidence of the cholinergic action of motor axon collaterals on Renshaw cells was obtained by the difficult technique of intra-arterial injection into the spinal cord (Fig. 2) as pioneered by Holmstedt and Skoglund (1953). Acetylcholine was very effective in exciting most Renshaw cells. The effect was enhanced by prior treatment with eserine and depressed by prior dihydro-β-erythroidine. Nicotine was a most potent stimulator.

As would be expected these pharmacological properties of Renshaw cells exactly matched the pharmacological findings on antidromic inhibition, as studied by the IPSP's of motoneurons. For this reason it was concluded that the antidromic inhibition of motoneurons was sufficiently explained by the Renshaw cell system (Fig. 1A). The earlier suggestions of electrical field effects from the antidromically activated motoneurons seem no longer to be acceptable.

The initial publication was in the Australian Journal of Science in October 1953. The complete publication included a more extensive series of investigations and also the intra-arterial injections. It was submitted to the Journal of Physiology on June 22, 1954. It was unbelievable to receive in Canberra a notice of acceptance within 10 days-just about the time of return air transport in those days. As I discovered much later, the reason was that the manuscript was received by Dr. Grace Eggleton at University College, London. She immediately handed it to Bernard Katz and next morning he returned the bulky manuscript with his judgment-"accept as is". One wishes for such treatment these days!

I think Dr. Koketsu will agree that this Renshaw cell paper should become a classic. Sir Henry Dale was most attracted by the demonstration of an identical chemical transmission from peripheral and central branches of motor axons. This provides the most striking example of what I then termed Dale's Principle, in accord with the writings of Dale (1952). A further theoretical development was proposed when a little later it was demonstrated that the so-called direct inhibition (Lloyd, 1946) was not direct, there being an interneuron on the Ia inhibitory pathway to the motoneuron (Fig. 1A). This was also the case with the inhibitory pathway of Ib and cutaneous inputs. Hence it was proposed (Eccles, 1957, page 213) that any one transmitter substance always has the same synaptic action, i.e., excitatory or inhibitory, at all synapses on nerve cells.

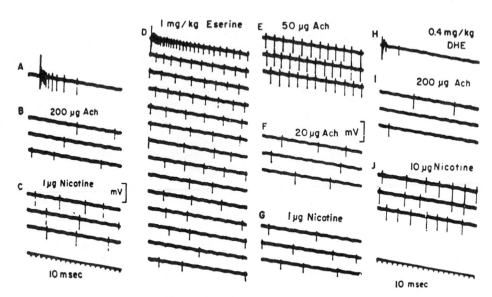

Fig. 2   Responses of another Renshaw cell. There was no spontaneous discharge. (A) is response to a single antidromic volley in L7 ventral root, while (B) and (C) each show three successive sweeps at the height of the responses evoked by intra-arterial injection of 200 µg of acetylcholine and 1 µg of nicotine, respectively. Several minutes after the intravenous injection of 1.0 mg eserine/kg, the response (A) was changed to (D), while (E), (F) and (G) show, respectively, three successive records at the heights of the responses evoked by the intra-arterial injections of 50 µg acetylcholine, 20 µg acetylcholine and 1 µg nicotine. Records (H), (I), and (J) were obtained during the maximum of the depression produced by the intravenous injection of 0.4 mg dihydro-β-erythroidine hydrobromide/kg, (H) being evoked by the antidromic volley and (I) and (J) by the intra-arterial injections of 200 µg acetylcholine and 10 µg nicotine, respectively (Eccles, Eccles, and Fatt, 1956).

According to this principle, any one class of nerve cells will function exclusively either in an excitatory or in an inhibitory capacity at all of its synaptic endings, i.e., there are functionally just two types of nerve cells, excitatory and inhibitory. The Renshaw cells, the group Ia intermediate neurons, and the other intermediate neurons on the inhibitory pathways for group Ib and cutaneous impulses would be examples of neurons that were exclusively inhibitory in function, and which consequently may be termed "inhibitory neurons." This generalization for synaptic organization in the central nervous system drew much criticism, but that has been long since forgotten. Now it is so generally accepted that it is regarded as a fact in neuronal design! The historical struggle of less than 30 years ago is completely unremembered. Even the concept of the Renshaw cell as a neuronal element drew heavy criticism despite the overwhelming evidence for its existence with precise location as indicated in Fig. 3. The inhibitory pathway as indicated in Fig. 3 is interesting for another reason. It provides the first example in the mammalian central nervous system of a synapse operated by an identified transmitter substance, in this case, acetylcholine working in a nicotinic manner.

More recently there have been several studies accurately locating Renshaw cells by tracer techniques with confirmation of the originally reported location. Moreover, there has been confirmation of all the original major findings. Nevertheless the Renshaw cells retain an enigmatic atmosphere with their unique intense and prolonged response. They provide a rare example of a powerful nicotinic action of ACh in the central nervous system. Our original investigations led us to conclude that the inhibitory action of the Renshaw cell system had no specific functional meaning. It seemed to function as a diffuse feed-back inhibitory system that was strangely spotty in its distribution.

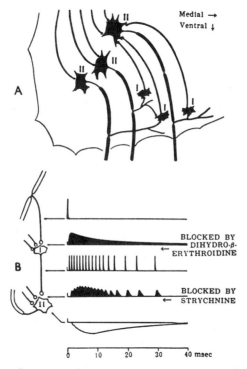

Fig. 3. A. Sketch of proposed neuron system in ventral horn of spinal cord. Collaterals are given off by motor axons before they leave the spinal cord with interneurons (I). The axons of these interneurons proceed dorsally and laterally and make contact with motoneurons (II), which, by this system, are inhibited. Reflexly active afferents are shown descending onto the motoneurons from the dorsal direction.

B. Diagram summarizing the postulated sequence of events from the antidromic impulse in motor axons to inhibition of motoneurons. All events are plotted on same time scale, and the corresponding histological structures are shown to the left (note indicator arrows). The five events are from above downwards: (1) impulse in axon collateral; (2) time course of acetylcholine liberated at axon collateral terminal; (3) repetitive discharge in interneuron; (4) time course of inhibitory transmitter substance liberated at

(continued)

193

Fig. 3 (continued)
interneuronal terminal; (5) hyperpolarization set up in motoneuron by inhibitory synaptic action. Note additional synapses
for convergent pathways both on interneuron and motoneuron (see
figure 3, A). The summation of the synaptic action of several
converging interneurons onto a motoneuron is responsible for
smoothing the latter part of the motoneuron hyperpolarization.

It has not been possible to recount all of the details of the Renshaw
cell story, but I do like to think of it as being dramatic and to be of
heuristic interest. Doubtless in the progress of the neurosciences there
will be played out comparable romantic stories. I hope so. I am particularly happy that, the name of Renshaw will be immortalized by these unique
nerve cells that he discovered just before his tragic death. I am even
more happy to present this story of our Renshaw cell adventure to Dr.
Karczmar, an inimitable adventurer.

References

Dale, H.H., Transmission of effects from nerve endings. London: Oxford
University Press, 1952.

Eccles, J.C., Physiology of Nerve Cells. Baltimore: Johns Hopkins Press,
1957.

Eccles, J.C., Eccles, R.M. & Fatt, P., Pharmacological investigations on
a central synapse operated by acetylcholine. J. Physiol. 131,
154-169, 1956.

Eccles, J.C., Fatt, P. & Koketsu, K., Cholinergic and inhibitory synapses
in a central nervous pathway. The Austral. Journal of Science 16,
50-54, 1953.

Eccles, J.C., Fatt, P. & Koketsu, K., Cholinergic and inhibitory synapses
in a pathway from motor-axon collaterals to motoneurons. J.
Physiol. 126, 524-562, 1954.

Holmstedt, B. & Skoglund, C.R., The action on spinal reflexes of
dimethylamido-ethoxy-phosphoryl cyanide, "Tabun", a cholinesterase
inhibitor. Acta physiol. scand. 29, suppl. 106, 410-427, 1953.

Lloyd, D.P.C., Facilitation and inhibition of spinal motoneurons. J.
Neurophysiol. 9, 421-438, 1946.

Renshaw, B., Influence of discharge of motoneurons upon excitation of
neighbouring motoneurons. J. Neurophysiol. 4, 167-183, 1941.

Renshaw, B., Central effects of centripetal impulses in axons of spinal
ventral roots. J. Neurophysiol. 9, 191-204, 1946.

THE BLOCKADE OF OPEN CHANNEL OF ACETYLCHOLINE RECEPTOR IS

RESPONSIBLE FOR SELECTIVE BLOCKADE OF NICOTINIC TRANSMISSION

Vladimir I. Skok

Department of the Autonomic
Nervous System Physiology
Bogomoletz Institute of Physiology
Kiev-24, USSR

ABSTRACT

Hexamethonium, a selective ganglionic blocker, at its lowest effective concentration exhibits the open-channel blockade of nicotinic acetylcholine (ACh) receptors in sympathetic ganglion neurones, with no signs of their competitive blockade. This is evidenced by the facts that 1) hexamethonium shortens in a voltage-dependent manner the apparent mean channel lifetime estimated from the excitatory postsynaptic current (EPSC) decay and from the ACh noise analysis as well as from the analysis of single channel activity, and 2) the hexamethonium-induced reduction of the ACh current amplitude is enhanced by the preliminary opening of the ACh-gated channels.

The rate constants that characterize binding of hexamethonium, pirilenum and some other selective ganglionic blockers to an open ACh-gated channel correlates with their ganglion-blocking activities, in contrast to what is observed in the effects of competitive ganglionic blockers tubocurarine and trimethaphan. This observation suggests that selective ganglionic blockade produced by some compounds is due to an open-channel blockade while in other cases it is due to a competitive mechanism. The selective blockade of open channel can be observed in different types of synapses. It is suggested that the site in the ACh-gated open channel that binds selective blockers normally binds Ca^{2+} ions.

INTRODUCTION

It has long been known that the ionic channels of electrically excitable membrane can be selectively blocked by certain compounds which bind to a channel in its open state. The classical examples are local anaesthetics at sodium channels (Strichartz, 1973; Hille et al., 1975) and tetraethylammonium at potassium channels (Armstrong, 1971; Armstrong and Hille, 1972).

The open-channel blockade was also observed in chemically excitable membrane (Blackman, 1970; Adams, 1976; Ascher et al., 1978; Colquhoun et al., 1979; Rang, 1981). However, because of the great variety of the drugs that can block chemically gated channels in their open state (local anaesthetics, barbiturates, bis-quaternary ammonium compounds, alkaloids etc.), this type of blockade was commonly thought to be less selective than the classical competitive blocking mechanism (Ascher et al., 1978, 1979; Karlin et al., 1983). In this work, evidence is presented that the open channel blockade may be highly selective and may determine the selective blockade of synaptic transmission.

THE MECHANISM OF OPEN CHANNEL BLOCKADE

The first evidence that the blockade of chemically gated channels in their open state may be related to a selective blockade of synaptic transmission was obtained from the comparison of the effects produced by two drugs, hexamethonium and tubocurarine, on fast excitatory post-synaptic current (EPSC) recorded from rabbit superior cervical ganglion neurones (Selyanko et al., 1981). Although tubocurarine is about five times more potent than hexamethonium in inducing the blockade of synaptic transmission through sympathetic ganglia (Grob, 1967; Bowman and Webb, 1972), the hexamethonium-induced blockade is more selective, as this compound is effective in the ganglia in much lower concentrations than in other cholinergic junctions, including those possessing nicotinic acetylcholine receptors (AChRs), particularly in skeletal neuro-muscular junction (Paton and Zaimis, 1949; Barlow and Zoller, 1964). In contrast, tubocurarine is about 4 times more effective in the neuro-muscular junction than in the sympathetic ganglion (Guyton and Reeder, 1950).

The effect of hexamethonium on EPSC is shown in Fig. 1. Hexamethonium (1.10^{-5} M) shortens the decay of EPSC leaving it a single exponential (Fig. 1, A, B, D), while not decreasing the EPSC amplitude (Fig. 1, D); the decrease in the EPSC amplitude can be observed only at higher concentrations of the drug, and is not voltage-dependent at resting membrane potential level (Fig. 1, E). The shortening of the EPSC decay by hexamethonium is voltage-sensitive (Fig. 1, C). In contract, tubocurarine (1.10^{-5} M) exhibits almost no shortening of EPSC decay, except in strongly hyperpolarized cell, but markedly reduces the amplitude of EPSC in a nonvoltage dependent manner at resting membrane potential level (Selyanko et al., 1981).

In power spectrum of the ACh-induced membrane current hexamethonium shortens exactly the same kinetic component that corresponds to the EPSC decay time constant, as is shown in Fig. 2 (Skok et al., 1983; Derkach et al., 1983).

Hexamethonium (1.10^{-5} M) also reduces the amplitude of the ACh current induced in the sympathetic neurones by short (20 ms) iontophoretic application of ACh from a micropipette, and this effect is enhanced by preceding application of ACh in paired-pulse experiments (Skok et al., 1983).

These results indicate that hexamethonium shortens the time the ACh-gated channels stay open and that this effect is use-and voltage-dependent. Both characteristics are commonly considered as the signs of open channel blockade. This blockade can be described by a model (Steinbach, 1968; Adams, 1976):

$$ A + R \underset{k_{-1}}{\overset{k_{+1}}{\rightleftharpoons}} AR \underset{\alpha}{\overset{\beta}{\rightleftharpoons}} AR^* + B \underset{k^*_{-B}}{\overset{k^*_{+B} [B]}{\rightleftharpoons}} AR^* B, \quad (1) $$

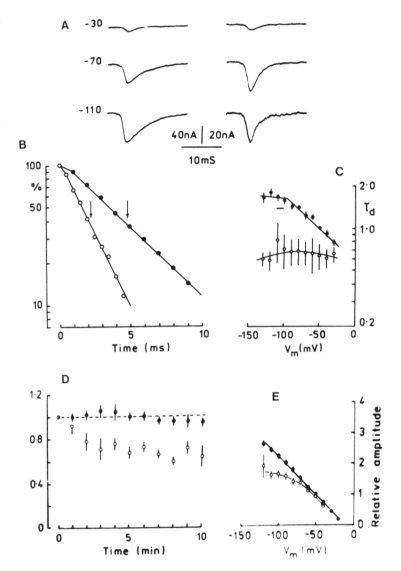

Fig. 1. The effect of hexamethonium (1.10^{-5}M) on excitatory postsynaptic currents (EPSCs) recorded from the rabbit
superior cervical ganglion neurones. A. EPSCs recorded
at different membrane potentials (indicated in mV beside
each trace) in normal solution (left) and in the presence
of hexamethonium (right). B. Semilogarithmic plot of the
normalized amplitude of the EPSCs shown in A as a function
of time, in normal solution (●) and in the presence of
hexamethonium (○). Membrane potential –70 mV. Arrows
indicate the decay time constants (τ_d); control was 4.8
ms, in hexamethonium it was 2.3 ms. C. Voltage dependence
of τ_d. Semilogarithmic plot of τ_d (normalized with
respect to its value at –50 mV) against membrane potential
in normal solution (●) and in the presence of hexamethonium (○).   The absolute normal τ_d value was 4.5 ±

(continued)

Fig. 1 (continued)

0.3 ms at −80 mV. Points are means of S.E.M. for 3 observations in C, and for 6 observations in D and E (Derkach et al., 1983; Skok et al., 1984). D. Amplitude (●) and τ_d (o) of the EPSC recorded at −50 mV, as a function of time after the onset of perfusion with hexamethonium. Amplitudes are normalized with respect to that at zero time (Skok et al., 1983). E. EPSC amplitude as a function of membrane potential in normal solution (●) and in the presence of hexamethonium (o). Amplitudes are normalized with respect to that in normal solution at −50 mV (modified from Selyanko et al., 1981).

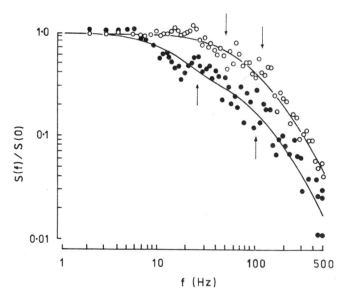

$\bullet$ NS : $T_1 = 1.5$ ms; $T_2 = 10.6$ ms;

$\circ$ 0.01 mM C_6: $T_1 = 1.2$ ms; $T_2 = 3.2$ ms.

Fig. 2. The spectral density of ACh-induced current fluctuations recorded from the rabbit superior cervical ganglion neurones as a function of frequency, in control solution (●) and in a solution containing 1.10^{-5} M hexamethonium (O). Each spectrum was obtained by subtraction of the spectrum without ACh from the spectrum in the presence of

(continued)

Fig. 2 (continued)
ACh. Each line through the data points represents the sum of two Lorentzian functions:

$$S(f) = S_1(0)/(1 + (f/f_1)^2) + S_2(0)/(1 + (f/f_2)^2) \; ,$$

where f_1 and f_2 are the cut-off frequencies at which the corresponding asymptotic spectral densities $S_1(0)$ and $S_2(0)$ decrease to one-half. The values of f_1 and f_2 (indicated by arrows) were 107 Hz and 15 Hz in control solution, and 128 Hz and 51 Hz in a solution containing hexamethonium, respectively. The values of channel lifetime τ_1 and τ_2 as obtained from the equations $\tau_1 = 1/2\pi f_1$, and $\tau_2 = 1/2\pi f_2$, were 1.5 ms and 10.6 ms in control solution, and 1.2 ms and 3.2 ms in a solution containing hexamethonium, respectively. It is assumed that the two lifetimes pertain to noninteracting channel populations with the same unit currents (Skok et al., 1983).

---

where A is an agonist, R is a postsynaptic receptor, B is a blocking agent in concentration [B], AR, AR* and AR*B are agonist-receptor complexes with closed, open and open-blocked channel, respectively, and k_{+1}, k_{-1}, β, α, k_{+B}, k_{-B} are the corresponding rate constants.

Both the EPSC decay time constant and the corresponding kinetic component obtained from the power spectrum analysis of the ACh noise recorded from sympathetic ganglion neurones correspond to apparent rather than to a true mean time the ACh-gated channels stay open, or channel lifetime (Derkach et al., 1985; see Colquhoun and Sakmann, 1983). It can be suggested that the apparent mean channel lifetime is a total time the complex AR $\rightleftharpoons$ AR* exists following single occupancy of R by A. During this time, about 5 transfers between AR and AR* can be observed (at room temperature). This results in a burst of about 5 channel openings, each single opening corresponding to one separate AR* state followed by appearance of single channel current, while each interval between two successive openings within the burst corresponds to one separate AR state. Thus, if the model (1) is correct, one should expect B to shorten each single channel opening and the burst but not each single channel closing.

In order to check this suggestion, the effect of heptamethonium on single ACh-gated channel activity was studied in rat superior cervical ganglion neurone (Derkach et al., 1985) using the cell-attached patch-clamp technique (see Hamill et al., 1981). Heptamethonium was used because of its high k^*_{-B} value, when compared with that in hexamethonium, and high voltage-dependence of both k^*_{+B} and k^*_{-B} when compared with that in other fast-dissociating open channel blockers (Skok et al., 1984). The former property allowed to observe single channel activity even during continuous presence of heptamethonium in patch pipette, while the latter property allowed to enhance the open channel blockade exerted by heptamethonium using hyperpolarization of patch membrane.

Mean durations of single opening, single closing and burst in single channel activity were estimated as decay time constants of corresponding distribution curves. For estimation of burst duration, the shortest closed-time was ignored (Derkach et al., 1986).

Fig. 3 and Table 1 illustrate the results obtained. Heptamethonium markedly shortened the bursts of openings and each single opening, and this effect was enhanced by increased concentration of the drug. Single closings and the amplitudes of single-channel currents were not affected, in agreement with the above model (1).

The open channel blockade is not the only type of blocking effect produced by heptamethonium. It can also block closed channel of AChR. This effect is evidenced by the fact that the hyperpolarizing voltage step applied a few milliseconds ahead of the appearance of EPSC decreases the amplitude of EPSC in the presence of 1.10^{-4} heptamethonium. This

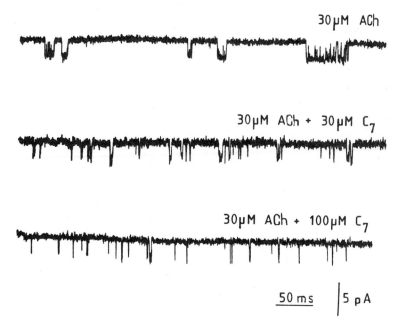

30 μM ACh

30 μM ACh + 30 μM C_7

30 μM ACh + 100 μM C_7

50 ms   5 pA

Fig. 3.   Single channel currents recorded with a pipette that contained ACh only (30 μM) or ACh and heptamethonium (30 μM or 100 μM). Records were obtained from three different patches.

decrease of the EPSC amplitude is not observed in the absence of heptamethonium or in the presence of heptamethonium but at longer intervals between the hyperpolarizing step and EPSC (Selyanko et al., 1982). This effect is also not observed if pentamethonium, a drug which exhibits marked competitive effect (see below), is used instead of heptamethonium. The latter observation suggests that the closed channel blockade is probably not identical in its mechanism to a competitive blockade.

RELATION BETWEEN THE OPEN CHANNEL BLOCKADE AND THE
TRANSMISSION BLOCKADE

Simple theoretical considerations predict that the blockade of transmitter-gated open channels in postsynaptic membrane should result in at least partial blockade of synaptic transmission. Reduction of the time the transmitter-gated channels stay open is expected to decrease the electric charge carried by EPSC. This in turn should reduce the level to which the postsynaptic membrane discharges by EPSC, or the amplitude of excitatory postsynaptic potential, to a level subthreshold for the postsynaptic spike initiation, thus causing the blockade of synaptic transmission. Therefore, one should expect that the drug which blocks the channel opened by a transmitter should also block the synaptic transmission. But until recently it has remained unknown whether this can be a mechanism for a selective transmission blockade.

One of the ways to answer this question was to see whether the open channel blocking potencies of most selective blocking drugs correlate with their transmission-blocking potencies. The apparent rate constant of the blocker binding to an open channel, k_{+B}^*, and the affinity constant, $K_B^* = k_{+B}^*/k_{-B}^*$, can be used as the quantitative characteristics of the channel-blocking potency. The values of k_{+B}^* and k_{-B}^* can be estimated from the following equations, in agreement with the model (1):

$$k_{+B}^* = [(\tau'_d)^{-1} - \tau_d^{-1}] \cdot [B]^{-1}, \qquad (2)$$

$$k_{-B}^* = \tau_r^{-1}, \qquad (3)$$

where τ_d and τ'_d are the EPSC decay time constants measured in the absence and in the presence of B, respectively, and τ_r is the time constant of the restoration of second ACh response observed in the paired-pulse experiment mentioned above as an interval between two ACh applications. The equation (2) can be used only if k_{+B}^* [B] is much higher than k_{-B}^*. That this condition is fulfilled is evidenced by the fact that the EPSC decay remains single exponential in the presence of B.

Table 2 and Fig. 4 illustrate the relation between k_{+B}^* or K_B^*, on one hand, and ganglion-blocking potencies, on the other hand, for several compounds. The compounds used belong to different chemical groups: symmetrical (tetra-, penta-, hexa- and heptamethonium) and non-symmetrical (trimethylammonium - tetramethylene - isopropylammonium, or IEM-1119), bis-quaternary ammonium compounds and a monocationic tertiary amine, pirilenum. Four of these compounds are selective ganglion-blocking drugs (penta- and hexamethonium, IEM-1119 and pirilenum). Tetra- and heptamethonium were used to compare their effects with those of structurally related IEM-1119 and hexamethonium. The characteristics of tubocurarine effects mentioned above are also shown. To estimate the competitive activity of the drugs used, their non-voltage-dependent effect on the amplitude of EPSC was analysed. The ganglion-blocking activities of the drugs studied were taken from the works of Skok et al., (1984), and Paton and Zaimis (1949; shown in brackets in Table 2). The ganglion-blocking activity of tubocurarine was estimated by Bowman and Webb (1972). All values characterizing the competitive and ganglion-blocking activities are expressed as relative to those in hexamethonium. The EPSC was recorded at -50 mV and 35-37° C.

It has been found that the EPSC amplitude-reducing effect in one group of the compounds studied differs markedly in its voltage dependence from that in other compounds. The hyperpolarization that corresponds to e-fold increase the effect ranges from 219 mV to 264 mV in IEM-1119, tetra- and pentamethonium, while it is only 61 mV in hexamethonium and 52 mV in heptamethonium (Skok et al., 1984). This suggests that the former three compounds reduce the EPSC amplitude through classical competitive effect, while the latter two compounds probably block closed channel. For other compounds listed in Table 2 and Fig. 4 the voltage dependence of the EPSC amplitude-reducing activities was not studied.

Fig. 4 illustrates the statistically significant correlation (r=0.97) between k_{+B}^* and ganglion-blocking activity of all compounds tested (tubocurarine is not included). The correlation between K_B^* and ganglion-blocking activities is statistically non-significant. No correlation has been

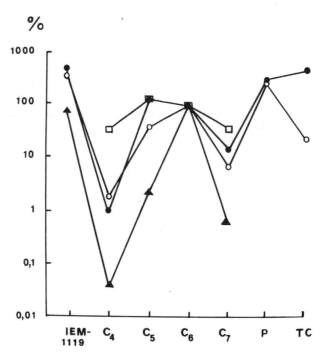

Fig. 4.   Comparison of the ganglion-blocking activity with the channel-
          blocking and competitive activities of IEM-1119, tetramethonium
          (C_4), pentamethonium (C_5), hexamethonium (C_6), heptamethonium
          (C_7), pirilenum (P) and tubocurarine (TC) indicated at abscissa.
          Ordinate, the forward rate constant k^*_{+B} of binding of a blocker
          to an open channel (●), the affinity constant $K^*_B = k^*_B/k^*_{-B}$ (▲),
          the ganglion-blocking activity (o) and the EPSC amplitude-
          blocking activity (□). Values are relative to those for C_6
          (100%; see Table 2).

observed between the EPSC amplitude-reducing activities and ganglion-blocking activities (except in pentamethonium).

Table 2 and Fig. 4 suggest that the rate the blocking agent binds to the open channel is much more important for selective blockade of synaptic transmission than competition of the blocking agent with a transmitter for the channel-gating site. The only exceptions are tubocurarine and, to a lesser extent, pentamethonium, as one could already expect from the results mentioned above. The fact that the k_{-B}^* is less important for the transmission blockade than k_{+B}^* is probably due to much small differences in k_{-B}^* values than k_{+B}^* values, in the time scale of the intervals

Table 1

Effect of Heptamethonium on Single AChR Channel
Activity

Pipette solution contained	Single-channel current (pa)	Single closing (ms)	Single opening (ms)	Burst of openings (ms)
ACh (30 μM) (n = 4)	2.2±0.01	0.15±0.02	2.62±0.11	8.54±1.22
ACh (30 μM) and heptamethonium (30 μM) (n = 4)	2.0±0.07	0.12±0.02	1.00±0.05	1.55±0.13

Table 2

Characteristics of Channel-Blocking and Ganglion-Blocking Effect of Antagonists

Compound	1 k_{+B}^* x $10^6 M^{-1} s^{-1}$	2 k_{-B}^* s^{-1}	3 Reduction of EPSC amplitude%	4 Ganglion-blocking activity%
IEM-1119	27.00±16.10 (n=4)	0.22±0.06 (n=8)	-	470
Tetramethonium (C_4)	0.12±0.04	1.80±0.70	33±5	1(2)
Pentamethonium (C_5)	2.60±0.45 (n=7)	0.62±0.14 (n=4)	115±8 (n=4)	140(80)
Hexamethonium (C_6)	7.30±2.10 (n=6)	0.06±0.01 (n=5)	100±17 (n=6)	100(100)
Heptamethonium (C_7)	0.56±0.16 (n=4)	0.52±0.09 (n=6)	39±5 (n=4)	15(10)
Pirilenum	16.67±6.60 (n=3)	-		280
Tubocurarine	2.0	-		537

Columns 1 and 2 show the values of k_{+B}^* and k_{-B}^* (Selyanko et al., 1984). Columns 3 and 4 show the activities of the drugs relative to that in C_6 to decrease the amplitude of EPSC at concentration 1.10^{-4} M (Selyanko and

Derkach, unpublished) and to block ganglionic transmission, correspondingly. The ganglion-blocking activities shown in brackets were taken
from Paton and Zaimis (1949) while those shown without brackets were from
Skok et al., (1984).

between the subsequent preganglionic stimuli used in transmission-testing
experiments (10 s^{-1}).

The close correlation between k^*_{+B} and ganglion-blocking activities
for tetra-, penta-, hexa- and heptamethonium is supported by the results
obtained by Gurney and Rang (1984) from rat submandibular ganglia. However, the authors did not find such correlation for longer-chain bis-
quaternary ammonium compounds (which are not selective ganglion-blockers).

The facts that the ganglion-blocking activities of some selective
ganglion-blockers correlate with their open-channel blocking activities
and that they block open channels at lower concentrations than are needed
for the competitive effect suggests that their selective transmission-
blocking effect is due to a chemical sensitivity of their open channel
rather than their channel-gating site ("recognition center"). At concentrations higher than those producing open channel-blocking effect some
ganglion-blocking compounds may exhibit mixed effects, open channel-
blocking and, in addition, other effects (hexamethonium). Other compounds
even at high concentrations produce pure competitive effects (trimethaphan: see Ascher et al., 1979; Bobrishev and Skok, unpublished observations).

OPEN CHANNEL BLOCKADE IN OTHER SYNAPSES

A question arises whether the selective blockade of the open channel
can be observed in the synapses other than the synapses in autonomic
ganglia, and whether it can determine there the selective blockade of
synaptic transmission.

Although the effect of tubocurarine on the end-plate, a selective
blocker of neuromuscular transmission in skeletal muscles, is mixed
(competitive and open-channel blocking), its predominant effect at concentration lower than 4.10^{-7} M is competitive (Colquhoun et al., 1979;
Colquhoun and Sheridan, 1982). Steroid anaesthetics, barbiturates and
anti-malarial drugs exhibit here an open channel blockade, but their
blocking effects can be observed only at comparatively high concentrations and are not selective (Adams, 1976; Adams and Feltz, 1980; Gillo
and Lass, 1984).

In contrast to nicotinic neuromuscular transmission in vertebrates,
nicotinic cholinergic interneuronal and neuromuscular transmission in
invertebrates can be selectively blocked through the open-channel blocking mechanism. Hexamethonium is a selective blocker of one type and
tubocurarine of another type of interneuronal transmission in molluscs
achieved via the open channel blockade (Ascher et al., 1978). The same
mechanism has been found in the effect of chlorisondamine, pempidine,
mecamylamine and decamethonium in crayfish neuromuscular transmission
(Lingle, 1983 a, b).

Glutamate receptors in insectal neuromuscular junction can be
selectively blocked by δ-phylanthotoxin (Clark et al., 1982) and by
large-size derivatives of penthamethonium (Magazanik et al., 1984). Both
groups of compounds are powerful open-channel blockers. The same mechanism was suggested for the effects of picrotoxin in GABA receptors, the

effects of strychnine in glycine receptors and the effect of pentobarbital in glutamate receptors in mammalian cultured spinal neurones (Barker, 1972), as well as for the apamin-induced blockade of non-cholinergic and non-adrenergic transmission in smooth muscle (Vladimirova and Shuba, 1978; Banks et al., 1979).

Thus, the open-channel blockade occurs in different types of synapses. However, the contribution of the open-channel blockade to selective blockade of synaptic transmission differs markedly from one type of synapses to another. The reasons for this variability are not yet clear. The end-plate channels which are least susceptible to open-channel blockade possess the shortest mean apparent lifetime. This time, if measured as the end-plate current decay time constant, is 0.3 ms at $39^{\circ}C$ and 1.0 ms at $23^{\circ}C$ in the mouse at the holding membrane potential between -65 mV and -80 mV (Dreyer et al., 1976), and about 1.0 ms in the frog (see Colquhoun, 1979).

This is much less than in those channels where the open channel blockade is more effective (see below). On the other hand, the channels responsible for faster component of biexponential EPSC decay in rat parasympathetic ganglion (6.2 ms at -80 mV and $30^{\circ}C$) are blocked by hexamethonium at higher k_{+B}^{*} (17.9 x 10^6 M^{-1} s^{-1}) than those responsible for slower component (20.0 ms), which are blocked at lower k_{+B} (10.3 x 10^6 M^{-1} s^{-1}: Gurney and Rang, 1984). The k_{+B}^{*} value for hexamethonium in the rabbit sympathetic ganglion (7.3 x 10^6 M^{-1} s^{-1} at -80 mV and $34-37^{\circ}C$: Skok et al., 1984) is similar to that in the molluscan ganglion (7.5 x 10^6 M^{-1} s^{-1} at -80 mV and $12^{\circ}C$: Ascher et al., 1978 b), although the mean apparent channel lifetime in the former case is much shorter (4.5 ms to 5.0 ms: Derkach et al., 1983) than in the latter (27 ms: Ascher et al., 1978 a). These results suggest that although the lowest sensitivity of open channel to blocking drug may be somehow related to very short channel lifetime (0.3 ms to 1.0 ms), there is no clear correlation between these channel properties at longer lifetimes.

The fact that acetylcholine- and glutamate-gated channels which are both permeable to sodium and potassium ions can be selectively blocked by different compounds implies that the sensitivity of the open channels to blocking compounds is not related to their ion selectivities.

An intriguing question is what might be the physiological significance in normal channel activity of a site binding the channel-blocking drugs. One possibility is that the open-channel blockade itself plays no role in normal synaptic transmission (Peper et al., 1982). Another possibility is that this site may normally bind divalent ions. This is consistent with the hypothesis that the duration of channel open state is normally determined by the affinity of an open channel to divalent permeable ions (Ascher et al., 1978 a; Marchais and Marty, 1979). There is evidence that calcium ions play an important role in normal functioning of nicotinic AChR. Each AChR molecule normally binds calcium ions, and releases them as a result of an interaction with ACh (Eldefrawi et al., 1975; Chang and Neumann, 1976). Moreover, several sites in the nicotinic AChR molecule are similar in structure with calcium binding sites of other proteins, and these sites overlap with those tentatively binding selective AChR blockers (Skok, 1985). Ca-binding sites have been found in the ionic channel of the molluscan neuronal AChR (Chemeris et al., 1982; Slater et al., 1984).

Mean apparent channel lifetime is increased by raised $[Ca]_o$ in those AChR channels which are susceptible to open-channel blockade by hexamethonium (autonomic and molluscan ganglion neurones: Marty, 1980; Rang, 1981; Selyanko et al., 1985; Connor et al., 1985) and is non-sensitive to raised $[Ca]_o$ in the end-plate AChR channels which are in-sensitive to open-channel blockade by hexamethonium (Bregestovski et al., 1979, Kuba and Takeshita, 1983). In the rabbit sympathetic ganglion, k_{+B}^* for hexamethonium is strongly decreased by increased $[Ca]_o$ (Selyanko et al., 1985). These data suggest that selective AChR open-channel blockers may bind to the sites which normally bind calcium ions. Sites which normally bind Mg^{2+} ions were found in the open channels of glutamate receptors (Mayer et al., 1984; Nowak et al., 1984).

One more possibility is that an open-channel blocker may bind to the sites that normally bind the transmitter which gates the channel. That ACh may bind to the nicotinic AChR open channel causing an open-channel blockade has been suggested by numerous observations (Sakmann et al,, 1980; Colquhoun and Sakmann, 1983; Sine and Steinbach, 1984). The concentration of ACh necessary to produce such blocking effect (about 1.10^{-4} M: Colquhoun and Ogden, 1984; Sine and Steinbach, 1984) is comparable to that in the synaptic cleft (Kuffler and Yoshikami, 1975).

REFERENCES

Adams, P.R., 1976, Drug blockade of open end-plate channels. J. Physiol. 260:531-552.
Adams, P.R., and Feltz, A. 1980, Quinacrine (mepacrine) action at frog end-plate. J. Physiol. 306:261-281.
Armstrong, C., 1971, Interaction of tetraethylammonium ion derivatives with the potassium channels of giant axons. J. Gen. Physiol. 58:413-437.
Armstrong, C., and Hille, B., 1972, The inner quaternary ammonium ion receptor in potassium channels of the node of Ranvier. J. Gen. Physiol. 59:388-400.
Ascher, P., Marty, A., and Neild, T.O., 1978a, Life-time and elementary conductance of the channels mediating the excitatory effects of acetylcholine in Aplysia neurones.
Ascher, P., Marty, A., and Neild, T.O., 1978b, The mode of action of antagonists on the excitatory response to acetylcholine in Aplysia neurones. J. Physiol. 278:207-235.
Ascher, P., Large, W.A., and Rang, H.P., 1979, Studies of the mechanism of action of acetylcholine antagonists on rat parasympathetic ganglion cells. J. Physiol. 295:139-170.
Banks, B.E.C., Brown, C., Burgess, G.M., Burnstock, G., Claret, M., Cocks, T.M., and Jenkinson, D.H., 1979, Apamine blocks certain neurotransmitter-induced increases in potassium permeability. Nature. 282:415-417.
Barker, J.L., 1975, CNS depressants: effects on post-synaptic pharma-cology. Brain Research. 92:35-55.
Barlow, R.B., Zoller, A., 1964, Some effects of long-chain polymethylene bis-onium salts on junctional transmission in the peripheral nervous system. Brit. J. Pharmacol. 23:131-510.
Blackman, J.C., 1970, Dependence on membrane potential of the blocking action of hexamethonium at a sympathetic ganglionic synapse. Proc. Univ. Otago Med. Sch. 48:4-5.
Bowman, W.C., and Webb, S.W., 1972, Neuromuscular blocking and ganglion blocking activities of some acetylcholine antagonists in the cat. J. Pharmac. Pharmacol. 24:762-772.
Bregestovski, P.D., Miledi, R., and Parker, I., 1979, Calcium conductance of acetylcholine-induced end-plate channels. Nature. 279:638-639.
Chang, H.-W., Neumann, E., 1976, Dynamic properties of isolated acetyl-choline receptor and chemical mediators. Kinetic studies by acetylcholine binding. Proc. Nat'l. Acad. Sci. USA. 73:3364-3368.

Chemeris, N.K., Kazachenko, V.N., Kislov, A.N., and Kurchikov, A.L.,
    1982, Inhibition of acetylcholine responses by intracellular
    calcium in Limnea stagnalis neurones. J. Physiol. 323:1-19.
Clark, R.B., Donaldson, P.L., Gration, K.A.F., Lambert, J.J., Piek, T.,
    Ramsey, R., Apanjer, W., and Usherwood, P.N.R., 1982, Block of
    Locust muscle glutamate receptors by δ-philanthotoxin occurs
    after receptor activations. Brain Research. 24:105-114.
Colquhoun, D., 1979, The link between drug binding and response: theories
    and observations, in: The Receptors. A Comprehensive Treatise.
    Ed. R.D. O'Brien, vol. 1:93-141, Plenum Press, New York.
Colquhoun, D., and Ogden, D.C., 1984, Evidence from single-channel record-
    ing of channel block by nicotinic agonists at the frog neuro-
    muscular junction. J. Physiol. 353:90P.
Colquhoun, D., and Sakmann, B., 1983, Bursts of openings in transmitter-
    activated ion channels. in: Single-Channel Recording. p. 345-
    364, Sakmann, B., and Neher, E., ed., Plennum Press, New York.
Colquhoun, D., and Sheridan, R.E., 1982, The effect of tubocurarine com-
    petition on the kinetics of agonist action on the nicotinic
    receptor. Br. J. Pharmacol. 75:77-86.
Connor, E.A., Neel, D.S., and Parsons, R.L., 1985, Influence of the
    extracellular ionic environment on ganglionic fast excitatory
    postsynaptic currents. Brain Research. 339:227-235.
Derkach, V.A., Selyanko, A.A., and Skok, V.I., 1983, Acetylcholine-
    induced current fluctuations and fast excitatory post-synaptic
    currents in rabbit sympathetic neurones. J. Physiol. 336:511-526.
Derkach, V.A., North, R.A., Selyanko, A.A., and Skok, V.I., 1986, Single
    channels activated by acetylcholine in rat cervical ganglion.
    In press.
Dreyer, F., Muller, K.-D., Peper, K., and Sterz, R., 1976, The m_1 omo-
    hyoideus of the mouse as a convenient mammalian muscle prepara-
    tion. A study of junctional and extrajunctional acetylcholine
    receptors by noise analysis and cooperativity. Pflügers Archiv.
    367:115-122.
Eldefrawi, M.E., Eldefrawi, A.T., Penfield, L.A., O'Brein, R.D., and
    Campen, E., 1975, Binding of calcium and zinc to the acetylcholine
    receptor purified from Torpedo californica. Life Sciences. 16:
    925-935.
Gillo, B., and Lass, Y., 1984, The mechanism of steroid anaesthetic
    (alphxalone) block of acetylcholine-induced ionic currents. Br.
    J. Pharmacol. 82:783-789.
Grob, D., 1967, Neuromuscular blocking drugs. in: Physiological Pharma-
    cology. III/C 389-460, Root, W.S., and Hofman, W.S., ed.,
    Academic Press, New York.
Gurney, A.M., and Rang, H.P., 1984, The channel-blocking action of
    methonium compounds on rat submandibular ganglion cells. Br. J.
    Pharmacol. 82:623-642.
Guyton, A.C., Reeder, R.C., 1950, Quantitative studies on the autonomic
    actions of curare. J. Pharmacol. Exp. Ther. 98:188-194.
Hamill, O.P., Marty, A., Neher, E., Sakmann, B., and Sigworth, F.J., 1981,
    Improved patch-clamp techniques for high-resolution current record-
    ing from cells and cell-free membrane patches. Pflügers Arch.,
    391:85-100.
Hille, B., Courtney, K., and Dum, R., 1975, Rate and site of action of
    local anaesthetics in myelinated nerve fibres. in: Molec.
    mechanisms of Anaesthesia. Progress in Anesthesiology.
Karlin, A., Cox, R., Kaldany, R.-R., Lober, P., and Holtzmanman, E.,
    1983, The arrangement and functions of the chains of the acetyl-
    choline receptor of Torpedo electric tissue. in: Molecular
    Neurobiology. Cold Spring Harbor Symposia on Quantitative Biology.
    48:1-8.

Kuba, K., and Takeshita, S., 1983, On the mechanism of calcium action on the acetylcholine receptor-channel complex at the frog end-plate membrane. Jap. J. Physiol. 33:931–944.

Kuffler, S.W., and Yoshikami, D., 1975. The number of transmitter molecules in a quantum: an estimate from iontophoretic application of acetylcholine at the neuromuscular synapse. J. Physiol. 251:465–484.

Lingle, Ch., 1983, Blockade of cholinergic channels by chlorisondamine on a crustacean muscle. J. Physiol. 339:395–417.

Lingle, Ch., 1983, Different types of blockade of crustacean acetylcholine-induced currents. J. Physiol. 339:419–437.

Magazanik, L.G., Antonov, S.M., and Gmiro, V.E., 1984. Kinetics and pharmacological blockade of glutamate-activated postsynaptic ion channels. Biol. Membr. 1:130–140 (in Russ.)

Marchais, D., and Marty, A., 1979, Interaction of permeant ions with channels activated by acetylcholine in Aplysia neurones. J. Physiol. 297:9–45.

Marty, A., 1980, Action of calcium ions on acetylcholine-sensitive channels in Aplysia neurones. J. Physiol. 76:523–527, Paris.

Mayer, M.L., Westbrook, G.L., and Guthrie, P.B., 1984, Voltage-dependent block by Mg^{2+} of NMDA responses in spinal cord neurones. Nature. 309:261–263.

Nowak, L., Bregestowski, P., and Ascher, P., 1984, Magnesium gates glutamate-activated channels in mouse central neurones. Nature. 307:462–465.

Paton, W.D.M., and Zaimis, E.J., 1949, The pharmacological actions of polymathylene bistrimethylammonium salts. Br. J. Pharmacol. 4:381–400.

Rang, H.P., 1981, The characteristics of synaptic currents and responses to acetylcholine of rat submandibular ganglion cells. J. Physiol. 311:23–55.

Sakmann, B., Patlak, J., and Neher, E., 1980, Single acetylcholine activated channels show burst-kinetics in presence of desensitizing concentrations of agonist. Nature. 286:71–73.

Selyanko, A.A., Derkach, V.A., and Skok, V.I., 1981, Effects of some ganglion-blocking agents on fast excitatory postsynaptic currents in mammalian sympathetic ganglion neurones. in: Adv. Physiol. Sci. 4:329–342, Physiology of Excitable Membranes (ed. J. Salanki).

Selyanko, A.A., Derkach, V.A., and Skok, V.I., 1982, Voltage-dependent actions of short-chain polymethylene bis-trimethylammonium compounds on sympathetic ganglion neurone. J. Auton. Nerv. System, 6:13–21.

Selyanko, A.A., Kerkach, V.A., and Skok, V.I., 1985, The effect of Ca^{2+} ions on the channel-blocking action of hexamethonium in sympathetic ganglion. Proceedings of the USSR Academy of Sciences. 284:225–228, (in Russian).

Sine, S.M., and Steinbach, J.H., 1984, Agonists block currents through acetylcholine receptor channels. Bio. Phys. J., 46:277–283.

Skok, V.I., 1986, Channel-blocking mechanism ensures specific blockade of synaptic transmission. Neuroscience, 17:1–9.

Skok, V.I., Selyanko, A.A., and Derkach, V.A., 1983, Channel-blocking activity is a possible mechanism for a selective ganglionic blockade. Pflügers Archiv. 398:169–171.

Skok, V.I., Selyanko, A.A., Derkach, V.A., Gmiro, V.E., and Lukomskaya, N.Ya., 1984, The mechanisms of ganglion-blocking action of bisammonium compounds. Neirophysiology, 16:46–52.

Slater, N.T., Carpenter, D.O., Haas, H.L., and David, J.A., 1984, Blocking kinetics at excitatory acetylcholine responses on Aplysia neurons. Biophys. J. 45:24–25.

Steinbach, A.B., 1968, A kinetic model for the action of xylocaine on
     receptors for acetylcholine. J. Gen. Physiol. 52:162-180.
Strichartz, G., 1973, The inhibition of sodium currents in myelinated
     nerve by quaternary derivatives of lidocaine. J. Gen. Physiol.
     62:37-54.
Vladimirova, I.A., and Shuba, M.F., 1978, Strychnine, hydrastine and
     apamin effect on synaptic transmission in smooth muscle cells.
     Neirophysiology, 10:295-299.

SYNAPTIC MECHANISMS FOR LONG-TERM POTENTIATION IN SYMPATHETIC GANGLIA

Donald A. McAfee, Clark A. Briggs, Richard E.
McCaman, and David G. McKenna

Division of Neurosciences
Beckman Research Institute of the City of Hope
Duarte, CA 91010

INTRODUCTION - How we study synaptic plasticity.

It is now accepted by neurobiologists and behaviorists alike that one process essential to adaptive behavior is the modulation of synaptic efficacy. This interconnecting link between neurons is clearly the site of multitudinous mechanisms that either regulate the release of neurotransmitters from presynaptic terminals or the efficacy of their reception at the postsynaptic receptor and membrane.

Of these various mechanisms the ones of particular interest to the behaviorist are those that are "use-dependent". That is, those mechanisms which cause changes in synaptic efficacy as a result of the synapse itself being activated. One well known example of such a use-dependent process is posttetanic potentiation (PTP). Induced by a few seconds of repetitive preganglionic stimulation, PTP may enhance transmission 2-3 fold and decay with a time constant of about 5 minutes. Most often studied at the skeletal neuromuscular junction, the phenomenon of PTP has been demonstrated at several vertebrate synapses ranging from autonomic ganglia (Barrett and Magleby, 1976; Zengel et al. 1980) to spinal neurons (Hirst et al., 1981) and cerebral cortex (McNaughton, 1982).

Recent studies in the CNS, especially in the hippocampus, have uncovered not only PTP, but a much more persistent potentiation lasting hours and, in some cases, indefinitely (Bliss and Lomo, 1973). This long-term potentiation (LTP) is also induced by a few seconds of repetitive stimulation, but unlike PTP it is Ca-dependent. LTP may also be induced by stimulus paradigms styled after classical conditioning techniques (Barrionuevo and Brown, 1983). Thus, the CNS location of the phenomenon and the clearly adaptive network supporting its induction, have led many investigators to herald LTP as a fundamental element in the process of learning and memory (Teyler and Discenna, 1984; Swanson et al., 1982).

Unfortunately, the extensive physiological and neurochemical complexities of the CNS have limited the progress in uncovering the cellular mechanisms underlying LTP. However, long-term changes in synaptic efficacy have also been observed in other, more simplified synaptic structures including the crayfish neuromuscular junction (Baxter et al., 1985), Aplysia pedal ganglion (Walters and Byrne, 1985), and the vertebrate sym-

Table 1.   Use-Dependent Potentiation of Transmission

Rabbit Superior Cervical Ganglion 23°C	Average Time Constant
FACILITATION I	50 msec
FACILITATION II	500 msec
AUGMENTATION	15 sec
POSTTETANIC POTENTIATION	150 sec
LONG-TERM POTENTIATION (RAT)	100 minutes

pathetic ganglion (Dunant and Dolivo, 1968; Brown and McAfee, 1982). The superior cervical sympathetic ganglion (SCG) is especially suitable for studies of synaptic efficacy (Larrabee and Posternak, 1952; McAfee, 1982). There are well defined input (preganglionic) and output (postganglionic) nerves. The tissue can be maintained in vitro for a day or more. The rodent ganglia are of a size suitable for combined electrophysiological and biochemical studies. Finally, the sympathetic ganglion has long been known to have several mechanisms governing long-term changes in synaptic excitability (Kuba and Koketsu, 1978).

Preganglionic stimulation results in a potent and rapid nicotinic cholinergic response and a slower muscarinic cholinergic EPSP. Over the last several years we have characterized a number of use-dependent responses in this tissue (Table 1). In collaboration with Dr. Karl Magleby, we were able to demonstrate at least four posttetanic processes in the rabbit superior cervical ganglion which had properties nearly identical to those in the frog neuromuscular junction (Zengel et al., 1980). For example,

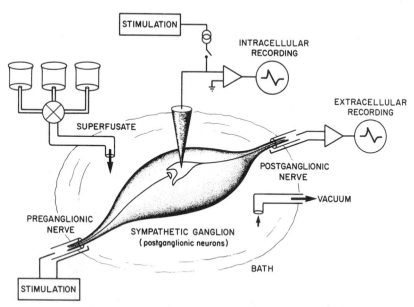

Figure 1. The experimental preparation. This schematic diagram of the superior cervical ganglion in vitro illustrates the arrangement of bipolar stimulating and recording electrodes, of an intracellular microelectrode, and the provisions for admitting physiological salines of various compositions.

they were Ca-independent, and some were modified by Sr and Ba ions. Subsequently, and in collaboration with Dr. Thomas Brown, we were able to demonstrate a much more persistent potentiation of nicotinic transmission in response to a brief preganglionic tetanic stimulus (Brown and McAfee, 1982). This phenomenon lasted for hours or indefinitely, and was Ca-dependent (Briggs et al., 1985a). We have labelled it LTP because of its similarity to the well studied CNS process.

The characteristics and mechanism of this form of LTP have been the main subject of our more recent investigations. As we will demonstrate below, LTP appears to arise as the result of increased release of acetylcholine, and may be a process dependent upon cyclic AMP.

ELECTROPHYSIOLOGICAL CHARACTERIZATION OF LTP

Extracellular recordings are easily effected with isolated rat superior cervical ganglia. Bipolar suction electrodes on the preganglionic (cervical sympathetic) nerve and on the postganglionic (internal carotid) nerve are suitable for stimulation and for the recording of compound action potentials. In addition, the sucrose gap technique allows the recording of membrane potential changes from a large population of postganglionic neurons, including slow potentials and summated EPSP's subthreshold for action potential generation (McAfee, 1982). Figure 1 schematically depicts the arrangement of the preparation for the study of synaptic efficacy.

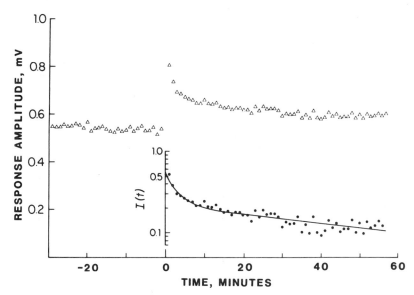

Figure 2. PTP and LTP. This is a plot of the amplitude of the postganglionic compound action potential in response to single preganglionic test stimuli presented every 60 sec. It illustrates the two component decay of enhanced transmission following a 20 Hz for 20 sec preganglionic tetanic stimulus (time = 0). The inset shows the fit of a double exponential model to the decay of potentiation (I(t) = the difference between posttetanic and control responses relative to the control amplitude). Accordingly, the fast component, PTP, decayed with a time constant of 2.5 minutes, while the slow component, LTP, decayed with a time constant of 105 minutes.

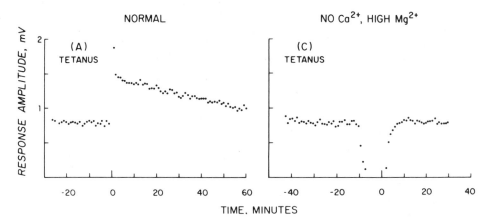

Figure 3. LTP is Ca-dependent. As in Figure 2, this plot of the postganglionic response to test stimuli demonstrates that preganglionic tetany was effective in inducing LTP when the Ca in the Locke solution was 2.2 mM but not when Ca was omitted.

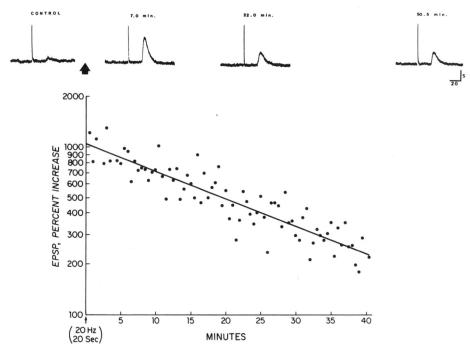

Figure 4. LTP of single neuron EPSP's. The oscillograph traces are selected intracellular records of EPSP's from a single neuron at various times before and after preganglionic tetany (20 Hz/20 sec). The plot of the potentiation of the EPSP illustrates the logarithmic nature of the decay with a time constant of 35 min.

When the preganglionic nerve is stimulated with single shocks at 60 sec intervals, the amplitudes of the postganglionic responses are constant for several hours. These postsynaptic responses are made submaximal either by submaximal stimulation, by stimulation of part of a divided preganglionic nerve, or by weak curarization. Under these conditions a brief preganglionic tetany enhances subsequent postganglionic responses to preganglionic test stimuli for several hours (Figure 2). Nicotinic cholinergic responses are enhanced and atropine does not antagonize this long-term potentiation. Because there is evidence that the muscarinic response can be independently enhanced by such treatments (Libet and Tosaka, 1970; Libet et al., 1975; Volle, 1966), we have included atropine in all of our bathing solutions. Thus, our results are confined to observations of nicotinic cholinergic transmission.

LTP can be induced by stimulus trains ranging from 5 Hz for 5 seconds to 200 Hz for 1 second. Even depolarization for 3 min with 50 mM KCl will enhance transmission for hours. However, such potentiation depends upon the presence of Ca in the bathing medium during the induction of LTP (Figure 3). Increasing the temperature increases the duration of LTP such that at 33°C there is usually no discernable decay of the potentiation over several hours.

PTP can be clearly distinguished from LTP in the data plotted in Figure 2 and in other experiments. Not only does PTP decay 10-fold more quickly than LTP, but it is not very sensitive to reduced Ca in the bathing medium (Zengel et al., 1980). Furthermore, the time constant for PTP decreases as the temperature is raised, whereas the time constant for LTP increases.

Intracellular records of nicotinic EPSP's generated by preganglionic stimulation also show LTP following tetanic stimulation (Figure 4). Unlike experiments utilizing extracellular measurements in which LTP of the population response could always be observed, intracellular measurements from single neurons failed to demonstrate LTP in about 35% of the experiments.

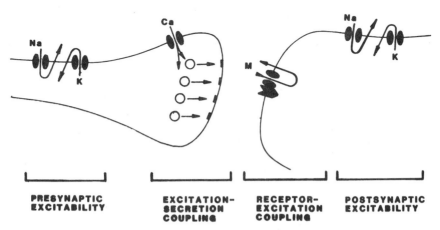

PRESYNAPTIC
EXCITABILITY

EXCITATION-
SECRETION
COUPLING

RECEPTOR-
EXCITATION
COUPLING

POSTSYNAPTIC
EXCITABILITY

Figure 5.   Determining the locus of LTP. This schematic diagram
summarizes the various targets of experiments designed
to uncover the synaptic mechanism generating LTP.

PRESYNAPTIC VS POSTSYNAPTIC LOCUS - ELECTROPHYSIOLOGICAL EVIDENCE

The enhanced synaptic efficacy which we observed could result from either of four general processes (Figure 5): 1. Increased <u>preganglionic excitability</u>. 2. Increased <u>excitation-secretion coupling</u>. 3. Increased <u>receptor-excitation coupling</u>. 4. Increased <u>postsynaptic excitability</u>.

<u>Preganglionic excitability</u>. Our first approach was to determine if preganglionic stimulation produced a residual excitation of the preganglionic nerve. During submaximal stimulation hyperexcitability could result in recruitment of subliminally excited preganglionic axons. However, the amplitude of the preganglionic volley monitored by a third suction electrode on the preganglionic trunk was not augmented during LTP. In addition, we employed supermaximal stimulation to preclude recruitment, but in the presence of 75 uM curare to produce a submaximal postsynaptic response. Even under these conditions preganglionic tetany produced LTP of the postganglionic response.

<u>Postganglionic excitability</u>. Another approach is to avoid presynaptic stimulation altogether, and to determine if direct electrical activation of the postganglionic neuron would induce LTP. Antidromic activation by stimulation of the postganglionic nerve does not induce LTP when tested by extracellular measurements (data not shown). However, it is not clear to what extent antidromically propagated action potentials actually invade the soma-dendritic membrane of the postganglionic neurons. A more certain experiment is to employ intracellular techniques where the excitability of a single postganglionic neuron can be studied. Direct stimulation of the postganglionic neuron through the microelectrode does not induce LTP even though synaptic tetany does (Figure 6). Furthermore, the input impedance of the postganglionic neuron is not affected by the various LTP paradigms suggesting that the passive properties of the postganglionic neuron membrane are not affected in a use-dependent fashion.

<u>Receptor-excitation coupling</u>. We next tested the idea that activation of the nicotinic receptor, rather than membrane depolarization, enhanced receptor-excitation coupling. In one approach, we induced LTP in a ganglion, waited several hours for it to decay away and then bathed the ganglion in media containing the nicotinic antagonist, hexamethonium. This procedure completely blocked postsynaptic responses to preganglionic

A   B   C

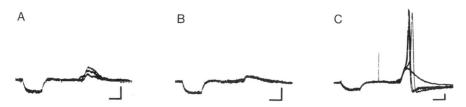

Figure 6.   LTP is not induced by postsynaptic stimulation. A. Three superimposed traces of test EPSP's recorded with an intracellular microelectrode. B. Responses (two traces) 5 minutes after direct tetanic stimulation through the microelectrode (20 Hz/20 sec) to the postganglionic neuron. C. Responses 40 minutes after tetanic stimulation to the preganglionic nerve. Calibration: 5 mV and 20 msec.

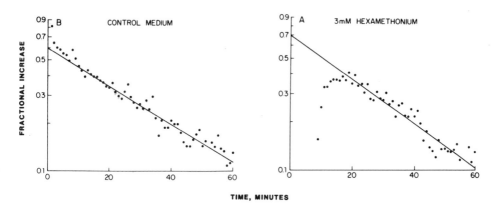

Figure 7. LTP is not induced by nicotinic excitation. The left
    panel is a logarithmic plot of postganglionic responses
    to test stimuli (1/min) following preganglionic tetanic
    stimulation (20 Hz/20 sec). The right panel is similar
    data from the same ganglion after the postganglionic
    responses were completely blocked by hexamethonium (3
    mM). The hexamethonium was washed out immediately
    following the second tetanic stimulation and the suc-
    ceeding recovery of the postganglionic response exceeded
    the pre-hexamethonium control levels. The responses
    then decayed with a time constant (31 min) similar to
    that generated in the absence of hexamethonium (36 min,
    left panel).

stimulation, but when the hexamethonium was washed out immediately
following a second preganglionic tetany the test responses were clearly
potentiated. Furthermore, this potentiation decayed with a time constant
similar to that observed when the ganglion was conditioned in the absence
of nicotinic blockade (Figure 7). This observation indicates that
postganglionic activity in general and nicotinic receptor activation in
particular is not required for LTP.

Carbachol was used to directly activate the nicotinic receptor (10 uM
to 1 mM for 5 min). This procedure resulted in a large depolarization of
the postganglionic neurons but, unlike treatment with high K^+, there was
no subsequent long-term potentiation of the postganglionic response to
test stimulation (Briggs et al., 1985a). Under these conditions, carbachol is likely to depolarize the postsynaptic membrane, whereas, K^+ will
depolarize both pre- and postsynaptic membrane (Brown et al., 1972).

Even though receptor blockade does not prevent LTP, and receptor activation does not induce LTP, it is still possible that the receptor responses are somehow enhanced by preganglionic tetany. Using intracellular
techniques we measured nicotinic responses to preganglionic test impulses
and to directly applied nicotinic agonists ejected from an adjacent
microelectrode (Figure 8). Preganglionic tetanic stimulation enhanced the
synaptic responses but not the responses to direct application of the
nicotinic agonist dimethylphenylpiperazinium (DMPP).

We conclude, therefore, that the conditioning tetanus inducing LTP
does not increase the postsynaptic membrane excitability or the efficacy
of nicotinic receptor activation. Indeed, it would appear that the
postganglionic neuron need not even be activated in any manner. We therefore hypothesize that LTP is due to a presynaptic process resulting in a

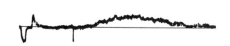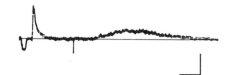

Figure 8. LTP is not accompanied by enhanced nicotinic reception.
The lefthand trace is a record of the postganglionic
intracellular potentials in response first to a single
preganglionic stimulus and then a bolus of DMPP solution
(30 uM), pressure ejected from a micropipette containing
30 uM DMPP. The righthand trace results from the same
paradigm but 70 minutes after preganglionic tetany (20
Hz/20 sec). Note that the EPSP in response to a single
preganglionic test stimulus was enhanced (LTP) by the
tetany, but that the depolarizing response to the direct
application of a nicotinic agonist, DMPP, was not
enhanced. Calibration: 10 mV and 200 msec.

sustained and enhanced release of acetylcholine. That is, LTP is the
result of increased <u>excitation-secretion coupling</u>.

PRESYNAPTIC VS POSTSYNAPTIC LOCUS - DIRECT MEASURE OF ACH

The most direct approach to test the excitation-secretion coupling
hypothesis is to incubate the ganglion in a small volume of Locke solution
and then to periodically collect this bathing medium for assay of released
acetylcholine (Briggs et al., 1985b). Provision was made to simultaneously stimulate and record from the ganglion while in a 50 ul bath.
Physostigmine, a cholinesterase inhibitor, was present to preserve the
released acetylcholine for subsequent assay.

Initial observations demonstrated that acetylcholine is spontaneously
released (0.2 pmol/5 min) without any preganglionic stimulation. However,
when stimulated once every 5 sec (0.2 Hz) the release of acetylcholine was
at least three-times the unstimulated spontaneous rate. A brief period of
preganglionic tetany resulted in a large release of acetylcholine which
did not decay back to the pretetanic levels within an hour (Figure 9).
Simultaneously, the postganglionic responses (0.2 Hz) to the preganglionic
test stimuli were enhanced.

When single test impulses are delivered at 5 minute intervals an
insignificant amount of acetylcholine is added to that already being spontaneously released. Again, the conditioning stimulus to the preganglionic
nerve (20 Hz/20 sec) evoked a large release of acetylcholine, but under
these conditions the release relaxed back to the pretetanic spontaneous
rate (Figure 10). Nevertheless, the postganglionic test responses
generated at 5 minute intervals exhibited LTP following the tetany.

The content of acetylcholine in rat ganglia homogenized following the
induction of LTP was not elevated. Other investigators have observed a
rebound increase in acetylcholine content of feline ganglia following an
hour or more of repetitive stimulation (Birks, 1977; Collier et al.,
1983). They have suggested that the enhanced release following long stimulus periods results from such increased content. However, it is not
clear that such a mechanism also operates in rat sympathetic ganglia
(Briggs et al., 1985b; Sacchi et al., 1978). We conclude therefore, that
the conditioning tetanus enhances evoked release and not spontaneous
release. It appears that ganglionic LTP results from an increase in
excitation-secretion coupling.

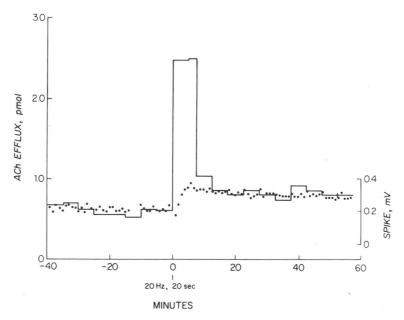

Figure 9. Evoked release of ACh shows LTP. The ganglion was mounted in
stimulating and recording electrodes and maintained in a 50 ul
bath of Locke solution containing physostigmine (20 uM). The
bath was exchanged at five minute intervals and assayed for ACh.
Test stimuli were delivered at 5 sec intervals and evoked release
of ACh at a rate of about twice the spontaneous release.
Preganglionic tetany (20 Hz/20 sec) evoked substantial release of
ACh. Both the ACh release and the action potentials were potentiated 60 min later.

OVERVIEW OF MECHANISM

Figure 11 is a schematic summary of the various processes at the
synapse which can be regulated to modulate synaptic efficacy. We have
identified LTP in sympathetic ganglia as a use-dependent process. However, this does not mean that it is not a receptor-mediated process in the
ganglion or elswhere. "Use" of the synapse could result in release of an
agonist which feeds back onto the terminal to regulate transmitter
release.

This hypothetical substance could be released from the same synapse
activated by the stimulus (homosynaptic), from another type of preganglionic terminal (heterosynaptic), from the postganglionic neuron
(recurrent), from an interneuron, or from non-neuronal tissue. The observation that LTP, unlike other forms of posttetanic potentiation, is Ca-
dependent supports the idea of a released agonist. Since LTP is not
blocked by cholinergic antagonists, such a substance must be other than
acetylcholine.

There is considerable evidence for catecholamine transmission in the
ganglion. Indeed, other investigators have argued that catecholamines
induce long-term potentiation in frog sympathetic ganglia (Kuba et al.,
1981; Kumamoto and Kuba, 1983). We can confirm that beta-adrenergic stimulation enhances synaptic transmission for hours. However, while the
effect of isoproterenol is blocked by propranolol, the effect of preganglionic tetany is not (Figure 12). Therefore, neurogenic LTP, if
receptor mediated, must be induced by a noncholinergic, nonadrenergic

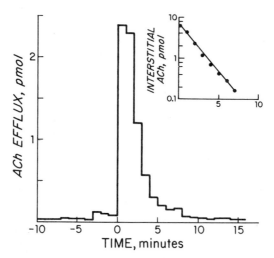

Figure 10. Spontaneous release of actylcholine does not show LTP. As
in Figure 8, the sympathetic ganglion was incubated in 50 ul of
physostigmine containing Locke solution. The solution was
exchanged every 5 minutes and assayed for acetylcholine. At zero
time the preganglonic nerve was stimulated at 20 Hz for 20 sec,
evoking a large release of acetylcholine which decayed to control
levels ($t\frac{1}{2}$ = 1.2 min) as a single exponential function (inset).
Thus spontaneous release of acetylcholine is not potentiated by
the conditioning stimulation. However, single preganglionic test
stimuli at -10,-5, 15 and 30 minutes indicated that the tetanus
did indeed induce LTP.

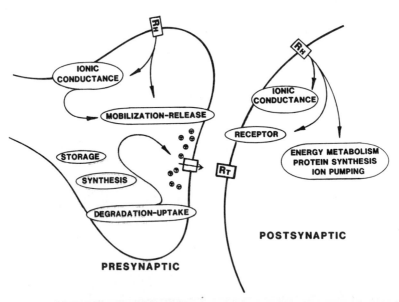

Figure 11. A summary diagram depicting various processes whose regulation
would modulate synaptic efficacy.

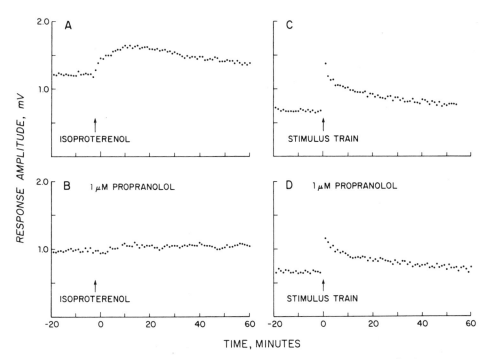

Figure 12. Neurogenic LTP is not beta-adrenergic. Transient exposure to isoproterenol (3 uM) induces a long-lasting
potentiation of responses to presynaptic test stimuli
presented at 60 sec intervals (upper left). This
effect of isoproterenol was blocked by propranolol
(lower left). However, the effect of preganglionic
tetany, which also induces LTP (upper right), is not
blocked by propranolol (lower right).

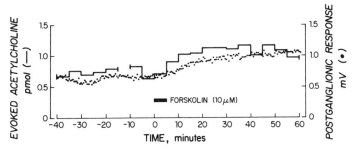

Figure 13. Forskolin may induce LTP. Acetylcholine release and
responses to test stimuli were simultaneously measured
from a ganglion incubated in a 50 ul bath. A 5 minute
exposure to forskolin resulted in a long-lasting potentiation of both release and synaptic response.

substance. This substance X may, however, share a mechanism in common with the beta-agonist -- an intracellular second messenger.

The best known second messenger for catecholamines is cyclic AMP. Accordingly, we tried a number of approaches to test the idea that cyclic AMP could mediate the effect of released substance X. Preganglionic stimulation (10 Hz) augments cyclic AMP in a Ca-dependent fashion, and in a noncholinergic, nonadrenergic fashion. This increase is potentiated by phosphodiesterase inhibitors. Neurogenic LTP is mimicked by exogenous 8-bromo-cyclic AMP and its duration appears to be increased by theophylline. In addition, the adenylate cyclase activator, forskolin, induces a long-lasting potentiation of compound action potentials and release of acetylcholine (Figure 13). Thus it seems plausible that LTP is induced by the release of an unknown agonist, possibly a peptide which acts via cyclic AMP.

SUMMARY

We hypothesize that LTP results from the sustained enhanced release of acetylcholine which follows a brief preganglionic tetany. We propose that the effect of the conditioning tetany may be to evoke the release of some substance, possibly a peptide, which activates a receptor-coupled adenylate cyclase. Cyclic AMP presumably catalyzes the phosphorylation of a protein that regulates some presynaptic process to increase excitation-secretion coupling. Such a model has been articulated for the CNS of Aplysia (Schwartz and Kandel, 1982; Walters and Byrne, 1985), and may even be applicable to the CNS of vertebrates. Beta-adrenergic transmission, known to increase cyclic AMP synthesis, has also been reported to mediate or regulate LTP in the hippocampus (Bliss et al., 1983; Hopkins and Johnston, 1984; but see Dunwiddie et al., 1982). Furthermore, hippocampal LTP is reported by some to result from enhanced release of excitatory neurotransmitter (Dolphin et al., 1982; Skrede and Malthe-Sorensson, 1981). Regardless of how general the ganglion model is for cerebral LTP, an important question remains: What is the role of LTP in autonomic function? Is it possible that LTP functions to enhance stress responses to cardiovascular crises? The answers to such questions remain for studies in vivo of the modulation of ganglionic efficacy.

ACKNOWLEDGEMENTS

The authors wish to recognize Judith Stetzler for expert technical assistance and Sharyn Webb for aid in preparation of this manuscript. This research was supported by grants from NIH, NSF, and the American Heart Association.

REFERENCES

Barrett, E.F., and Magleby, K.L., 1976, Physiology of cholinergic transmission, in: "Biology of Cholinergic Function", A.M. Goldberg and I. Hanin, eds., Raven Press, New York.

Barrionuevo, G., and Brown, T.H., 1983, Associative long-term potentiation in hippocampal slices, Proc. Natl. Acad. Sci. USA, 80:7347.

Baxter, D.A., Bittner, G.D., and Brown, T.H., 1985, Quantal analysis of long-term synaptic potentiation, Proc. Natl. Acad. Sci USA, (in press).

Birks, R.I., 1977, A long-lasting potentiation of transmitter release related to an increase in transmitter stores in a sympathetic ganglion, J. Physiol. 271:847.

Bliss, T.V.P., and Lomo, T., 1973, Long-lasting potentiation of synaptic transmission in the dentate area of the anaesthetized rabbit following stimulation of the perforant path, J. Physiol. 232:331.

Bliss, T.V.P., Goddard, G.V., and Riives, M., 1983, Reduction of long-term potentiation in the dentate gyrus of the rat following selective depletion of monoamines, J. Physiol. 334:475.

Briggs, C.A., Brown, T.H., and McAfee, D.A., 1985a, Neurophysiology and pharmacology of long-term potentiation in the rat sympathetic ganglion, J. Physiol. 359:503.

Briggs, C.A., McAfee, D.A., and McCaman, R.E., 1985b, Long-term potentiation of synaptic acetylcholine release in the rat superior cervical ganglion, J. Physiol. in press.

Brown, D.A., Brownstein, M.D., and Scholfield, C.N., 1972, Origin of the after-hyperpolarization that follows removal of depolarizing agents from the isolated superior cervical ganglion of the rat, Br. J. Pharmacol. 44:651.

Brown, T.H., and McAfee, D.A., 1982, Long-term synaptic potentiation in the superior cervical ganglion, Science 215:1411.

Collier, B., Kwok, Y.N., and Welner, D.A., 1983, Increased acetylcholine synthesis and release following presynaptic activity in a sympathetic ganglion, J. Neurochem. 40:91.

Dolphin, A.C., Errington, M.L., and Bliss, T.V.P., 1982, Long-term potentiation of the perforant path in vivo is associated with increased glutamate release, Nature 297:496.

Dunant, Y., and Dolivo, M., 1968, Plasticity of synaptic functions in the exised sympathetic ganglion of the rat, Brain Res. 10:272.

Dunwiddie, T.V., Roberson, N.L., and Worth, T., 1982, Modulation of long-term potentiation. Effects of adrenergic and neuroleptic drugs, Pharmacol. Biochem. Behav. 17:1257.

Hirst, G.D., 1981, Post-tetanic potentiation and facilitation of synaptic potentials evoked in cat spinal motoneurones, J. Physiol. 321:97.

Hopkins, W.F., and Johnston, D., 1984, Frequency-dependent noradrenergic modulation of long-term potentiation in the hippocampus, Science 226:350.

Kandel, E.R., and Schwartz, J.H., 1982, Molecular biology of learning: modulation of transmitter release, Science 218:433.

Kuba, K., and Koketsu, K., 1978, Synaptic events in sympathetic ganglia, Prog. in Neurobiol. 11:77.

Kuba, K., Kato, E., Kumamoto, E., Koketsu, K., and Hirai, K., 1981, Sustained potentiation of transmitter release by adrenaline and dibutyryl cyclic AMP in sympathetic ganglia, Nature 291:654.

Kumamoto, E., and Kuba, K., 1983, Sustained rise in ACh sensitivity of a sympathetic ganglion induced by post-synaptic electrical activities, Nature 305:145.

Larrabee, M.G., and Posternak, J.M., 1952, Selective action of anesthetics on synapses and axons in mammalian sympathetic ganglia, J. Neurophysiol. 15:91.

Libet, B., Kobayashi, H., Tanaka, T., 1975, Synaptic coupling into the production and storage of a neuronal memory trace, Nature 258:155.

Libet, B., and Tosaka, T., 1970, Dopamine as a synaptic transmitter and modulator in sympathetic ganglia: A different mode of synaptic action, Proc. Natl. Acad. Sci. USA 67:667.

McAfee, D.A., 1982, The superior cervical ganglion: Physiological considerations, in: "Progress in Cholinergic Biology", I. Hanin and A.M. Goldberg, eds., Raven Press, New York.

McNaughton, B.L., 1982, Long-term synaptic enhancement and short-term potentiation in rat fascia dentata act through different mechanisms, J. Physiol. 324:249.

Sacchi, O., Consolo, S., Peri, G., Prigioni, I., Ladinsky, H., and Perri, V., 1978, Storage and release of acetylcholine in the isolated superior cervical ganglion of the rat, Brain Res. 151:443.

Skrede, K.K., and Malthe-Sorenssen, D., 1981, Increased resting and evoked release of transmitter following repetitive tetanization in hippocampus: a biochemical correlate to long-lasting synaptic potentiation, Brain Res. 208:436.

Swanson, L.W., Teyler, T.J., and Thompson, R.F., 1982, Hippocampal long-term potentiation: Mechanisms and implications for memory, Neurosci. Res. Prog. Bull. 20:613.

Teyler, T.J., and Discenna, P., 1984, Long-term potentiation as a candidate mnemonic device, Brain Res. Rev. 7:15.

Volle, R.L., 1966, Modification by drugs of synaptic mechanisms in autonomic ganglia, Pharmacol. Rev. 18:839.

Walters, E.T., and Byrne, J.H., 1985, Long-term enhancement produced by activity-dependent modulation of Aplysia sensory neurons, J. Neurosci. 5:662.

Zengel, J.E., Magleby, K.L., Horn, J.P., McAfee, D.A., and Yarowsky, P.J., 1980, Facilitation, augmentation, and potentiation of synaptic transmission at the superior cervical ganglion of the rabbit, J. Gen. Physiol. 76:213.

MODULATION BY NEUROTRANSMITTERS OF THE NICOTINIC TRANSMISSION
IN THE VERTEBRATES

Kyozo Koketsu

Kurume University
67 Asahi-machi, Kurume 830, Japan

In the course of cholinergic nicotinic transmission, acetylcholine (ACh) is released from presynaptic membrane when an action potential arrives at the cholinergic nerve terminals. ACh released from presynaptic membrane crosses by diffusion the narrow synaptic cleft and reaches the subsynaptic membrane which is a part of postsynaptic membrane. At the subsynaptic membrane ACh binds with the nicotinic ACh receptor which is endowed with a specific and characteristic protein structure. Binding of ACh with specific binding sites of the ACh receptor induces a sudden molecular conformational change of the receptor protein, resulting in an opening of ionic channels which are imbedded in the protein structure of ACh receptor. Opening of the ionic channel causes an influx of extracellular Na^+ and a simultaneous outflux of intracellular K^+. Consequently, the postsynaptic ionic current (excitatory postsynaptic current; EPSC) carried by Na^+ and K^+ initiates the nicotinic excitatory postsynaptic potential (EPSP).

Neuromuscular and ganglionic transmissions constitute well-known examples of typical nicotinic transmission. The end-plate potential (EPP) and the fast excitatory postsynaptic potential (fast EPSP) are nicotinic excitatory postsynaptic potentials (EPSPs) generated in the course of neuromuscular and ganglionic transmission, respectively. Efficiency of nicotinic transmission is represented by the size of the nicotinic EPSPs. The size of EPSP is determined by 1) the amplitude of the EPSC that is, either the end-plate current (EPC) or the fast EPSC in the case of neuromuscular or ganglionic transmission, respectively, and 2) the resting membrane potential and conductance of postsynaptic membrane. The amplitude of EPSC is determined by 1) the amount of ACh released from cholinergic nerve terminals and 2) the sensitivity of the subsynaptic membrane (the ACh receptor) to ACh. Altogether, the size of EPSP, i.e., the efficiency of nicotinic transmission is determined by 1) the amount of ACh released, 2) the sensitivity of subsynaptic membrane, and 3) resting membrane potential and conductance (Koketsu and Karczmar, 1985). EPSPs are modulated by the changes in any of these three factors. These three factors are all modulated by the action of neurotransmitters other than ACh.

As to the first mechanism, the phenomenon of the modulation of the amount of transmitter released from presynaptic nerve terminals has been originally described by J.C. Eccles as he proposed the concept of the presynaptic inhibition in the central nervous system (Eccles, 1964). Subsequently, it was demonstrated that the amount of ACh released from cholinergic nerve terminals is modulated by the action of ACh as well as of many other neurotransmitters. Such a modulation may be termed the presynaptic modulation.

The second concept, that of the modulation of the sensitivity of subsynaptic membrane has been introduced more recently by Koketsu and his collaborators (Koketsu, 1981, 1984; Karczmar et al. 1968). In the case of nicotinic transmission, it was amply demonstrated that the sensitivity of subsynaptic membrane is modulated by the actions of many neurotransmitters other than ACh (Koketsu, 1981, 1984). Such a modulation may be termed the postsynaptic modulation.

Finally, the modulation of the resting membrane potential and conductance of postsynaptic membrane was described in this laboratory and by others (see Koketsu and Akasu, 1985). The size of an EPSP is modulated by other EPSPs and by inhibitory postsynaptic potentials (IPSPs) which are induced simultaneously at the same postsynaptic membrane. These EPSPs or IPSPs cause the change in the resting membrane potential and the conductance of postsynaptic membrane, and thereby modulate the EPSP under observation. Indeed, this constitutes the best known mechanism among those underlying the modulation of the size of an EPSP.

The present communication deals with recent experimental results obtained in our studies of the modulatory effects of neurotransmitters

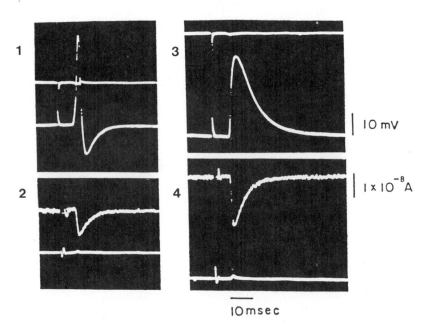

10 msec

Fig. 1.   Records 1 (action potential) and 3 (EPP) were obtained by means of the current-clamp in a bullfrog sympathetic ganglion cell and a frog sartorius muscle fiber, respectively; records 2 (fast EPSC) and 4 (EPC) were obtained by means of the voltage-clamp procedure from a bullfrog sympathetic ganglion cell and a frog sartorius muscle fiber, respectively. Upper and lower traces in each record are current and voltage recordings, respectively.

on the three factors determining the size of the EPPs and the fast
EPSPs. EPPs and fast EPSPs were recorded by intracellular
microelectrodes from end-plate and ganglion cells, respectively. The
EPC and fast EPSC were recorded by means of the voltage-clamp method
(see Fig. 1). Motor nerve-sartorius muscle preparation of frog (<u>Rana
nigromaculata</u>) and lumbar sympathetic ganglia of bullfrog (<u>Rana
catesbeiana</u>) were used in these studies of neuromuscular and ganglionic
transmission, respectively.

1) Modulation of ACh Release

That ACh is acting directly on cholinergic nerve terminals was
suggested by Koketsu and Nishi (1968) who demonstrated a depolarization
of preganglionic nerve terminals via the <u>nicotinic</u> action of ACh. This
finding was confirmed by Ginsborg (1971). No direct evidence was as yet
provided via the measurement of either ACh liberated from the terminal
or the quantal content, to show that the release of ACh is modulated by
the nicotinic action of ACh (see Ginsborg and Guerrero, 1964; Nishi,
1970). On the other hand, that ACh release from preganglionic nerve
terminals is modulated by the <u>muscarinic</u> action of ACh was demonstrated
directly by Koketsu and Yamada (1982). In this experiment it was shown
that the muscarinic action of ACh which caused no depolarization of
cholinergic nerve terminals reduced the quantal content of fast EPSPs
(see Fig. 2).

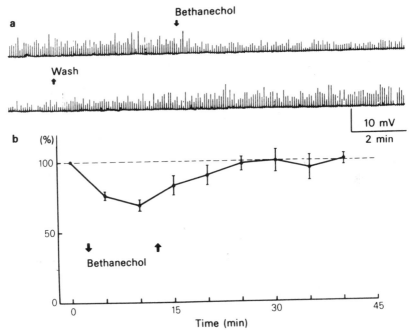

Fig. 2   (a) Effect of bethanechol (10μM) on fast EPSPs in a low
          Ca^{2+}-high Mg^{2+} solution. Arrows indicate the period when
          bethanechol was present in the bathing solution. (b)
          Effect of bethanechol (10μM) on the mean quantal content
          of the fast EPSPs. Ordinate scale shows the percentage
          change in the mean quantal content of fast EPSPs; mean
          values are shown and vertical lines indicate S.E. of the
          mean (n=17). Arrows indicate the period of application
          of bethanechol (Koketsu and Yamada, 1982).

Gamma - aminobutyric acid (GABA) which appears to be the neurotransmitter responsible for presynaptic inhibition, was found to depolarize the membrane of preganglionic nerve terminals (Koketsu et al., 1974). Koketsu et al. (o.c.) suggested that GABA inhibits ACh release from preganglionic nerve terminals without affecting ACh sensitivity of the subsynaptic membrane of ganglion cells. This suggestion was confirmed subsequently (Kato et al., 1978), as GABA was observed to decrease significantly the quantal content of fast EPSPs (see Fig. 3). However, presynaptic inhibitory action of GABA may not depend on depolarization of cholinergic nerve terminals (Kato and Kuba, 1980).

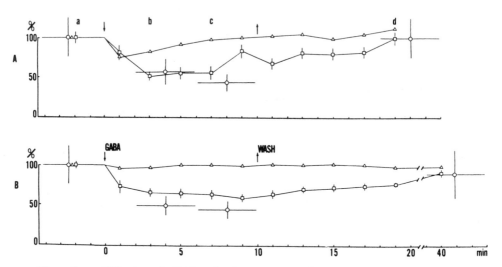

Fig. 3   Effects of GABA   (A,0.1mM; B,1mM) on fast EPSP amplitude
(□), quantal content of fast EPSP (C) and membrane
resistance (▲). The ordinates represent percent changes
of each parameter.   Each square with vertical bars
denotes the mean amplitude and the S.E. of 24 fast EPSPs
recorded for 2 min.   Quantal contents were calculated by
the variance method from 43 fast EPSPs recorded for the
time interval shown by the horizontal bars.   Vertical
bars for open circles are the S.E.s of quantal content.
GABA (0.1 mM) was applied to the ganglion cell in the
experiment shown in A.   Thirty minutes after the
experiment shown in A, the same ganglion cell was treated
again with GABA (1 mM) as shown in B. Note that GABA did
not change the membrane resistance while it reduced
markedly the quantal content (Kato et al., 1978).

It has been known for a long time that catecholamines may facilitate ACh release from cholinergic nerve terminals at the neuromuscular junction (Jenkinson et al., 1968; Kuba, 1970; Kuba and Tomita, 1971), whereas catecholamines depress ACh release in the ganglia (Christ and Nishi, 1971a, b; Dun and Nishi, 1974). However, a marked and sustained facilitation of ACh release by catecholamines was described by Kuba et al., 1981 (Fig. 4). Thus, catecholamines may exert both facilitatory and depressant actions on ACh release (Koketsu, 1981;

Koketsu et al., 1982a). Concentration-dependent dual action was also observed with regard to 5-hydroxytryptamine (5-HT) and histamine. It appears that ACh release is facilitated by relatively small concentrations of these amines, whereas it is depressed with relatively high concentrations (Hirai and Koketsu, 1980; Yamada et al., 1982). Such a dual action of 5-HT is shown in Fig. 5. Dun and Karczmar (1981) have reported, on the other hand, that 5-HT depresses monophasically the ACh release in mammalian sympathetic ganglia.

ACh release from cholinergic nerve terminals is known to be modulated by the action of adenosine triphosphate (ATP). In case of neuromuscular transmission, adenosine and its derivatives were reported to decrease the amount of ACh released from motor nerve terminals (Ginsborg and Hirst, 1972; Ribeiro and Walker, 1975). Similarly, Nakamura et al. (1974) suggested that ATP may decrease ACh release from preganglionic nerve terminals. This suggestion was supported by the demonstration that the quantal content of the fast EPSP was markedly depressed by ATP (Akasu et al., 1982, 1983a; see also Silinsky and Ginsborg, 1983). The membrane of preganglionic nerve terminals is markedly depolarized by ATP, suggesting that the reduction of ACh release from cholinergic nerve terminals may be due to depolarization of nerve terminals (Akasu et al., 1982, 1983a).

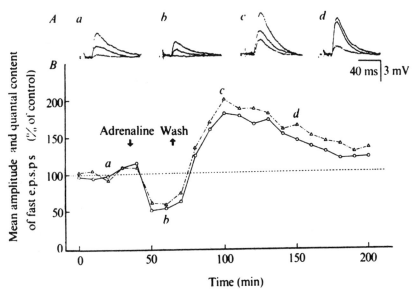

Fig. 4   A, effects of epinephrine (adrenaline, 100μ M) on the fast EPSPs recorded in a low Ca^{2+}-high Mg^{2+} solution. The amplitude of the fast EPSPs in each condition fluctuated in a quantal manner. B, time course of the adrenaline action. Each point represents the mean amplitude (O) or quantal content (Δ) calculated from 200 fast EPSPs. Quantal contents before application of adrenaline ranged from 1.6 to 2.0. Downward and upward arrows indicate the beginning and end, respectively, of the application of adrenaline. The duration of the 'after-potentiation' of the fast EPSP by adrenaline
(continued)

Fig. 4 (continued)
        observed in this cell was apparently shorter than that
        induced by dibutyryl cyclic AMP in another cell (not
        shown). However, this difference seems to be mainly due
        to the variability of cell responses, and not to the
        specificity of the stimulating agents. In fact, a much
        longer potentiation (approximately 5h) by adrenaline was
        seen in other cells. The points a, b, c and d in B
        correspond to a, b, c and d in A, respectively (Kuba et
        al., 1981).

Polypeptides such as substance P or luteinizing hormone releasing
hormone (LH-RH) which are the putative neurotransmitters for the late
slow EPSP of sympathetic ganglion cells, were found to exert a biphasic
action on ACh release, as their low concentrations increase it markedly
while higher concentrations block it (Akasu et al., 1983c).

The mechanism underlying the modulation of the release of ACh from
presynaptic nerve terminals by neurotransmitters is not entirely
clarified. Several mechanisms may be, however, suggested. It is well
known that the release of ACh is triggered by an increase of
intracellular Ca^{2+} concentration which occurs when an action potential
invades nerve terminal membrane. Thus, Ca^{2+} concentration could be a
target of the modulatory effect of a neurotransmitter on ACh release.
For example, a neurotransmitter may modulate action potential-generated
influx of Ca^{2+} by changing the g_{Ca} or other ionic conductances, such as
g_K, or it may modulate the intracellular Ca^{2+} metabolism which mobilizes
intracellularly-stored Ca^{2+}.

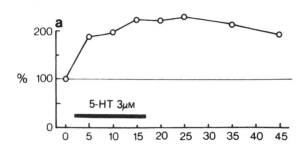

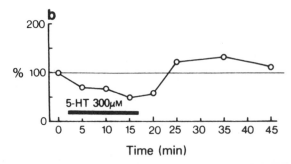

Fig. 5   Effects of 5-hydroxytryptamine (5-HT) on the mean quantal
          content of fast EPSP recorded from bullfrog sympathetic
          ganglion. Abscissae show the percentage change in the
          quantal content of fast EPSP and each circle indicates
                                                         (continued)

Fig. 5 (continued)
the mean quantal content calculated by the variance method. 5-HT at a concentration of $3\mu M$ (1) and $300\mu M$ (b) was added to the perfusate for 15 min. as indicated by the bars (Hirai and Koketsu, 1980).

2) Modulation of ACh Sensitivity of the ACh-Receptor.

The sensitivity of the subsynaptic membrane, i.e., nicotinic ACh receptors to ACh can be estimated by the amplitude of the ACh potential which is induced when a fixed amount of ACh is directly applied to the subsynaptic membrane. Since the amplitude of the ACh potential is the function of the amplitude of ACh current and the resting membrane potential (and conductance), the exact index of the sensitivity of the nicotinic ACh receptor is represented by the amplitude of ACh current which can be measured by voltage-clamp technique.

It is well known that the sensitivity of the nicotinic ACh receptor is inhibited by pharmacological actions of many drugs, chemical and toxins. Indeed, both neuromuscular and ganglionic transmission are depressed or blocked by many substances which are known as nicotinic antagonists or blockers. On the other hand, substances that facilitate the nicotinic transmission by increasing the sensitivity of nicotinic ACh receptors (Kaibara et al., 1978) seem to be available as well. Since all these substances are exogenous, they may be termed as exogenous antagonists or sensitizers.

In the field of physiology, the concept that the sensitivity of the nicotinic ACh receptor could be inhibited or facilitated by actions of endogenous substances, such as neurotransmitters or neurohormones, was proposed by Koketsu and his collaborators (Koketsu, 1981, 1984). The concept states that the sensitivity of the nicotinic ACh receptor can be modulated by actions of many kinds of neurotransmitters under physiological conditions. The mechanism underlying the modulation of the sensitivity of nicotinic ACh receptors by neurotransmitters has been analysed in our laboratory. Interestingly, mechanisms seem to be essentially similar to those of exogenous nicotinic antagonists known in the field of pharmacology. For example, the mode of inhibitory action of neurotransmitters on the nicotinic ACh receptor sensitivity could be divided into two types, namely competitive and non-competitive types, which has been well known in exogenous nicotinic antagonists. Neurotransmitters which inhibit or facilitate the sensitivity of the nicotinic ACh receptor may be termed as endogenous antagonists or sensitizer, respectively.

The possibility that 5-HT might depress the sensitivity of nicotinic ACh receptors was originally suggested by Colomo et al. (1968). This suggestion was confirmed by a recent experiment in which the effect of 5-HT on the dose-response relation between ACh concentration and ACh current was analyzed with respect to end-plate and sympathetic ganglion cells (Akasu et al., 1981a). The sigmoid log dose-response relation was shifted in parallel to the right by 5-HT suggesting that apparent dissociation constant (K_m) for the ACh receptors is increased by 5-HT (see Fig. 6). It was thus concluded that 5-HT might decrease the affinity of ACh to nicotinic ACh receptors, as does d-TC as it blocks the nicotinic transmission in a competitive manner (Akasu et al., 1981a). Similar observations were made with regard to histamine (Ohta et al., 1984).

The depression of the sensitivity of nicotinic ACh receptors by catecholamines was first demonstrated by Koketsu et al. (1982a, b). They showed that the dose-response curve of ACh currents was shifted downward in the presence of catecholamines, suggesting that catecholamines decrease the maximum response (V_{max}) without significantly changing K_m. It was thus concluded that action of catecholamines on the nicotinic transmission is of a non-competitive type (Koketsu et al., 1982a, b). It was also found that polypeptides such as LH-RH and substance P exert similar non-competitive depressant action on the sensitivity of nicotinic ACh receptors (Akasu et al., 1983b, d). The experimental results obtained with LH-RH are shown in Fig. 7.

The sensitivity of nicotinic ACh receptors can be modulated not only by depressant actions of endogenous antagonists but also by facilitatory actions of endogenous sensitizers, such as ATP. The possibility that ATP may facilitate the sensitivity of nicotinic ACh receptors was first pointed out in experiments carried out with frog skeletal muscle end-plate (Ewald, 1976). Detailed analysis of the facilitatory actions of ATP on the nicotinic transmission was made in our laboratory (see Fig. 8) with respect to sympathetic ganglion cells and muscle end-plate (Akasu et al., 1981b; Akasu and Koketsu, 1985). It was also shown that the potentiation of ACh currents by ATP is not due to the anticholinesterase action of ATP. Kinetic analysis of the effect of ATP on the dose-response curve suggested that ATP may increase the ACh sensitivity without changing the affinity (K_m) of ACh for the receptor sites (Akasu et al., 1981b; Akasu and Koketsu, 1985).

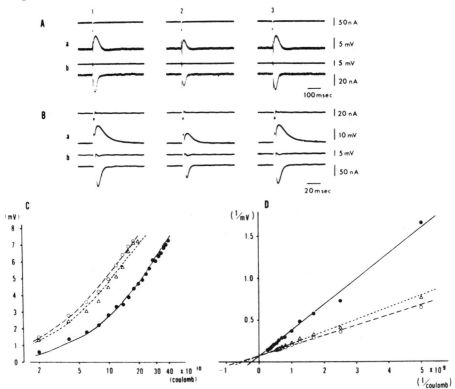

Fig. 6   Depression of the sensitivity of nicotinic ACh receptors by 5-HT (300 μM). Effects of 5-HT on ACh potential produced by iontophoretic application of ACh as well as ACh currents recorded by means of voltage-clamp procedure are shown in A and B; the records were obtained from a bullfrog sympathetic ganglion cell and a frog skeletal muscle cell, respectively. In the records of panel A,
(continued)

Fig. 6 (continued)

two pairs (a and b) of recordings obtained from a single
ganglion cell are shown. The top pair of recordings (a)
represents the iontophretic current (1st tracing) and the
acetylcholine potential (2nd tracing), while the bottom
pair (b) indicates resting membrane potential change (or
its absence) during clamping (1st tracing) and the ACh
current (2nd tracing). Again, in the records of panel B,
two pairs (a and b) of recordings obtained from a single
muscle cell are shown. The top pair of recordings (a)
represents, again, the iontophoretic current and the
acetylcholine potential, while the bottom pair (b)
indicates the resting membrane potential change (or its
absence) during clamping and the ACh current. Records 1,
2 and 3 were taken before, during and after bath-
application of 5-HT which was applied for 5 min in both A
and B. The resting membrane potentials were -60 mV for
the ganglion cell (A) and -90 mV for the muscle cell (B);
they were clamped at the original potential level. It
should be noted that no significant deflection of the
membrane potential occurred during the generation of ACh
current. C and D were obtained from a single sympathetic
ganglion cell (resting membrane potential: -62 mV). C
represents the log dose-response relation between amount
of ACh applied iontophoretically and peak amplitude of
ACh potentials. Open and closed circles represent
recordings obtained before and during a bath-application
of 5-HT, respectively, and open triangles--those obtained
20 min after withdrawal of 5-HT. D is the double-
reciprocal plot constructed from C by assuming $n_H=1$
(Akasu et al., 1981a).

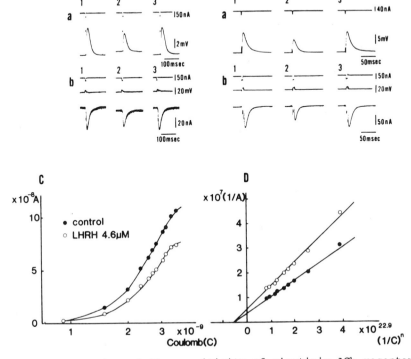

Fig. 7   Depression of the sensitivity of nicotinic ACh receptors
(continued)

Fig. 7 (continued)
    by LH-RH (4.6 μM). ACh potentials (records a in A and B)
    and ACh currents (records b in A and B) were obtained
    from a bullfrog sympathetic ganglion cell (A) and a frog
    sartorius muscle end-plate (B). Top and second traces of
    the records indicate the electrical current used for
    iontophoretic application of ACh and membrane potential
    change, respectively. The three tracings of records b
    indicate the iontophoretic current (top tracing), resting
    membrane potential change (or its absence) during
    clamping (2nd tracing), and ACh current obtained by the
    voltage clamp procedure (3rd tracing). Records 1, 2 and
    3 were taken before, during and after bath-application of
    LH-RH (4.6 μM) which was applied for 10 min in both A and
    B. The resting membrane potentials were -55 mV (A,
    ganglion cell) and -85 mV (B, muscle cell); the clamp was
    applied at these membrane potential levels. C: the log-
    dose relationship between the amount of ACh (expressed in
    terms of iontophoretic current charge in coulombs;
    abscissa) and peak amplitude of ACh currents
    (ordinate). Closed and open circles illustrate results
    obtained before and during bath-application of LH-RH
    (4.6 μM) to frog skeletal muscle end-plate, respective-
    ly. D: kinetic analysis by double reciprocal plot
    constructed from C by assuming Hill number (n) of 2.7.
    Note that LH-RH (2.6 μM) markedly depressed the maximum
    response of the dose-response curve, while it did not
    significantly affect the K_m (Akasu et al., 1983b).

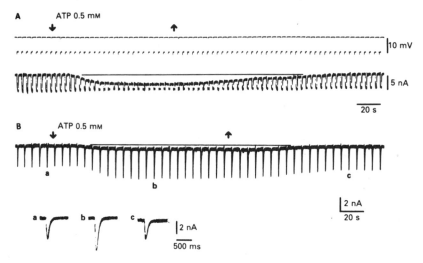

Fig. 8   Effect of ATP (0.5 mM) on the membrane conductance (A)
          and the nicotinic receptor sensitivity (B) of voltage-
          clamped ganglion cells. Records were obtained from the
          same ganglion cell held at -50 mV (A) and -60 mV (B).
          (A) ATP was applied to the superfusing solution between
          arrows. Instantaneous hyperpolarizing command potentials
          (upper trace) were applied to measure conductance changes
          during ATP application. Lower trace indicates the
          membrane current. (B) Carbachol-induced currents were
          produced by repeated (at 0.2 Hz) iontophoretic
                                                       (continued)

Fig. 8 (continued)
application of carbachol pulses (20 nA for 40 ms) to the
ganglion cell. Oscilloscope records a-c were taken at
times indicated on tracing B (Akasu and Koketsu, 1985).

The nicotinic ACh receptor is a macromolecular protein complex that
contains, as its components, the receptor and the channel; it may be
referred to as the receptor-ion channel complex (RICC). Combination of
ACh with specific binding sites of receptor structure leads to opening
of ion channels by a sudden conformational change in the RICC. This
reaction may be expressed as follows:

$$A + R \xrightleftharpoons[k_2]{k_1} AR \xrightleftharpoons[\beta]{\alpha} AR^* \qquad (1)$$

where A and R are ACh and RICC, respectively, and AR and AR^* represent
the closed and the open confirguration of the ion channel,
respectively. K_1, k_2, α, and β are the velocity constants for the
specific processes. Nicotinic EPSC or ACh current is directly
proportional to AR^*.

The ACh current (I) recorded experimentally may be expressed as
follows:

$$I = \underline{a} \cdot N \cdot I_s \qquad (2)$$

where $\underline{a}$ is probability that the ion channel is opened, N is total number
of functioning channels of the RICC to which ACh is being bound and I_s
is ion current passing through a single open channel. I_s may be
expressed as follows:

$$I_s = G_s (E - V) \qquad (3)$$

where G_s is single channel conductance and E and V are the equilibrium
potential of ACh current and resting membrane potential, respectively.

Equations 1-3 predict that a number of mechanisms are available for
the neurotransmitter modulation of the ACh current (I). According to
equation 1 and assuming constant values for A and R, a neurotransmitter
may change the affinity of ACh (k_1/k_2), resulting in the change of AR
and, consequently, of N (eq. 2). Also, a neurotransmitter may change
the value of R by activating "sleeping" or "unavailable" RICCs. A
neurotransmitter may change the probability ($\underline{a}$ in eq. 2; α / β in eq. 1)
of finding the functioning channels in the open state. Finally,
according to equation 3, when V (voltage-clamp condition) remains
constant, a neurotransmitter may change the value of G_s or E by changing
the intracellular ionic concentration.

3) Modulation of Postsynaptic Membrane Potential and Conductance.
It is well known that the slow EPSP, late slow EPSP and slow IPSP
of the sympathetic ganglia are evoked in the postsynaptic ganglion cell
membrane when preganglionic nerves are stimulated (see Fig. 9). The
EPSPs and IPSPs induced not only changes in the membrane potential but
also that in the membrane conductance. Consequently, the fast EPSP is
either facilitated or depressed by these EPSPs and IPSPs in the course
of the nicotinic transmission. The identification of the
neurotransmitters which are responsible for inducing these EPSPs and
IPSPs is not complete as yet. Nevertheless, there is strong evidence
showing that ACh, catecholamines and some polypeptides are the putative
neurotransmitters responsible for initiating these postsynaptic
potentials.

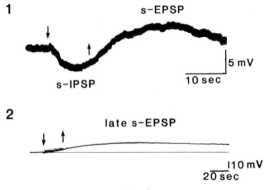

Fig. 9   A slow IPSP followed by a slow EPSP (record 1) and a late
          slow EPSP (record 2) recorded by means of intracellular
          microelectrode from a bullfrog sympathetic ganglion
          cell.   Repetitive stimulation (30/sec) was applied to
          presynaptic nerves between downward and upward arrows;
          record 1 was obtained in the presence of nicotine, and
          record 2 in the presence of nicotine and atropine.

In addition to these neurotransmitters, there are other neurotransmitters or related substances which directly act on the ganglion cell membrane changing the membrane potential and/or conductance; these neurotransmitters are the 5-HT, histamine, ATP, GABA, etc. (see Koketsu and Akasu, 1985).

Summary

Efficiency of the nicotinic transmission is represented by the amplitude of the nicotinic postsynaptic responses, such as the fast EPSPs or EPPs. The amplitude of the nicotinic EPSPs is determined by 1) the amount of ACh released from cholinergic nerve terminals, 2) the sensitivity of nicotinic ACh receptors which are located at the subsynaptic membrane, to ACh, and 3) the resting membrane potential and conductance of the postsynaptic membrane. All these three factors which determine the efficiency of the nicotinic transmission are modulated by the actions of neurotransmitters and putative neurotransmitters. This paper describes the experimental results from this laboratory that support these concepts; a discussion of the mechanisms underlying these modulatory actions of neurotransmitters is provided.

References

Akasu, T., Hirai, K. and Koketsu, K., 1981a.   5-Hydroxytryptamine
    controls ACh-receptor sensitivity of bullfrog sympathetic ganglion
    cells. Brain Res., 211:217-220.

Akasu, T., Hirai, K. and Koketsu, K., 1981b. Increase of acetylcholine-receptor sensitivity by adenosine triphosphate: a novel action of ATP on ACh-sensitivity. Br. J. Pharmacol., 74:505-507.

Akasu, T., Hirai, K. and Koketsu, K., 1982. Modulatory effect of ATP on the release of acetylcholine from presynaptic nerve terminals in bullfrog sympathetic ganglia. Kurume Med. J., 29:75-83.

Akasu, T., Hirai, K. and Koketsu, K., 1983a. Modulatory actions of ATP on nicotinic transmission in bullfrog sympathetic ganglia. In: "Physiology and Pharmacology of Adenosine Derivatives". J.W. Daly, Y. Kuroda, J.W. Phillis, H. Shimizu and M. Ui, eds., Raven Press, New York.

Akasu, T., Kojima, M. and Koketsu, K., 1983b. Luteinizing hormone-releasing hormones modulates nicotinic ACh-receptor sensitivity in amphibian cholinergic transmission. Brain Res., 279:347-351.

Akasu, T., Kojima, M. and Koketsu, K., 1983c. Modulatory effect of luteinizing hormone-releasing hormone and substance P on the nicotinic transmission in bullfrog sympathetic ganglia. J. Physiol. Soc. Japan, 45:418.

Akasu, T., Kojima, M. and Koketsu, K., 1983d. Substance P modulates the sensitivity of the nicotinic receptor in amphibian cholinergic transmission. Br. J. Pharmacol., 80:123-131.

Akasu, T. and Koketsu, K., 1985. Effect of adenosine triphosphate on the sensitivity of the nicotinic acetylcholine-receptor in the bullfrog sympathetic ganglion cell. Br. J. Pharmacol., 84:525-531.

Christ, D.D. and Nishi, S., 1971a. Site of adrenaline blockade in the superior cervical ganglion of the rabbit. J. Physiol., 213:107-117.

Christ, D.D. and Nishi, S., 1971b. Effects of adrenaline on nerve terminals in the superior cervical ganglion of the rabbit. Br. J. Pharmacol., 41:331-338.

Colomo, F., Rahamimoff, R. and Stefani, E., 1968. An action of 5-hydroxytryptamine on the frog motor end-plate. Eur. J. Pharmacol., 3:272-274.

Dun, N.J. and Karczmar, A.G., 1981. Evidence for a presynaptic inhibitory action of 5-hydroxytryptamine in a mammalian sympathetic ganglion. J. Pharmacol. Exp. Ther. 217:714-718.

Dun, N.J. and Nishi, S., 1974. Effects of dopamine on the superior cervical ganglion of the rabbit. J. Physiol., 239:155-164.

Eccles, J.C., 1964. "The Physiology of Synapses", Springer-Verlag, Berlin.

Ewald, D.A., 1976. Potentiation of postjunctional cholinergic sensitivity of rat diaphragm muscle by high-energy-phosphate adenine nucleotides. J. Membr. Biol., 29:47-65.

Ginsborg, B.L., 1971. On the presynaptic acetylcholine receptors in sympathetic ganglia of the frog. J. Physiol., 216:237-246.

Ginsborg, B.L. and Guerrero, S., 1964. On the action of depolarizing drugs on sympathetic ganglion cells of the frog. J. Physiol., 172:189-206.

Ginsborg, B.L. and Hirst, G.D.S., 1972. The effect of adenosine on the release of the transmitter from the phrenic nerve of the rat. J. Physiol., 224:629-645.

Hirai, K. and Koketsu, K., 1980. Presynaptic regulation of the release of acetylcholine by 5-hydroxytryptamine. Br. J. Pharmacol., 70:499-500.

Jenkinson, D.H., Stamenovic, B.A. and Whitaker, B.D.L., 1968. The effect of noradrenaline on the end-plate potential in twitch fibres of the frog. J. Physiol., 195:743-754.

Kaibara, K., Kuba, K., Koketsu, K. and Karczmar, A.G., 1978. The mode of action of fluoride ions on neuromuscular transmission in frogs. Neuropharmacology, 17:335-339.

Karczmar, A.G., Koketsu, K. and Soeda, S., 1968. Possible reactivating and sensitizing action of neuromyally acting agents. Int. J. Neuropharmacol., 7:241-252.

Kato, E. and Kuba, K., 1980. Inhibition of transmitter release in bullfrog sympathetic ganglia induced by γ-aminobutyric acid. J. Physiol., 298:271-283.

Kato, E., Kuba, K. and Koketsu, K., 1978. Presynaptic inhibition by -aminobutyric acid in bullfrog sympathetic ganglion cells. Brain Res., 153:398-402.

Koketsu, K., 1981. Electropharmacological actions of catecholamine in sympathetic ganglia: Multiple modes of actions to modulate the nicotinic transmission. Jpn. J. Pharmacol. (Suppl.), 31:27-28.

Koketsu, K., 1984. Modulation of receptor sensitivity and action potentials by transmitters in vertebrate neurones. Jpn. J. Physiol., 34:945-960.

Koketsu, K. and Akasu, T., 1985. Postsynaptic modulation. In: "Autonomic and Enteric Ganglia", A.G. Karczmar, K. Koketsu and S. Nishi, eds., pp. 273-295, Plenum Press, N.Y.

Koketsu, K., Akasu, T., Miyagawa, M. and Hirai, K., 1982a. Modulation of nicotinic transmission by biogenic amines in bullfrog sympathetic ganglia. J. Auton. Nerv. Syst., 6:47-53.

Koketsu, K. and Karczmar, A.G., 1985. General concepts of ganglionic transmission and modulation. In: "Autonomic and Enteric Ganglia", A.G. Karczmar, K. Koketsu and S. Nishi, Eds., pp. 63-77, Plenum Press, N.Y., 1985.

Koketsu, K., Miyagawa, M. and Akasu, T., 1982b. Catecholamine modulates nicotinic ACh-receptor sensitivity. Brain Res., 236:487-491.

Koketsu, K. and Nishi, S., 1968. Cholinergic receptors at sympathetic preganglionic nerve terminals. J. Physiol., 196:293-310.

Koketsu, K., Shoji, T. and Yamamoto, K., 1974. Effects of GABA on presynaptic nerve terminals in bullfrog (Rana catesbiana) sympathetic ganglia. Experientia, 30:382-383.

Koketsu, K. and Yamada, M., 1982. Presynaptic muscarinic receptors inhibiting active acetylcholine release in the bullfrog sympathetic ganglion. Br. J. Pharmacol., 77:75-82.

Kuba, K., 1970. Effects of catecholamines on the neuromuscular junction in the rat diaphragm. J. Physiol., 211:551-570.

Kuba, K., Kato, E., Kumamoto, E., Koketsu, K. and Hirai, K., 1981. Sustained potentiation of transmitter release by adrenaline and dibutyryl cyclic AMP in sympathetic ganglia. Nature, Lond., 291:654-656.

Kuba, K. and Tomita, T., 1971. Noradrenaline action on nerve terminal in the rat diaphragm. J. Physiol., 217:19-31.

Nakamura, M., Hayashi, H., Hirai, K. and Koketsu, K., 1974. Effect of ATP on sympathetic ganglion from bullfrogs. Jpn. J. Pharmacol. (Suppl.), 42:134.

Nishi, S., 1970. Cholinergic and adrenergic receptors at sympathetic preganglionic nerve terminals. Fed. Proc., 29:1957-1965.

Ohta, Y., Ariyoshi, M. and Koketsu, K., 1984. Histamine as an endogenous antagonist of nicotinic ACh-receptor. Brain Res., 306:370-373.

Ribeiro, J.A. and Walker, J., 1975. The effects of adenosine triphosphate and adenosine diphosphate on transmission at the rat and frog neuromuscular junctions. Br. J. Pharmacol., 54:213-218.

Silinsky, E.M. and Ginsborg, B.L., 1983. Inhibition of acetylcholine release from preganglionic frog nerves by ATP but not adenosine. Nature, Lond., 305:327-328.

Yamada, M., Tokimasa, T. and Koketsu, K., 1982. Effects of histamine on acetylcholine release in bullfrog sympathetic ganglia. Eur. J. Pharmacol., 82:15-20.

NICOTINIC RECEPTORS ON VAGAL NERVE TERMINALS IN THE ATRIUM

S. Nishi, H. Higashi, K. Odawara and K. Ikeda

Department of Physiology, Kurume University School of

Medicine, Kurume, Japan

The presence of presynaptic receptors on cardiac sympathetic nerve terminals, which control the release of norepinephrine, has been described by various investigators (see Starke, 1977; Westfall, 1977; Lokhandwala, 1979). In contrast there has been no report of presynaptic receptors at the vagal (parasympathetic) nerve terminals in the heart. This paper reports that the vagal postganglionic nerve terminals in the atrium of the guinea-pig are endowed with nicotinic receptors and that activation of these receptors results in the facilitation of acetylcholine (ACh) release from the nerve terminals (Odawara and Nishi, 1980). It will be also reported that the terminal nicotinic receptors are quite similar in pharmacological characteristics to the extrasynaptic nicotinic receptors on the postganglionic neuron soma.

EFFECTS OF NICOTINE ON ATRIAL CONTRACTION

Nicotine has long been characterized as having two phases of action on the heart, initially negative and subsequently positive chrono- and inotropic effects (Giotti, 1954; Trendelenburg, 1960; Leaders and Long, 1962; Chiang and Leaders, 1965; Khan, Mantegazza and Piccinini, 1965; Barnett and Benforado, 1966; Long and Gross, 1966; Bhagat, Robinson and West, 1967; Chiang and Leaders, 1968). Examples of such nicotinic actions are shown in Fig. 1. As seen in Fig. 1A, nicotine (0.2 mM) applied to a guinea-pig atrial strip which was electrically driven at 120 beats/min caused a marked inhibition of contractions which was followed by a long-lasting augmentation. A similar effect was observed on spontaneously beating atrial strips (Fig. 1B) in which nicotine reduced the amplitude as well as the frequency of contractions before it exerted the augmentative action. The nicotine-induced enhancement has been elucidated to be due to the action of norepinephrine liberated from sympathetic nerve terminals by the applied nicotine (see Lokhandwara, 1979). It has been generally assumed that the mechanism of the nicotine-induced inhibition of the atrium is due to the activation of nicotinic receptors located on the intramural ganglion cells; this activation leads to the liberation of ACh and to inhibition of atrial contractions (Giotti, 1954; Leaders and Long, 1962; Chiang and Leaders, 1965; Khan, Mantegazza and Piccinini, 1965; Long and Gross, 1966). Atropine abolished the nicotine-induced inhibition of atrial contractions.
        The inhibitory action of nicotine on the atrium was examined to determine whether it was indeed due to activation of nicotinic receptors

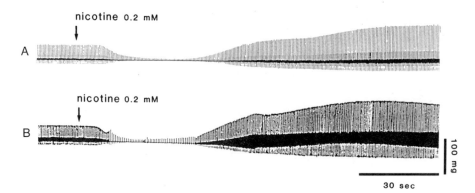

nicotine 0.2 mM

A

nicotine 0.2 mM

B

100 mg

30 sec

Fig. 1. Nicotine-induced changes of atrial contractions. (A)
Electrically driven contractions of an isolated
guinea-pig atrial strip. (B) Spontaneous contractions
of another atrial strip. Nicotine (0.2 mM) was
applied continuously beginning at the arrow.

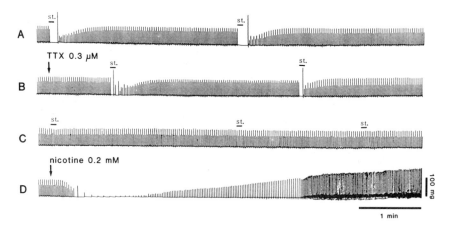

st.   st.

A

TTX 0.3 µM   st.   st.

B

st.   st.   st.

C

nicotine 0.2 mM

D

100 mg

1 min

Fig. 2. Effect of nicotine on atrial contractions following
application of tetrodotoxin. (A-D) Continuous records
of spontaneous contractions of an isolated guinea-pig
atrial strip with the left and right vagal nerves
intact. Vagal nerves were stimulated at each bar
(marked by st.) with 1 msec current pulses at 20 Hz
for 5 sec. Tetrodotoxin (TTX, 0.3 µM) was added to
the perfusing solution at the arrow on record B.
Nicotine (0.2 mM) was added at the arrow on record D.

on the ganglion cell bodies by observing the atrial effect of nicotine
after the blockade of nerve conduction by tetrodotoxin.

NICOTINE ACTIONS AFTER TETRODOTOXIN

As illustrated in Fig. 2, the spontaneous contractions of the
isolated atrium were markedly inhibited following stimulation (st.) of
both the left and right vagus nerves innervating the atrium. This vagal
inhibition gradually decreased during the application of tetrodotoxin
(TTX, 0.3 µM), and disappeared in about 10 min. Nicotine (0.2 mM)
applied at this time was still able to produce the inhibition and

subsequent augmentation of atrial contractions, as markedly as before tetrodotoxin treatment. Parenthetically, TTX (0.3 µM) abolished the action potentials of guinea-pig cardiac ganglion cells in a few min. It appears, therefore, that nicotine can exert its action after blockade of the nerve conduction. This implies that nicotine acts directly on the postganglionic nerve terminals via the appropriate receptors and liberates ACh which then inhibits atrial contractions by activating muscarinic receptors on the muscle fibers.

PHARMACOLOGICAL CHARACTERISTICS OF NICOTINIC RECEPTORS AT VAGAL NERVE TERMINALS

The minimal effective concentration of nicotine which produced the negative inotropic effect was approximately 50 µM, and the ED50 of nicotine-induced inhibition was approximately 0.6 mM. The negative inotropic action of nicotine was antagonized by ganglionic blocking drugs, and the order of blocking potency appeared to be d-tubocurarine (ED50: 0.21 µM), hexamethonium (0.51 µM), pentamethonium (0.63 µM) and decamethonium (1.03 µM). These antinicotinic agents also antagonized the vagal inhibition with the same order of potency as above but with a much weaker effectiveness. In the case of bisquaternary blocking agents, the ED50 for blocking the vagal inhibition appeared to be 150 to 300 times that for decreasing the nicotinic inhibition of atrial contractions. Such findings indicate that the inhibition of atrial contractions by bath applied nicotine is primarily due to activation of terminal nicotinic receptors since the inhibition is eliminated by 1 uM hexamethonium which has little effect on nicotinic ganglionic transmission.

It should be added that during the course of this experiment it was observed that propranolol, a beta-adrenergic blocking drug, depressed the effect of nicotine on atrial contractions, reversibly and dose-dependently.

COMPARISON BETWEEN NICOTINIC RECEPTORS AT THE NERVE TERMINALS AND SOMATA

The findings in the preceding section indicate that the nicotinic receptors at the vagal nerve terminals differ in certain aspects from the nicotinic receptors at the neuron somata. To examine such a possibility, the effects of propranolol and ganglionic blocking agents on the nicotinic responses of the cardiac intramural ganglion cells were studied.

Propranolol markedly depressed the nicotinic ACh-potential, ionophoretically induced, while it only slightly depressed the fast EPSP (nicotinic in nature) elicited by focal stimulation, as illustrated in Fig. 3. When the fast EPSP was elicited in a hyperpolarized cell (e.g., -80 mV), a hump was observed on the falling phase of the EPSP near its peak. Thus the falling phase had an initial fast decay phase, a hump and a slow decay phase. The latter phase had a time constant of about 15 msec. Propranolol (5-10 µM) eliminated the hump and the slow decay phase, leaving only the fast phase with a time constant of 5 to 8 msec. Thus the EPSP was considerably shortened by propranolol.

The order of blocking potency for the ganglionic blocking drugs in depressing the ACh-potential appeared to be the same as that observed for the decrease in the nicotine-induced inhibition of atrial contraction; d-tubocurarine (ED50: 3.2 µM), hexamethonium (7.1 µM), pentamethonium (8.5 µM) and decamethonium (15.8 µM). The same order of potency of the blocking drugs was also found for their depressant actions on the fast EPSP, but the ED50 of each drug for depressing the fast EPSP was 10 to 30 times higher than that for decreasing the ACh-potential.

The selective depression of the ACh-potential by propranolol and the characteristic difference between the ACh-potential and the fast EPSP in their susceptibilities to ganglionic blocking agents suggest that there

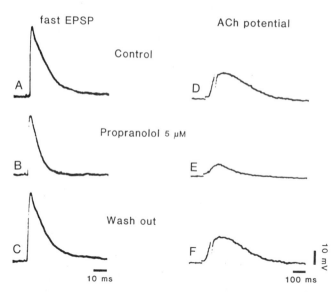

Fig. 3. Effect of propranolol on the nicotinic responses of
intramural ganglion cells in the isolated guinea-pig
atrial strip. (A-C) Fast EPSPs of a neuron were
elicited at a membrane potential of -80 mV by single
focal stimuli. (D-F) Resposes (ACh-potentials) of
another neuron at a resting membrane potential of -52
mV were induced by ionophoretic application of ACh by
pulses of 0.1 μA with a duration of 30 msec. Records
were taken intracellularly before (A and D) and 5 min
after (B and E) the addition of propranolol to the
perfusing solution and 15 min after (C and F) washing
out propranolol.

are extrasynaptic nicotinic receptors in addition to the subsynaptic
nicotinic receptors. Propranolol might specifically depress the
ionophore or an allosteric site of the extrasynaptic receptor. The hump
and the slow decay phase of the fast EPSP might be formed by activation
of the extrasynaptic receptors by the liberated ACh, and the short-
lasting EPSP remaining in the presence of propranolol might be generated
by activation of the subsynaptic receptors. Furthermore, the resemblance
of the terminal nicotinic receptors to the somatic extrasynaptic
nicotinic receptors in the susceptibility to propranolol and also their
higher sensitivity to ganglionic blocking agents than the subsynaptic
receptors indicate that the terminal nicotinic receptors are similar to
the somatic extrasynaptic receptors.

MECHANISM UNDERLYING THE LIBERATION OF ACh BY NICOTINE

It is reasonable to assume that activation of terminal nicotinic
receptors produces a depolarization of the presynaptic membrane that
liberates ACh. If the activated receptors were to become permeable to Ca
ions, in addition to Na and K ions, similar to the end-plate membrane
(Takeuchi, 1963); the liberation of ACh from the vagal nerve terminal
would be substantially facilitated. It is well established that ACh
liberation from cholinergic nerve terminals is dependent on the entry of
Ca ions (Katz and Miledi, 1965).
Fig. 4A shows that the ACh-potential could be induced in a solution
in which the Na ions of the Krebs solution were iso-osmotically

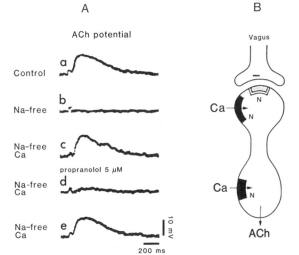

Fig. 4. ACh-potentials of an intramural ganglion cell in the isolated guinea-pig atrial strip. Records a and b were taken before and 5 min after the perfusing Krebs solution was switched to a solution in which all the Na ions were replaced with Tris. Record C was taken 8 min after perfusing with a Krebs solution in which the Na ions were substituted with Ca ions. Records d and e were taken 5 min after addition of propranolol (5 μM) to the Na-free Ca solution and 13 min after washing out propranolol with the Na-free Ca solution. (B) This is a schematic drawing of the subsynaptic (dotted) and extrasynaptic (black) nicotinic receptors on the neuron soma and the nicotinic receptor (black) at the axon terminal, with arrows showing Ca entry and ACh liberation.

substituted with Ca ions. The ACh-potential in the Ca medium was markedly depressed and shortened by propranolol (5 μM). The results indicate that the ACh-potential in the Ca medium was generated primarily by activation of the extrasynaptic ACh receptors and that the activated extrasynaptic receptor membrane became permeable to Ca ions. Based on the similarity of the nicotinic receptors on the neuron soma and its axon terminals, as mentioned above, it would be expected that the terminal receptors would also become permeable to Ca ions during activation by ACh (Fig. 4B). The resultant entry of Ca ions into the axoplasm would effectively facilitate the liberation of ACh by the terminal membrane depolarization brought about primarily by an increased membrane conductance to Na and K ions (Takeuchi and Takeuchi, 1960).

CONCLUSIONS

These results suggest that the atrial inhibition by nicotine is mainly due to activation of nicotinic receptors at the vagal postganglionic nerve terminals and that the vagal postganglionic neuron somata possess subsynaptic as well as extrasynaptic nicotinic receptors. The latter become permeable to Ca ions when activated by ACh. The terminal nicotinic receptors may have similar characteristics. The entry of Ca ions through the activated nicotinic receptor membrane of the terminals would facilitate the liberation of ACh. It is, as yet, difficult to speculate on the physiological significance of the excitatory nicotinic receptors at the vagal postganglionic nerve terminals, because ACh has multiple sites of action in the heart. It is known that the ACh liberated from the vagal nerve terminals effectively reaches the sympathetic nerve terminals (see Lokhandwara, 1979). It would be reasonable to assume, therefore, that the liberated ACh reaches the sites on the vagal terminals more easily than on the sympathetic terminals and facilitates the ACh liberation. This would provide an additional mechanism for the predominance of vagal influence over sympathetic influence on the heart.

REFERENCES

Barnett, A., and Benforado, J. M., 1966, The nicotinic effects of choline esters and of nicotine in guinea-pig atria, J. Pharmacol. Exp. Ther., 152:29.

Bhagat, B., Robinson, I. M., and West, W. L., 1967, Mechanism of sympathomimetic responses of isolated guinea-pig atria to nicotine and dimethylphenylpiperazinium iodide, Br. J. Pharmacol., 30:470.

Chiang, T. S., and Leaders, F. E., 1965, Mechanism for nicotine and DMPP on the isolated rat atria-vagus nerve preparation, J. Pharmacol. Exp. Ther., 149:225.

Chiang, T. S., and Leaders, F. E., 1968, Dissociation between the initial negative and the secondary positive chronotropic and inotropic effects of nicotine in rat atria, Arch. Int. Pharmacodyn. Ther., 172:347.

Giotti, A., 1954, Interaction of nicotine and eserine, ephedrine, atropine, hexamethonium and adrenaline in isolated guinea-pig auricles, Br. J. Pharmacol., 9:15.

Katz, B., and Miledi, R., 1965, The effect of calcium on acetylcholine release from motor nerve endings, Proc. R. Soc. B, 161:496.

Khan, M., Mantegazza, P., and Piccinini, F., 1965, Effect of low temperatures on the responses of guinea-pig isolated atria to nicotine and to sympathetic and parasympathetic stimulation, Br. J. Pharmacol., 25:119.

Leaders, F. E., and Long, J. P., 1962, Mechanism of the positive chronotropic response to nicotine, J. Pharmacol. Exp. Ther., 137:206.

Lokhandwala, M. F., 1979, Presynaptic receptor systems on cardiac sympathetic nerves, Life Sci., 24:1823.

Long, J. P., and Gross, E. G., 1966, Studies on the auricular stimulating action of nicotine, Arch. Int. Pharmacodyn. Ther., 161:30.

Odawara, K., and Nishi, S., 1980, The nicotinic receptors at the vagal efferent nerve terminals in the atrium, Proc. Internat. Union Physiol. Sci., 14:618.

Starke, K., 1977, Regulation of noradrenaline release by presynaptic receptor systems, Rev. Physiol. Biochem. Pharmacol., 77:1.

Takeuchi, N., 1963, Effects of calcium on the conductance change of the end-plate membrane during the action of transmitter, J. Physiol. (Lond.), 167:141.

Takeuchi, A., and Takeuchi, N., 1960, On the permeability of end-plate membrane during the action of the transmitter, J. Physiol. (Lond.), 154:52.

Trendelenburg, U., 1960, The action of histamine and 5-hydroxytryptamine on isolated mammalian atria, J. Pharmacol. Exp. Ther., 130:450.

Westfall, T. C., 1977, Local regulation of adrenergic neurotransmission, Physiol. Rev., 57:659.

MUSCARINIC RECEPTOR ACTIVATION UNDERLYING THE SLOW INHIBITORY
POSTSYNAPTIC POTENTIAL (S-I.P.S.P.) AND THE SLOW EXCITATORY
POSTSYNAPTIC POTENTIAL (S-E.P.S.P.)

P. Shinnick-Gallagher, K. Hirai and J.P. Gallagher

Department of Pharmacology
University of Texas Medical Branch
Galveston, TX 77550

INTRODUCTION

Subtypes of muscarinic receptors were initially proposed
by Birdsall and colleagues based on the different affinity
states for agonists and for the selective muscarinic antagonist, pirenzepine (Birdsall et al., 1978; Hammer et al.,
1980). Biochemical and physiological analyses of subtypes of
muscarinic receptors have been unable to compare receptors at
the same site or location but mediating functionally different
events.

Parasympathetic ganglia lying on top of the cat urinary
bladder possess two functionally different synaptic potentials
mediated through muscarinic receptors (Gallagher et al., 1982),
the s-i.p.s.p. and s-e.p.s.p. We examined in detail the
characteristics of the muscarinic slow potentials, particularly the s-i.p.s.p., and compared the muscarinic receptors
underlying slow synaptic inhibition and slow synaptic
excitation on the same parasympathetic neuron.

RESULTS AND DISCUSSION

The cholinergic potentials recorded in bladder parasympathetic ganglia in response to preganglionic nerve stimulation can be mimicked by acetylcholine (ACh) applied iontophoretically (Figure 1). The time course of the slow
response is longer than that resulting from nerve stimulation,
probably reflecting a larger amount of ACh release from the
iontophoretic pipette. This sequence of events is similar to
that recorded in amphibian and certain mammalian sympathetic
ganglia (see reviews Nishi, 1974; Kuba and Koketsu, 1978; see
also Libet, 1970; Weight and Votava, 1971; Weight and Padjen,
1973; Cole and Shinnick-Gallagher, 1980, 1981, 1984; Horn and
Dodd, 1981; Dodd and Horn, 1983). Amphibian parasympathetic
ganglia appear to be different since they possess only a
f-e.p.s.p. and a s-i.p.s.p. (Hartzell et al., 1977).

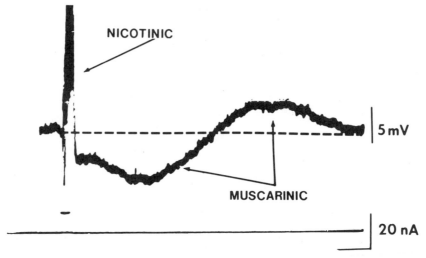

Fig. 1. Nicotinic and muscarinic receptor activation following
ACh iontophoresis. A series of iontophoretic pulses
(10 Hz for 1 sec) were applied to a cell not treated
with antagonists. A sequence of three potentials,
the fast depolarization resulting in action potential
firing (peaks cut off), a slow hyperpolarization and
finally a slow depolarization could all be recorded.
The slow potentials in this cell were not masked by
the presence of action potentials (from Griffith, Wm.,
Ph.D. dissertation).

Types of cholinergic slow potentials

In bladder parasympathetic ganglia different sequences of
muscarinic slow potentials are recorded in different cells on
stimulating the preganglionic nerve trunk (Figure 2). Some
cells exhibited only one of the muscarinic slow potentials
whereas other cells have both responses. No slow potentials
were observed in about 8% of the cells. Since these latter
neurons exhibited resting potentials of -55mV or > and could
fire direct action potentials in response to cathodal current
injection, they appeared not be be damaged (Griffith et al.,
1980). These muscarinic slow potentials were usually elicited
with repetitive stimulation of 40 Hz for 250 msec to 1 sec;
however, slow potentials can also be observed with a single
stimulus pulse.

Because of the relative paucity of cells having only a
s-e.p.s.p. it has not been possible to analyze the membrane
mechanism of action of the s-e.p.s.p. in these parasympathetic
neurons. We investigated in more detail the mechanism of
action of the muscarinic s-i.p.s.p.

The s-i.p.s.p., a Ca^{++}-dependent K^+ conductance

Membrane conductance is increased during the s-i.p.s.p.
(Figure 3). Electrotonic potentials resulting from anodal
current passed across the membrane are decreased in amplitude
during a s-i.p.s.p. indicating an increase in membrane con-

246

ductance (15 ± 2%, n=12; Fig 3A). This change in membrane
conductance is sufficient enough to shunt the membrane such
that directly evoked action potentials are blocked during the
s-i.p.s.p. (Figure 3B).

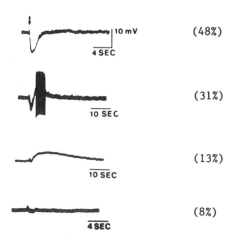

(48%)

(31%)

(13%)

(8%)

Fig. 2. Different types of intracellularly recorded slow
potentials. The arrow indicates the onset of train
stimulation (40 Hz for 1 sec). All tracings are
recorded after nicotinic receptor blockade (C_6,
500μM); (from Griffith, Wm.; Ph.D. dissertation).

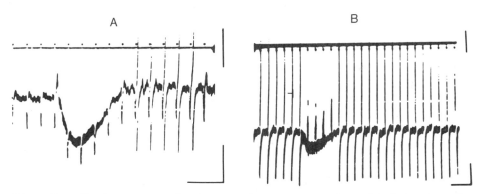

Fig. 3. Membrane conductance change associated with the slow
potentials. A. Downward deflections indicate
electrotonic potentials. During the nerve-evoked
s-i.p.s.p., a decrease in the size of the anelectro-
tonic pulses can be recorded. An increase in membrane resistance as well as action potential firing
occurs during the s-e.p.s.p. (calibration: 5mV x 1
sec, 1 nA). B. Direct action potentials were elicited
through the recording electrode (peaks cut off) and
the increase in membrane conductance during the
s-i.p.s.p. blocked the action potentials (calibration:
5 mV x 1 sec, 1 nA). A and B train stimulation is
40 Hz for 1 sec.

We have reported previously that the s-i.p.s.p. and ACh induced hyperpolarization are decreased in amplitude with membrane hyperpolarization, nulled around -100mV, and reversed polarity on further hyperpolarization. The hyperpolarization induced by muscarine applied in a pressure pulse is enhanced in a low K^+ (0.47 mM) solution and depressed in high K^+ (20 mM) suggesting K^+ ion mediates the s-i.p.s.p. (Figure 4). Furthermore, the reversal potential for the s-i.p.s.p. is shifted to the right in a Nernstian fashion in a high K^+ (20mM) solution (Gallagher et al., 1982). These data indicated that the s-i.p.s.p. was mediated by an increase in K conductance. The ionic mechanism of the muscarinic action of ACh underlying the s-i.p.s.p. in these parasympathetic ganglia is similar to that reported in amphibian sympathetic (Horn and Dodd, 1983) and parasympathetic (Hartzell et al., 1977) as well mammalian sympathetic (Cole and Shinnick-Gallagher, 1984) ganglia.

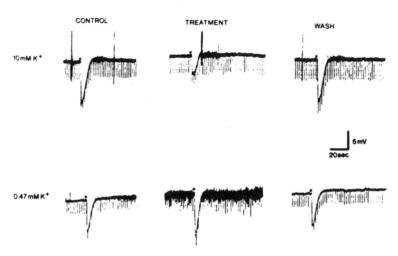

Fig. 4. The muscarine-induced hyperpolarization is dependent on extracellular K^+ concentration. Muscarine (100μM) was applied to a parasympathetic neuron in a pressure pulse (10 psi, 50 msec; dot) in control Krebs solution (left traces) and 5 min after adding Krebs solution having altered extracellular K^+ concentrations (middle traces). Right traces indicate muscarine hyperpolarizations 5 mins after washing with control Krebs solution. Resting membrane potential was held at -57mV (top records) and -60mV (bottom records).

We futher analyzed the s-i.p.s.p. in parasympathetic neurons by characterizing pharmacologically the potassium channels underlying the s-i.p.s.p. Three potassium channel antagonists blocked the muscarine or ACh-induced hyperpolarization, namely, barium (100μM), an antagonist of several different K^+ conductance mechanisms, intracellular cesium, also a blocker of numerous outward K currents, and 4-aminopyridine (4-AP) an antagonist of the A-current, a transient outward potassium current, and other outward currents.

The calcium dependency of the muscarine hyperpolarization was tested directly using low Ca or Ca-free media and Ca antagonists. Initially, we observed that the muscarinic hyperpolarization persisted for 30 min in a low Ca media (Figure 5) when synaptic transmission, the s-i.p.s.p., was completely blocked in 5 min under similar conditions (not shown). Subsequently, we found that the muscarinic hyperpolarization was blocked in a Ca^{2+}-free solution and by treatment with Ca^{2+} antagonists Mn^{2+}, Co^{2+} and Cd^{2+} (Nakamura et al., 1985). These data clearly demonstrated that the muscarinic hyperpolarization was a Ca-dependent K conductance.

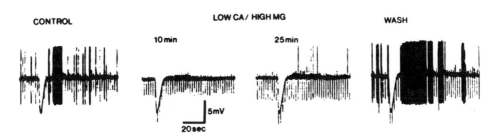

Fig. 5. Effect of low Ca/high Mg on the muscarine hyperpolarization. Muscarine (100 µM) was applied in a pressure pulse (10 p.s.i., 50 msec) in control Krebs solution and in Krebs solution containing 0.25mM Ca and 3.56mM Mg. Right record indicates muscarine hyperpolarization 5 min after washing with control Krebs solution. Resting membrane potential was held at -55mV throughout.

Interestingly, antagonists of calcium-dependent K currents ($I_{K,Ca}$) in other autonomic neurons, namely tetraethylammonium (TEA) (Adams et al., 1982; Galvan and Sedlmeir, 1985; Belluzzi et al., 1985) and apamin, the neurotoxin from bee venom (Figure 6; Pennefather et al., 1985) did not block the ACh hyperpolarization produced by puff application (2M, 20 p.s.i., 100 msec) or s-i.p.s.p. recorded in the presence of hexamethonium (0.5mM) in cat bladder parasympathetic ganglia. These data suggested that the s-i.p.s.p. recorded from cat parasympathetic ganglia may be mediated through a K channel not of the calcium-dependent type.

Other experiments using intracellular injection of EGTA, a chelator of calcium, and TMB-8 (1-10 µM), a blocker of Ca influx and Ca release from sarcoplasmic reticulum, supported the notion that the s-i.p.s.p. was mediated by a calcium dependent K conductance. Both treatments depressed and/or completely blocked the s-i.p.s.p. and muscarinic hyperpolarization. Furthermore, intracellular injection of Ca induced a hyperpolarization which mimicked the s-i.p.s.p. recorded in the same neuron (Figure 7). Altogether these data indicate that the s-i.p.s.p. is mediated by a Ca^{++}-dependent K conductance, which does not appear to be similar to the conductances associated with classical voltage-activated Ca^{++}-dependent K^+ currents (I_K,Ca).

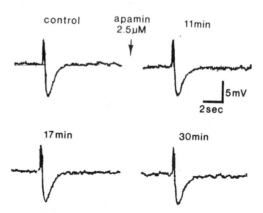

Fig. 6.   Apamin (2.5 μM) does not block the s-i.p.s.p. S-i.p.s.p.s were elicited by stimulating the preganglionic nerve trunk (40 Hz, 250 msec). Apamin was added to the Krebs solution as indicated (arrow). Resting potential = -60mV throughout.

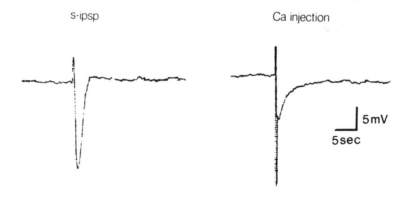

Fig. 7.   Comparison of time course of s-i.p.s.p. and a Ca-induced hyperpolarization. S-i.p.s.p. is evoked by stimulating the preganglionic nerve trunk at 40 Hz for 1 sec. Ca (2M, $CaCl_2$) was injected (5nA; 100 msec) through one barrel of a double-barrelled microelectrode; the other barrel was used for recording. Resting membrane potential = -60mV.

Muscarinic receptors underlying the s-i.p.s.p. and s-e.p.s.p.

Initially, muscarinic receptors were divided into sub-types based on the different affinities of agonists in the cerebral cortex (Birdsall et al., 1978). We tested whether a variety of muscarinic agonists could selectively activate either hyperpolarization or depolarization in cat parasympathetic neurons (Table 1). Superfusion of muscarinic agonists at 1μM concentration induced hyperpolarizations and depolarizations. Because of the small number of cells having only a s-e.p.s.p. (<10%) it was not possible to compare the ED_{50}'s of the agonists on depolarizations in the absence of hyperpolarizations. It was apparent, however, that the agonists do not discriminate between muscarinic excitation and muscarinic inhibition in parasympathetic neurons.

Table 1.

COMPARISON OF MEMBRANE EFFECTS OF MUSCARINIC AGONISTS

	Hyperpolarization	Depolarization
	mV	mV
Muscarine	(10/11)	(1/11)
1 μM	6.5±4.6	1
n = 11		
MCN-343	(13/13)	(6/13)
1 μM	7.2±5.5	2.6±1.7
n = 13		
Oxotremorine	(13/13)	(4/13)
1 μM	5.4±3.2	1.8±0.85
n = 13		
Pilocarpine	(14/17)	(12/17)
1 mM	4.9±2.8	3.1±2.4
n = 17		
ACh	(9/10)	(7/10)
1 μM	6.8±3.7	1.4±0.8
n = 10		
nerve stim.	(19/19)	(10/19)
n = 19	12.3±4.4	2.1±1.1

Data obtained in presence of 1 mM hexamethonium. Nos. in parenthesis represent fraction of cells responding.

Analysis of the s-i.p.s.p. requires the use of nicotinic antagonists to eliminate the recording of the nicotinic f-e.p.s.p., which obscures or interferes with the recording of s-i.p.s.p. We compared the effects of hexamethonium (C_6), d-tubocurarine (d-Tc), mecamylamine (Mec), nicotine (N), and TEA on the hyperpolarizations induced by muscarine (100μM) applied in a pressure pulse. At a low concentration (10μM) the classical nicotinic antagonists, C_6, N, d-Tc and Mec, had no effect on a muscarine hyperpolarization. However, at higher concentrations (100-300μM) these antagonists depressed (25 to 65%; figure 8) the muscarinic hyperpolarization. d-TC (300μM) completely blocked the muscarine hyperpolarization. In recent experiments we found that TEA (1mM) did in fact block a hyperpolarization produced by pressure application of muscarine (100μM, 10 p.s.i., 50 msec) and the s-i.p.s.p., recorded in the presence of mecamylamine (10μM). This concentration of mecamylamine completely blocked f-e.p.s.p.'s. Other nicotinic ganglionic blocking agents, particularly gallamine, have been used to classify subtypes of muscarinic receptors (Mitchelson, 1984). Thus, it is possible that the site of action of TEA (1mM) in antagonizing the muscarine hyperpolarization may be at the receptor level.

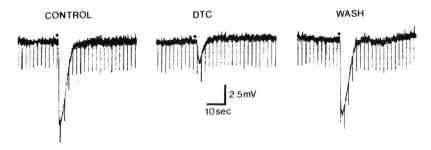

CONTROL   DTC   WASH

2.5mV
10sec

Fig. 8. Effect of d-tubocurarine (d-TC) on the muscarine-
induced hyperpolarization. Muscarine (100µM) was
applied (dot) in a pressure pulse (10 p.s.i., 50
msec) in control Krebs solution, 5 min after adding
d-TC (100µM) to the Krebs solution and 5 min after
washing with control Krebs solution. Resting membrane potential = -53mV throughout.

Subtypes of muscarinic receptors have also been classified on the basis of their ability to bind the muscarinic
antagonist, pirenzepine (Hammer et al., 1980). We examined
pirenzepine to test whether it could discriminate between
the muscarinic receptors underlying synaptic inhibition and
synaptic excitation in parasympathetic neurons.

We tested the effect of pirenzepine on the concentration-
response relationship for muscarine (Figure 9). Pirenzepine
shifted the concentration-response curve to the right indicating competitive inhibition. Based on this and other data,
the pA_2, the antagonist affinity value, determined for
pirenzepine was 8.7. This value is close to the pA value
of 8.4 for pirenzepine determined for the muscarine depolarization in rat sympathetic ganglia (Brown et al., 1980).
These data though preliminary suggest that the s-i.p.s.p.
in parasympathetic ganglia is mediated by an M_1-receptor
which is similar to the receptor underlying the s-e.p.s.p. in
rat sympathetic ganglia. This data together with our findings
with various muscarinic antagonists suggest that both the
s-i.p.s.p. and s-e.p.s.p. are mediated through M_1 receptors
and that pirenzepine can not distinguish between the muscarinic receptors mediating muscarinic excitation and muscarinic inhibition in autonomic neurons.

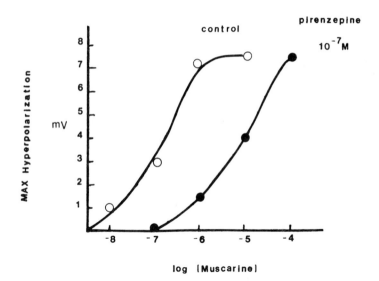

Fig. 9.   Pirenzepine shifts the concentration-response relationship for muscarine in a competitive manner.
dl-Muscarine was applied in the superfusing Krebs
solution in the presence (solid circles) and
absence (open circles) of pirenzepine (0.1μM).
Resting membrane potential was held at -65mV
throughout.

Bibliography

Adams, P.R., Brown, D.A. and Constanti, A. 1982. M-currents
    and other potassium currents in bullfrog sympathetic
    neurones. J. Physiol. (Lond.) 330: 537-572.
Belluzzi, O., Sacchi, O. and Wanke, E. 1985. Identification
    of delayed potassium and calcium currents in the rat sym-
    pathetic neurone under voltage clamp. J. Physiol. (Lond.)
    358: 109-129.
Birdsall, N.J.M., Burgen, A.S.V. and Hulme, E.C. 1978. The
    binding of agonists to brain muscarinic receptors.
    Molec. Pharmacol. 14: 723-736.
Brown, D.A., Forward, A. and Marsh, S. 1980. Antagonist
    discrimination between ganglionic and ileal muscarinic
    receptors. Br. J. Pharmacol. 71: 362-364.
Cole, A.E. and Shinnick-Gallagher, P. 1980. Alpha-
    adrenoceptor and dopamine receptor antagonists do not
    block the slow inhibitory postsynaptic potential in sym-
    pathetic ganglia. Brain Res., 187, 226-230.
Cole, A.E. and Shinnick-Gallagher, P. 1981. Comparison of
    receptors mediating the catecholamine hyperpolarization

and slow inhibitory postsynaptic potential in sympathetic ganglia. J. Pharmacol. Exp. Ther., 217: 440-444.

Cole, A.E. and Shinnick-Gallagher, P. 1984. Muscarinic inhibitory transmission in mammalian sympathetic ganglia mediated by increased potassium conductance. Nature 307: 270-271.

Dodd, J. and Horn, J.P. 1983. Muscarinic inhibition of sympathetic C neurones in the bullfrog. J. Physiol. (Lond.) 334: 271-291.

Gallagher, J.P., Griffith, W.H. and Shinnick-Gallagher, P. 1982. Cholinergic transmission in cat parasympathetic neurones. J. Physiol. (Lond.) 332: 96-109.

Galvan, M. and Sedlmeir, C. 1984. Outward currents in voltage-clamped rat sympathetic neurones. J. Physiol. (Lond.) 356: 115-133.

Griffith III, Wm. H. 1980. The Physiology and Pharmacology of a Mammalian Parasympathetic Ganglion. Ph.D. Dissertation. University of Texas, Galveston, TX.

Griffith, W.H., Gallagher, J.P. and Shinnick-Gallagher, P. 1980. An intracellular investigation of the cat vesical pelvic ganglion (VPG). J. Neurophysiol. 43: 343-354.

Hammer, R., Berrie, C.P., Birdsall, N.J.M., Burgen, A.S.V. and Hulme, E.C. 1980. Pirenzepine distinguishes between different subclasses of muscarinic receptors. Nature 283: 90-92.

Hartzell, H.C., Kuffler, S.W., Stickgold, R., Yoshikami, D. 1977. Synaptic excitation and inhibition resulting from direct action of acetylcholine on two types of chemoreceptors on individual amphibian parasympathetic neurones. J. Physiol (Lond.) 271: 817-846.

Hirai, K., Nakamura, T., and Shinnick-Gallagher, P. and Yoshimura, M. Slow inhibitory potential mediated by a calcium-dependent potassium conductance in cat bladder parasympathetic ganglia. Submitted.

Horn, J.P. and Dodd, J. 1981. Monosynaptic muscarinic activation of K^+ conductance underlies the slow inhibitory postsynaptic potential in sympathetic ganglia. Nature. 292: 625-627.

Kuba, K. and Koketsu, K. 1978. Synaptic events in sympathetic ganglia. Prog. Neurobiol. 11: 77-169.

Libet, B. 1970. Generation of slow inhibitory and excitatory postsynaptic potentials. Fed. Proc. 29: 1945.

Mitchelson, F. 1984. Heterogeneity in muscarinic receptors: evidence from pharmacologic studies with antagonists. TIPS, Supp.: 12-16.

Nishi, S. 1974. Ganglionic Transmission. In: The Peripheral Nervous System, ed. J.I. Hubbard, pp. 225-255, Plenum Press.

Pennefather, P., Lancaster, B. and Adams, P.R. and Nicoll, R.A. 1985. Two distinct Ca-dependent K currents in bullfrog sympathetic ganglion cells. Proc. Natl. Acad. Sci. 82: 3040-3044.

Ramey, G. and Lazdunski. M. 1984. The coexistence in rat muscle cells of two distinct classes of Ca^{2+}-dependent K^+ channels with different pharmacological properties and different physiological functions. Biochem. Biophys. Res. Comm. 118: 669-674.

Weight, F.F. and Votava, J. 1970. Slow synaptic excitation in sympathetic ganglion cells: Evidence for synaptic inactivation of potassium conductance. Science 170: 755.

ALTERATION OF THE GANGLIONIC FAST EPSC BY ANTICHOLINESTERASE DRUGS OR

PROTEASE TREATMENT

R.L. Parsons, D.S. Neel, A.B. MacDermott[*] and E.A. Connor[†]

Dept. of Anatomy & Neurobiology, College of Medicine
The University of Vermont, Burlington, VT 05405
[*]Neurophysiology Lab, NINCDS-NIH
Bethesda, MD 20205
[†]Dept. of Neurobiology, Stanford University, Stanford, CA 94305

INTRODUCTION

Vertebrate autonomic ganglia have proven to be useful model systems for electrophysiological studies of both voltage-dependent and chemically-gated membrane conductances (2, 19). We have used amphibian autonomic ganglia to analyze the basic biophysical and pharmacological properties of nicotinic, cholinergic-gated responses at a vertebrate neuronal synapse (7, 10, 21). Our results have demonstrated that the ganglionic fast excitatory postsynaptic current (EPSC) differs from the more extensively studied muscle end-plate synaptic current (EPC) in its time course, voltage dependence, and response to a number of pharmacological interventions (7-11, 21).

In an earlier study, we initiated experiments to investigate the role of acetylcholine removal by cleft cholinesterase on the EPSC time course (21). Our results suggested that complex changes in EPSC characteristics occurred in the presence of two commonly used anticholinesterase (anti-AChE) agents, neostigmine and physostigmine. Further, particularly in the case of physostigmine, the alterations in EPSC time course could not be explained simply on the basis of anticholinesterase action (21). Multiple actions of many different anti-AChE drugs on muscle EPCs have recently been reported (3, 12-15, 17, 18, 22). Consequently, in this study, we have compared the influence of three different anti-AChE drugs (neostigmine, physostigmine, and methane sulfonal fluoride) to that of protease treatment on the ganglionic EPSC. Our results demonstrate that all of these treatments have multiple effects on the ganglionic EPSC.

MATERIALS AND METHODS

All experiments were done "in vitro" using B cells of the VIII, IX, and X sympathetic ganglia from the bullfrog, Rana catesbeiana, maintained in a HEPES-buffered solution (mM: NaCl 120, KCl 2.5, $CaCl_2$ 1.8, HEPES 1.0; pH = 7.3). Stock solutions of all three drugs (neostigmine bromide, Sigma Chemical Co.; physostigmine sulfate, Calbiochem; methane sulfonal fluoride (MSF), Eastman) and protease (type IV or type VII, Sigma Chemical Co.) were made up daily and diluted just prior to use.

Individual cells were voltage-clamped using a two-electrode voltage clamp as described previously (7, 21). Individual EPSCs were collected during constant preganglionic stimulation ($\sim$0.4Hz), digitized, averaged, and analyzed for peak current amplitude and decay time course.

Control and enzyme-treated preparations were analyzed ultrastructurally. Paired untreated and enzyme-treated ganglion preparations were fixed with a combination of 2% para- and 2.5% glutaraldehyde in Millonig's phosphate buffer (pH 7.2; 0.06M). The ganglia were fixed for 12 hours and processed for epon embedding by standard protocols. Ultrathin sections were stained with uranyl acetate and lead citrate and examined using a JEOL 100CX II electron microscope.

RESULTS

Characteristics of the Ganglionic Fast EPSC in Control Preparations:

In control ganglion cells, the EPSC rises to a peak value within a few milliseconds and decays exponentially over most of its time course. The peak EPSC amplitude is only a few nA in cells voltage-clamped to -50mV, i.e. $\sim$-6.0nA at 20-23°C. Figure 1A illustrates an action potential elicited by preganglionic stimulation and recorded in an unclamped cell with resting potential of -55mV. Figure 1B is an example of an averaged EPSC recorded after voltage clamping the membrane potential to -70mV. A semilogarithmic plot of the decay, superimposed on the data points above the current trace, demonstrates that the EPSC decay is exponential. In this example the decay τ is 5.6ms.

Peak current amplitude and decay τ are voltage-dependent, both increasing with hyperpolarization. The peak EPSC amplitude-membrane voltage relation is linear in the negative voltage range -30mV to -100mV as indicated in Figure 1C. In some cells there is a deviation from this linear relationship at positive voltages. The reversal potential for the EPSC is $\sim$-5.0mV. The decay τ has a small negative voltage dependence as illustrated in Figure 1D.

The EPSC size either with single stimuli or following repetitive stimulation can vary from a few to tens of nAs in cells voltage-clamped at a given voltage. However, there is no correlation between EPSC decay τ and EPSC size. Therefore, the decay τ is voltage-dependent but not influenced by EPSC amplitude (7, 20, 21).

EPSC decay τ is temperature dependent, τ increasing as the temperature is reduced from 23°C to 10°C. The temperature dependence of τ is illustrated in Figure 2 where the natural logarithm of τ is plotted as a function of temperature. The estimated Q_{10} of τ is $\sim$3. The temperature dependence of EPSC amplitude in these same cells was slightly less, having a Q_{10} of 1.7.

Neostigmine, MSF, and Protease-treatment Produce Similar Alterations in EPSC Decay

Table I summarizes the changes in EPSC characteristics occurring in the presence of neostigmine (1 x 10^{-5}M) or following treatment with either 10mM MSF (for 60 min.) or 0.01-0.05% protease (60-120 min.). With each treatment, EPSC decay was significantly slowed and, in some cells from each group, the EPSC decay time course became non-exponential. When present, this deviation from a single exponential was more apparent at hyperpolarized potentials. In the neostigmine-treated preparations the EPSC prolongation and deviation from an exponential decay often progressed with time. An example of this time dependent alteration in EPSC decay in the case of neostigmine-treated cells is shown in Figure 3. During pro-

256

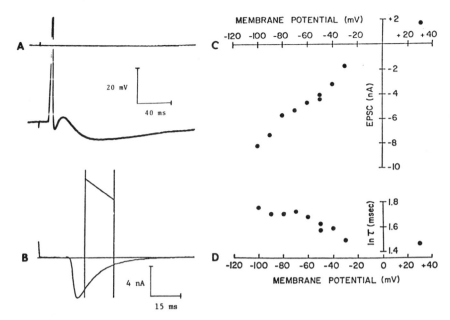

Figure 1.   Records which illustrate characteristics of nicotinic transmission in control preparations. A, an indirectly-stimulated
action potential recorded at -55mV. B, an EPSC recorded with
the membrane potential voltage-clamped to -70mV. The peak current amplitude was -5.3nA and the decay time constant was 5.6ms
(temp. = 20°C). C, the peak current amplitude of averaged EPSCs
is plotted as a function of membrane voltage. The EPSC reversal
potential for this cell was 0 mV. D, the ln τ-voltage relation
for the same cell has a coefficient of voltage dependence of
-0.0033mV^{-1}. Modified from Connor et al. (1983).

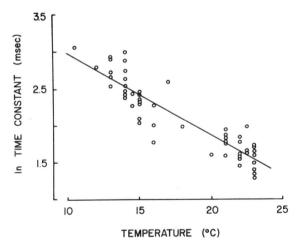

Figure 2.   Logarithm of EPSC τ values from 53 cells voltage-clamped to
-50mV as a function of temperature. The slope of the linear
regression line drawn through the data points indicates the
strong temperature dependence of EPSC decay τ which has a Q_{10} of
$\sim$ 3. Reproduced from the Journal of General Physiology (1980)
75: 39-60 by copyright permission of the Rockefeller Univ. Press.

Table I. Comparison of EPSC alteration by anticholinesterase agents and protease treatment.

Condition	EPSC size	EPSC decay characteristics	EPSC decay voltage dependence
Control	Small; ∿6nA at -50mV (22-23°C)	exponential with $\tau \sim$ 5ms at -50mV (22-23°C)	small negative voltage dependence (-0.0039 ± 0.0015*)
Neostigmine (1 x 10⁻⁵M)	Small increase (15-20%) in some experiments	EPSC prolonged (∿140%) for cells exposed for 20-60 minutes) and decay non-exponential in some cells, especially at hyperpolarized potentials (i.e. -100mV)	Similar to control (-0.0042+ 0.0030)
Protease treatment (0.01-0.05% for 1-2 hrs)	Increased (∿190%, with 0.05% protease treatment)	EPSC prolonged (∿150% 0.05% protease treatment) and decay non-exponential in some cells, especially at hyperpolarized potentials	Similar to control (-0.0034 + 0.0016)
MSF pretreatment (10mM for 1 hr)	Decrease in EPSC size (∿40%)	EPSC prolonged (∿170%); decay non-exponential in some cells, especially at hyperpolarized potentials	Similar to control (-0.0044 + 0.0030)
Physostigmine 1-5 x 10⁻⁶M	Small increase (10-20%) in some experiments	EPSC prolonged (∿140%); decay exponential	Similar to control (-0.0031 + 0.0027)
Physostigmine 1-10 x 10⁻⁵M	Concentration dependent decrease in EPSC size	EPSC prolonged; decay time course exhibits two exponential components. Both fast and slow component time constants exhibit concentration dependence	Slow component time constant (τ_s) generally increases with hyperpolarization; fast component time constant (τ_f) exhibits no consistent dependence on voltage

*Value represents mean ± S.D.

tease exposure the prolongation of EPSC decay also occurred progressively with time and often continued after replacing the protease containing solution with control solution (Figure 4). Generally, with shorter treatments, the EPSC decay time course remained exponential, whereas, after longer treatment duration, the decay phase noticeably deviated from a single exponential function. In contrast, after a one hour pretreatment in MSF, the EPSC decay was prolonged by ∿170% and in four experiments did not appear to change further over a two hour period. Example records which illustrate the alteration in the EPSC decay following

MSF treatment are shown in Figure 5. Although EPSC decay was noticeably slowed by each of these three different treatments, the decay retained its voltage dependence for currents obtained between -50 and -100mV and the estimated coefficient of the voltage dependence was similar to that of control cells (Table I) (20, 21).

Although the alteration in EPSC decay time course was quite similar, EPSC amplitude was not uniformly influenced by neostigmine, MSF or protease treatment. In experiments with neostigmine, EPSC size was not consistently changed, i.e. in some preparations there was a small increase; in others no noticeable change in EPSC amplitude. In contrast, following pretreatment with protease, there was a consistent increase in EPSC amplitude and after exposure to MSF, a marked decrease in amplitude. In spite of the different effects on EPSC amplitude, the shape of the peak EPSC-voltage relationship and reversal potential was similar in cells following each of these treatments to that obtained in untreated cells.

Protease and other enzyme treatments are thought to physically remove the esterase from the synaptic cleft at the motor end-plate. Further, protease treatment produces a progressive dysjunction at the neuromuscular junction as the motor nerve terminals separate from the muscle end-plate region (4, 5, 16). We observed in other experiments that ganglionic transmission remained following protease treatments (0.01-0.1%) of much longer

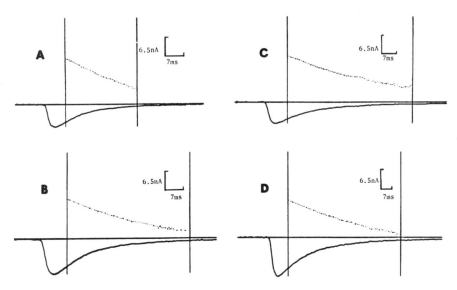

Figure 3. Averaged EPSCs from different cells in one ganglion preparation illustrating the progressive prolongation of current decay time course during exposure to 1 x 10^{-5}M neostigmine. EPSCs were recorded in cells voltage-clamped to -90mV at 15°C. Logarithmic current values are presented above each trace. A, an averaged control EPSC. B-D, averaged EPSCs recorded after 15, 30, and 50 min. of exposure to neostigmine. Reproduced from the Journal of General Physiology (1980) 75: 39-60 by copyright permission of the Rockefeller University Press.

duration (3-4 hrs) than used in the present study to investigate changes
in EPSC size and decay time course. Control and protease-treated preparations were examined ultrastructurally to assess whether synaptic contact
regions appeared to be altered by enzyme exposure. EPSCs were recorded
from these same protease-treated preparations to ensure that ganglionic
transmission remained and that the EPSC was prolonged. The results
obtained indicated that following protease treatments (0.01-0.05% up to
two hours) large empty spaces exist between individual ganglion cells due
to the reduction of collagen fibers and other intercellular matrix materials. Protease treatment also produced vacuolation in processes of the
ganglionic satellite cells causing alteration in the normal lamellar
organization of these processes ensheathing the postganglionic neurons.
However, areas of synaptic contact and the cellular membranes of individual ganglion cells appear normal. There was no evidence of any separation of preganglionic fiber terminals and ganglion cells. Similar resting
potential and action potential amplitude values were obtained in unclamped
cells before and after enzyme treatments. Further, there was no noticeable difference between the values of the holding currents needed to voltage clamp enzyme treated cells or untreated cells. Both observations
suggest that the ganglion cells remain in good condition following enzyme

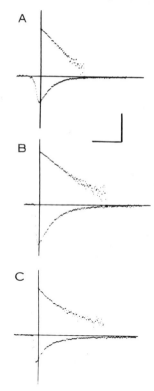

Figure 4.   Time dependent prolongation of EPSC decay following 0.01%
            protease pretreatment (2 hrs). Logarithmic current values are
            presented above each trace. A, an averaged EPSC from a cell
            prior to protease exposure. B and C, averaged EPSCs obtained
            from two other cells in this ganglion 74 min. and 101 min. after
            protease removal. Records were obtained at -50mV and 22°C.
            Calibration: vertical axis = 5nA for A and B, 10nA for C;
            horizontal axis = 10 ms.

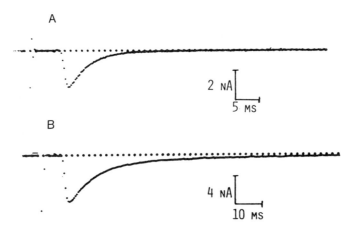

A

2 NA⌐
       5 MS

B

4 NA⌐
        10 MS

Figure 5. Averaged EPSCs from two different cells voltage-clamped to -50mV
in the same ganglion illustrating the prolongation of the current
decay time course following MSF treatment. A, an averaged EPSC
from a control cell. B, an averaged EPSC recorded in another
cell following exposure to 10mM MSF. T = 22°C.

exposure. Figure 6 illustrates the ultrastructural changes present after
a 1.5 hour exposure to 0.05% protease. Example records, obtained from
this ganglion, which demonstrate the alteration in EPSC time course occurring after protease treatment are presented in Figure 7. In these
examples, the EPSC decay remained exponential. However, the decay of
EPSCs recorded from other cells in this preparation deviated noticeably
from an exponential function.

The Alteration in EPSC Decay in Physostigmine-treated Cells Differed from
that seen with the Other Treatments

Physostigmine produced concentration dependent alterations in EPSC
size and decay time course. However, the pattern of EPSC alteration in
physostigmine differed from that observed with the other treatments. With
the lowest concentrations of physostigmine studied, $1-5 \times 10^{-6}$M, EPSC
decay was consistently slowed, but for most currents the decay time course
could still be adequately fitted by a single exponential function. Interestingly, this prolongation occurred consistently at warm temperatures
(22-24°) but was diminished at cooler temperatures (~ 14°C). The results
from four experiments presented in Table II illustrate the consistent
slowing of EPSC decay by 10^{-6}M physostigmine at 24°C and lack of effect
at 14°C. Also, at this concentration, there was no noticeable change in
peak EPSC amplitude from that measured in control cells prior to
physostigmine application.

In the presence of $1-5 \times 10^{-5}$M physostigmine, EPSC decay was slowed
further and the decay phase was no longer a single exponential but
rather had two distinct exponential components; an initial fast component
with a time constant (τ_f) less than that of control EPSCs and second

261

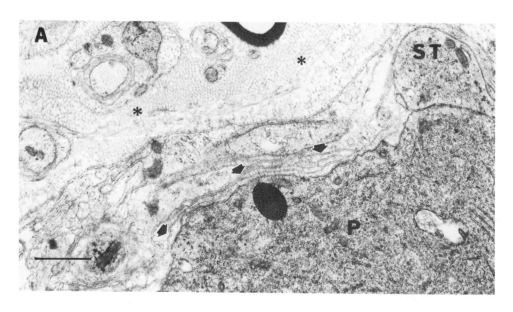

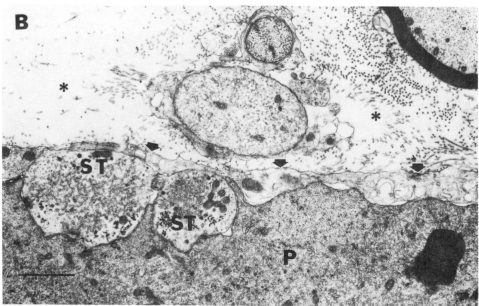

Figure 6. Electron microscopic detail of frog sympathetic ganglion preparations. A, untreated, and B, protease treated. Sympathetic
postganglionic neurons (P), preganglionic synaptic terminals (ST),
satellite cell processes (arrowheads), and extracellular matrix
(*) are shown. Note in B, the protease exposure reduced the
amount of extracellular matrix and produced vacuolation in
satellite cell processes. Synaptic terminal profiles remained
in contact with the ganglion neurons. Bar equals 1.0μm.

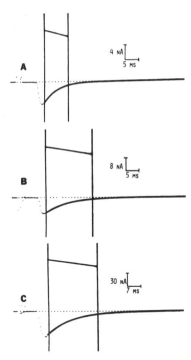

Figure 7. Averaged EPSCs from three different cells voltage-clamped to -50mV
in the 0.05% protease-treated ganglion which was examined ultrastructurally. A, a control EPSC. B and C, EPSCs recorded 53 min.
and 120 min. after protease removal. A linear fit to the ln of
the decay phase between the vertical cursor lines is shown above
each trace. In all three examples the decay phase could be well
described by an exponential function even after protease treatment
when the peak current value was large as in example C.

Table II. Temperature dependence of EPSC prolongation by 1.3×10^{-6}M
physostigmine.

Experiment	Condition*	decay τ (14°C)	decay τ (24°C)	Number of cells/group
1	control	14.1	4.6	(4)
	physostigmine	13.1	6.2	(7)
2	control	10.8	3.4	(4)
	physostigmine	9.1	5.2	(4)
3	control	11.3	3.5	(6)
	physostigmine	10.4	4.9	(7)
4	control	11.2	2.7	(5)
	physostigmine	11.2	4.3	(6)
Mean $\pm$ SD	control	11.9 $\pm$ 1.5	3.6 $\pm$ 0.8	
	physostigmine	11.0 $\pm$ 1.7	5.2 $\pm$ 0.8	

*Cells were voltage-clamped to -50mV.

263

much slower component with a time constant (τ_s) considerably greater than that of control EPSCs. The decay τ of both components depended on physostigmine concentration; τ_f decreasing with concentration and τ_s increasing with concentration. Table III illustrates the effect of increasing the physostigmine concentration five-fold from 1×10^{-5}M to 5×10^{-5}M on the two decay components and the ratio of the amplitudes of the fitted exponential components, I_s/I_f, in cells voltage-clamped to -75mV. Example records which illustrate this concentration dependent alteration in EPSC time course by physostigmine in three different cells voltage-clamped to -75mV are presented in Figure 8.

Table III. Concentration-dependent alteration in EPSC decay at -75mV

Physostigmine concentration	EPSC Amplitude	τ_f	τ_s	I_s/I_f +	Number of cells
(μm)	(nA)	(msec)	(msec)		
0	11.9 ± 1.3	6.8 ± 0.7*	--	--	6
10	11.4 ± 2.0	5.1 ± 0.4	25.9 ± 6.3	0.33 ± 0.06	5
50	7.2 ± 0.9	3.8 ± 0.2	29.8 ± 2.8	0.23 ± 0.04	6

+Amplitudes of exponential components extrapolated to the beginning of the EPSC
*Control current decay fit as single exponential
Results expressed as mean ± SEM

The influence of membrane potential on the fast and slow decay components of physostigmine-treated cells was studied over the voltage range -50 to -100mV. In most cells exposed to either 1×10^{-5}M or 5×10^{-5}M physostigmine the fast component time constant decreased with hyperpolarization. However, in a few cells there appeared to be no consistent change in τ_f with hyperpolarization. In contrast, the time constant of the slow component (τ_s) of EPSCs from physostigmine-treated cells increased with hyperpolarization (Table IV).

Physostigmine (1×10^{-5}M) did not alter the shape of the peak EPSC-voltage relationship or the EPSC reversal potential. Figure 9 is a current-voltage plot of a control cell and a second cell from the same ganglion exposed to 1×10^{-5}M physostigmine.

With concentrations of physostigmine $\geq 7.5 \times 10^{-5}$M, the EPSC amplitude was depressed and the decay was prolonged even more. In some cases the decay time course appeared to have more than two components; however because of the small size of these EPSCs, the decay time course often could not be analyzed accurately.

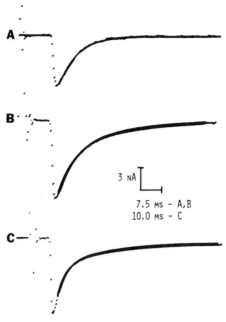

3 NA

7.5 MS - A,B
10.0 MS - C

Figure 8. Averaged EPSCs from three different cells voltage-clamped to -75mV, which illustrate the concentration dependent alteration in EPSC decay time course by physostigmine. The decay phase of each current was fit with a computer generated function: a single exponential function for trace A and a two component exponential function for traces B and C. A, an averaged control EPSC with the decay τ equal to 5.9 msec. B, an averaged EPSC recorded in 1×10^{-5}M physostigmine. The two decay component time constants were 5.2ms and 20.3ms and the I_s/I_f ratio was 0.43. C, an averaged EPSC recorded in 5×10^{-5}M physostigmine. The two decay component time constants were 3.9ms and 32.6ms and the I_s/I_f ratio was 0.33.

Table IV. Voltage-dependent alteration of EPSC decay in 5×10^{-5}M physostigmine.

Voltage (mV)	τ_f (msec)	τ_s (msec)	I_s/I_f	Number of cells
-50	4.2 ± 0.1*	25.6 ± 3.3	0.37 ± 0.07	6
-75	3.8 ± 0.2	29.8 ± 2.8	0.23 ± 0.06	6
-100	3.8 ± 0.2	39.8 ± 8.6	0.17 ± 0.02	6

*Mean ± SEM

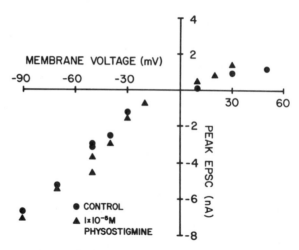

Figure 9. A comparison of the peak current-voltage relationship for two different cells from the same ganglion which illustrates that the reversal potential for the EPSC is not altered by 1×10^{-5}M physostigmine.

DISCUSSION

The addition of neostigmine, pretreatment with MSF, or exposure to protease produced a marked prolongation of the EPSC although the EPSC decay time course retained a voltage dependence similar to that of control cells. Inhibition of cholinesterase, by itself, should increase the acetylcholine concentration in the synaptic cleft immediately following evoked release and slow the rate of transmitter removal. An increase in EPSC amplitude and slowing of the EPSC decay phase would be consistent with these effects. EPSC size was not changed in a consistent manner by neostigmine, MSF, or protease treatment. However, with multiquantal evoked currents, changes in EPSC amplitude can result from either an alteration in the kinetics of transmitter release or postsynaptic sensitivity to acetylcholine. The results of the present study do not provide evidence to distinguish between these possibilities.

In many cells, following either MSF, neostigmine, or protease treatment, the EPSC decay time course deviated from a single exponential. This deviation of the decay phase from an exponential function and the time dependence of the prolongation observed in many experiments with neostigmine suggests that the prolongation of decay is not simply due to esterase inhibition. Dreyer et al. (12) reported previously that several hours of exposure to neostigmine were required for its full effect to develop at the motor end-plate. It was suggested that this prolonged time course reflected a slow action of neostigmine on the membrane micro-environment surrounding the receptor-channel complex. The deviation of the EPSC decay time course from an exponential did not result simply from an increase in the cleft acetylcholine concentration immediately following release. A much larger increase in ESPC amplitude can occur in 10μM 4-aminopyridine-treated (4-AP) preparations (5-fold increase) with the EPSC decay remaining well described by an exponential function. Further, the time constant of EPSC decay for cells exposed to 4-AP is similar to that of control cells; illustrating again that the EPSC decay time course is independent of EPSC amplitude (11). The anti-AChE actions of neostigmine and MSF are well documented (14, 17). Unfortunately, to our knowledge no information has been reported which indicates whether enzyme treatments reduce esterase activity in ganglion preparations. However, no interruption of ganglionic transmission was observed with protease treatment and from both physiological criteria (i.e., rise time of the EPSC) and anatomical evidence, there was no indication of any physical separation in the region of synaptic contact between preganglionic fibers and postganglionic cells. Therefore, cleft AChE may be protected from enzymatic influence in ganglia. Consequently, the similarity between the alteration of the EPSC decay following protease treatment to that seen in neostigmine- and MSF-treated cells only provides an indirect indication that AChE may be removed or its activity reduced following protease treatment. We tentatively conclude, therefore, in addition to any presumed anti-AChE actions, that all three treatments most likely have additional pharmacological actions which alter the properties of nicotinic receptor-channel gating in ganglia.

The alteration in EPSC time course in physostigmine-treated cells was different from that seen with either neostigmine- or MSF-treatment, but was similar in many respects to that characteristic of atropine-treated cells (7). In physostigmine-treated ($1-5 \times 10^{-5}$M) cells, the EPSC decay exhibited two distinct exponential components which became more obvious with increasing concentration and membrane hyperpolarization. In contrast, the decay of EPSC from neostigmine or MSF-treated cells did not exhibit clear fast and slow components. However, if the decay time course of EPSCs from MSF- or neostigmine-treated cells was fitted as the sum of two exponential components, both component time constants were greater than that of the values of τ obtained from control cell EPSCs prior to treatment. For instance, in two experiments with MSF treatment, the value of τ at -50mV in eight control cells was 5.2 ± 0.4 ms (m $\pm$ SEM, 22°C). The EPSC decay in 15 cells from these same two ganglia voltage-clamped to -50mV was markedly prolonged after MSF treatment. When the decay phase of these EPSCs was fitted by the sum of two exponential components; the two time constants were 7.3 ± 0.3 ms and 41.1 ± 2.2 ms. The concentration- and voltage-dependent effects of physostigmine on the two EPSC decay time constants and the I_s/I_f ratio is consistent with the open channel blockade model proposed for atropine and local anesthetics on end-plate and ganglionic nicotinic channels (1, 7, 9, 23). Consequently, we suggest that at least part of the alteration in EPSC decay time course by physostigmine can be accounted for by the following scheme:

$$nACh + R + P \xleftarrow{K_D} ACh_n R + P \underset{\alpha}{\overset{\beta}{\rightleftharpoons}} ACh_n R^* + P \underset{F}{\overset{G}{\rightleftharpoons}} ACh_n R^*P$$

where R represents the receptor-channel complex; $ACh_n R^*$, the open conducting state; p, physostigmine; and $ACh_n R^*P$, the blocked, non-conducting state (23).

The alteration in EPSC size and decay observed previously in atropine-treated preparations was more dramatic than the present study with physostigmine-treated cells. This difference may arise in part because partial inhibition of AChE by physostigmine most likely would, by itself, prolong EPSC decay. Because of this, the effects of physostigmine on EPSC characteristics were quantitated over a limited concentration range. The interpretation of results obtained at any higher concentrations are hindered further as physostigmine's anti-AChE action increases progressively in this concentration range (6). It was apparent, however, from qualitative observations that the splitting of the decay time course and the decrease in size became more dramatic as the concentration of physostigmine was increased (21). Therefore, we conclude that a significant component of the physostigmine-induced inhibition of ganglionic transmission can be attributed to a blockade of activated nicotinic channels. Recently, Fiekers (14) has demonstrated that physostigmine also blocks acetylcholine-activated muscle end-plate channels and further, that this blockade occurs after inhibition of AChE by MSF treatment.

In summary, the results presented here suggest that anti-AChE agents have complex actions on receptor-channel gating in autonomic ganglion cells as demonstrated recently for muscle end-plate receptor-channel complexes (3, 12-15, 17, 18, 22).

ACKNOWLEDGMENTS

We thank Dr. Richard Kriebel and Mr. Allen Angel for the preparation of the electron micrographs. This work was supported by U.S. Public Health Service Grants NS-14552 and NS-19880 and a MDA grant to R.L. Parsons.

REFERENCES

1. Adams, P.R. (1976) Drug blockade of open end-plate channels. J. Physiol. 260: 531-552.
2. Adams, P.R. (1982) Voltage-dependent conductances of vertebrate neurons. Trends Neurosci. 5: 116-119.
3. Akaike, A., Ikeda, S.R., Brookes, N., Pascuzzo, G.J., Rickett, D.L. and Albuquerque, E.X. (1984) The nature of the interactions of pyridostigmine with the nicotinic acetylcholine receptor ionic channel complex. II. Patch clamp studies. Mol. Pharmacol. 25: 102-112.
4. Betz, W. and Sakmann, B. (1971) Dysjunction of frog neuromuscular synapses by treatment with proteolytic enzymes. Nature New Biol. 232: 94-95.
5. Betz, W. and Sakmann, B. (1973) Effects of proteolytic enzymes on function and structure of frog neuromuscular junction. J. Physiol. 230: 673-688.
6. Brzin, M., Tennyson, V.M. and Duffy, P.E. (1966) Acetylcholinesterase in frog sympathetic and dorsal root ganglia. A study by electron microscopic cytochemistry and microgasometric analysis with the magnetic diver. J. Cell Biol. 31: 215-242.
7. Connor, E.A., Levy, S.M. and Parsons, R.L. (1983) Kinetic analysis of atropine-induced alterations in bullfrog ganglionic fast synaptic currents. J. Physiol. 337: 137-158.
8. Connor, E.A., Neel, D.S. and Parsons, R.L. (1985) Influence of the extracellular ionic environment on ganglionic fast excitatory postsynaptic currents. Brain Research. In Press.
9. Connor, E.A. and Parsons, R.L. (1983) Procaine alters fast excitatory postsynaptic current decay in amphibian sympathetic ganglia. Br. J. Pharmac. 78: 293-299.
10. Connor, E.A. and Parsons, R.L. (1983) Analysis of fast excitatory postsynaptic currents in bullfrog parasympathetic ganglion cells. J. Neurosci. 3: 2164-2171.
11. Connor, E.A. and Parsons, R.L. (1984) Alteration of the fast excitatory postsynaptic current by barium in voltage-clamped amphibian sympathetic ganglion cells. Br. J. Pharmac. 83: 31-42.
12. Dreyer, F., Walther, C. and Peper, K. (1976) Junctional and extrajunctional acetylcholine receptors in normal and denervated frog muscle fibres. Pflugers Arch. 366: 1-9.
13. Fiekers, J.F. (1985) Concentration-dependent effects of neostigmine on the end-plate acetylcholine receptor channel complex. J. Neurosci. 5: 502-514.

14. Fiekers, J.F. (1985) Interactions of edrophonium, physostigmine, and methane sulfonyl fluoride with the snake end-plate acetylcholine receptor-channel complex. J. Pharmacol. exp. Therap. In press.
15. Goldman, M.M. and Narahashi, T. (1974) Effects of edrophonium on end-plate currents in frog skeletal muscle. Eur. J. Pharmacol. 25: 362-371.
16. Hall, Z.W. and Kelly, R.B. (1971) Enzymatic detachment of end-plate acetylcholinesterase from muscle. Nature New Biol. 232: 549-557.
17. Kordas, M., Brzin, M. and Majcen, Z. (1975) A comparison of the effect of cholinesterase inhibitors on end-plate current and on cholinesterase activity in frog muscle. Neuropharmacology 14: 791-800.
18. Kordas, M. (1977) On the role of junctional cholinesterase in determining the time course of the end-plate current. J. Physiol. 270: 133-150.
19. Kuba, K. and Koketsu, K. (1978) Synaptic events in sympathetic ganglia. Progr. Neurobiol. 11: 77-169.
20. Kuba, K. and Nishi, S. (1979) Characteristics of fast excitatory postsynaptic current in bullfrog sympathetic ganglion cells. Pflugers Arch. 378: 205-212.
21. MacDermott, A.B., Connor, E.A., Dionne, V.E. and Parsons, R.L. (1980) Voltage-clamp study of fast excitatory synaptic currents in bullfrog sympathetic ganglion cells. J. gen. Physiol. 75: 39-60.
22. Pascuzzo, G.J., Akaiki, A., Maleque, M.A., Shaw, K., Aronstam, R.S., Rickett, D.L. and Albuquerque, E.X. (1984) The nature of the interactions of pyridostigmine with the nicotinic acetylcholine receptor-ionic channel complex. I. Agonist, desensitizing and binding properties. Mol. Pharmacol. 25: 92-101.
23. Ruff, R.L. (1977) A quantitative analysis of local anesthetic alteration of miniature end-plate currents and end-plate current fluctuations. J. Physiol. 264: 89-124.

ROLE OF ACETYLCHOLINE IN THE CEREBRAL CORTEX

K. Krnjević

Anaesthesia Research and Physiology Departments
McGill University
Montréal (Québec), Canada

INTRODUCTION

Acetylcholine (ACh) has been considered a possible central synaptic transmitter for some 50 years (Dale, 1938). What kind of role cholinergic synapses might play in brain function is a topic that has long fascinated Alexander Karczmar (e.g. Karczmar, 1969; 1973). It is therefore entirely appropriate to review here briefly what we know about cholinergic action in the cerebral cortex.

Overall it can be said that ACh has a predominantly muscarinic modulatory action, which is particularly effective as a facilitator of responses evoked by fast acting excitatory transmitters, and which is mediated by a selective depression of K^+ or Cl^- outward currents that normally limit the firing of cortical neurons. As a result, in the presence of ACh, cortical neurons give much stronger and more prolonged responses to various inputs. The evidence that supports this statement has come from electrophysiological studies summarized below.

Before proceeding further, it is necessary to mention that there is now little doubt that cholinergic fibres indeed release ACh in the cortex (MacIntosh and Oborin, 1953; Collier, 1977; Dudar, 1977). These fibres are probably of exclusively telencephalic origin, their cell bodies being situated in the basal region of the forebrain (Shute and Lewis, 1963; Krnjević and Silver, 1965, 1966; Lewis et al., 1967; Fibiger, 1982; Mesulam et al., 1983; E. McGeer (this volume)). Albeit quite well established for nearly 20 years, this projection has received far more attention in the last few years since the discovery that degeneration of these cholinergic fibres is the most striking (if perhaps not exclusive) pathological feature in the brain of patients suffering from Alzheimer-type senile dementia (Bowen et al., 1976; Whitehouse et al., 1982). Inevitably, this suggests that ACh is somehow especially involved in memory and other cognitive functions mediated by the cerebral cortex.

MODULATORY ACTION OF ACh ON CORTICAL NEURONS

1. Extracellular studies

A. Muscarinic Excitation. That ACh might have a special kind of

271

action in the cortex first became apparent when microiontophoretic
applications were combined with extracellular single unit recording

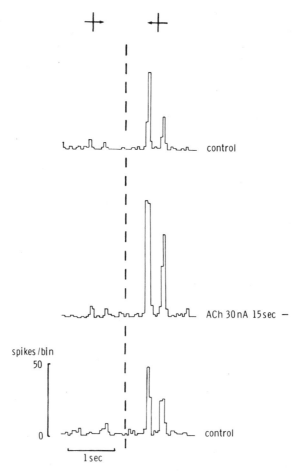

Figure 1

ACh enhances response of a cat's cortical neuron to visual stimulus.
Peristimulus time histograms show averaged responses to series of
consecutive movements of an optimally-oriented bar of light, forwards and
backwards over the receptive field. Upper record, initial control
responses; middle, during ACh iontophoretic application; lower, recovery.
(Figure 2 in Sillito and Kemp (1983)).

(Krnjević and Phillis, 1963a; Spehlmann, 1963). Many cortical cells showed
an increase in firing, having a relatively slow onset and long duration –
especially when compared with the strikingly rapid effect produced by
glutamate and other excitatory amino acids. An important feature was the
pronounced muscarinic character of this action (Krnjević and Phillis,
1963b) – confirmed by most later observers (e.g. Stone, 1972; Sillito and
Kemp, 1983). In this respect, it was markedly different from the action of
ACh on Renshaw cells, at that time the only well known central
cholinoceptive neurons (Eccles et al., 1954, see J.C. Eccles in the present
volume). But this kind of slow muscarinic excitation subsequently proved to
be much more prevalent throughout the CNS, on closer examination being
shown even by Renshaw cells (Curtis and Ryall, 1966).

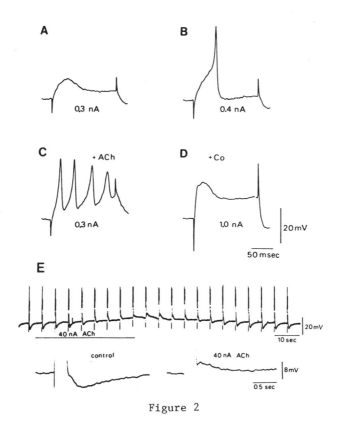

Figure 2

ACh facilitates Ca^{2+}-action potentials of tetrodotoxin-treated hippocampal
pyramidal cells in culture. A,B injections of sub- and suprathreshold
depolarizing current pulses. C, in presence of ACh (10^{-5} M) previously
subthreshold pulse elicits repetitive firing, which was blocked by 2 mM
cobalt (D), even when much stronger depolarizing current was injected. E,
depression of post-spike hyperpolarizations by ACh applied
iontophoretically; in lower traces, loss of after-hyperpolarization is
illustrated at faster sweeps and higher amplification. (From Figs. 1 and 6
in Gähwiler, 1984).

273

B.   Facilitation of cell firing. It was early recognized that the action of ACh is quite labile, greatly depending on the general level of excitability of cortical cells: thus it was rather easily depressed or even abolished by deeper anaesthesia, arterial hypotension and possibly hypoxia. But even when ACh was unable to elicit firing of a neuron, it could be shown to markedly facilitate the firing evoked by other agents, such as glutamate, or by various synaptic inputs (Krnjević and Phillis, 1963b; Krnjević et al., 1971b). Fig. 1 provides a clear illustration of the increased response of a visual cortex neuron to a specific visual signal. A significant aspect of this action of ACh – emphasized by Sillito and Kemp (1983) – is that the enhanced discharge shows no loss of its directional selectivity; if anything ACh further increases the signal-to-noise ratio. As a rule there is also a facilitation of after-discharges, so that responses become not only more intense but are also prolonged. Hence, it was proposed that by generating a state of enhanced responsiveness, the cholinergic innervation could be responsible for a general activation of cortical function ("arousal"), resulting in increased awareness: this was ascribed especially to the prolongation of responses (Krnjević, 1967), which may be essential for the laying down of short-term memory traces and conscious processes (Libet, 1973).

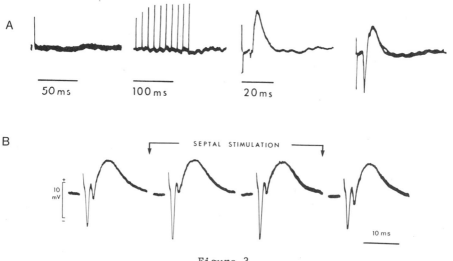

Figure 3

Medial septal stimulation facilitates hippocampal population spikes in rats under urethane. A, from left to right traces show: neither a single (1), nor a tetanic stimulus (2) applied to medial septum evoked marked responses in CA1; but a predominantly inhibitory response (large positive field) was evoked by commissural stimulus alone (3), which was greatly altered (4) when preceded by septal tetanus (as in second trace, ending 20 ms before commissural stimulus): positive wave is much reduced and a large negative population spike appears (part of Fig. 4 in Krnjević and Ropert, 1982). B, similar septal stimulation can also potentiate antidromic responses evoked in CA3 by fimbrial stimulation. Note large increase in antidromic (very short latency) population spike when conditioned by brief septal tetani (from Fig. 4 in Dalkara et al., 1985). A similar action is produced by local applications of ACh at the site of recording and is believed to be due to enhancement of ephaptic excitation.

Mechanism of ACh action

This could be analyzed only by direct recording of changes in membrane
potentials and conductances evoked by ACh.

Intracellular studies

The first systematic recordings (Krnjević et al., 1971b) revealed a
mode of action that differed greatly from the fast nicotinic depolarizing
action that had been extensively studied at the muscle end plate (Del
Castillo and Katz, 1956) and which was evidently caused by a selective
enhancement of Na^+ and K^+ conductance (Takeuchi, 1963). In the first
place, the depolarizing effect of ACh in cortical neurons was relatively
weak, slow and prolonged. Moreover, quite consistently there was no
evidence of an associated increased in conductance, but rather a tendency
(variable but consistent) for the membrane conductance to diminish: as a

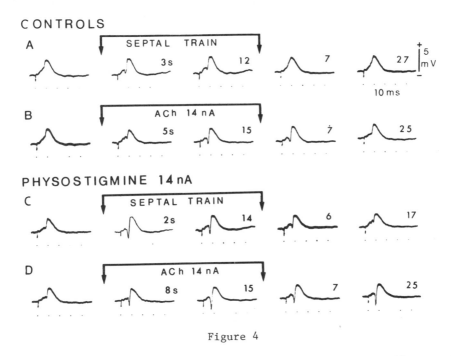

Figure 4

Pharmacological evidence that the septal facilitatory action illustrated in
Fig. 3A is mediated by release of ACh from septo-hippocampal fibres. In
control traces A-B, first records at left show positive wave evoked by
single commissural stimulus. A small negative population spike appeared
when commissural shock was given (A) 20 ms after a septal tetanus (10
pulses at 100 Hz) or (B) in conjunction with iontophoretic release of ACh
(for 15 s). Times at which records were obtained after start and end of
conditioning procedures are indicated in seconds. Traces C and D show much
greater and prolonged potentiation of population spikes by identical septal
trains of ACh applciations during simultaneous iontophoretic release of an
anticholinesterase agent (physostigmine) in hippocampus. These actions of
physostigmine were fully reversible (from Fig. 10 in Krnjević and Ropert,
1982).

result, the real or extrapolated reversal potential for the action of ACh was at a highly negative level (close to −90 mV and therefore consistently more hyperpolarized than the resting potential). This was strong evidence that ACh depresses the conductance for an ion with a relatively negative equilibrium potential, most probably K^+, because Cl^- injections into the cells – sufficient to produce major shifts of IPSP reversal potential – did not change the reversal potential for the effect of ACh.

In addition to the inactivation of a resting K conductance, there was a slowing down of repolarization after action potentials, which enhanced repetive firing and after-discharges. This indicated a further action of ACh, tending to depress the delayed phase of K outward current involved in post-spike depression of excitability. In keeping with the idea that K+ channels are the predominant sites of action of ACh was the finding that Ba^{2+} – which has long been known as an almost universally effective blocker of K^+ channels – has a remarkably similar (that is ACh-like) excitatory effect on cortical neurons, though not mediated by muscarinic receptors (Krnjević et al., 1971a).

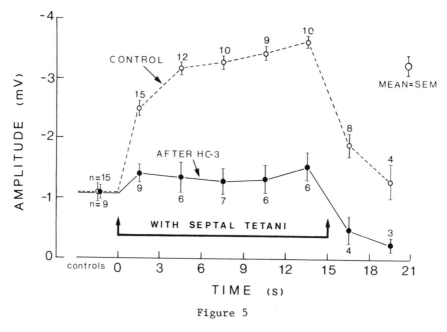

Figure 5

Further evidence that this septal facilitatory action is mediated by a cholinergic mechanism is its marked depression after intraventricular injection of hemicholinium-3 (HC-3, a selective blocker of choline uptake and therefore of ACh synthesis). Open circles, mean amplitudes of population spikes before and during facilitation by conditioning septal tetani (10 pulses at 70 Hz, preceding commissural stimulus by 30 ms). Closed circles, corresponding data recorded 30–45 minutes after injecting 15 µg HC-3 into lateral ventricle (from Fig. 3 in Glavinović et al., 1983).

These results were confirmed in a number of later studies, both on cortical (Woody et al., 1978; Benardo and Prince, 1982) and on a variety of other central neurons (Zieglgänsberger and Reiter, 1974; Bernardi et al., 1976; Crepel and Dhanjal, 1982). A good example of the facilitation of inward currents – in this case of Ca^{2+}-spikes is given in Fig. 2: these records, from a hippocampal cell in vitro, were obtained in the presence of tetrodotoxin; they also demonstrate the disappearance of the after-hyperpolarization (Gähwiler, 1984).

The finding that intracellular Ca^{2+} activates K currents (Meech, 1972; Krnjević and Lisiewicz, 1972) later led to speculation that ACh might act indirectly by lowering intracellular free Ca^{2+} (Krnjević, 1977). This could happen either by a reduction in Ca^{2+} influx or an enhancement of intracellular Ca^{2+} sequestration. As will be discussed in more detail below, there is now significant evidence that, at least in some cells, ACh acts in such an indirect manner.

Voltage clamp studies

More precise information about the muscarinic effects of ACh has been obtained more recently by voltage-clamping nerve cells. In the first place, this has led to the identification of previously unsuspected sub-types of K^+ currents. A major advance – particularly for cholinergic studies – was Brown and Adams' (1980) discovery in frog sympathetic ganglia of a K^+ current that was both muscarine- and voltage-sensitive (accordingly named the M-current). An important point is that this current is activated by relatively small depolarizations from the resting level and shows no voltage-dependent inactivation: hence it acts as a highly effective brake on excitation. Its susceptibility to block by ACh therefore provides a powerful means of modulating firing in response to any depolarizing inputs. In later work, a basically similar M-current was demonstrated, also by voltage-clamping, in hippocampal neurons in vitro (Halliwell and Adams, 1982).

An exclusive action of ACh on the M-current, however, cannot be reconciled with evidence, from more than one laboratory, that ACh also depresses the post-spike hyperpolarization, notably in hippocampal slices (Benardo and Prince, 1982; Cole and Nicoll, 1983) – as well as in some peripheral autonomic neurons (Morita et al., 1982) – in general agreement with the original observations on cortical cells (Krnjević et al., 1971b). A further reinvestigation by voltage clamp has indeed now uncovered at least one component of the Ca^{2+}-activated K current in frog ganglia that is depressed by ACh (P. Adams, this volume). Whether the M current is directly antagonized by ACh (as originally proposed by Brown and Adams, 1980) or only indirectly through changes in Ca influx (Belluzzi et al., 1985) remains to be established; perhaps both types of action operate, in various combinations, in different cells.

Indirect actions of ACh

A most important effect is the regulation of transmitter release. It has long been known that ACh depresses its own release via presynaptic muscarinic receptors (e.g. Szerb, 1978). More recently it has become clear that it can also greatly reduce the release of other transmitters. The best electrophysiological evidence for this kind of action has been obtained in the hippocampus.

The first indication was that when ACh is applied in the dendritic layer – where excitatory synapses are concentrated – it depresses EPSPs by a presynaptic action (Hounsgaard, 1978). In the stratum pyramidale, where inhibitory synapses predominate, there is an opposite effect, that is disinhibition, resulting in increased firing (Krnjević et al., 1980; Ben-Ari et al., 1981; Valentino and Dingledine, 1981; Haas, 1982). Particularly compelling evidence of this mechanism has been obtained in cultures of hippocampal neurons, where ACh greatly reduces the quantal content of IPSPs, an action that could not be explained otherwise than by an interference with transmitter (GABA) release (Segal, 1983).

Although ACh can thus have opposite muscarinic effects, disfacilitatory at dendritic synapses and disinhibitory at perisomatic synapses, the principal action of septal cholinergic activation on CA1 and CA3 pyramidal cells is to enhance population spikes (Figs. 3-5), a major part of this effect being probably mediated by disinhibition (Krnjević and Ropert, 1982). These observations, however, do not exclude the possibility of a selective disfacilitatory cholinergic action by a specific septal cholinergic projection to dendritic excitatory synapses. Comparable indirect – disinhibitory or disfacilitatory – effects of ACh may also occur in the neocortex, but they have not yet been demonstrated directly.

CONCLUSIONS

So far, the best defined actions of ACh in the cortex – including the hippocampus – tend to diminish both intrinsic and extrinsic mechanisms that normally keep excitation under firm control. The intrinsic mechanisms are basically K^+ conductances, that are either voltage and/or Ca^{2+}-dependent, which can generate very substantial outward currents of K^+, and so sharply limit the depolarizing action of excitatory synapses. Equally (and in situ perhaps even more) important is the powerful extrinsic control exerted by both tonic and phasic inhibitory inputs: the best known are mediated by GABA and therefore activate especially a Cl^- conductance, which powerfully opposes depolarization (some K^+-mediated slower IPSPs may also be evoked by GABA acting on different receptors (Newberry and Nicoll, 1985)).

By removing these brakes on depolarization, ACh tends to enhance firing in response not only to synaptic but also to electrical inputs, such as the sharp, passive electrical (ephaptic) interactions that are particularly prominent between the densely packed hippocampal pyramidal cells (Taylor and Dudek, 1982). This allows much stronger, highly synchronized firing of the pyramidal cells – for example during antidromic activation (Fig. 3B) (Dalkara et al., 1985) – and greatly accelerates the recruitment of inactive cells during seizure discharges. Finally, by reducing post-spike depression, ACh facilitates firing in bursts and after-discharges. A reduction of outward currents is probably essential for the generation of major Ca^{2+} influx into cortical neurons (Stafstrom et al., 1985), that may well be the trigger for the initiation of intracellular processes needed to lay-down memory traces and to create awareness.

ACKNOWLEDGMENTS

The author's research receives continuing financial support from the Canadian Medical Research Council.

REFERENCES

Belluzzi, O., Sacchi, O., and Wanke, E., 1985, Identification of delayed potassium and calcium currents in the rat sympathetic neurone under voltage clamp, J. Physiol., 358:109-129.
Benardo, L.S., and Prince, D.A., 1982, Cholinergic excitation of mammalian hippocampal pyramidal cells, Brain Res., 249:315-331.

Ben-Ari, Y., Krnjević, K., Reinhardt, W., and Ropert, N., 1981,
    Intracellular observations on the disinhibitory action of
    acetylcholine in the hippocampus, Neuroscience, 6:2475-2484.
Bernardi, G., Floris, V., Marciani, M.G., Morocutti, C., and Stanzione, P.,
    1976, The action of acetylcholine and L-glutamic acid on rat caudate
    neurons, Brain Res., 114:134-138.
Bowen, D.M., Smith, C.B., White, P., and Davison, A.N., 1976,
    Neurotransmitter-related enzymes and indices of hypoxia in senile
    dementia and other abiotrophies, Brain, 99:459-496.
Brown, D.A., and Adams, P.R., 1980, Muscarinic suppression of novel
    voltage-sensitive K^+ current in a vertebrate neurone. Nature,
    283:673-676.
Cole, A.E, and Nicoll, R.A., 1983, Acetylcholine mediates a slow synaptic
    potential in hippocampal pyramidal cells, Science, 221:1299-1301.
Collier, B., 1977, Biochemistry and physiology of cholinergic transmission,
    in: "Handbook of Physiology, Section I: The Nervous System", Volume 1,
    Part 1, J.M. Brookhart, V.B. Mountcastle, E.R. Kandel, and S.R. Geiger,
    eds., American Physiological Society, Bethesda, Maryland, pp. 463-492.
Crepel, F., and Dhanjal, S.S., 1982, Cholinergic mechanisms and
    neurotransmission in the cerebellum of the rat. An in vitro study.
    Brain Res., 244:59-68.
Curtis, D.R., and Ryall, R.W., 1966, The excitation of Renshaw cells by
    cholinomimetics, Exp. Brain Res., 2:49-65.
Dale, H.H., 1938, Acetylcholine as a chemical transmitter of the effects of
    nerve impulses, J. Mt. Sinai Hosp., 4:401-429.
Dalkara, T., Krnjević, K., Ropert, N., and Yim, C.Y., 1985, Chemical
    modulation of ephaptic activation of CA3 hippocampal pyramids,
    Neuroscience.
Del Castillo, J., and Katz, B., 1956, Biophysical aspects of neuromuscular
    transmission, Progr. Biophys., 6:121-170.
Dudar, J.D., 1977, The role of the septal nuclei in the release of
    acetylcholine from the rabbit cerebral cortex and dorsal hippocampus
    and the effect of atropine, Brain Res., 129:237-246.
Eccles, J.C., Fatt, P., and Koketsu, K., 1954, Cholinergic and inhibitory
    synapses in a pathway from motor-axon collaterals to motoneurones, J.
    Physiol., 126:524-562.
Fibiger, H.C., 1982, The organization and some projections of cholinergic
    neurons of the mammalian forebrain, Brain Res. Reviews, 4:327-388.
Gähwiler, B.H., 1984, Facilitation by acetylcholine of tetrodotoxin-
    resistant spikes in rat hippocampal pyramidal cells, Neuroscience,
    11:381-388.
Glavinović, M., Ropert, N., Krnjević, K., and Collier, B., 1983,
    Hemicholinium impairs septo-hippocampal facilitatory action,
    Neuroscience, 9:319-330.
Haas, H.L., 1982, Cholinergic disinhibition in hippocampal slices of the
    rat. Brain Res., 233:200-204.
Halliwell, J.V., and Adams, P.R., 1982, Voltage-clamp analysis of
    muscarinic excitation in hippocampal neurons, Brain Res., 250:71-92.
Hounsgaard, J., 1978, Presynaptic inhibitory action of acetylcholine in
    area CA1 of the hippocampus, Exp. Neurol., 62:787-797.
Karczmar, A.G., 1969, Quelques aspects de la pharmacologie des synapses
    cholinergiques et de sa signification centrale, Actualités
    Pharmacologiques, 28:293-338.
Karczmar, A.G., 1973, The chemical coding via the cholinergic system: its
    organization and behavioral implications, in: "Neurohumoral coding of
    brain function", R.P. Drucker-Colin and R.D. Myers, eds., Plenum
    Press, New York, pp. 399-418.
Krnjević, K., 1967, Chemical transmission and cortical arousal,
    Anesthesiology, 28:100-105.
Krnjević, K., 1977, Control of neuronal excitability by intracellular
    divalent cations: a possible target for neurotransmitter actions, in:

"Neurotransmitter Function: Basic and Clinical Aspects", W.S. Field, ed., Symposia Specialists Press, Miami, Florida, pp. 11-26.

Krnjević, K., and Lisiewicz, A., 1972, Injections of calcium ions into spinal motoneurons, J. Physiol., 225:363-390.

Krnjević, K., and Phillis, J.W., 1963a, Iontophoretic studies of neurones in the mammalian cerebral cortex, J. Physiol., 165:274-304.

Krnjević, K., and Phillis, J.W., 1963b, Pharmacological properties of acetylcholine-sensitive cells in the cerebral cortex. J. Physiol., 166:328-350.

Krnjević, K., Pumain, R., and Renaud, L., 1971a, Effect of Ba^{2+} and tetraethylammonium on cortical neurones. J. Physiol., 215:223-245.

Krnjević, K., Pumain, R., and Renaud, L., 1971b, The mechanism of excitation by acetylcholine in the cerebral cortex, J. Physiol., 215:247-268.

Krnjević, K., Reiffenstein, R.J., and Ropert, N., 1980, Disinhibitory action of acetylcholine in the hippocampus, J. Physiol., 308:73-74P.

Krnjević, K., and Ropert, N., 1982, Electrophysiological and pharmacological characteristics of facilitation of hippocampal population spikes by stimulation of the medial septum, Neuroscience, 7:2165-2183.

Krnjević, K., and Silver, A., 1965, A histochemical study of cholinergic fibres in the cerebral cortex, J. Anat. (Lond.), 99:711-759.

Krnjević, K., and Silver, A., 1966, Acetylcholinesterase in the developing forebrain, J. Anat. (Lond.), 100:63-89.

Lewis, P.R., Shute, C.C.D., and Silver, A., 1967, Confirmation from choline acetylase analyses of a massive cholinergic innervation to the rat hippocampus, J. Physiol., 191:215-224.

Libet, B., 1973, Electrical stimulation of cortex in human subjects, and conscious sensory aspects, Handb. Sensory Physiol., Springer-Verlag, Berlin, 2:743-790.

MacIntosh, F.C., and Oborin, P.E., 1953, Release of acetylcholine from intact cerebral cortex, Abst. XIX Int. Physiol. Congr., Montréal, pp. 580-581.

Meech, R.W., 1972, Intracellular calcium injection causes increased potassium conductance in Aplysia nerve cells, Comp. Biochem. Physiol., 42A:493-499.

Mesulam, M.-M., Mufson, E.J., Wainer, B.H., and Levey, A.I., 1983, Central cholinergic pathways in the rat: an overview based on an alternative nomenclature (Ch1-Ch6). Neuroscience, 10:1185-1201.

Morita, K., North, R.A., and Tokimasa, T., 1982, Muscarinic agonists inactivate potassium conductance of guinea-pig myenteric neurones, J. Physiol., 333:125-139.

Newberry, N.R., and Nicoll, R.A., 1985, Comparison of the action of baclofen with γ-aminobutyric acid on rat hippocampal pyramidal cells, J. Physiol., 360:161-85.

Segal, M., 1983, Rat hippocampal neurons in culture: responses to electrical and chemical stimuli, J. Neurophysiol., 50:1249-1264.

Shute, C.C.D., and Lewis, P.R., 1963, Cholinesterase-containing systems of the brain of the rat, Nature (Lond.), 199:1160-1164.

Sillito, A.M., and Kemp, J.A., 1983, Cholinergic modulation of the functional organization of the cat visual cortex, Brain Res., 289:143-155.

Spehlmann, R., 1963, Acetylcholine and prostigmine electrophoresis at visual cortical neurons, J. Neurophysiol., 26:127-139.

Stafstrom, C.E., Schwindt, P.C., Chubb, M.C., and Crill, W.E., 1985, Properties of persistent sodium conductance and calcium conductance of layer V neurons from cat sensorimotor cortex in vitro, J. Neurophysiol., 53:153-170.

Stone, T.W., 1972, Cholinergic mechanisms in the rat somatosensory cerebral cortex, J. Physiol., 225:485-499.

Szerb, J.C., 1978, Characterization of presynaptic muscarinic receptors in central cholinergic neurons, in: "Cholinergic Mechanisms and Psychopharmacology, Advances in Behavioural Biology", Vol. 24, D.J. Jenden, ed., Plenum Press, New York, pp. 49-60.

Takeuchi, N., 1963, Some properties of conductance changes at the end-plate membrane during the action of acetylcholine, J. Physiol., 167:128-140.

Taylor, C.P., and Dudek, F.E., 1982, Synchronous neural afterdischarges in rat hippocampal slices without active chemical synapses, Science, 218:810-812.

Valentino, R.J., and Dingledine, R., 1981, Presynaptic inhibitory effect of acetylcholine in the hippocampus, J. Neuroscience, 1:784-792.

Whitehouse, P.J., Price, D.L., Struble, R.G., Clark, A.W., Coyle, J.T., and DeLong, M.R., 1982, Alzheimer's disease and senile dementia: loss of neurons in the basal forebrain, Science, 215:1237-1239.

Woody, C.D., Swartz, B.E., and Gruen, E., 1978, Effects of acetylcholine and cyclic GMP on input resistance of cortical neurons in awake cats, Brain Res., 158:373-395.

Zieglgänsberger, W., and Reiter, C., 1974, A cholinergic mechanism in the spinal cord of cats, Neuropharmacol., 13:519-527.

ACTIONS OF ACETYLCHOLINE ON SPINAL MOTONEURONS

Z.G. Jiang and N.J. Dun

Loyola University of Chicago, Stritch School of Medicine
Department of Pharmacology
2160 South First Avenue
Maywood, IL 60153

INTRODUCTION

The evidence that acetylcholine (ACh) is a chemical transmitter in the vertebrate peripheral nervous system is unequivocal. A transmitter and/or modulator role of ACh in the vertebrate central nervous system is less well established (cf. Karczmar, 1967; Krnjevic, 1974). The most extensively investigated central cholinergic synapses are those on Renshaw cells of the spinal cord where ACh was shown to be the excitatory transmitter released from collateral branches of spinal motoneurons (Eccles et al., 1954; 1956; Curtis and Eccles, 1958). The effect of ACh on the motoneuron itself is not well understood. Recent studies with antibodies raised against choline acetyltransferase (CAT) revealed in addition to CAT-containing motoneurons, the presence of CAT-containing small diameter neurons as well as fibers in the ventral horn (Kimura et al., 1981; Houser et al., 1983; Borges and Iversen, 1986). In fact, CAT-immunoreactive boutons appeared to abut on motoneurons suggesting that ACh may exert a transmitter and/or modulator role at these neurons (Borges and Iversen, 1986). In an effort to provide a pharmacological basis for a possible transmitter or modulator function of ACh in the ventral horn, the actions of ACh on motoneurons and on spinal synaptic transmission were investigated using thin spinal cord slices as stable intracellular recordings can be maintained for hours in this preparation.

MATERIALS AND METHODS

Sprague-Dawley rats 10-15 days old were used in this study. The procedures used in obtaining thin transverse (400-500 μm) slices of thoracolumbar spinal cord from neonatal rats have been described earlier (Ma and Dun, 1985, 1986). The slices with ventral and dorsal rootlets were transferred to the recording chamber and continuously superfused with a Krebs solution saturated with 95% O_2 and 5% CO_2; the temperature of the solution was maintained at $34 \pm 0.5^{\circ}C$. Intracellular recordings were obtained from neurons situated in the ventral horn by means of glass microelectrodes filled with 3M K acetate; the impedance of the microelectrodes varied between 30 and 100 MΩ. Electrical stimulation of the ventral and dorsal rootlets was accomplished via concentric bipolar electrodes positioned close to the respective rootlets. Signals were

amplified via a WPI 707A preamplifier and displayed on either a Nicolet
Digital Oscilloscope or a Gould pen recorder. Signals stored in the
Nicolet Digital Oscilloscope were later retrieved, processed and plotted on
a Hewlett Packard Plotter.

RESULTS

Identification of Motoneurons

Ventral horn neurons were identified as motoneurons by the appearance
of an all-or-none spike potential or initial segment action potential
following the stimulation of ventral rootlets (Fig. 1). In a total of 127
impaled ventral horn neurons, 76 neurons exhibited antidromic spikes. To
ascertain that the antidromically activated neuron was a motoneuron, the
conduction velocity of antidromic spike was calculated according to

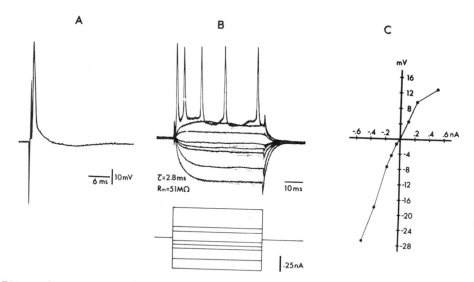

Figure 1. Membrane properties of a type I motoneuron in the neonatal rat
spinal cord slice. A: antidromic spike following stimulation of
ventral rootlets. B: depolarizing and hyperpolarizing
electrotonic potentials elicited by graded current pulses. C:
voltage-current relationship obtained from B. The V/I curve
showed a normal rectification when the cell was depolarized. The
axonal conduction velocity was estimated to be 45 m/s for this
motoneuron.

the method described by Blight and Someya (1985). Two types of motoneurons
could be distinguished on the basis of their conduction velocities and
membrane properties. The first type (47 of 58 motoneurons), referred to
herein as type I, exhibited low input resistance, short time constant and
high conduction velocity. The remaining motoneurons (type II) had higher
input resistance, longer time constant and slower conduction velocity.
Representative recordings obtained from type I and type II neurons are
shown in Figs. 1 and 2, respectively. The membrane properties of these two
types of motoneurons are summarized in Table 1. These two types of
motoneurons may correspond to the α and γ motoneurons that were described
in situ by Eccles (1964).

ACh Depolarizations

Applied either by superfusion (0.1-1 mM) or by pressure ejection (100 mM ACh, 3-30 ms pulse duration, 40 psi, tip diameter 5-10 μm), ACh caused a depolarization in 58 of the 76 motoneurons examined. In the large majority of motoneurons sampled (46 of 58), the ACh depolarization was relatively slow in onset and reached the peak in 15-40 sec. A biphasic response, i.e., a brisk depolarization followed by a slow response, was noted in 5 motoneurons (Fig. 5). Finally, ACh caused a fast depolarization in 3 motoneurons (Fig. 4). Pharmacological studies revealed that the slow and

Table I

Membrane Properties of Two Types of Spinal Motoneurons

	Type I Cell (n = 47)	Type II Cell (n = 11)
Resting Potential (mV)	-65.7 ± 4.8	-62.7 ± 7.9
Action Potential (mV)	76.0 ± 8.3	74.2 ± 9.9
Conduction Velocity (m/s)	$41 - 66*$ (n = 8)	$12 - 30*$ (n = 4)
Input Resistance (MΩ)	21.6 ± 6.3 (7.5 - 54)	109 ± 52.8 (40 - 186)
Time Constant (ms)	3.0 ± 0.6 (1.7 - 4.5)	7.8 ± 0.96 (5.2 - 9.3)

* Calculated at the temperature of $34 \pm 0.5^{\circ}C$.
Values in parentheses represent the range

fast ACh depolarizations were blocked, respectively, by atropine and by either d-tubocurarine (d-Tc) or hexamethonium. On the other hand, a combination of atropine and d-Tc were needed to completely eliminate the biphasic response. Both the slow and fast depolarizations were enhanced by low concentrations (< 0.1 μM) of physostigmine.

Muscarinic Depolarizations

The slow depolarization induced by ACh was principally muscarinic in nature as the responses were antagonized completely by atropine (0.1 - 1μ M). The muscarinic depolarization recorded in 8 of the 10 motoneurons tested were not affected by low Ca solution, whereas the response was slightly depressed in the remaining two cells; this indicated that in the majority of motoneurons the response was due to a direct activation of motoneuron muscarinic receptors. The muscarinic depolarization was associated with an increase in membrane resistance (15 - 18%) in 12 of the 18 cells tested (Fig. 3). In the remaining 6 motoneurons, the depolarization was not accompanied by a detectable change in membrane resistance. The muscarinic depolarization was attenuated upon conditioning hyperpolarization and nullified at the membrane potential of -70 to -108 mV (mean $\pm$ SD = -91 ± 12.2 mV, n = 9). In three experiments the recording electrode had relatively low resistance (< 30 MΩ); thus, it was possible to pass into the cell large enough current to hyperpolarize the membrane potential to levels more negative than -100 mV. In these three cases, a reversal of the polarity of muscarinic depolarizations was not observed.

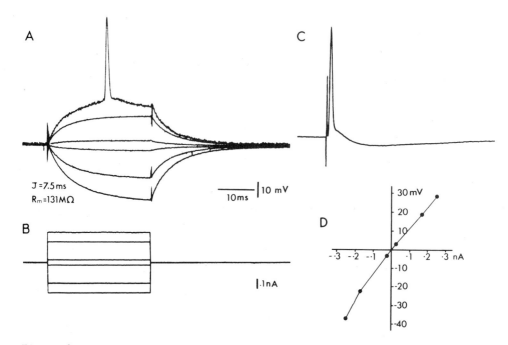

Figure 2. Membrane properties of a type II motoneuron. Graded hyperpolarizing and depolarizing electrotonic potentials (A) elicited by graded current pulses (B). An action potential appeared when sufficiently large depolarizing current was injected into the soma. C: an antidromic spike evoked by stimulation of the ventral rootlets. The conduction velocity of the motor axon was calculated to be 20 m/s. Graph D shows the voltage-current relationship of the data obtained from A and B. The resting potential of this motoneuron was -69 mV. The input resistance (Rm) and time constant (τ) was 131 MΩ and 7.5 ms, respectively.

Nicotinic Depolarizations

ACh caused a fast depolarization (0.2 - 4 sec peak time) with a short lasting duration (1.8 - 15 sec) in 3 motoneurons. As the depolarization was not blocked by atropine or tetrodotoxin (Fig. 4), but was sensitive to d-Tc (50 μM) and hexamethonium (0.1 mM), it appeared to be nicotinic in nature. The nicotinic depolarization was associated with a small decrease (10 - 20%) in membrane resistance and the response was enhanced by conditioning hyperpolarization (Fig. 4). The extrapolated reversal potential of the nicotinic depolarization varied between -30 and -10 mV in the 3 cells examined.

Biphasic Responses

A biphasic response was observed in 8 motoneurons as in this case a fast rising and rapidly decaying depolarization was followed by a slower and longer lasting response (Fig. 5). The first and second phase of the response were reversibly eliminated by d-Tc and atropine, respectively, indicating that the response was due to the activation of nicotinic and muscarinic receptors.

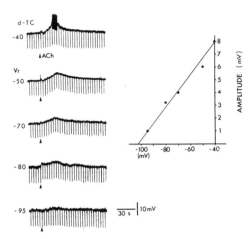

Figure 3. The voltage dependence of the ACh muscarinic depolarizations in a motoneuron. d-Tc (10 μM) was added to the Krebs solution throughout the experiment. Hyperpolarizing currents were injected into the cell to shift the membrane potential to a desired level as indicated by numerals to the left of each tracing. The resting potential (Vr) was -50 mV. The graph on the right was plotted with the data from the tracings on the right. The null potential was about -100 mV for this particular motoneuron.

ATROP+TTX

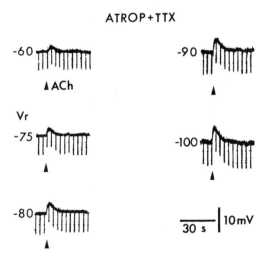

Figure 4. Nicotinic receptor mediated depolarizations in a type II motoneuron. The response was not blocked by atropine (1 μM) and tetrodotoxin (TTX, 0.2 μM). Note that the depolarization was faster in onset and shorter lasting as compared to that shown in Fig. 3. The membrane resistance was decreased by about 10% during the response. Conditioning depolarization and hyperpolarization from the resting potential (Vr) reduced and enhanced the amplitude of ACh potential, respectively. D-tubocurarine (10 μM) completely blocked the ACh response after 10 min application (not shown).

The occurrence of different types of cholinergic responses appeared to relate to the type of the motoneurons generating the response. Table 2 summarizes the frequency of occurrence of nicotinic, muscarinic, or biphasic type of cholinergic response in type I vs. type II motoneurons. Clearly, muscarinic depolarizations occurred most frequently in type I motoneurons, whereas type II motoneurons exhibited a high incidence of biphasic cholinergic responses.

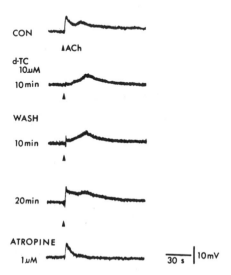

Figure 5. ACh induced a biphasic response in a type II motoneuron in a rat spinal cord slice. Note that in control recording, ACh ejection elicited a fast rising and decaying potential followed by a slow depolarization. The initial phase was reversibly blocked by d-tubocurarine; whereas, the second phase was completely abolished by atropine within 10 min.

Table 2

Excitatory Action of ACh on Motoneurons

	Group I Cells	Group II Cells
Numbers of Cells Tested	27*	11*
Muscarinic Depolarization	18	1
Nicotinic plus Muscarinic Depolarizations	2	6
Nicotinic Depolarization	1	2
No Response	6	2

* Chi-square test, $p < 0.05$

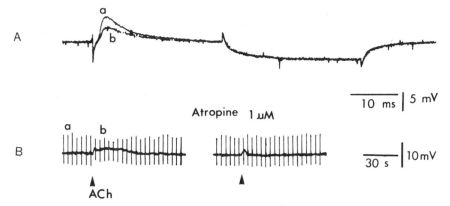

Figure 6. Depolarization and suppression of EPSPs by ACh in a motoneuron. A: superimposed recordings of EPSPs before (a) and after (b) ACh. EPSPs were evoked by stimulation of dorsal rootlets. The hyperpolarizing electrotonic potentials showed no apparent change after ACh. B: chart recordings of EPSPs (small upward deflections) and hyperpolarizing electrotonic potentials (small downward deflections). Pressure ejection of ACh (arrowheads) caused a depolarization and a reduction of EPSP amplitude. Atropine effectively blocked both the depolarization and synaptic depression caused by ACh.

Suppression of Excitatory Postsynaptic Potentials By ACh

In addition to its depolarizing effect, ACh was found to depress excitatory post-synaptic potentials (EPSPs) evoked by stimulation of the dorsal rootlets in 8 of the 12 motoneurons investigated. The depression was not due to membrane depolarization induced by ACh as returning the membrane potential to the resting level did not restore the EPSP amplitude (Jiang and Dun, 1986). The depolarization as well as the synaptic depression caused by ACh was effectively prevented by pretreating the slice with atropine but not with d-Tc (Fig. 6).

The depolarization induced by pressure ejection of glutamate was not appreciably affected by ACh in 3 motoneurons tested. Furthermore, superfusion of the slices with strychnine (1 µM) and/or bicuculline (1 µM) did not modify the inhibitory action of ACh on the EPSPs. Collectively, the results suggest that ACh depresses synaptic transmission by a presynaptic mechanism as it activates presynaptic muscarinic receptors thus reducing the release of the transmitter (Jiang and Dun, 1986).

DISCUSSION

Our results show that the cholinergic action on the spinal ventral horn neuron, whether post or presynatpic, is exerted mainly via muscarinic receptors. Two such actions were demonstrated: first, a majority of motoneurons was excited by ACh primarily via muscarinic receptors; only a small portion of motoneurons being activated by nicotinic stimulation; second, ACh depressed synaptic transmission in motoneurons by acting at a presynatpic muscarinic site (Jiang and Dun, 1986).

The excitatory muscarinic effect on the motoneurons observed here is consistent with the early studies that demonstrated that the injection of ACh into the spinal cord circulation increases motor discharges and the effects are blocked by atropine (Bulbring and Burn, 1941; Calma and Wright, 1944). However, the site of action of ACh could not be determined in these earlier studies. The present study indicates that this site in question is the motoneuron; furthermore, as the ACh-induced depolarization generally was not affected by low Ca solution, the response was due to the direct action of ACh on the motoneurons. The responses in a small portion of motoneurons were depressed, but never completely eliminated by low Ca, suggesting that in addition to depolarizing motoneurons directly, exogenously applied ACh may also stimulate nearby excitatory interneurons.

Interestingly, the muscarinic and nicotinic depolarization induced by ACh in motoneurons bear strong resemblance to the respective responses evoked in autonomic ganglia. The nicotinic depolarization elicited in motoneurons was found to be associated with a decrease in membrane resistance and it was increased by membrane hyperpolarization; these features are similar to those of the nicotinic depolarization observed in the autonomic neurons which is primarily due to an increase of membrane conductance to Na and K (Koketsu, 1969; Nishi, 1974). Whether or not an analogous mechanism is involved in the nicotinic depolarization of the motoneuron remains to be verified. Similarly, the muscarinic depolarization of the motoneurons was accompanied in most cases by an increase of input resistance and it was attenuated by hyperpolarization, these findings being compatible with the notion that the muscarinic depolarization of the motoneurons is due to the inactivation of K conductance as has been suggested for the peripheral ganglion cells (Weight and Votava, 1970; Kuba and Koketsu, 1976; Brown and Adams, 1980). The same mechanism seems to underlie central muscarinic depolarization as in the case of cortical neurons (Krnjevic et al., 1971) and hippocampal cells (Dodd et al., 1981). However, the muscarinic depolarization in a number of motoneurons was not associated with a clear change of membrane resistance; in this case, the response was relatively independent of the membrane potential. A change in membrane resistance during muscarinic depolarization may not be detected, despite an increase and/or decrease of ionic conductance, if the active sites are located on the dendrites, far away from the recording site in the soma. Alternatively, the possibility cannot be ruled out that the muscarinic activation may cause membrane conductance change with respect to several ions; this would not result in any net change of membrane resistance. In this context, Kuba and Koketsu (1976) reported that muscarinic depolarization in a portion of bullfrog ganglion cells was not associated with a clear change in membrane resistance, as this depolarization was probably caused by a change of membrane permeability to several ions including Na, K and Ca. A similar conclusion was reached with respect to the muscarinic depolarization of the rat hippocampal cells (Segal, 1982). Finally, the possible involvement of second messengers, such as cyclic GMP, in the mediation of muscarinic depolarization that is apparently not associated with any conductance change in the rabbit sympathetic neurons should also be kept in mind (Hashiguchi et al., 1982; Karczmar and Dun, 1985).

Still another finding concerning the occurrence in the motoneurons of muscarinic and nicotinic responses must be emphasized: type I motoneurons appeared to be activated exclusively via muscarinic receptors, whereas type II motoneurons seem to be endowed with both nicotinic and muscarinic receptors. The physiological implication of this differential distribution of muscarinic and nicotinic receptors in these two types of motoneurons and of its relation to α and γ motoneurons (Eccles, 1964) remains to be investigated.

A second action of ACh on the motoneurons was demonstrated at this time. This action consisted of a depression of EPSPs evoked by stimulation of dorsal rootlets. The depression of EPSPs may be attributed to a presynaptic effect of ACh resulting in a reduction of transmitter liberation. First, while depressing the EPSPs, the depolarization induced by the putative transmitter glutamate in the spinal cord (Fonnum, 1984) was not appreciably affected by ACh. Second, ACh remained effective in depressing the EPSPs in the presence of strychnine and bicuculline; if the depression was due to a release of inhibitory transmitters glycine and GABA from spinal interneurons that could be activated by ACh, the depression of EPSPs should have been antagonized by strychnine and bicuculline. In this connection, extensive literature indicates the presence of muscarinic receptors in the peripheral autonomic nerve endings and the activation of these receptors leads to a diminution of ACh or norepinephrine release (Kilbinger, 1984). An analogus mechanism may indeed be present in the presynaptic endings abutting upon the motoneurons of the spinal cord. Our finding that ACh may exert an inhibitory and an excitatory effect via two different sites is significant as it may explain the contradictory results reported in a number of early studies concerning the action of ACh on motoneurons (Curtis et al., 1966; Weight and Salmoiraghi, 1966).

In conclusion, our results indicate that a large number of motoneurons are endowed with excitatory muscarinic receptors while a few may exhibit nicotinic receptors. In addition, there is evidence for the presence of inhibitory muscarinic receptors situated in nerve endings that are presynaptic in relation to the motoneurons. In conjunction with the demonstration of CAT-containing fibers and interneurons in the ventral horn (Borges and Iversen, 1986) these findings raise the possibility that ACh released from collateral fibers of motoneurons or from cholinergic interneurons may regulate motoneuron activity via both pre and postsynaptic mechanisms.

REFERENCES

Blight, A.R. and Someya, S., 1985, Depolarizing afterpotentials in myelinated axons of mammalian spinal cord, Neuroscience, 15:1-12.

Borges, L.F. and Iversen, S.D., 1986, Topography of choline acetyltransferase immunoreactive neurons and fibers in the rat spinal cord, Brain Res., 362:140-148.

Brown, D.A. and Adams, P.R., 1980, Muscarinic suppression of a novel voltage-sensitive K^+ current in a vertebrate neurone, Nature, 283:673-676.

Bulbring, E. and Burn, J.H., 1941, Observations bearing on synaptic transmission by acetylcholine in the spinal cord, J. Physiol. (Lond.), 100:337-368.

Calma, I. and Wright, S., 1944, Action of acetylcholine, atropine and eserine on the central nervous system of the decerebrate cat, J. Physiol. (Lond.), 103:93-102.

Curtis, D.R. and Eccles, R.M., 1958, The excitation of Renshaw cells by pharmacological agents applied electrophoretically, J. Physiol. (Lond.), 141:435-445.

Curtis, D.R., Ryall, R.W. and Watkins, J.C., 1966, The action of cholinomimetics on spinal interneurones, Expl. Brain Res., 2:97-106.

Dodd, J., Dingledine, R. and Kelly, J.S., 1981, The excitatory action of acetylcholine on hippocampal neurones of the guinea pig and rat maintained in vitro, Brain Res., 207:109-127.

Eccles, J.C., 1964, "The Physiology of Synapses," Springer, Berlin.

Eccles, J.C., Eccles, R.M. and Fatt, P., 1956, Pharmacological investigations on a central synapse operated by acetylcholine, J. Physiol. (Lond.), 131:154-169.

Eccles, J.C., Fatt, P. and Koketsu, K., 1954, Cholinergic and inhibitory synapses in a pathway from motor axon collaterals to motoneurones, J. Physiol. (Lond.), 126:524-562.

Fonnum, F., 1984, Glutamate: a neurotransmitter in mammalian brain, J. Neurochem., 42:1-11.

Hashiguchi, T., Kobayashi, H., Tosaka, T. and Libet, B., 1982, Two muscarinic depolarizing mechanisms in mammalian sympathetic neurons, Brain Res., 242:378-382.

Houser, C.R., Crawford, G.D., Barber, R.P., Salvaterra, P.M. and Vaughn, J.E., 1983, Organization and morphological characteristics of cholinergic neurons: an immunocytochemical study with a monoclonal antibody to choline acetyltransferase, Brain Res., 266:97-119.

Jiang, Z.G. and Dun, N.J., 1986, Presynaptic suppression of excitatory postsynaptic potentials in rat ventral horn neurons by muscarinic agonists, submitted.

Karczmar, A.G., 1967, Neuromuscular pharmacology, Ann. Rev. Pharmacol., 7:241-276.

Karczmar, A.G., and Dun, N.J., 1985, Pharmacology of synaptic ganglionic transmission and second messengers, in: "Autonomic and Enteric Ganglia: Transmission and Its Pharmacology," A.G. Karczmar, K. Koketsu, and S. Nishi, eds., Plenum Press, New York.

Kilbinger, H., 1984, Presynaptic muscarine receptors modulating acetylcholine release, Trends in Pharmacol. Sci., 5:103-105.

Kimura, H., McGeer, P.L., Peng, J.H. and McGeer, E.G., 1981, The central cholinergic system studied by choline acetyltransferase immunohistochemistry in the rat, J. Comp. Neurol., 200:151-201.

Koketsu, K., 1969, Cholinergic synaptic potentials and the underlying ionic mechanisms, Federal Proceedings, 28:101-131.

Koketsu, K. and Yamada, M., 1982, Presynaptic muscarinic receptors inhibiting active acetylcholine release in the bullfrog sympathetic ganglion, Br. J. Pharmacol., 77:75-82.

Krnjevic, K., 1974, Chemical nature of synaptic transmission in vertebrates, Physiol. Rev., 54:418-540.

Krnjevic, K., Pumain, R. and Renaud, L., 1971, The mechanism of excitation by acetylcholine in the cerebral cortex, J.Physiol. (Lond.), 215:247-268.

Kuba, K. and Koketsu, K., 1976, Analysis of the slow excitatory postsynaptic potential in bullfrog sympathetic ganglion cells, Jap. J. Physiol., 26:647-664.

Ma, R.C. and Dun, N.J., 1985, Vasopressin depolarizes lateral horn cells of the neonatal rat spinal cord in vitro, Brain Res., 348:36-43.

Ma, R.C. and Dun, N.J., 1986, Excitation of lateral horn neurons of the neonatal rat spinal cord by 5-hydroxytryptamine, Develop. Brain. Res., 24:89-98.

Nishi, S., 1974, Ganglionic transmission, in: "The Peripheral Nervous System," J.I. Hubbard, ed., Plenum Press, New York.

Segal, M., 1982, Multiple actions of acetylcholine at a muscarinic receptor studied in the rat hippocampal slice, Brain Res., 246:77-87.

Weight, F.F. and Votava, J., 1970, Slow synaptic excitation in sympathetic ganglion cells: evidence for synaptic inactivation of potassium conductance, Science, 170:755-758.

Weight, F.F. and Salmoiraghi, G.C., 1966, Responses of spinal cord interneurons to acetylcholine norepinephrine and serotonin administered by microelectrophoresis, J.P.E.T., 153:420-427.

AN EEG INVESTIGATION OF THE ASCENDING CHOLINERGIC PATHWAYS

Vincenzo G. Longo, Arsenia Scotti de Carolis, Stefano

Sagratella and Tarcisio Niglio

Istituto Superiore di Sanità, Rome, Italy

In the present paper are reported the results of an investigation on the influence on the cerebral electrical activity (EEG) of the stimulation and destruction of the cholinergic nuclei of the basal forebrain in the rabbit.

The presentation will be divided into three sections: the first deals with the results of the electrical stimulation of various subcortical areas; the second with the administration of drugs; the third with chemical destruction of the basal forebrain centers.

Effects of the electrical stimulation of the basal forebrain

Since the basal forebrain nuclei have been considered as the anterior extension of the reticular formation, we have undertaken a study on the effects on the cortical electrical activity of the stimulation of the regio innominata (R.I.), compared to that of the mesencephalic reticular formation (M.R.F.).

High frequency stimulation (250 Hz) of either region induces an electrocortical arousal. The intensity of the stimulus necessary to induce an EEG arousal of equivalent duration is 2-3 times higher for the R.I. compared to the M.R.F. (Fig. 1). Low frequency stimulation (5-10 Hz) of the R.I. gives rise to a recruiting response in the anterior sensori-motor cortex; this response is not elicitable upon stimulation of the M.R.F. (Fig. 2).

Effects of drugs

SCH 23390. When Shute and Lewis (1967) published their original work on the ascending cholinergic projections from the reticular nuclei to the forebrain, they described a dorsal and a ventral tegmental pathway. Later investigations indicated that the ventral pathway probably corresponded to a dopamine-containing projection system. We have therefore advanced the hypothesis that the difference in threshold we found in the experiments concerning the stimulation of M.R.F. and R.I. was due to the fact that two different systems (cholinergic and dopaminergic) were stimulated in the case of M.R.F., while only the cholinergic one was involved in the stimulation of the R.I. We have therefore administered SCH 23390, a blocker of the central dopamine receptors of the D_1 type (Iorio et al., 1983), trying to re-establish the balance between the two types of stimulation. The results indicated however that the drug

(0.1-3mg/kg i.v.) has a blocking effect on the EEG arousal which is
exerted equally with respect to the two types of stimulation.

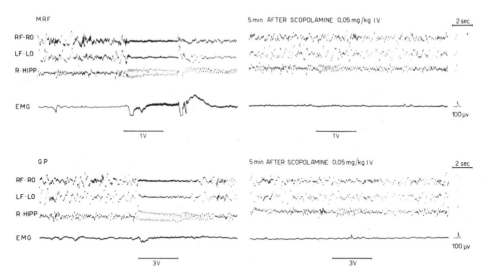

Fig. 1.   Effects of the electrical stimulation of the M.R.F. (upper
           record) and of the R.I. (lower record) on the EEG of the rabbit.
           The bar indicates the application of the stimulus.   The activa-
           tion of the record is obtained with different stimulus intensi-
           ties which are considerably higher for the R.I.   Note also the
           spasm of the neck muscles induced by the stimulation of the
           reticular formation.   The administration of scopolamine blocks
           the response to both stimulations.   Stimulus parameters: 250 Hz,
           0.1 m sec.   Leads: RF-RO: right anterior sensorimotor cortex-
           optic cortex; LF-LO: left anterior sensorimotor cortex-optic
           cortex; R HIPP: right dorsal hippocampus; EMG: electromyogram
           of the neck muscles.

Effects of scopolamine.   Scopolamine was administered in doses of 0.05-0.1
mg/kg i.v.   The drug raised the threshold of the arousal EEG response to
the high frequency electrical stimulation of the M.R.F. and of the R.I.
It did not influence the recruiting response.   These data confirm and
extend to the R.I. previous results obtained in ours(Longo, 1966) and in
other laboratories (Fig. 1).

Effects of hemicholinium-3 (HC-3).   This drug blocks the uptake of
choline by the cholinergic nerve terminals.   This limitation of acetylcholine (ACh) synthesis leads to a diminution of whole brain levels of the
neurotransmitter.

     In our experiments HC-3 was administered into the cerebral ventricles
of the rabbit and into the R.F.M. and R.I., in doses of 50-500 μg.

     Immediately after the administration of 125 μg of the drug into the
cerebral lateral ventricles, a cortical and subcortical desynchronization was noticed, followed after about 1 hour by a generalized slowing
and a blockade of the arousal reaction to external stimulation.   The
same effects were obtained by administering the drug into the M.R.F. or
into the R.I.   In order to ascertain if the depletion of brain ACh was
responsible for these changes, some of these animals were treated with

eserine, which reduced the amplitude of the slow waves but failed to
induce the desynchronization of the record or the return of the response
to the acoustical stimuli.

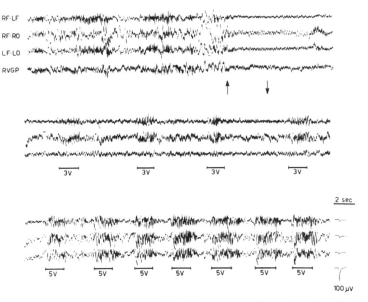

Fig. 2.   Recruiting response after low frequency electrical stimulation
          of the R.I. of the rabbit.
          Upper record.   Concomitant with the spindles in the cortical
          leads, waves at the same frequency are noticed in the R.I.
          Between the arrows a vibro acoustical stimulus is applied.
          Middle record.   Electrical stimulation (3 V, 10 Hz, 0.5 msec) of
          the R.I. elicits the appearance of the recruiting response in the
          ipsilateral cortex.
          Lower record.   The recruiting spreads to the contralateral
          cortex when the intensity of stimulation is increased to 5 V.
          Leads: RF-LF: anterior sensorimotor cortex; RF-RO: right
          anterior sensorimotor cortex-optic cortex; LF-LO: left
          anterior sensorimotor cortex-optic cortex; RVGP: right regio
          innominata.

     Some additional experiments were performed, in which the drug in
concentrations of 1 and 2.5% in water was applied to the cortex.   No
significant modifications of the record were observed.   With the higher
concentration cortical seizures appeared one hour after the application.
It should be noticed in this regard that animals treated intraventricularly with the highest doses (250-500 µg) showed convulsions.

Effects of chemical destruction of the basal forebrain
AF64A (ethylcholine mustard aziridinium).   This choline analog has been
often used as a tool for developing animal models of central cholinergic
hypofunction (Fisher and Hanin, 1980).   Intrastriatal injection of AF64A
produces a persistent reduction in biochemical processes required for
cholinergic transmission.   AF64A was tested in rabbits with chronically
implanted electrodes in order to follow the progression of the EEG
changes and eventually the recovery.   Unilateral lesions were used since
they made it possible to compare damaged and intact hemispheres in the
same animals.   The drug was administered into the R.I. of one side and
the records were obtained from 24 hours up to 45 days after treatment.
The minimal dose which induced EEG changes was 60 nmol.   These changes

appeared 3-7 days after the treatment and were localized ipsilaterally to the injected side. They consisted of a generalized slowing of the cortical waves, disappearance of the spindles and blockade of the arousal reaction to external stimuli (Fig. 3). Behaviorally, in the first days the animals were depressed, their muscle tonus was diminished, and there was a loss of weight; these changes disappeared in about one week, when the EEG changes were at their maximum. Return of the EEG to normal usually took 3 weeks, although in one case treated with 150 nM the changes lasted up to 45 days.

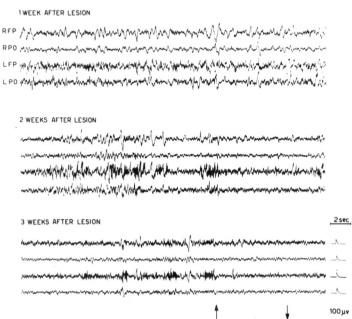

Fig. 3.   Modifications of the EEG record after injection of AF64A (150 nmol) into the right R.I. in a rabbit bearing chronically implanted electrodes.
One week after the treatment (upper record) the electrocorticogram corresponding to the lesioned side is rich in slow waves, spindles are absent. The spindles are always absent two (middle record) and three weeks after treatment. Between arrows: vibroacoustical stimulation.
Leads: RFP: right anterior-posterior sensorimotor cortex; RPO: right posterior sensorimotor-optic cortex; LFP: left anterior-posterior sensorimotor cortex; LPO: left posterior sensorimotor-optic cortex.

These changes were seen only after administration of the drug into the R.I. Intracerebroventricular administration of doses up to 150 nM elicited only a slowing of the EEG lasting for 4-5 days, while injection into the M.R.F. was not followed by significant changes of the electrocorticogram.

In the animals showing disappearance of the spindles in the cortex ipsilateral to the injected site, drugs which are known to induce synchronization of the EEG were administered. Scopolamine, pentobarbital and clonidine did not cause the spindles to reappear in the cortex ipsilateral to the lesioned side (Fig. 4). On the other hand, eserine lost its "desynchronizing" power. Upon topical application into the cortex, the drug did not affect the record. However, 30-40 minutes after deposition of a 2.5% solution, EEG seizures occurred.

The anatomical post mortem examinations showed that the lesions that appeared mainly when the high doses were administered, extended well behind the R.I. and in some instances included the thalamic nuclei. The question therefore arises if these changes are due to the destruction of the R.I., or involve as well other structures. Moreover, as the high doses of the drug were employed, it can be hypothesized that other neurotransmitter systems, in addition to the cholinergic system, are involved in the changes which have been described.

Effects of HC-3 on a passive avoidance task in rats. Behaviorally, HC-3, injected intracerebrally or into the cerebral ventricles, has been found to impair learning of a conditioned avoidance response in rats and mice. We have examined the effects of HC-3 administered into the left and right basal globus pallidus of the rat in doses of 20 μg. Training consisted of administering a 2 sec foot shock on entry into the dark compartment of a two-compartment box. Control rats retested 1, 2 and 24 hr later showed a median latency of entry of 240 sec. Administration of HC-3 30 minutes before training produced a significant reduction in latency of entry on retesting, compared to vehicle treated controls. The results with this drug resembled these obtained with scopolamine, 1 mg/kg i.p.

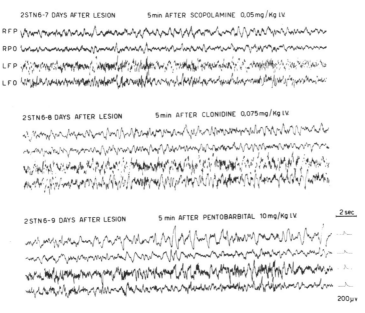

Fig. 4. Effects of drugs on the EEG of a rabbit treated with 150 nmol of AF64A into the R.I. After treatment with various "synchronizing" drug the spindles appear only in the cortex contralateral to the lesioned side. Leads: as in Fig. 3.

The role of a cholinergic input in the control of neocortical electrical activity has been emphasized in the joint studies of this laboratory and of that of Loyola University (Longo, 1966; Karczmar et al., 1970); the present investigation has provided further evidence as to the significance of this input. In particular we have shown that one functional result of unilateral lesions of the R.I. is the disappearance of the spindles in the ipsilateral cortex. Two other changes observed in the course of these experiments are probably dependent on the elimination of the cholinergic input to the cortex: one is the blockade of the arousal reaction and the other is the lack of effect of eserine on the EEG.

These results suggest a potential use of EEG recording in designing animal models for psychiatric and neurological diseases involving the cholinergic system, such as Alzheimer's dementia.

REFERENCES

Fisher, A., and Hanin, I., 1980, Choline analogs as potential tools in developing selective animal models of central cholinergic hypofunction, Life Sci., 27:1615.

Iorio, L.C., Barnett, A., Leitz, F.H., Houser, V.P., and Korduba, C.A., 1983, SCH 23390, A potential benzodiazepine antipsychotic with unique interaction on dopaminergic systems. J. Pharmac. Exp. Ther., 226:462.

Karczmar, A.G., Longo, V.G., and Scotti de Carolis, A., 1970, A pharmacological model of paradoxical sleep: the role of cholinergic and monoamine systems, Physiol. and Behavior, 5:175.

Longo, V.G., 1966, Behavioral and electroencephalographic effects of atropine and related compounds. Pharmacol. Rev., 18:965.

Shute, C.C.D., and Lewis, P.R.V., 1967, The ascending cholinergic reticular system: neocortical, olfactory and subcortical projections, Brain, 90:497.

ACTIVATION AND BLOCKADE OF THE NICOTINIC AND GLUTAMATERGIC SYNAPSES BY

REVERSIBLE AND IRREVERSIBLE CHOLINESTERASE INHIBITORS

Edson X. Albuquerque, Yasco Aracava[1], Mamdouh Idriss[2],
Bernhard Schönenberger[3], Arnold Brossi[3] and Sharad S. Deshpande

Department of Pharmacology and Experimental Therapeutics
University of Maryland School of Medicine
Baltimore, MD 21201 U.S.A.

INTRODUCTION

The nicotinic acetylcholine receptor-ionic channel (AChR)[4] of the neuromuscular junction, particularly that from <u>Torpedo</u> electric tissue, is the best characterized of all receptors. It has been functionally isolated, and the topographic arrangement of the polypeptide subunits and the amino acid composition have been detailed (Klymkowsky et al., 1980; Karlin et al., 1983; Noda et al., 1983; Sakmann et al., 1985). The involvement of some of these subunits in the binding sites for drugs has been determined biochemically and electrophysiologically (Krodel et al., 1979; Horn et al., 1980; Karlin, 1980; Aguayo et al., 1981; Spivak and Albuquerque, 1982; Changeux et al., 1984; Wan and Lindstrom, 1984). In addition to the sites that recognize ACh and other agonists and also specifically bind the snake venom α-bungarotoxin (α-BGT), the AChRs have several other sites, presumably located at the ionic channel moiety, to

This research was supported by the United States Army Research and Development Command Contract DAMD-17-84-C-4219.
[1]On leave of absence from the Departament of Pharmacology, Institute of Biomedical Sciences, University of São Paulo, 05508, São Paulo, Brazil.
[2]Permanent address: Division of Entomology, Faculty of Agriculture, University of Alexandria, Alexandria, Egypt.
[3]Permanent address: Laboratory of Chemistry, National Institute of Diabetes and Digestive and Kidney Diseases, Bethesda, MD, 20892.
[4]Abbreviations used: ACh, acetylcholine; AChR, acetylcholine receptor-ion channel complex; AP, action potential; α-BGT, α-bungarotoxin; ChE, cholinesterase; AChE, acetylcholinesterase; DFP, diisopropylfluorophosphate; EDP, edrophonium; EPC, endplate current; EPSC, excitatory postsynaptic current; EPSP, excitatory postsynaptic potential; ETiM, extensor tibialis muscle; FTiM, flexor tibialis muscle; MEPC, miniature endplate current; NEO, neostigmine; PHY, physostigmine; PYR, pyridostigmine; TTX, tetrodotoxin; τ_{EPC} and τ_{EPSC}, decay time constant of the EPC and EPSC, respectively.

which agents can bind and thereby allosterically modify neuromuscular transmission (Changeux et al., 1984). These sites bind to a class of ligands, known as noncompetitive blockers of the nicotinic receptor, which comprise a large variety of drugs with distinct pharmacological activities such as local anesthetics, phencyclidine and perhydrohistrionicotoxin (see Spivak and Albuquerque, 1982).

Investigations of the insect neuromuscular synapse revealed a lack of action of ACh and several other cholinergic agonists and antagonists (Colhoun, 1963; McDonald et al., 1972), although there is strong evidence that cholinergic transmission is present in central synapses of arthropods (Corteggiani and Serfaty, 1939; Tobias et al., 1946; Colhoun, 1958). Indeed, neither α-BGT nor α-Naja toxin affected the transmission in the insect neuromuscular junction (Idriss & Albuquerque, unpublished results). At arthropod neuromuscular synapses, the transmitter involved in the excitatory process seems to be L-glutamate (Usherwood and Grundfest, 1965; Usherwood and Machili, 1968; Faeder and O'Brien, 1970). The features of the insect central and peripheral synapses that control their suscep- tibility to ChE inhibitors are not clear. The relationship between the toxicity of the ChE inhibitors and their neurophysiological or neuro- chemical actions in insects has not been well established. The inhibition of ChE in vertebrates is reported to cause asphyxiation. However, it is still unknown why many anti-ChE agents are more toxic to insects than to vertebrates (Hollingworth, 1976) and how the inhibition of ChE in insects leads ultimately to death.

In addition to well known anti-ChE properties of carbamates at the cholinergic synapses which have been studied in detail by Karczmar and colaborators (Karczmar and Ohta, 1981; Karczmar and Dun, 1985), recent studies carried out in our laboratory have demonstrated that pyridostigmine interacts directly with sites on the neuromuscular AChR macromolecule (Pascuzzo et al., 1984; Akaike et al., 1984). Studies with a number of reversible and irreversible inhibitors of ChE have shown that, in addition to direct actions on the nicotinic AChR complex (Shaw et al., 1985; Aracava and Albuquerque, 1985), these agents interact with the pre- and postsynaptic components of the insect glutamatergic neuromuscular synapses (Idriss and Albuquerque, 1985b; Idriss et al., 1986; Rao et al., 1986). The importance of direct interactions of the ChE inhibitors with the nicotinic AChR has also been demonstrated in the studies determining the protection afforded by carbamates against the irreversible ChE inhibitors (Deshpande et al., 1986). This hypothesis was reinforced by the fact that physostigmine in its stereoisomeric (+) form, which is 100- fold less potent to block ChE than the natural (-) isomer, was able to provide similar protection against lethal doses of the organophosphate (OP) compounds. The purpose of the present investigation is therefore to unveil the direct actions of the reversible ChE inhibitors, physostigmine (PHY), neostigmine (NEO), edrophonium (EDP), pyridostigmine (PYR) and the irreversible organophosphate anti-ChE agents methylphosphonofluoridic acid 1,2,2-trimethylpropyl ester (soman), methylphosphonofluoridic acid 1- methylethylester (sarin), dimethylphosphoramidocyanidic acid, ethyl ester (tabun), diisopropylaminoethylmethylphosphonothiolate (VX) and diiso- propylfluorophosphate (DFP) on neuromuscular transmission of the frog and insect. In addition, the results from the protection studies using carbamates and some non anti-ChE agents in the prophylaxis against poisoning by OP compounds are presented.

MATERIALS AND METHODS

Preparations and Solutions

Frog Nerve-Muscle Preparations. Sciatic nerve-sartorius muscle preparations of the frog Rana pipiens were used for the studies of EPCs and for fluctuation analysis. Frog Ringer's solution had the following composition (mM): NaCl 116, KCl 2, $CaCl_2$ 1.8, Na_2HPO_4 1.3, NaH_2PO_4 0.7. The solution was saturated with pure oxygen and had a pH of 7.0 ± 0.1. For EPC experiments, the preparations were pretreated with 400-600 mM glycerol to disrupt excitation-contraction coupling while tetrodotoxin (TTX, 0.3 µM) was added to the bathing medium to prevent twitching during noise analysis experiments. All experiments were conducted at room temperature (22-24°C).

Locust Nerve-Muscle Preparations. FTiM and ETiM of adult Locusta migratoria were dissected according to the technique previously described by Hoyle (1955). The physiological solution had the following composition (mM): NaCl 170, KCl 10, NaH_2PO_4 4, Na_2HPO_4 6 and $CaCl_2$ 2. This solution had a pH of 6.8. To decrease the muscle twitch, the preparation was treated with glycerol (150 mM) and the physiological solution was modified by reducing $CaCl_2$ concentration to 0.8 mM, and by addition of 10 mM $MgCl_2$. For the noise analysis experiments, the concentration of Ca^{2+} was further decreased to 0.2 mM. To minimize receptor desensitization, the preparations were pretreated with 1 µM concanavalin-A for 30 min (Mathers and Usherwood, 1976). All experiments were carried out at room temperature (22-24°C).

Isolation of Muscle Fibers for Single Channel Recordings. Single fibers were isolated from the interosseal and lumbricalis muscles of the largest toe of the hind foot of the frog Rana pipiens. The physiological solution used was the frog Ringer's solution mentioned earlier. After careful dissection, the muscles were treated with collagenase (Type I, Sigma; 2 hrs) followed by protease (Type VII, Sigma; 20-30 min). During the protease treatment, the isolation of the fibers was achieved by application of a stream of the solution from a Pasteur pipette. Single fibers were stored overnight at 5°C in a solution containing bovine serum albumin (0.5 mg/ml). The details of this technique are described elsewhere (Allen et al., 1984).

Electrophysiological Techniques

EPC and EPSC Recording and Analysis. The voltage-clamp technique used to evaluate the transient currents generated by nerve stimulation was similar to that described by Takeuchi and Takeuchi (1959) and modified by Kuba et al. (1974). Glass microelectrodes filled with 3 M KCl and having resistances of 3-5 MΩ were routinely used for intracellular recording and current injection. Frog EPC or locust excitatory postsynaptic current (EPSC) waveforms were sent on-line to the computer (PDP 11/40 or 11/24) at a digitizing rate of 10 KHz. The decay phase (80-20%) was fit by a single exponential (linear regression on the logarithms of the data points) from which the decay time constant (τ_{EPC} or τ_{EPSC}) was determined.

Fluctuation Analysis. EPC or EPSC fluctuations were induced either by ACh microiontophoresis (micropipettes filled with 3 M ACh) or by bath application of monosodium L-glutamate (15-100 µM) in frog and locust nerve-muscle preparations, respectively. The method for fluctuation analysis was similar to that described elsewhere (Anderson and Stevens, 1973; Pascuzzo et al., 1984). Segments of records obtained before (baseline) and during application of either ACh or L-glutamate were analyzed, and the resulting power density spectra provided single channel conductance (γ) and channel lifetime (τ_I) estimates.

Patch-Clamp Recording and Data Analysis. The isolated muscle fibers were secured in the recording chamber using an adhesive mixture of parafilm and paraffin oil (30%:70%) (See Allen et al., 1984). The bath and the pipettes were filled with a HEPES-buffered solution consisting of (mM): NaCl 115, KCl 2.5, $CaCl_2$ 1.8 and HEPES 3, and the pH was adjusted to 7.2. TTX (0.3 µM) was added to prevent the fibers from contracting. Single channel currents were recorded using patch-clamp technique (Hamill et al., 1981). Micropipettes were prepared in two stages from borosilicate capillary glass (A & M Systems), and after heat polishing they had inner diameter of 1-2 µm and resistance of 8-10 MΩ when filled with HEPES solution. All drug solutions were filtered through a Millipore filter (0.2 µm) before use. An LM-EPC-7-patch-clamp system (List-Electronic, West Germany) was used to record the single channel currents. The experimental data were filtered at 2-3 KHz by a second-order Bessel low-pass filter and sent to the computer at digitizing rate of 10-12.5 KHz from FM tape. Histograms of total current amplitude and channel-open, closed and burst times were provided by an automated computer analysis program. A channel was considered open when data points exceeded a set number of standard deviations from the baseline (usually corresponding to 50% of the unitary channel conductance). Similar criteria were used for channel closure so that the intervals between consecutive closures defined channel open time. It should be noted that a "flicker" or departure from the open state that exceeded the threshold for closure, terminated an open event, regardless the duration of the gap. However, a burst was terminated only if such a closure lasted longer than 6.4 or 8 msec. Thus, bursts may be composed of several openings, and may have appearance of long open events chopped into many segments by flickers. The details of these analyses were described elsewhere (Akaike et al., 1984). All recordings were performed at 10°C.

Protection Studies

Lethality Determination: Female Wistar rats (200-220 g, 3 months old) were pretreated with a mix of a given carbamate and atropine sulphate (0.5 mg/kg). The carbamates studied were: (-) PHY sulphate (0.1 mg/kg), (+) PHY salicylate (0.1-0.5 mg/kg), NEO bromide (0.2 mg/kg), PYR bromide (0.4 mg/kg). In studies using (-) PHY, (±) mecamylamine hydrochloride (1-4 mg/kg) was added to the pretreatment regimen. These drugs were injected intramuscularly (0.1 ml/100 g body wt) 30 min prior to subcutaneous injection of a lethal dose of sarin (0.13 mg/kg) or VX (0.05mg/kg; minimum lethal dose = 0.015 mg/kg). All the drugs were dissolved in 0.9% NaCl solution. Lethality was recorded for 24-hr period post-challenge, and the surviving animals were further observed for up to 10 days.

Tissue ChE Determination: Blood was collected from the tail vein of rats anesthetized with ether, and the soleus muscles and brain tissues (cerebral hemispheres) were removed after decapitation. Blood ChE and muscle and brain acetylcholinesterase (AChE) were analyzed using the modified Ellman (1961) procedure. Protein determination was carried out according to the method of Lowry et al. (1951) using bovine serum albumin as a standard.

Drugs and Toxins

ACh chloride, (-) PHY sulphate, NEO bromide, EDP chloride, DFP, atropine sulphate, concanavalin-A, and monosodium L-glutamate were purchased from Sigma Chemical Co., (±) mecamylamine hydrochloride from Merck, Sharp and Dohme Research Labs, and TTX from Sankyo Co., Japan. PYR bromide, sarin, soman, tabun and VX were provided by the U.S. Army Medical Institute of Chemical Defense. (+) PHY was prepared by routes published in J. Nat. Prod. 48:878-893, 1985. α-BGT and α-Naja toxin were provided by Dr. M.E. Eldefrawi (Univ. Maryland). All the stock solutions were stored at -25°C and diluted to desired concentrations with the physiological solutions prior to use.

Statistical Analysis

Statistical analysis of the data was performed using student's t test and p values < 0.05 were considered significant.

RESULTS

Effects of the Reversible and Irreversible ChE Inhibitors on the Endplate Currents Elicited at the Frog Neuromuscular Junction

The ChE inhibition at the endplate region by carbamates as well as OP compounds resulted in potentiation of muscle twitch, and increased EPC peak amplitude and prolongation of τ_{EPC}. Figure 1 shows the anti-ChE effects of (-) PHY on the EPCs which were apparent at concentrations ranging between 0.2 to 2 μM. Similar effects were seen with other carbamates and OP compounds (Figs. 3 and 4), except (+) PHY, which did not alter the properties of the EPC in a way expected from ChE inhibition (Fig. 2). This finding was confirmed by the determination of ChE activity in homogenates of both brain and soleus muscles of rats using the optical isomers of PHY. As shown in Table 1, relative to (-) PHY, (+) PHY was about 90-fold less potent in inhibiting brain ChE while a 225-fold difference was found in muscle ChE activity.

In addition, at high concentrations, all ChE inhibitors studied produced depression of peak amplitude and decrease in τ_{EPC} which suggested direct interactions of these agents with the postsynaptic AChR. These blocking effects became discernable with (-) PHY at concentrations > 2 μM (Fig. 1). More interestingly, (+) PHY, although devoid of significant anti-ChE activity at the neuromuscular junction, produced blocking effects similar to those of the natural isomer (Fig. 2). The depression of the EPC amplitude occurred without affecting the linearity of the current-voltage relationship observed under control conditions. τ_{EPC} was shortened in a voltage- and concentration-dependent manner, i.e. the blocking effect was more pronounced at hyperpolarized potentials inducing

Table 1. Effect of Natural (-) and Optical Isomer (+) PHY on the Inhibition of Cholinesterase in Rat Brain and Soleus Muscle.

Tissue	IC_{50} (µM)		$\dfrac{IC_{50}\ (+PHY)}{IC_{50}\ (-PHY)}$
	(-) PHY	(+) PHY	
Brain	3.6	316	90
Soleus muscle	2.0	450	225

Activity of ChE was determined in the homogenate of respective tissues by Ellman procedure at 22°C.

a progressive loss in the voltage sensitivity of the EPC decay as the concentration of the drug was increased. According to the sequential model for open channel blockade (see Discussion Section), the unblocking reaction of an "irreversible" blocker is considered to be too slow to contribute to the EPC decay. This yields a single exponential decay and a linear decrease of τ_{EPC} with increasing drug concentration. At a

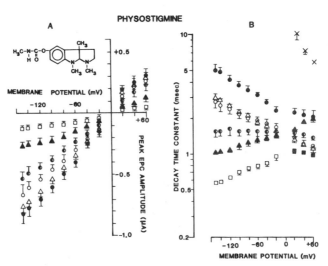

Fig. 1 Effects of (-) PHY on the peak amplitude and decay time constant of the EPCs. Relationship between the EPC peak amplitude and the membrane potential (A) and voltage sensitivity of τ_{EPC} (B) under control conditions and in the presence of PHY. (◯) control, (●) 0.2, (△) 2, (◐) 20, (▲) 60, and (☐) 200 µM PHY. At 200 µM PHY, and at membrane potentials between +20 and +60 mV, ■ and X represent the τ of the fast and slow phases of EPC decays, respectively. Each point is the mean ± SEM of 8 to 24 surface fibers from 2-6 muscles. Inset: Chemical structure of PHY. (From Shaw et al., 1985).

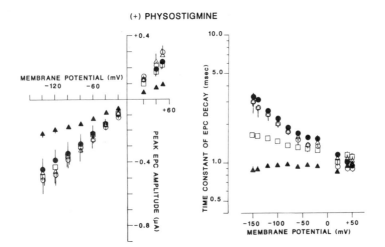

Fig. 2 Effects of (+) PHY on the peak amplitude (A) and
decay time constant (B) of the EPCs. (○) Control,
(●) 0.2, (△) 2, (□) 20 and (▲) 60 μM (+) PHY.

voltage range of −20 to −150 mV and in the presence of any concentration
of (−) PHY tested, the EPC decay was a single exponential function of
time. Consistent with the predictions of the model mentioned above, a
linear plot of $1/\tau_{EPC}$ vs. drug concentration and an exponential voltage
dependence of the rate constant of the blocking reaction (k_3) were
observed. However, when the membrane potential was shifted to more
positive potentials in the presence of concentrations of PHY higher than
100 μM, double exponential decays became discernible (Shaw et al.,
1985). With (+) PHY (up to 60 μM), the decay phase of the EPC remained a
single exponential function of time at all membrane potentials tested.

Soman, sarin, VX, tabun and DFP, in addition to their alterations of
EPCs due to ChE inhibition, produced blocking effects which became more
evident at high concentrations of these drugs. Previously, Kuba et al.
(1973; 1974) have shown that the irreversible ChE inhibitor DFP at
relatively high concentrations was able to interact with the AChR and
induce an open channel blockade. Lower concentrations of DFP (< 1 mM)
caused little effect. The effects of DFP on the AChR, in contrast to its
ChE inhibition, were completely reversible upon washing the nerve-muscle
preparation for about 60 min. In Figures 3 and 4, the effects of two
other OP compounds, VX and soman, are illustrated. Compared to DFP, these
agents, as well as tabun and sarin, disclosed blockade of the EPCs at much
lower doses. At concentrations > 1 μM they induced a dose-dependent
decrease in τ_{EPC}, although the decay was still prolonged relative to
control conditions. On the EPC peak amplitude, at 0.1 μM, both VX and
tabun produced a marginal increase, but a marked decrease was observed at
concentrations of 1-100 μM. This depression of the EPC amplitude was more
pronounced with hyperpolarization, so that, in contrast to control
conditions, a nonlinear current-voltage relationship was observed.
However, no time-dependent effect was produced by these agents at any
concentration used. While τ_{EPC} was not decreased beyond control values,
the EPC peak amplitude was markedly depressed. A more detailed analysis
of VX actions revealed that this pattern was not seen on the miniature

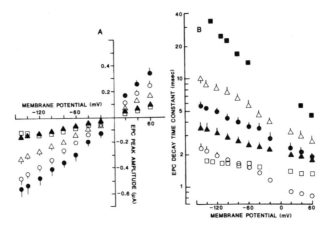

Fig. 3 Concentration- and voltage-dependent action of VX
on EPC peak amplitude (A) and τ_{EPC} (B). ($\bigcirc$)
control, ($\bullet$) 0.1, ($\triangle$) 1, ($\blacktriangle$) 10, and ($\square$)
100 µM VX. In B, the symbols ($\square$) and ($\blacksquare$)
represent the τ of the fast and slow components
of EPC decay, respectively, in the presence of
100 µM VX. Each point is the mean ± SEM of 6-15
surface fibers from at least four muscles.

endplate currents (MEPCs). At similar concentrations used to study EPCs,
VX produced depression of both MEPC peak amplitude and τ_{MEPC} which did
not exceed control values. These findings raised the question of whether
these irreversible anti-ChE agents might have presynaptic actions, by
reducing the quantal release of the transmitter. Indeed, while the
spontaneous transmitter release was increased (as shown by increase in
MEPC frequency), VX decreased quantal content during nerve stimulation.

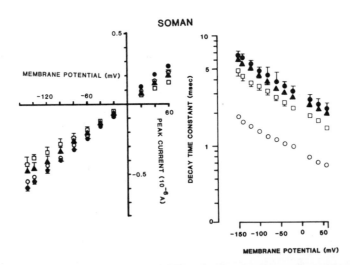

Fig. 4 Effects of soman on the endplate currents. (A) EPC
peak amplitude and (B) τ_{EPC}. Symbols are: ($\bigcirc$),
control; ($\bullet$), 0.1; ($\blacktriangle$), 1; and ($\square$), 10 µM soman.

Effects of Reversible and Irreversible ChE Inhibitors on Single Channel
Currents

The actions of carbamate ChE inhibitors, NEO, EDP, PHY in its (-) and
(+) forms and the OP compound, VX, were evaluated on single channel
currents activated by ACh at the perijunctional region of the frog interosseal and lumbricalis muscle fibers. The negligible presence of ChE in
these fibers and their suitability for patch-clamp recordings (Allen et
al., 1984; Shaw et al., 1985) have enabled the studies of the direct
interactions of these anti-ChE agents with the postsynaptic AChR. Cell-
attached recordings were performed using a patch pipette filled with a
solution containing ACh (0.3-0.4 μM) and a desired concentration of each
one of the ChE inhibitors under study.

The direct actions of VX on the single channel properties were
assessed using noise analysis and patch-clamp techniques. EPC fluctuation
analysis carried out in a preparation pretreated with DFP showed that VX
at 25 and 50 μM decreased channel lifetime (τ_I) to about 73% and 56% of
the control values, respectively. The effects of VX on single channel
properties were more clearly evaluated by direct recordings of the
elementary currents. Under control conditions, i.e. in the absence of
anti-ChE agent, ACh produced square-wave pulses with a conductance of
about 30 pS at 10°C (Fig. 5). VX induced alterations in the kinetics of
activation of the AChR without changing the single channel conductance
(Fig. 5). Mostly, the openings appeared as isolated short pulses which
denoted a more stable blocked state compared to NEO and EDP which induced
bursting-type events (see Fig. 7). Dose- and voltage-dependent shortening

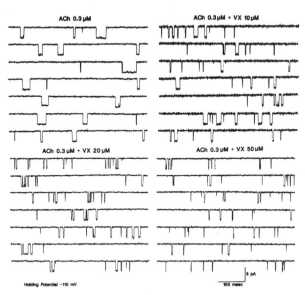

Fig. 5 Samples of ACh-activated channel currents in the
presence of various concentrations of VX.
Records were obtained from single muscle fibers
isolated from adult frog muscle under cell-
attached patch configurations. Potential was
held between -120 and -130 mV.

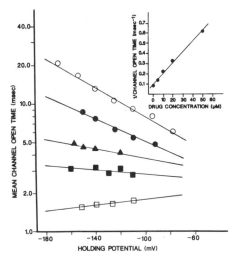

Fig. 6 Voltage- and concentration-dependent effects of
VX on the open channel times. Relationship
between the logarithm of the mean channel open
times and holding potentials from single
channel recordings obtained with ACh (0.3 µM)
either alone (◯) or together with 5 (●), 10
(▲), 20 (■) and 50 (☐) µM VX.

of mean channel open time (τ_o) was observed when VX was added at different
concentrations (1–50 µM) to the patch solution containing ACh (0.3 µM)
(Fig. 6). Consistent with the sequential model for open channel blockade
described in the Discussion Section (1), the blocking effects were more
pronounced at hyperpolarized potentials which resulted in a gradual loss
in the voltage sensitivity of τ_o with increasing concentrations of VX, and
(2) the plots of reciprocal of τ_o vs. concentration of the blocking agent
were linear up to 50 µM VX. Single exponential distribution of the
channel open times remained unchanged at all the concentrations of VX
tested. In contrast to OP compounds such as soman and most of carbamates
(see below), no agonist effect was detected for VX at concentrations up to
50 µM.

The carbamates NEO or EDP when added at concentrations ranging from
0.2 to 50 µM to the patch pipette solution containing ACh (0.3–0.4 µM),
produced typical bursts composed of many openings and closings (Fig. 7).
The alterations were kinetically consistent with the blockade of the open
state of the ionic channels described by the sequential model (Adler et
al., 1978; Neher and Steinbach, 1978). As illustrated for EDP, the
duration of the openings within a burst was decreased in a concentration-
dependent manner (Fig. 8A), such that linear plots between the reciprocal
of mean channel open time ($1/\tau_o$) and drug concentration were observed.
The distribution of the closed times showed two distinct components, one
fast due to the fast closings within a burst (blocked state) and a slow
component related to the interburst closed intervals. According to this
model, the mean of the fast component (τ_b) corresponds to the reciprocal
of the backward rate constant (k_{-3}) of the blocking reaction. The
analysis of the fast component showed that the number of fast closings was

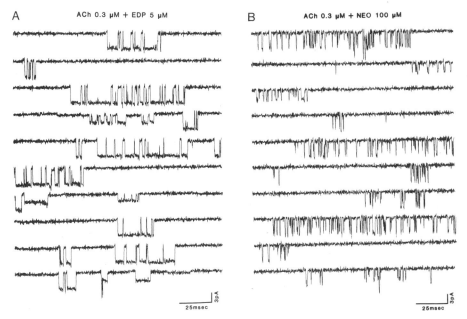

Fig. 7   Effects of edrophonium (A) and neostigmine (B) on ACh-activated
         channel currents. Pipette solution: ACh (0.3 μM) either plus EDP
         (5 μM) or NEO (100 μM). Holding potential: -140 mV.

increased and the duration prolonged in the presence of these blockers
compared to control conditions (Fig. 9).   The fast component, although
independent of concentration of the blocker, was prolonged with hyperpolarization, as predicted by the model (Fig. 8B).   These alterations in
the kinetics of AChR activation occurred without significant change in the
single channel conductance, which suggested a nonconducting blocked
state.   In contrast to PHY (see below), NEO and EDP disclosed agonistic

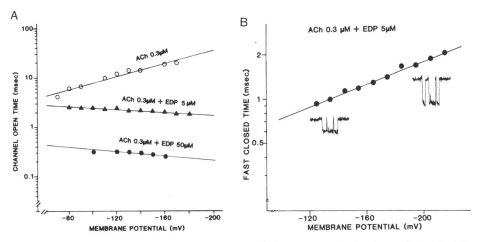

Fig. 8   Voltage-dependence of the open (A) and blocked times (B) of ACh-
         activated channels in the presence of edrophonium. Patch pipettes
         were filled with ACh (0.3 μM) either alone or together with
         different concentrations of EDP.

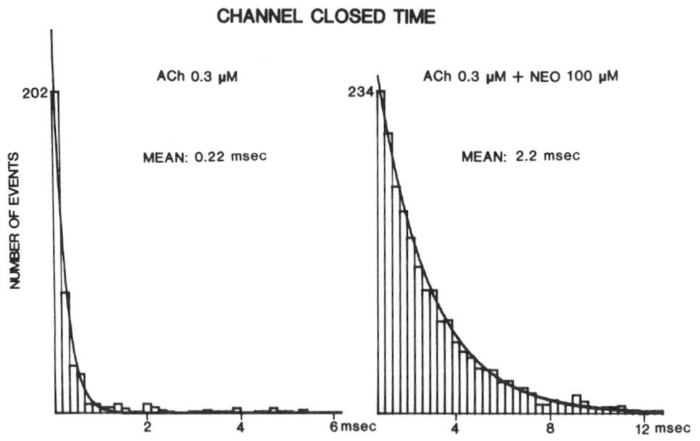

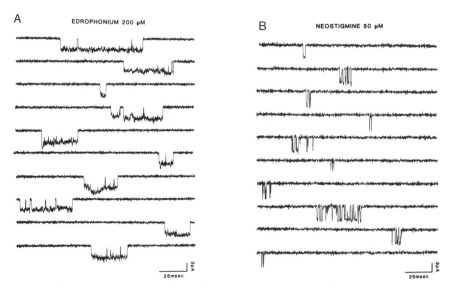

CHANNEL CLOSED TIME

ACh 0.3 µM

MEAN: 0.22 msec

202

NUMBER OF EVENTS

2   4   6 msec

ACh 0.3 µM + NEO 100 µM

MEAN: 2.2 msec

234

4   8   12 msec

Fig. 9 Histograms of fast closed (blocked) times of AChR activated by ACh in the presence of neostigmine.

action only at high concentrations (Fig. 10). NEO (> 50 µM) generated short channel openings which tended to appear in bursts. EDP (>200 µM), on the other hand, activated altered currents similar to those observed with (−) PHY (Fig. 13). EDP-activated currents rapidly disappeared at hyperpolarized potentials, but they could be recorded again after an interval at depolarizing potentials.

In the presence of (−) PHY (0.1-600 µM), the activation of ACh channels appeared as irregular and noisier currents interrupted by many short gaps (see Shaw et al., 1985 and Fig. 11). These events were induced

A   EDROPHONIUM 200 µM

B   NEOSTIGMINE 50 µM

3 pA
25 msec

3 pA
25 msec

Fig.10 Edrophonium- and neostigmine-activated channel currents. Single channel currents were activated from the perijunctional region of frog muscle fibers using a pipette containing only the desired ChE inhibitor. Holding potential: −140 mV.

at concentration as low as 0.1 µM and had a conductance similar to those
activated by ACh alone (30 pS). However, at concentrations of (-) PHY
>50 µM, these events became more evident, and a decrease in channel
conductance was observed (18 pS at 200 µM PHY) which was not further
changed at higher concentrations. The histograms of channel open times
disclosed a single exponential distribution at all the concentrations of
PHY tested and shortened mean channel open times up to 200 µM (-) PHY
(Fig. 12). In contrast to the predictions of the sequential model, the
plot of the reciprocal of this parameter vs. drug concentration showed a
partial saturation; indeed, no additional decrease in mean channel open
time was observed at higher concentrations of the agent. The analysis of
the fast closed times (briefer than 8 msec) revealed an increased number
of short closures within bursts in the presence of (-) PHY, but their
duration was not significantly changed. In addition, (-) PHY at concentrations as low as 0.5 µM acted as an agonist, activating channels with
conductance similar to that of ACh-activated currents (Fig. 13). The
distribution of the open times could be fit to a single exponential
function. Channel activation was suppressed by either α- BGT or α-Naja
toxin which suggested interactions with ACh recognition sites on the
AChR. High concentrations of (-) PHY (5-50 µM) induced a clear appearance
of those altered events recorded in the presence of (-) PHY together with
ACh. At concentrations higher than 50 µM, PHY generated channel openings
with lower conductance.

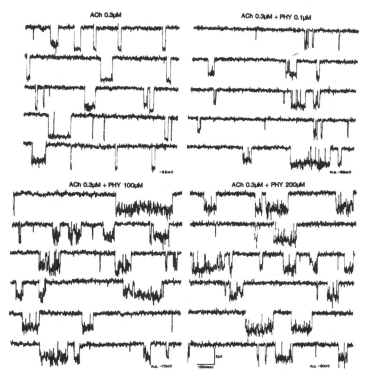

Fig.11 Samples of ACh-activated channel currents in the absence
       and presence of (-) physostigmine. Patch pipette
       containing ACh either alone or in combination with
       various concentrations of PHY. (From Shaw et al., 1985).

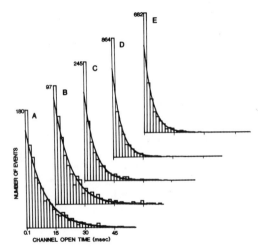

Fig.12 Open time histograms of channels activated by ACh
(0.3 μM) in the absence (A, 959 events) or
presence of (−) PHY at 0.1 (B, 474 events), 20
(C, 728 events), 200 (D, 1980 events) 600 (E,
1628 events) μM concentration. τ_o, determined
from the fit of distributions to a single exponential function, was: 9.1 (A), 7.6 (B), 5.2 (C),
4.0 (D), and 4.2 msec (E). (From Shaw et al.,
1985).

Preliminary studies using (+) PHY demonstrated that this isomer has
agonistic property on the nicotinic AChR. The activated ion channel had a
conductance similar to that opened by ACh. In contrast to the natural
PHY, (+) isomer (10 μM) activated square-wave pulses with fewer short gaps
during the open state of the channels. Although the currents activated by
(+) PHY were more similar to those elicited by ACh, the duration of the

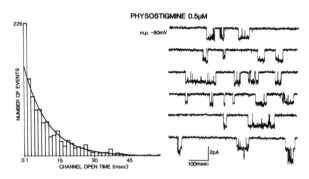

Fig.13 Samples of currents activated by (−) PHY and
corresponding open time histogram. Histogram
contains 1088 events, and τ_o was 9.6 msec as
determined from the fit to a single exponential
function. (From Shaw et al., 1985).

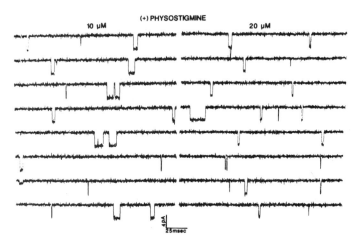

Fig.14 (+) Physostigmine-activated channel currents. Holding potential: -120 mV.

open state was much shorter with a mean of 4 msec instead 10 msec, at a holding potential of -120 mV (Fig. 14). This finding suggested that an interaction of carbamates with the nicotinic AChR may be involved in the antagonism of the toxic effects of OP compound since (+) PHY despite its negligible anti-ChE activity offered significant protection to animals exposed to irreversible ChE inhibitors (see below).

Pre- and Postsynaptic Effects of the Anti-ChE Agents on the Locust Glutamatergic Neuromuscular Junction

The reversible and irreversible ChE inhibitors were studied on locust neuromuscular junctions using either ETiM or FTiM. Any possible interference of the CNS with the nerve-muscle preparation was eliminated by cutting N5 1 mm from the metathoracic ganglion. When the locust FTiM was exposed to (-) PHY at a concentration $\geqslant$ 40 μM in locust physiological solution for 15 min, repetitive episodes of spontaneous EPSPs and muscle action potentials (APs) followed by silent periods were recorded. This spontaneous activity was blocked by decreasing external Ca^{2+} concentration ($[Ca^{2+}]_o$) to $\leqslant$ 0.2 mM or by washing off the anti-ChE for 60 minutes (Albuquerque et al., 1985; Idriss and Albuquerque, 1985b; Idriss et al., 1986).

All irreversible ChE inhibitors used, VX, DFP and tabun, induced spontaneous firing previously described for PHY. The effect of $[Ca^{2+}]_o$ on this phenomenon was studied in detail. Using normal $[Ca^{2+}]_o$ (2 mM), spontaneous firing of APs and EPSPs followed by silent periods was recorded after a 15-min exposure of locust muscle to DFP (0.5 mM). Reduction of $[Ca^{2+}]_o$ to 0.8 mM abolished the muscle APs but not EPSPs. A further reduction in $[Ca^{2+}]_o$ to 0.2 mM blocked both APs and EPSPs. Similar effects were observed with VX which at 10 μM concentration induced a typical cyclic pattern of bursts and silent periods in the presence of 0.8 mM $[Ca^{+2}]_o$ and 10 mM $[Mg^{+2}]_o$. Superfusion of the muscle with a solution of TTX (0.3 μM) blocked the spontaneous repetitive EPSPs and APs

315

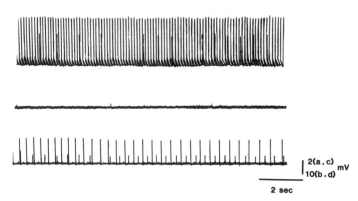

Fig.15 Effect of tetrodotoxin on spontaneous activity recorded from FTiM treated with tabun. A: small miniature EPSCs recorded under control conditions at 2 mM $[Ca^{2+}]_o$; B: APs recorded after 20-min exposure to tabun (20 μM); C: record after exposure to tabun (20 μM) plus TTX (0.3 μM); and D: record after 60-min wash with tabun alone. Membrane potential: -50 mV.

induced by an irreversible anti-ChE agent (Fig. 15). TTX-induced blockade of EPSPs and APs was reversible upon 60-min washing with a toxin-free solution containing only the anti-ChE agent. The possible involvement of cholinergic receptors in this phenomenon was tested (Fulton and Usherwood, 1977). Treatment of locust muscles with either α-BGT or α-Naja toxin (10 μg/ml) did not block the spontaneous EPSPs produced by ChE inhibitors. The effect of atropine on this phenomenon was also tested. Although this agent produces muscarinic blocking effects at pico- to nonomolar range, atropine at concentrations as high as 10 μM did not suppress the presynaptic effects of the anti-ChE agents studied. When used at very high concentrations (> 20 μM), atropine had direct effects on the glutamate-induced EPSC.

In addition to presynaptic action, both carbamate and OP agents interacted postsynaptically at locust neuromuscular synapses. The plot of the EPSC amplitude vs. membrane potentials between -60 to -130 mV was linear under control conditions (Fig. 16). VX (10 μM) produced a decrease in τ_{EPSC} and depression of the peak amplitude of the EPSC which was more pronounced at hyperpolarized potentials, therefore inducing a marked nonlinearity in the current-voltage relationship. Similar effects were observed with DFP (1 mM), which produced a significant voltage-dependent depression of the peak amplitude and shortening of the EPSC decay. On the other hand, PHY (0.5-1 mM) caused a significant depression of the EPSC peak amplitude, but did not significantly change τ_{EPSC}. These effects of VX, DFP and PHY on the EPCs were reversible upon washing the preparation. Tabun, on the other hand, although it produced a marked effect at the presynaptic nerve terminal (Fig. 15), did not alter the EPSCs.

The effects of VX on the glutamate-activated single channel currents were determined from noise analysis experiments performed in the locust

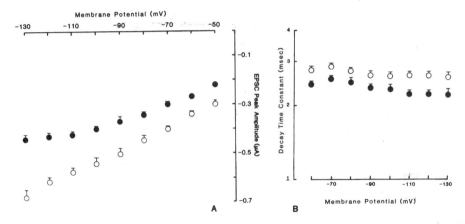

Fig.16 Effects of VX on the locust EPSCs. (A) current-voltage relationship; (B) τ_{EPSC}. Each point represents the mean ± S.D. of EPSCs recorded from the same group of FTiM fibers before ($\bigcirc$, 4-7 EPSCs) and after 10 µM VX ($\bullet$, 20-35 EPSCs).

neuromuscular preparation. Monosodium L-glutamate (100-150 µM) was applied via the bathing medium in the absence and in the presence of VX (10 µM). VX, at a holding potential of -47 mV, decreased channel lifetime from 1.7 to 1.2 msec (Idriss et al., 1986).

Physostigmine as a Pretreatment Drug Against Toxicity by Irreversible ChE Inhibitors

Among the carbamates tested, the (-) PHY disclosed the greatest efficacy against lethal doses of OP compounds. All the animals receiving 0.13 mg/kg sarin died within 15 min. However, (-) PHY (0.1 mg/kg) administered 30 min prior to injection of a lethal dose of sarin provided marked protection (Table 2; see Deshpande et al., 1986). This protecting effect was further enhanced by a coadministration of atropine (0.5 mg/kg) which by itself reduced the secretions but did not prevent lethality. NEO and PYR even at higher doses alone or in combination of atropine showed practically no protection effect. The levels of ChE in blood, soleus muscle and brain tissues of rats receiving the mixture of (-) PHY and atropine prior to a lethal dose of sarin are shown in Table 3. This pretreatment protected 100% of the animals which showed a significant increase in AChE level in the muscle and brain tissue in comparison to those receiving sarin alone. However, when the rats received a multiple lethal dose of sarin (0.65 mg/kg), the pretreatment of these animals even with higher higher dose of (-) PHY and atropine was ineffective in preventing lethality in spite of almost similar level of ChE inhibition seen in rats protected against 0.13 mg/kg sarin. This finding confirmed the implication of the direct effects of OP compounds described earlier in the overall toxicity of the irreversible ChE inhibitors. The hypothesis involving the direct effects of the carbamates on the postsynaptic AChR rather than ChE inhibition in the protection offered by carbamates against

317

Table 2. Effect of Physostigmine, Neostigmine and Pyridostigmine on
Survival of Rats Injected with a Lethal Dose of Sarin.

Preatreatment[a] drug	Carbamate dose (mg/kg)	# Survived / # Injected	Percent Survival[b]
None[c]	--	0/66	0
Atropine[d]	--	0/18	0
(-) PHY	0.1	26/36	72
(-) PHY plus atropine	0.1	24/25	96
NEO	0.2	2/12	17
NEO plus atropine	0.2	1/8	12
PYR	0.4	3/19	16
PYR plus atropine	0.4	4/15	27

[a]The pretreatment drug mixture was injected subcutaneously 30 min
prior to subcutaneous injection of a lethal dose (0.13 mg/kg) of
sarin.
[b]All the animals were observed for 24 hr for lethality.
[c]These rats received only a lethal dose of sarin.
[d]When present alone or mixed with carbamates the dose of atropine
was 0.5 mg/kg.

OP poisoning could be more clearly assessed using (+) PHY which has negligible ChE inhibitory activity (Table 1). As shown in Table 4, (+) PHY
when coadministered with atropine 0.5 mg/kg was very effective in
protecting rats against a lethal dose of sarin. The above hypothesis was
further strengthened by the results from the studies using mecamylamine, a

Table 3. Cholinesterase Levels in the Brain and Soleus Muscles of
Rats Treated with Physostigmine and Atropine and
Subsequently Receiving a Lethal Dose of Sarin.

Preatreatment[a] (mg/kg)	Sarin (mg/kg)	% ChE inhibition[b]			% of Survival
		Blood	Muscle	Brain	
Control (None)	--	0	0	0	100
None	0.13	87	71	97	0
None	0.65	88	82	98	0
(-) PHY (0.1) plus atropine	0.13	71	32	56	100
(-) PHY (0.2) plus atropine	0.65	50	42	62	0

[a]The preatreatment drugs were administered 30 min prior to injection
of sarin. The dose of atropine was 0.5 mg/kg.
[b]In muscle and brain AChE activity was determined.

Table 4. Effects of (+) and (−) Optical Isomers of PHY on Protection of Rats against Lethal Effects of Sarin (0.13 mg/kg).

Pretreatment[a]	Dose (mg/kg)	Percent Survival[b]
None	—	0
(−) PHY	0.1	100
(+) PHY	0.1	47
	0.3	81
	0.5	87

[a]The pretreatment drug mixture also contained atropine (0.5 mg/kg).
[b]Observation period for recording lethality was 24 hr.

ganglionic competitive antagonist with no significant effect on ChE activity. Mecamylamine significantly enhanced the protection offered by (−) PHY against multiple lethal doses of VX (0.05 mg/kg) (Table 5). It should be pointed out that mecamylamine by itself was not effective in protecting the animals against OP poisoning. The effectiveness of mecamylamine may be based on its direct interactions with the cholinergic synapses of both peripheral and central nervous systems. Although being a competitive antagonist at the ganglia, mecamylamine at the neuromuscular AChR acted as a powerful ion channel blocker via noncompetitive mechanisms (Varanda et al., 1985).

DISCUSSION

The present study demonstrated that the ChE inhibitors PHY, DFP and VX have direct effects on the postsynaptic endplate interacting with the sites on the nicotinic AChR. Such effects have been suggested previously, for various anti-ChE agents, by several investigators (Kuba et al., 1973, 1974; Pascuzzo et al., 1984; Akaike et al., 1984; Shaw et al., 1985; Aracava and Albuquerque, 1985; Fiekers, 1985; Albuquerque et al., 1985). Our studies based on voltage-clamped EPCs, single channel recordings and noise spectral analysis have revealed that the actions of the carbamate and OP anti-ChE agents on the AChR are manifested in several ways which include enhancement of receptor desensitization, open channel blockade, and in some cases, agonistic activity. The electrophysiological findings have been corroborated by biochemical studies (Sherby et al., 1985) which demonstrated that PHY, PYR and NEO act as agonists as well as noncompetitive blockers. PHY, PYR and NEO induced potentiation of AChR desensitization most likely due to their agonist action (Shaw et al., 1985; Sherby et al., 1985; Akaike et al., 1984). In addition, we have evidence indicating that the actions of both carbamates and OP compounds are not restricted to cholinergic synapses. On the glutamate-mediated neuromuscular junction of locusts, these agents produced a marked increase in transmitter release.

Table 5. Effects of (-) Physostigmine and Mecamylamine Pretreatment on Survival of Rats Receiving a Lethal Dose of VX.

Pretreatment[a]	Dose (mg/kg)	#Survived #Injected	Percent Survival[b]
None	--	0/10	0
(±) Mecamylamine	4.0	0/6	0
(-) PHY	0.1	7/15	47
(±) Mecamylamine and (-) PHY	4.0 0.1	12/12	100

[a]Pretreatment solution also containing atropine (0.5 mg/kg) was administered 30 min before injection of VX (0.05 mg/kg). Minimal 100% lethal dose of VX was 0.015 mg/kg.
[b]Observation period for recording lethality was 24 hr.

The direct actions of the carbamates may have clinical implications considering their use as therapeutic drugs in some cholinergic disorders and as prophylactic agents against poisoning by irreversible ChE inhibitors. Indeed, the results provided by the protection studies disclosed a great variability in effectiveness among the carbamates in prophylaxis against OP poisoning (Meshul et al., 1985; Deshpande et al., 1986). The pretreatment regimen including the natural PHY and atropine was able to protect almost all the animals subjected to a lethal dose of sarin (0.13 mg/kg). The same mixture tested against multiple lethal doses of VX (0.05 mg/kg; LD_{100} = 0.015mg/kg) protected 50% of the animals. Interestingly, this protection against VX was markedly enhanced when mecamylamine (a non anti-ChE agent, a ganglionic competitive antagonist and a noncompetitive antagonist at the neuromuscular AChR) was included in the prophylactic regimen against VX (Table 5). These findings strongly suggested an additional mechanism rather than ChE inhibition underlying the antagonism between reversible and irreversible inhibitors. This hypothesis was further strengthened by the preliminary results of protection studies using (+) PHY. This isomer is about 100-fold less potent than the natural optical isomer in inhibiting ChE (Table 1). Nevertheless, (+) PHY was very effective in protecting animals against a lethal dose of sarin (Table 4). Under these circumstances, it was of fundamental importance to identify the molecular mechanisms underlying the effects of both reversible and irreversible ChE inhibitors on the pre- and postsynaptic membranes of the cholinergic as well as glutamatergic synapses.

On EPCs elicited at frog neuromuscular junction, most of anti-ChE agents showed two effects: at low concentrations, an increase in EPC amplitude and prolongation of τ_{EPC} which are indicative of ChE inhibition; at higher concentrations, a decrease in amplitude and τ_{EPC} suggestive of blockade of the open state of the channels. Most of the evidence for open channel blockade has been derived from the analysis of EPC decays (Ruff, 1977; Adler et al., 1978; Spivak and Albuquerque, 1982; Ikeda et al., 1984) and confirmed by single channel current recordings (Neher and

Steinbach, 1978; Aracava et al., 1984; Spivak and Albuquerque, 1985). A sequential model has been proposed to explain the experimental findings which can be expressed as follows:

$$\text{Diffusion} \uparrow$$

$$nA + R \underset{k_{-1}}{\overset{k_1}{\rightleftharpoons}} A_nR \underset{k_{-2}(V)}{\overset{k_2(V)}{\rightleftharpoons}} A_nR^* \underset{\underset{D}{\overset{k_{-3}(V)}{\swarrow}}}{\overset{\overset{D}{\searrow}\,k_3(V)}{\rightleftharpoons}} A_nR^*D$$

$$\downarrow$$
$$\text{Hydrolysis}$$

In this model R is the AChR macromolecule which interact with n molecules of the transmitter A to form an agonist-bound but nonconducting species, A_nR. This species undergoes a conformational change to a conductive state A_nR^*. A_nR^*D is the species blocked by the drug D and is assumed to have no conductance. k_3 and k_{-3} are the forward and backward rate constants for the blocking reactions, respectively, and V indicates the voltage sensitive steps. Under physiological conditions, τ_{EPC} is a measure of mean channel lifetime (Anderson and Stevens, 1973) and is dependent upon the rate constant k_{-2} which is described by the equation: $k_{-2} = B\,exp^{AV}$ (Magleby and Stevens, 1972). The binding of a drug to the open channel will accelerate the EPC decays as a consequence of shortening the duration of the channel open state which now egresses from A_nR^* via two routes (1) spontaneous closure towards A_nR and R and (2) by drug blockade which depends upon concentration of the blocking agent and the rate constant k_3. Due to opposing voltage dependence of the rate constants k_{-2} and k_3, the increase in drug concentration will produce an acceleration of EPC decays with a progressive loss in the voltage sensitivity of τ_{EPC}. In the case that k_3 and k_{-3} are comparable, the reverse reaction $A_nR^*D \longrightarrow A_nR^* + D$ will be significant enough to contribute to the EPC, thus yielding double exponential decays. On the other hand, if k_{-3} is negligible, the unblocking reaction is too slow to contribute to the EPC, and the decay will be single exponential function of time. Neglecting k_{-3} on the assumption that k_3 is $\gg k_{-3}$, EPC decay or channel open times will be shortened according to the following expression:- $(\tau_{EPC})^{-1}$ or $(\tau_o)^{-1} = k_{-2} + [D]\,k_3$. The discernment and interpretation of the alterations on EPCs, especially with anti-ChE agents, are sometimes difficult. In addition, under conditions of ChE inhibition, reduction of the number of free receptors by either a competitive blocker (α-BGT) or an agent which enhances desensitization will affect τ_{EPC} (Magleby and Stevens, 1972; Magleby and Terrar, 1975; Kordas, 1977). Thus, more clear evidences of open channel blockade are provided by direct recording of single channel currents.

The effects of (-) PHY on EPCs could mostly be described by the sequential model. A linear relationship between $1/\tau_{EPC}$ and (-) PHY concentration and a decrease in the voltage sensitivity of τ_{EPC} were observed. The double exponential decays observed in the presence of high concentrations of PHY as well as Met PHY, a quaternary analog of PHY, at positive potentials could not be fully explained by this model, most likely because these agents exhibit other effects on the nicotinic neuromuscular AChR (Shaw et al., 1985). The blocking effects of OP compounds on EPCs were also observed. However, due to strong anti-ChE effect, τ_{EPC} was not reduced beyond control levels (Figs. 3 and 4). Thus, patch-clamp technique was used in a preparation devoid of ChE activity to study the interactions of these anti-ChE agents with the nicotinic AChR at the single channel current level.

In a situation where k_{-3} and k_3 are comparable, the channel current, normally a rectangular pulse, is chopped into a burst of brief openings and closings. These current transitions are interpreted as blocking and unblocking of the channels by the drug. The burst is terminated when the open channel undergoes a conformational change towards its resting state. The duration of the openings within a burst (τ_o) is linearly shortened with increasing concentrations of the blocker and influenced by voltage according to the voltage-dependence of k_{-2} and k_3. The duration of the blocked state (τ_b), i.e. the intra-burst closings, is independent of concentration of the blocking agent and is governed by k_{-3} which has a voltage sensitivity opposite to that of k_3. Thus, hyperpolarization while shortening τ_o prolonged τ_b. NEO and EDP produced this type of blockade (Fig. 8). At a concentration range of 0.2-50 µM, both agents induced alterations in ACh-activated channel currents in a manner kinetically consistent with the sequential model. VX, on the other hand, produced a more stable blockade ($k_{-3} < k_3$) such that typical bursts were not discerned. Instead, the majority of recorded events appeared as well separated short pulses precluding any distinction between the blocked and normal closed or resting state (Fig. 5). (-) PHY, on ACh-activated channels, induced altered currents with irregular and increased noise during the open state. The analysis showed that the alterations induced by (-) PHY could not all be described by the sequential model. The plot of $1/\tau_o$ vs. (-) PHY concentration showed a departure from linearity towards a saturation which was complete at concentrations higher than 200 µM. This finding suggested the existence of processes other than an open channel blockade which is consistent with the biochemical studies (Sherby et al., 1985). Another interesting observation is that (-) PHY at concentrations above 300 µM was able to completely block the endplate current evoked by nerve stimulation, but single channel currents could be recorded in relatively high frequency at concentrations of PHY as high as 600 µM. Similarly to (-) PHY, it has been reported that ACh at high concentrations induces irregular and noisier currents during the open state coupled with lower conductance events which could be due to an open channel blockade (Sine and Steinbach, 1984). However, it is possible that many of the channels observed in the presence of ACh plus (-) PHY were activated by the carbamate itself since this agent was able to activate channels at very low concentrations of 0.1 µM.

Patch-clamp recordings were also useful to disclose the agonist property of certain anti-ChE agents and to reveal more subtle characteristics of the single channel currents. (-) PHY, PYR, NEO, EDP and the OP compound soman all act as weak agonists (Aracava and Albuquerque, 1985; Akaike et al., 1984; Albuquerque et al., 1984). Since the pretreatment with α-BGT blocked the activation of these channels, it is possible that these agents interact with the ACh recognition site. The channels opened by some of these agents are seen even at very low concentrations (e.g. 0.5 µM PHY). In contrast to the square shape typical of ACh-activated channel currents, (-) PHY-activated channels were characterized by a considerable amount of current noise during the open state. Channel conductance was similar to that of ACh-activated channels (~30 pS) at low concentrations of PHY and decreased to about 18 pS at concentrations higher than 50 μM. Recent studies carried out with (+) PHY showed that this optical isomer also has powerful agonist activity on the nicotinic AChR. However, channel currents activated by (+) PHY are quite different from those activated by the natural isomer. Short, well separated pulses with conductance similar to ACh-activated currents were generated by (+) PHY at a concentration range of 5-50 μM. NEO and EDP activated ionic channels only at high concentrations. EDP-activated channels resembled those of (-) PHY while NEO generated very short square-wave pulses with conductance similar or slightly lower than those activated by ACh. PYR, on the other hand, induced low-frequency openings with reduced conductance (~10-12 pS) (Akaike et al., 1984). Most likely, this agonist effect of PYR was important in the enhancement of AChR desensitization observed with this agent. In myoballs or in muscles, PYR in combination with ACh induced the appearance of channels with marked flickering but with no significant change in the τ_o (Akaike et al., 1984). The frequency of these channel openings changed as a function of time of exposure to both drugs. Over a period of 10 min the opening frequency was gradually decreased, and a 10 pS event which was rarely observed under control conditions (Hamill and Sakmann, 1981; Akaike et al., 1984) became predominant. Higher concentrations of PYR (200 μM) produced a biphasic effect on channel activation; initially there was an increase in channel openings and irregular waves of bursting activity, but this was followed by a marked decrease in the channel activation. The agonist, desensitizing and channel blocking actions of these carbamates have been confirmed by binding studies (Sherby et al., 1985). However, in these studies performed on AChR-rich membranes of the Torpedo electroplax, high concentrations of carbamates were required.

On the locust glutamatergic synapses, the most significant action of both carbamate and OP compounds occurs at the presynaptic nerve terminal. PHY, DFP and VX all induced an increase in transmitter release as evidenced by the generation of spontaneous EPPs and MEPPs. At normal $[Ca^{2+}]_o$ (2 mM), the increased transmitter release would result in EPPs large enough to trigger APs. McCann and Reece (1967) also recorded spontaneous muscle APs by injecting PHY (1 mM) into the fly abdomen. However, from their data it was difficult to discriminate whether the events observed resulted from the central or peripheral action, since the ganglia were maintained intact. It should be mentioned that in all the preparations used in the present study, the metathoracic ganglion which supplies the nerves to these muscles has been removed to eliminate any central cholinergic component. Therefore, all the effects registered in the presence of these agents might have resulted from their action on the nerve-muscle junction. The spontaneous activity did not arise from the interaction of anti-ChE agents with the nicotinic and/or muscarinic receptors at the presynaptic nerve terminal (Fulton and Usherwood, 1977), since neither nicotinic (α-BGT, α-Naja toxin and d-tubocurarine) nor muscarinic (atropine) antagonists could abolish these spontaneous events. In addition, superfusion of cholinergic agonist, i.e. ACh (5-10 mM), did not initiate any spontaneous activity, thus suggesting that cholinergic receptors are not involved. Instead, changes in external Ca^{2+} concentration deeply affected the presynaptic effect of anti-ChE agents, suggesting a phenomenon mediated by Ca^{2+} influx (Fig. 9). However, the primary target of these agents seemed to be Na^+ channels at the nerve terminal since the spontaneous activity was reversibly blocked by TTX. Similar increase in transmitter release has been observed in the mammalian neuromuscular transmission with the irreversible ChE inhibitors in particular (Laskowsky and Dettbarn, 1975; Deshpande, Idriss and Albuquerque, unpublished results).

In addition, these agents, except tabun, also interacted postsynaptically at locust neuromuscular synapse (Idriss et al., 1986). Both VX and DFP produced a shortening of the EPSC decays as well as a decrease in the peak amplitude, which indicated an effect on the ionic channel associated with the glutamate receptors. Recent studies of Idriss and Albuquerque (1985a) showed that certain noncompetitive antagonists of the nicotinic AChR such as phencyclidine, chlorisondamine, philanthotoxin and atropine also interacted with the glutamate receptor on the locust neuromuscular junction decreasing both EPSC peak amplitude and the τ_{EPSC}. These findings suggest certain similarities between the subunits comprising the ionic channels of the nicotinic and glutamate receptors.

In conclusion, the present study demonstrated that both reversible and irreversible anti-ChE agents, in addition to their enzyme-inhibitory property, have definite actions on the nicotinic AChR, viz. blocking the open ionic channel, enhancing desensitization, and acting as agonists of the AChR. Patch-clamp studies disclosed the agonist activity of some of these anti-ChE agents. We also showed that there is no binding site for PHY on the intracellular portion of the AChR since this agent did not produce any effects when applied to the cytoplasmic side under inside-out patch configuration. In addition, since similar effects were observed with the quaternary analog MetPHY, the charged form of these agents is most likely responsible for the interactions with the AChR (Shaw et al., 1985). These direct effects of ChE inhibitors on the AChR may play an important role in the efficacy of certain carbamates in prophylaxis against poisoning by OP compounds. This hypothesis may be extended to explain the actions of ChE reactivators since the studies carried out with 2-PAM and HI-6 disclosed direct interactions of these oximes with the nicotinic AChR (Rao et al., 1984). Furthermore, difficulties in counteracting some of the toxic effects of OP compound may be due to the direct effects of irreversible anti-ChE agents on both pre- and postsynaptic membranes. Finally, the studies performed on the locust nerve-muscle preparations revealed an important presynaptic effects of these drugs which promoted an increase in glutamate release via increase in Na^+ permeability at the nerve terminal. The postsynaptic blocking effects observed on the locust synapses raise the question of whether there is a similarity between the nicotinic and glutamatergic receptor-ionic channel macromolecules.

ACKNOWLEDGEMENTS

We wish to thank Ms. Mabel A. Zelle for the computer programming and Mrs. Barbara Marrow for her technical assistance. We would also like to express our gratitude to Prof. G.R. Wyatt for the generous supply of locusts and Dr. W.M. Cintra and M. Alkondon for providing some of their data on (+) PHY and organophosphate agents.

REFERENCES

Adler, M., Albuquerque, E.X., and Lebeda, F.J., 1978, Kinetic analysis of end plate currents altered by atropine and scopolamine, Mol. Pharmacol. 14: 514-529.

Aguayo, L.G., Pazhenchevsky, B., Daly, J.W, and Albuquerque, E.X. 1981, The ionic channel of the acetylcholine receptor. Regulation by sites outside and inside the cell membrane which are sensitive to quaternary ligands, Mol. Pharmacol. 29: 345-355.

Akaike, A., Ikeda, S.R., Brookes, N., Pascuzzo, G.J., Rickett, D.L., and Albuquerque, E.X., 1984, The nature of the interactions of pyridostigmine with the nicotinic acetylcholine receptor-ionic channel complex II. Patch clamp studies, Mol. Pharmacol. 25: 102-112.

Albuquerque, E.X., Akaike, A., Shaw, K.-P., and Rickett, D.L., 1984, The interaction of anticholinesterase agents with the acetylcholine receptor-ionic channel complex, Fundam. Appl. Toxicol. 4: S27-S33.

Albuquerque, E.X., Deshpande, S.S., Kawabuchi, M., Aracava, Y., Idriss, M., Rickett, D.L. and Boyne, A.F., 1985, Multiple actions of anticholinesterase agents on chemosensitive synapses: Molecular basis for prophylaxis and treatment of organophosphate poisoning, Fundam. Appl. Toxicol. 5: S182-S203.

Allen, C.N., Akaike, A., and Albuquerque E.X., 1984, The frog interosseal muscle fiber as a new model for patch clamp studies of chemosensitive- and voltage-sensitive ion channels: actions of acetylcholine and batrachotoxin, J. Physiol. (Paris) 79: 338-343.

Anderson, R., and Stevens, C.F., 1973, Voltage clamp analysis of acetylcholine produced end-plate current fluctuations at frog neuromuscular junction, J. Physiol. (Lond.), 235: 655-691.

Aracava, Y., Ikeda, S.R., Daly, J.W., Brookes, N., and Albuquerque, E.X., 1984, Interactions of bupivacaine with ionic channels of nicotinic receptor. Analysis of single-channel currents, Mol. Pharmacol. 26:304-313.

Aracava, Y., and Albuquerque, E.X., 1985, Direct interactions of reversible and irreversible cholinesterase (ChE) inhibitors with the acetylcholine receptor-ionic channel complex (AChR): Agonist activity and open channel blockade, Neurosci. Abstr. 11: 595.

Changeux, J.-P., Devillers-Thiéry, A., and Chemouilli, P., 1984, Acetylcholine receptor: an allosteric protein, Science 225: 1335-1345.

Colhoun, E.H., 1958, Acetylcholine in Periplaneta americana L. I. ACh levels in nervous tissue, J. Insect Physiol. 2: 117-127.

Colhoun, E.H., 1963, The physiological significance of ACh in insects and observations upon other pharmacologically active substances, Adv. Insect Physiol. 1: 1-41.

Corteggiani, E., and Serfaty, A., 1939, Acetylcholine et cholinesterase chez les insectes et les arachnidés, C R Soc. Biol. (Paris), 131: 1124-1126.

Deshpande, S.S., Viana, G.B., Kauffman, F.C., Rickett, D.L., and Albuquerque, E.X., 1986, Effectiveness of physostigmine as a pretreatment drug for protection of rats from organophosphate poisoning, Fundam. Appl. Toxicol. 6: 566-577.

Ellman, G.L., Courtney, K.D., Andres, V., Jr., and Featherstone, R.M., 1961, A new rapid colorimetric determination of acetylcholinesterase activity, Biochem. Pharmacol. 7: 88-95.

Faeder, I.R., and O'Brien, R.D., 1970, Responses of perfused isolated leg preparations of the cockroach Gromphadorhina portentosa to L-glutamate, GABA, picrotoxin, strychnine and chlorpromazine, J. Exp. Zool. 173: 203–214.

Fiekers, J.F., 1985, Concentration–dependent effects of neostigmine on the endplate acetylcholine receptor channel complex, J. Neurosci. 5: 502–514.

Fulton, B.P., and Usherwood, P.N.R., 1977, Presynaptic acetylcholine action at the locust neuromuscular junction, Neuropharmacology 16: 877–880.

Hamill, O.P., and Sakmann, B., 1981, Multiple conductance states of single acetylcholine receptor channels in embryonic muscle cells, Nature (Lond.) 294: 462–464.

Hamill, O.P., Marty, A., Neher, E., Sakmann, B., and Sigworth, F.J., 1981, Improved patch–clamp techniques for high–resolution current recording from cells and cell–free membrane patches, Pflügers Arch. 391: 85–100.

Hollingworth, R.M., 1976, The biochemical and physiological basis of selective toxicity. in: "Insecticide Biochemistry and Physiology", C.F. Wilkinson, ed., Plenum Press, New York, p. 431–506.

Horn, R., Brodwick, M.S., and Dickey, W.D., 1980, Asymmetry of the acetylcholine channel revealed by quaternary anesthetics, Science 210: 205–207.

Hoyle, G., 1955, The anatomy and innervation of locust skeletal muscle, Proc. Roy. Soc. London Ser. B 143: 281–292.

Idriss, M., and Albuquerque, E.X., 1985a, Phencyclidine (PCP) blocks glutamate–activated postsynaptic currents, FEBS Lett. 189: 150–156.

Idriss, M., and Albuquerque, E.X., 1985b, Anticholinesterase (Anti–ChE) agents interact with pre– and postsynaptic regions of the glutamatergic synapse, Biophys. Soc. Abstr. 47: 259a.

Idriss, M.K., Aguayo, L.G., Rickett, D.L., and Albuquerque, E.X., 1986, Organophosphate and carbamate compounds have pre– and post–junctional effects at the insect glutamatergic synapse, J. Pharmacol. Exp. Ther., submitted.

Ikeda, S.R., Aronstam, R.S., Daly, J.W., Aracava, Y. and Albuquerque, E.X., 1984, Interactions of bupivacaine with ionic channels of the nicotinic receptor. Electrophysiological and biochemical studies, Mol. Pharmacol. 26: 293–303.

Karczmar, A.G. and Dun, N.J., 1985, Pharmacology of synaptic ganglionic transmission and second messengers, in: "Autonomic and Enteric Ganglia: Transmission and Pharmacology", A.G. Karczmar, K. Koketsu, S. Nishi, eds., Plenum Press, New York, p. 297–337.

Karczmar, A.G. and Ohta, Y., 1981, Neuromyopharmacology as related to anticholinesterase action, Fundam. Appl. Pharmacol. 1: 135–142.

Karlin, A., 1980, Molecular properties of nicotinic acetylcholine receptors, in: "The Cell Surface and Neuronal Function", C.W. Cotman, G. Poste, and G.J. Nicolson, eds., Elsevier/North Holland Biomedical Press, New York, p. 191–260.

Karlin, A., Holtzman, E., Yodh, N., Lobel, P., Wall, J., and Hainfeld, J., 1983, The arrangement of the subunits of the acetylcholine receptor of Torpedo californica, J. Biol. Chem. 258: 6678–6681.

Klymkowsky, M.W., Heuser, J.E., and Stroud, R.M., 1980, Protease effect on the structure of acetylcholine receptor membranes from Torpedo californica, J. Cell Biol. 85: 823–838.

Kordas, M., 1977, On the role of junctional cholinesterase in determining the time course of the end-plate current, J. Physiol. (Lond.) 270: 133-150.

Krodel, E.K., Beckmann, R.A., and Cohen, J.B., 1979, Identification of local anesthetic binding site in nicotinic postsynaptic membranes isolated from Torpedo marmorata electric tissue, Mol. Pharmacol. 15: 294-312.

Kuba, K., Albuquerque, E.X., and Barnard, E.A., 1973, Diisopropylfluoro-phosphate: suppression of ionic conductance of the cholinergic receptor, Science 181: 853-856.

Kuba, K., Albuquerque, E.X., Daly, J., and Barnard, E.A., 1974, A study of the irreversible cholinesterase inhibitor, diisopropylfluoro-phosphate, on time course of end-plate currents in frog sartorius muscle, J. Pharmacol. Exp. Ther. 189: 499-512.

Laskowski, M.B., and Dettbarn, W.D., 1975, Presynaptic effects of neuro-muscular cholinesterase inhibition, J. Pharmacol. Exp. Ther. 194: 351-361.

Lowry, O.H., Rosebrough, M.J., Farr, A.L., and Randall, R.J., 1951, Protein measurement with the Folin phenol reagent, J. Biol. Chem. 193: 265-275.

Magleby, K.L., and Stevens, C.F., 1972, A quantitative description of end-plate currents, J. Physiol. (Lond.) 223: 173-197.

Magleby, K.L., and Terrar, D.A., 1975, Factors affecting the time course of decay of end-plate currents: A possible cooperative action of acetylcholine on receptors at the frog neuromuscular junction, J. Physiol. (Lond.) 244: 467-495.

Mathers, D.A., and Usherwood, P.N.R., 1976, Concanavalin A blocks desen-sitization of glutamate receptors on insect muscle fibers, Nature (Lond.) 259: 409-411.

McCann, F.V., and Reece, R.W., 1967, Neuromuscular transmission in insects: effect of injected chemical agents, Comp. Biochem. Physiol. 21: 115-124.

McDonald, T.J., Farley, R.D., and March, R.B., 1972, Pharmacological profile of the excitatory neuromuscular synapses of insect retractor unguis muscle, Comp. Gen. Pharmacol. 3: 327-338.

Meshul, C.K., Boyne, A.F., Deshpande, S.S., and Albuquerque, E.X., 1985, Comparison of the ultrastructural myopathy induced by anticholin-esterase agents at the endplate of rat soleus and extensor muscles, Exp. Neurol. 89: 96-114.

Neher, E. and Steinbach, J.H., 1978, Local anesthetics transiently block currents through single acetylcholine-receptor channels, J. Physiol. (Lond.) 277: 153-176.

Noda, M., Furutani, Y., Takahashi, H., Toyosato, M., Tanabe, T., Shimizu, S., Kikyotani, S., Kayano, T., Hirose, T., Inayama, S., Miyata, T. and Numa, S., 1983, Cloning and sequence analysis of calf cDNA and human genomic DNA encoding α-subunit precursor of muscle acetylcholine receptor, Nature (Lond.) 305: 818-823.

Pascuzzo, G.J., Akaike, A., Maleque, M.A., Shaw, K.-P., Aronstam, R.S., Rickett, D.L., and Albuquerque, E.X., 1984, The nature of the interactions of pyridostigmine with the nicotinic acetylcholine receptor-ionic channel complex I. Agonist, desensitizing and binding properties, Mol. Pharmacol. 25: 92-101.

Rao, K.S., and Albuquerque, E.X., 1984, The interactions of pyridine-2-aldoxime methiodide (2-PAM), a reactivator of cholinesterase, with the nicotinic receptor of the frog neuromuscular junction, Neurosci. Abstr. 10: 563.

Rao, K.S., Aracava, Y., Rickett, D.L., and Albuquerque, E.X., 1986, Noncompetitive blockade of the nicotinic acetylcholine receptor ion channel complex by an irreversible cholinesterase inhibitor, J. Pharmacol. Exp. Ther., submitted.

Ruff, R.L., 1977, A quantitative analysis of local anesthetic alteration of miniature end-plate currents and end-plate current fluctuations, J. Physiol. (Lond.) 264: 89-124.

Sakmann, B., Methfessel, C., Mishina, M., Takahashi, T., Takai, T., Kurasaki, M., Fujuda, K., and Numa, S., 1985, Role of acetylcholine receptor subunits in gating of the channel, Nature (Lond.) 318: 538-543.

Shaw, K.-P., Aracava, Y., Akaike, A., Rickett, D.L., and Albuquerque, E.X., 1985, The reversible cholinesterase inhibitor physostigmine has channel-blocking and agonist effects on the acetylcholine receptor-ion channel complex, Mol. Pharmacol. 28: 527-538.

Sherby, S.M., Eldefrawi, A.T., Albuquerque, E.X., and Eldefrawi, M.E., 1985, Comparison of the actions of carbamate anticholinesterases on the nicotinic acetylcholine receptor, Mol. Pharmacol. 27: 343-348.

Sine, S.M., and Steinbach, J.H., 1984, Activation of a nicotinic acetyl-choline receptor, Biophys. J. 45: 175-185.

Spivak, C.E., and Albuquerque, E.X., 1982, Dynamic properties of the nicotinic acetylcholine receptor ionic channel complex: activation and blockade. in: "Progress in Cholinergic Biology: Model Cholinergic Synapses", I. Hanin, and A.M. Goldberg, eds., Raven Press, New York, p. 323-357.

Spivak, C.E., and Albuquerque, E.X., 1985, Triphenylmethylphosphonium blocks the nicotinic acetylcholine receptor noncompetitively, Mol. Pharmacol. 27: 246-255.

Takeuchi, A., and Takeuchi, N., 1959, Active phase of frog's end-plate potential, J. Neurophysiol. 22: 395-411.

Tobias, J.M., Kollros, J.J., and Savit, J., 1946, Acetylcholine and related substances in the cockroach, fly and crayfish, and the effect of DDT, J. Cell. Comp. Physiol. 28: 159-182.

Usherwood, P.N.R., and Grundfest, H., 1965, Peripheral inhibition in skeletal muscle of insect, J. Neurophysiol. 28: 497-518.

Usherwood, P.N.R., and Machili, P., 1968, Pharmacological properties of excitatory neuromuscular synapses in the locust, J. Exp. Biol. 49: 341-361.

Varanda, W.A., Aracava, Y., Sherby, S.M., VanMeter, W.G., Eldefrawi, M.E., and Albuquerque, E.X., 1985, The acetylcholine receptor of the neuromuscular junction recognizes mecamylamine as a noncompeti-tive antagonist, Mol. Pharmacol. 28: 128-137.

Wan, K.K., and Lindstrom, J., 1984, Nicotinic acetylcholine receptor, in: "The Receptors" Vol. I., M.P. Conn, ed., Academic Press, New York, p. 377-430.

THE INVOLVEMENT OF ALKALINE EARTH CATIONS

IN THE CONTROL OF ACETYLCHOLINE RELEASE

Eugene M. Silinsky

Department of Pharmacology
Northwestern University Medical School
Chicago, Illinois 60611

INTRODUCTION

Neuroscientists allured by the mechanisms of transmitter secretion have at their disposal fortuitous electrophysiological deflections which allow a direct, moment to moment assay for acetylcholine (ACh) secretion. Specifically, the ratio of the amplitudes of the electrical events associated with neurally-evoked ACh release (end-plate potentials, EPPs) to the spontaneous potentials (miniature end-plate potentials, MEPPs) serves as a reliable estimate of the mean number of ACh quanta released synchronously by a nerve impulse (M, del Castillo and Katz, 1954). Extracellular Ca ions are essential for the process of evoked ACh release (for reviews see Katz, 1969; Silinsky, 1985). Specifically Ca must be equlibrated with a receptor near the external surface of the calcium channel prior to depolarization to support transmitter secretion. Depolarization, normally provided by the action potential, opens these voltage-sensitive calcium channels and Ca enters the nerve terminal cytoplasm down its electrochemical gradient. Once in the cytoplasm, Ca reduces a series of energy barriers and promotes ACh release.

Much as pharmacologists have learned about receptors for neurotransmitters by comparing the effects of a series of structurally related drug congeners, it has been possible to obtain information about the workings of nerve endings by comparing the effects of Sir Humphrey Davy's alkaline earth metal (Me) cation series on ACh release. The experimental and theoretical results to be summarized in this chapter suggest that nerve endings function as receptor-effector systems for Me species, with the initiation site near the calcium channel serving as the receptor and cellular Ca binding proteins serving as the sites of efficacy. Furthermore, the normal operating mode of the nerve terminal appears to be one that requires only a small proportion of the total number of Ca channels, in turn leaving most of the Ca entry sites 'spare'.

GENERAL OBSERVATIONS ON ALKALINE EARTH CATION PHARMACOLOGY

Fig. 1 compares the effects of two activators of ACh release, Ca and Sr ions, in the same fibre (Silinsky, 1981). Note that compared to Ca, which is the naturally occurring <u>full agonist,</u> Sr produces much lower maximum levels of M and requires higher concentrations to do so. Mg, which does not support M, is also a <u>competitive inhibitor</u> of Ca and Sr. In the simplest sense, this means that Mg produces a parallel shift to the right of the log [Me]-M curve for Ca or for Sr. For a more thorough appraisal of competitive inhibition as applied to studies on Me pharmacology, see Silinsky, 1981 (page 423) and Silinsky, 1985 (page 120). With respect to activation, Sr can support M by activating the same ion channel as Ca, yet produces a much lower maximal response; Sr is thus a <u>partial agonist</u> for synchronous, evoked ACh release (Meiri and Rahamimoff, 1971; Silinsky, 1981). The different maximal responses reflect the different <u>efficacies</u> of the activating cations, with the efficacy sequence being Ca>Sr>Mg.

The action of Ba ions will be noted as an aside here. Ba cannot support M (Miledi, 1966; Silinsky, 1977, 1978) but is capable of supporting the asynchronous discharge of enormous numbers of ACh quanta by nerve impulses. These electrophysiological effects of Ba are reminiscent of those evoked by a black widow spider bite. Thus, despite the absolute efficiency of Ba, it is evident that the absence of temporal harmony between each nerve action potential and quantal ACh release in Ba makes this cation a poor choice teleologically as the normal physiological mediator of depolarization-secretion coupling. The effects of Ba at cholinergic synapses are exceedingly complex and are summarized in Silinsky, 1985 (see sections II and III and Appendix B).

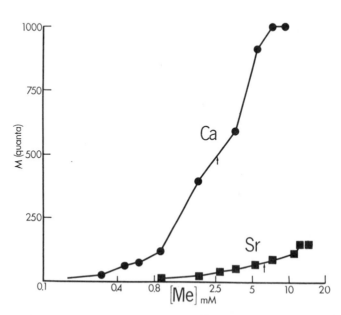

Fig. 1. Comparison of Ca and Sr on M in the same fibre. Each symbol represents the average response to a sufficient number of stimuli to reduce the coefficient of variation to less than 5%. Arrows indicate concentration that produces a half-maximal response. Preparation for this and all other figures was the cutaneous pectoris nerve-muscle preparation of the frog. Reprinted with permission from Silinsky, 1981.

WHAT IS RESPONSIBLE FOR THE DIFFERING EFFICACIES OF THE ALKALINE EARTH CATIONS?

One alluring suggestion is that different efficacies reflect the different mobilities of the Me species in the Ca channel (Meiri and Rahamimoff, 1971; Silinsky, 1978). While this may be valid in some instances, the results to be presented below suggest that when ACh release is promoted by delivering Me species to the cytoplasm using unilamellar lipid vesicles (liposomes) as a vehicle (and thus bypassing Ca channels), the selectivity sequence Ca>Sr>Mg is preserved. Fig. 2 shows the effects of Ca-containing liposomes and Mg-containing liposomes on EPPs (Kharasch, Mellow and Silinsky, 1982). Note that the control M (A) is increased several-fold by Ca containing liposomes (B). After restoring the lower level of release in the control solution (C), equimolar Mg-containing liposomes were applied and found to have no effect on ACh release (D). When the effects of equimolar Ca and Sr were compared in liposomes (Fig. 3), intracellular Ca was found to evoke much larger increases in synchronous ACh release (M) than intracellular Sr (Mellow, Perry and Silinsky, 1982). It is of interest that, in contrast to M, the effects of the cations in accelerating the ongoing MEPP frequency were equivalent. This is illustrated as insets in Fig. 3. (For details of the preparation of liposomes, controls against leakage of liposomal contents to the extracellular fluid, and further experiments with univalent and multivalent cations, see Rahamimoff, Meiri, Erulkar and Barenholz, 1978; Kharasch et al., 1981; Mellow et al., 1982).

As a consequence of the selectivity observed with liposomal cations, it was suggested that a Ca binding protein associated with a cellular aspect of the secretory apparatus is the site of efficacy with the efficacy sequence Ca>Sr>Mg reflecting the apparent intracellular affinity of the ion for the Me binding site (Silinsky, 1981, 1982). This suggestion was confirmed by studies on squid giant synapses, which revealed that differences in Me currents into nerve endings are not responsible for the differing abilities of the ions to support transmitter release (Augustine and Eckert, 1984).

THE MATHEMATICAL DESCRIPTION OF THE NERVE ENDING-SPARE CALCIUM BINDING SITES

The equations of pharmacological receptor theory were employed for determining the affinity constants and efficacies of the Me species (Silinsky, 1981; for derivations see Silinsky 1985). The results suggest that only a small proportion of the Ca channels (less than 10% in some instances) are needed to produce maximal levels of release in Ca, in turn leaving the majority unrequited or spare. For example, agents which irreversibly block Ca channels (lanthanum ions-Silinsky, 1981) or destroy putative Ca channels (antibodies-Lang, Newsome-Davis, Prior and Wray, 1984) produce a shift in the log [Ca]-M relationship to the right, and, where studied, without a change in maximum M. This is not surprising as the limiting substrate for maximal ACh output is likely to be beyond the Ca channel (e.g. available synaptic vesicles, active zones, Ca binding proteins, etc.). Thus, despite the irreversible occlusion of Ca channels, the reduction in M may be overcome by raising the extracellular Ca concentration and utilizing the spare channels. For the partial agonist Sr, there are no spare channels; Sr must use all its delivery sites to produce its maximum M. The ideas expressed thus far are summarized in the depiction of motor nerve terminals shown in Fig. 4. Note the external and internal openings of Ca channels, Ca binding proteins (bp) and synaptic vesicles in various stages of membrane association.

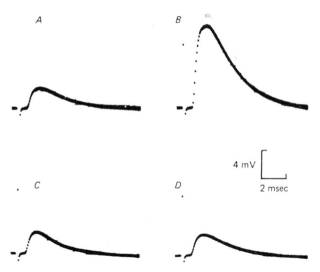

Fig. 2. Effects of Ca liposomes (B) and Mg liposomes (D) on evoked ACh release. A, C-control solution (0.4 mM Ca-1 mM Mg Ringer). Each EPP is a computer averaged response (see text) to stimuli presented at 0.5 Hz. M in control=3 (A), M in the presence of 80 mM calcium chloride-containing lipsomes=15 (B), M in recontrol solution =3.1 (C), M in the presence of 80 mM magnesium chloride-containing liposomes=2.9 (D). Reprinted with permission from Kharasch et al., 1981.

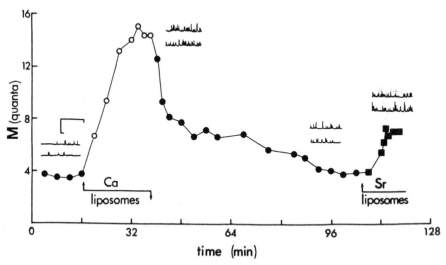

Fig. 3. Effects of Ca liposomes (open circles) and Sr liposomes (squares) on ACh release. Liposomes contained 80 mM strontium chloride or calcium chloride. Symbols show averaged M; insets show MEPP frequency at 16 min, 32 min, 88 min and 112 min. Whilst the maximum M in the presence of Ca liposomes was approximately twice that in equimolar Sr liposomes, the elevation in MEPP frequency was statistically-indistinguishable under the two conditions. Calibrations for MEPPs (insets) 3 mV, 1 sec.

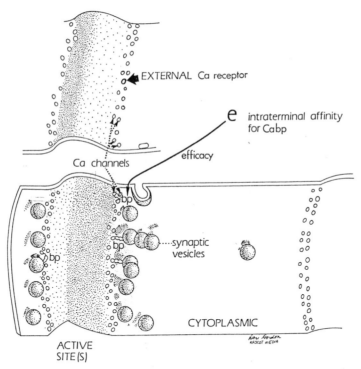

Fig 4. A schematic representation of the external and cytoplasmic surfaces of the motor nerve ending. For simplicity, the Ca binding protein (bp) is shown only for a few sites. Modified with permission from Silinsky, 1982.

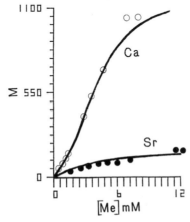

Fig. 5. A comparison of the experimental data with the theoretical curves drawn by computer. See text for details.

The [Me]-M curves for Ca and Sr may be reconstructed using the mathematical framework of receptor theory in conjunction with a simple sequential interaction model for a four site Ca binding protein. There are three parameters of interest to consider: 1) Me entry (This is described by a simple rectangular hyperbola-equation 1, Silinsky 1985). 2) The intracellular affinity of a strategic part of the releasing structure for Me. This is equivalent to the efficacy (see Fig. 4). Note that the effective intracellular Me concentration capable of promoting ACh secretion ([Me-eff]) is determined by the intracellular Me affinity. 3) The relationship between [Me-eff] and ACh secretion. This is described by an Adair-Pauling sequential interaction model for 4 sites. Fig 5 shows that the theoretical curves for Ca and Sr in the same fiber are in excellent agreement with the experimental results. The equation employed for the relationship between [Me-eff] and release is eqn 44a of Silinsky, 1985 using the same interaction factors but normalizing this equation of fractional release by the factor 1200 (the estimated number of releasing sites at this nerve ending). It should be noted that the Adair-Pauling equation serves as a 'decoder curve' for M regardless of whether Ca or Sr is the activating cation. Thus it is possible to calculate the external affinity and efficacies for either agonist and then accurately predict the complete [Me]-M relationship from eqn 44a of Silinsky, 1985. (See Silinsky, 1986 for use of this equation in predicting the inhibitory effects of adenosine on ACh release).

WHAT SUBCELLULAR SITES ARE RESPONSIBLE FOR CATION SELECTIVITY?

Fig. 6 illustrates the salient biophysical events implicated in the process of evoked transmitter release (see Silinsky 1985 for the original references). A shows a synaptic vesicle filled with ACh and attached to cytoskeletal elements (cs) through a docking protein (possibly Synapsin I (S1) in some but not all cholinergic synapses). The vesicle in Fig. 6A is resting about 50 angstroms away from the nerve terminal membrane (M). Once Ca has entered the cytoplasm through the voltage sensitive Ca channel (ch), it subsequently may bind selectively to a variety of Ca binding proteins in the synaptic vesicle membrane or the nerve terminal membrane. Ca may also merely screen fixed negative charges on vesicular and nerve terminal membranes — screening is a non-selective process that occurs without dehydration of the ion and is dependent only on cation valency and concentration, not the specific chemical properties of the ion. Acceleration of MEPP frequencies by Me species in liposomes is likely to occur via a screening process. Such Me screening or binding is required to reduce an electrostatic energy barrier between the membranes and to allow the vesicle to approach the nerve terminal from its initial resting position of 50 angstroms (Fig. 6A) to within 20 angstroms of the plasma membrane (B).

Fixed membrane charges have a high affinity for water and at distances of 20 angstroms and less, the hydration of vesicular and nerve terminal membranes is believed to be the most powerful impediment to membrane fusion. Charge neutralization by alkaline earth cations or substantial Ca-dependent membrane rearrangements (Fig. 6C) are required to reduce the hydration energy barrier. It should be noted that enzymatic processes have also been suggested to assist vesicular movement, e.g. contraction of the cytoskeleton propelling the vesicle to the nerve terminal much like the troponin - tropomyosin - actinomyosin complex in muscle contraction. Unfortunately, in the 100 microseconds allocated to intracellular Ca, only a 7 angstrom movement can occur by a contractile mechanism or any other enzyme catalyzed process unless a large battery of enzymes are coupled so that any one enzyme molecule need not have an unreasonably high turnover rate to promote ACh secretion. After dehydration and after the requisite membrane rearrangements whereby polar groups are neutralized or displaced

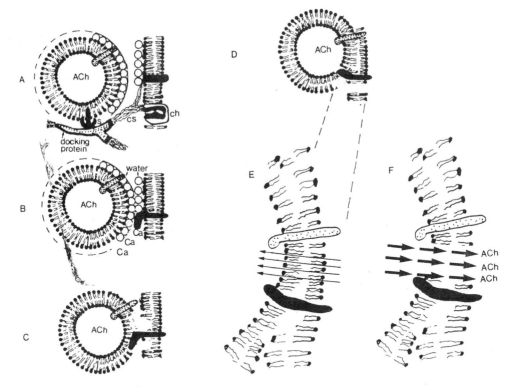

Fig. 6. Possible forces that control the exocytosis of ACh. A Ca binding protein in the plasma membrane (equivalent to bp in Fig. 5 and the Ca binding hands shown in Fig 7) is shown as a blackened structure. For further details see text. Reprinted with permission from Silinsky, 1985.

away from the approaching surfaces (Fig. 6C), the highly curved vesicle with adhering Ca (an energetically unfavorable state) flattens by fusing with the nerve terminal membrane (Fig. 6D). The unstable, newly formed bilayer ruptures (possibly by osmotic forces-E) and allows the exocytotic discharge of the neurotransmitter substance (Fig. 6F).

Wherein lie the sites of Me selectivity? As Ca, Sr and Mg are all capable of promoting the movement of the vesicle to within 20 angstroms (Heuser, 1977), it appears simplest to suggest that a plasma membrane Ca binding protein represents the site that distinguishes the chemical properties of one alkaline earth cation from another. In this regard the 'cartoon' of Fig. 7 depicts two strategic binding domains of a membrane Ca binding protein, each domain is a hand in the pair of hands (for precise details see Kretsinger, 1980). The Ca binding hands are equivalent to the Ca binding feet of Figs. 7 and 8A, Silinsky, 1985. In 7A, the unbound state, the middle fingers are extended; in this position the negatively-charged moieties would impede fusion of the negatively-charged vesicle with the plasmalemma. When Ca is bound (Fig. 7B), the middle finger encircles the Ca and the fixed negative charges are displaced away from prospective regions of fusion. The conformational change in a membrane Ca binding protein as illustrated in Fig. 7B might thus be predicted to favour transmitter release. The higher the affinity of the Me species, the lower the concentration required to overcome the energy barrier to exocytosis. It is of interest that many Ca binding proteins (e.g. troponin) appear to exhibit similar Me selectivity to the speculated Ca binding protein that controls transmitter release.

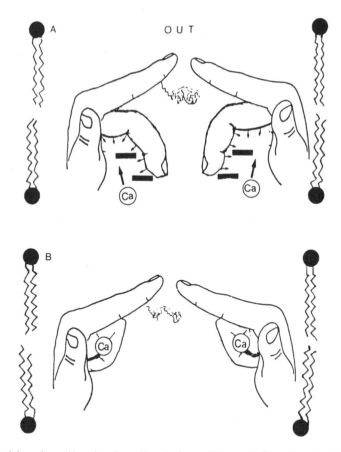

Fig. 7. A working hypothesis for the interaction of Ca with Ca binding proteins in the nerve terminal plasma membrane. Each Ca binding protein is made up of four binding domains (four hands). Only one pair of hands is illustrated in detail. Some liberty has been taken with the relative arrangements of the hands for the purposes of illustration. A. shows a membrane Ca binding protein activated by depolarization; the middle finger (the Ca binding region) has not bound Ca. The helical segments of the Ca binding domain are represented by the thumbs and forefingers. In B, Ca binding changes the conformation of the binding protein and reduces an energy barrier for transmitter release by repositioning the negatively charged moieties away from the region where the vesicle will subseqently fuse. From Silinsky, 1986 as modified by permission from Dr. R. H. Kretsinger.

Recently a controversy has developed concerning whether or not Ca entry is actually needed to promote transmitter release (Dudel, 1984; Zucker and Lando, 1986). It might be noted in concluding that if the Cabp is a) voltage sensitive and b) linked to Ca channel gating and Me entry (as has been suggested in Fig. 8A of Silinsky, 1985), then the theoretical descrepancies between the "Ca entry" and "voltage" models of transmitter release may be resolved.

This work was supported by a grant from the U.S.P.H.S. (NS 12782).

REFERENCES

Augustine, G.J., and Eckert, R., 1984, Divalent cations differentially support
     transmitter release at the squid giant synapse. J. Physiol. (London),
     346:257.
del Castillo, J., and Katz, B., 1954, Quantal components of the end-plate
     potential. J. Physiol. (London), 124:560.
Dudel, J., 1984, Control of quantal transmitter release at frog's motor nerve
     terminals. Pflugers. Arch. 402:225.
Heuser, J.E., 1977, Synaptic vesicle exocytosis revealed in quick-frozen frog
     neuromuscular junctions treated with 4-aminopyridine and given a single
     electrical shock. in: "Approaches to the Cell Biology of Neurons" W.M.
     Cowan, and J.A. Ferrendelli eds., Society for Neurosciences Symposium,
     Volume 2.
Katz, B., 1969, "The Release of Neural Transmitter Substances" The Sherrington
     Lectures X. Liverpool University Press, Liverpool, U.K.
Kharasch, E.D., Mellow, A.M., and Silinsky, E.M., 1981, Intracellular magnesium
     does not antagonize calcium-dependent acetylcholine secretion. J.
     Physiol. (London), 314:255.
Kretsinger, R.H., 1980, Crystallographic studies of calmodulin and homologs.
     Ann. N.Y. Acad. Sci., 356:14.
Lang, B., Newsome-Davis, J., Prior, C.,and Wray, D., 1984, Effect of passively
     transferred Lambert-Eaton myasthenic syndrome antibodies on the calcium
     sensitivity of transmitter release in the mouse. J. Physiol. (London),
     357:28P.
Meiri, U., and Rahamimoff, R., 1971, Activation of transmitter release by
     strontium and calcium ions at the neuromuscular junction. J. Physiol.
     (London), 215:709.
Mellow, A.M., Perry, B.D., and Silinsky, E.M., 1982, Effects of calcium and
     strontium in the process of acetylcholine release from motor nerve
     endings. J. Physiol. (London), 328:547.
Miledi, R., 1966, Strontium as a substitute for calcium in the process of
     transmitter release at the neuromuscular junction. Nature (London),
     212:1233.
Rahamimoff, R., Meiri, H., Erulkar, S.D., and Barenholz, Y., 1978, Changes in
     transmitter release induced by ion-containing liposomes. Proc. Natl.
     Acad. Sci.,U.S.A. 75:5214.
Silinsky, E.M., 1977, Can barium support the release of acetylcholine by nerve
     impulses? Brit. J. Pharmacol., 59:215.
Silinsky, E.M., 1978, On the role of barium in supporting the asynchronous
     release of acetylcholine quanta by motor nerve impulses. J. Physiol.
     (London), 274:157.
Silinsky, E.M., 1981, On the calcium receptor that mediates depolarization-
     secretion coupling at cholinergic motor nerve terminals.
     Brit. J. Pharmacol., 73:413.
Silinsky, E.M., 1982, Properties of calcium receptors that initiate
     depolarization-secretion coupling. Fed. Proc., 41:2172.
Silinsky, E.M., 1985, The biophysical pharmacology of calcium-dependent
     acetylcholine secretion. Pharmacol. Rev., 37:81.
Silinsky, E.M., 1986, Inhibition of transmitter release by adenosine: Are
     calcium currents depressed or are the intracellular effects of calcium
     impaired? Trends. Pharmacol. Sci., 6:(in press).
Zucker, R.S.,and Lando, L., 1986, Mechanism of transmitter release: voltage
     hypothesis and calcium hypothesis. Science, 231:574.

PHARMACOLOGY OF ACETYLCHOLINE ACTIVATED ION CHANNELS:

CONTEMPORARY APPROACHES

Toshio Narahashi

Department of Pharmacology
Northwestern University Medical School
Chicago, IL 60611

INTRODUCTION

It has long been known that certain guanidine compounds exert complex effects on synaptic and neuromuscular transmission. Guanidine itself increases transmitter release at the neuromuscular and synaptic junctions (Kusano, 1970; Otsuka and Endo, 1960; Teravainen and Larsen, 1975). More recently, the n-alkyl derivatives of guanidine have been found to block ion channels associated with the acetylcholine receptors in the end-plate (Watanabe and Narahashi, 1979).

Guanidine compounds are of special interest from the neurophysi-ological and neuropharmacological points of view for several reasons: First, the guanidine moiety in the tetrodotoxin and saxitoxin molecules is believed to play an important role in their highly specific and potent blocking action on the sodium channel (Hille, 1975; Ritchie and Rogart, 1977). Therefore, the study of channel block by guanidine compounds is expected to provide us with useful information about the topography of the channel. Second, since the structures of the n-alkylguanidines are relatively simple, a good structure-activity relationship is expected to be obtained. Third, methylguanidine is important clinically. A variety of neuropathological symptoms that occur during renal failure may be correlated with the accumulation of methylguanidine (Giovannetti et al., 1969).

In the course of experiments dealing with n-alkylguanidine block of end-plate ion channels, a few unique features have been unveiled as related to the question of current- vs voltage-dependent channel block and that of closed vs open channel block. This chapter gives a highlight of these findings (Farley et al., 1981; Vogel et al., 1984; Watanabe and Narahashi, 1979).

METHODS

The end-plate current (EPC) was measured with the sartorius muscle or cutaneous pectoris muscle preparations from the frog Rana pipiens using the two-microelectrode voltage clamp technique adapted to our laboratory (Deguchi and Narahashi, 1971) from the method originally developed by Takeuchi and Takeuchi (1959). Acetylcholine (ACh) was applied iontophoretically to the end-plate from a microelectrode filled with 1 M ACh chloride. The muscle preparations were pre-soaked in normal Ringer's

solution containing 2 M formamide to abolish muscle contraction (del
Castillo and de Motta, 1977). The formamide was washed out for a period
of 1 hour prior to experiments. The Ringer's solution used contained (in
mM): 115 NaCl, 5.4 KCl, 1.8 CaCl₂, and 2 N-2-hydroxyethylpiperazine-N'-
2-ethane-sulfonic acid (HEPES). The pH was adjusted to 7.3 with NaOH.
In some experiments, 1-2 μM d-tubocurarine was added to Ringer's solution
to reduce the size of the EPCs. This improved the space clamp condition
in the sartorius muscle preparation. All experiments were performed at a
room temperature of 20-22°C.

Single channel recording experiments were performed with gigaohm seal
patch clamp techniques (Hamill et al., 1981) as applied to the cultured
myotubes isolated from chick embryos. Both outside-out and inside-out
membrane patches were used. The external solution used had the following
composition (in mM): 120 or 360 CsCl, 2 BaCl₂ and 5 HEPES. The pH was
adjusted to 7.2. The internal solution used had the following composition
(in mM): 60-360 cesium salt and 5 HEPES. Fluoride, glutamate, or
chloride was used as the internal anion, and the pH was adjusted to 7.2.
The experiments were conducted at a temperature of 10-11°C.

PRESYNAPTIC STIMULATION AND POSTSYNAPTIC BLOCK

Shorter-chain n-alkylguanidines exerted a dual effect on neuromuscular
transmission. An example of an experiment is shown in Fig. 1 which
illustrates changes in end-plate potential (EPP) during application of 0.5
mM methylguanidine (record B) and after wash-out of the drug (records C and
D). The EPP amplitude was increased in methylguanidine. After washing the
amplitude was initially increased further but eventually decreased to the
control level. The complex changes in amplitude are due to a stimulation
of transmitter release that proceeds and is reversed slowly, and a block of
end-plate that proceeds and is reversed quickly. Thus the increase in EPP
amplitude in record B reflects a sum of presynaptic stimulation and
postsynaptic inhibition, the transient increase during wash-out is due to a
quick relief from end-plate block, and the eventual recovery reflects a
slow recovery from presynaptic stimulation.

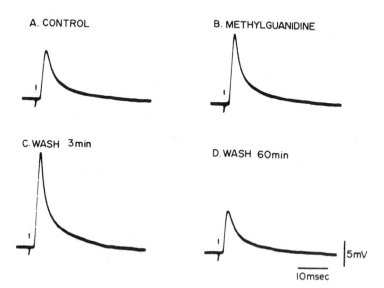

Fig. 1. The effects of methylguanidine on end-plate potential evoked by
nerve stimulation. A, control. B, after a 10-min exposure to 0.5 mM
methylguanidine. C, after washing with drug-free solution for 3 min.
Note a further increase in amplitude. D, reversal of methylguanidine's
effect after 60 min of washing. From Farley et al. (1981).

In order to see postsynaptic block more clearly, ACh was applied iontophoretically and the resultant ACh-induced current was measured as a function of membrane potential under voltage clamp conditions. Methylguanidine at a concentration of 0.5 mM suppressed the EPC in a unique manner (Fig. 2). The inward ACh currents evoked at membrane potentials ranging from -20 mV to -90 mV were suppressed by methylguanidine, whereas those evoked at more positive potentials ranging from -10 mV to +30 mV were unaffected. This experiment also suggests that methylguanidine block is either voltage-dependent or current-dependent. This problem will be explored in the following section.

VOLTAGE- VS. CURRENT-DEPENDENT BLOCK

Current-voltage relationship

In order to resolve the question as to whether methylguanidine block depends on the membrane potential or on the current flow, the current-voltage (I-V) relationship was examined in more detail. Figure 3 illustrates the I-V relationship before and during application of 3 mM methylguanidine in normal Ringer's solution containing 115 mM Na(A) and the I-V relationship before and during application of 3 mM methylguanidine and after washing with drug-free solution in Ringer's solution in which the sodium concentration was reduced to one-half of the normal or 57.5 mM(B). Unlike the experiment shown in Fig. 2, the peak amplitude of EPC is plotted. In normal Ringer's solution, the EPC amplitudes are decreased by methylguanidine in the potentials ranging from -10 mV to -90 mV in a manner similar to ACh current shown in Fig. 2. However, the EPC amplitudes in the positive potentials are increased by methylguanidine. This is due to stimulation of transmitter release described in the preceding section. The stimulation must have occurred in the negative potential range, but the effect was masked by a strong depressant action of the end-plate by methylguanidine.

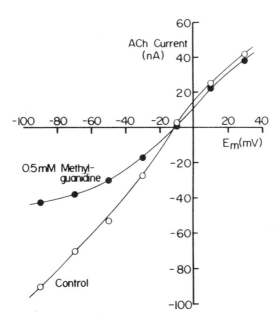

Fig. 2. Current-voltage relationship for iontophoretically induced acetylcholine currents at an end-plate before and during application of 0.5 mM methylguanidine. From Vogel et al. (1984).

When the external sodium concentration was decreased to one-half of the normal level, the reversal potential for EPCs was shifted from -7 mV to -28 mV. The most important point is that rectification of I-V curve in methylguanidine, which occurred at the EPC reversal potential (-7 mV) in normal sodium solution, occurred at the new reversal potential of -28 mV in 50% Na solution. This indicates that methylguanidine block of end-plate occurs in a manner dependent upon the direction of current flow rather than the membrane potential.

Conductance-voltage relationship

In order to illustrate the current dependence of block more clearly, the end-plate conductance (g) was calculated from the equation $g = EPC/(E_m-E_r)$, where E_m and E_r represent the membrane potential and the EPC reversal potential, respectively. The conductance was then normalized to the maximal value, and is plotted against the membrane potential in Fig. 4. It is clearly seen that a large change in conductance occurs at the respective reversal potential in normal and 50% Na solutions. This again supports the idea that methylguanidine block depends on the direction of current flow rather than the membrane potential.

Use-dependent block and recovery

Both block by methylguanidine and recovery from the block were affected by repetitive EPCs. EPCs were evoked by nerve stimulation at a frequency of 1/10 sec, and the membrane potential was changed either from -50 mV to +50 mV or from +50 mV to -50 mV. When the conditioning stimuli at -50 mV were followed by test stimuli at +50 mV in the presence of 3 mM methylguanidine, the amplitudes of test EPCs recovered gradually (Fig. 5, filled circles). Test EPCs at -50 mV following conditioning stimuli at +50 mV decreased gradually (Fig. 5, open circles). Control experiments without methylguanidine showed no change in EPC amplitude by the above protocols (Fig. 5, half-filled circles). These results indicate that repetitive outward EPCs at +50 mV relieve the methylguanidine block and that

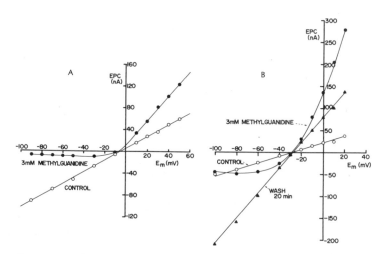

Fig. 3. Current-voltage relationships for nerve evoked end-plate currents before and during application of 3 mM methylguanidine, and after washing with drug-free solution. A, in Ringer's solution containing 115 mM Na. B, in Ringer's solution in which the Na concentration was reduced to one-half of the normal or 57.5 mM. After washout of drug, the I-V relation became linear, but had a steeper slope than that of the control, which reflects the persistence of the presynaptic stimulatory action of methylguanidine. From Vogel et al. (1984).

342

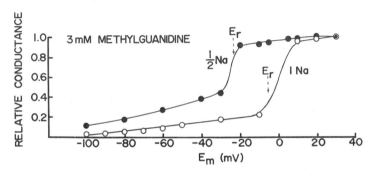

Fig. 4. Conductance during peak end-plate current plotted as a function of the membrane potential in the presence of 3 mM methylguanidine. 1 Na, normal Na concentration or 115 mM; 1/2 Na, Na concentration was reduced to one-half of the normal, or 57.5 mM. The conductance is normalized to the maximum value. From Vogel et al. (1984).

repetitive inward EPCs at -50 mV intensify the block. The relief from the block was found to depend on the number of outward EPCs and not on the frequency of EPCs. These observations provide evidence that the opening of end-plate channels is a prerequisite for the blocking or unblocking action to occur.

Mechanism of current-dependent block

Current-dependent block such as that observed with methylguanidine block of end-plate channels has been found in at least two other cases. Block of squid axon potassium channels by internally applied tetraethyl-ammonium (TEA) depends on the direction of current flow, only outward potassium currents being depressed (Armstrong, 1969, 1971). In contrast, paragracine, when applied internally to the squid axon, blocks the outward sodium currents without any effect on the inward sodium currents (Seyama et al., 1980). Methylguanidine resembles TEA and paragracine in that it blocks the ACh-activated channel only when current flows in the inward direction.

It appears that the binding of the methylguanidine molecule to a site in the channel depends strongly on the direction of current flow. The inward current strengthens the methylguanidine binding to the site, whereas the outward current weakens the binding. Another way of looking at this would be to assume that the inward current brings the molecule to the intrachannel site from outside causing a block, and that the outward current dislodges and sweeps away the molecule from the site causing an unblock.

The use dependence of methylguanidine block of ACh-activated channels appears to be similar to that of local anesthetic block of sodium channels (Courtney, 1975; Cahalan, 1978; Hille, 1977; Strichartz, 1973; Yeh, 1978, 1979). The use-dependent block of the sodium channels has been explained by assuming that the inactivation gate of the sodium channel can close with the drug molecule trapped inside the channel. Similarly, the methylguanidine-bound ACh-activated channel can close while trapping the drug molecule within the channel. The drug molecule can be released only when the channel is open and the current flows in outward direction. When the channel is open with inward current flowing, the drug molecule can enter the channel and bind to an intrachannel site. Therefore, the relief from the methylguanidine block depends on the number of EPCs evoked, not the frequency of EPCs. This model is in contrast to the conventional model for end-plate channel block (Neher and Steinbach,

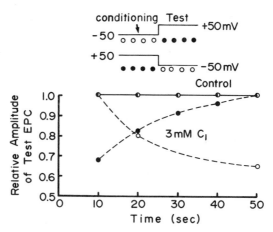

Fig. 5. Time course of end-plate current block development and recovery in 3 mM methylguanidine (C_1). The relative amplitude of the test EPC is plotted as a function of time following the last conditioning stimulus (see inset). Time course of block development at -50 mV is indicated by open circles; time course of relief of block at +50 mV is indicated by the filled circles. In the absence of drug (control), repetitive pulsing did not influence EPC amplitudes either at +50 or at -50 mV (half-filled circles). From Vogel et al. (1984).

1978; Ruff, 1977), in which the drug-bound channel is assumed not to be able to close.

OPEN VS. CLOSED CHANNEL BLOCK

Block of ACh-activated channels at their open state has been observed with a variety of chemicals including local anesthetics and their derivatives such as QX-222 and QX-314, decamethonium, amantadine, barbiturates, histrionicotoxin and TEA (Adams, 1976, 1977; Adams and Sakmann, 1978; Adler et al., 1979; Masukawa and Albuquerque, 1978; Neher and Steinbach, 1978). As described earlier in this chapter, n-alkylguanidines have been found to block the ACh-activated channels (Watanabe and Narahashi, 1979; Farley et al., 1981; Vogel et al., 1984). In contrast to shorter-chain n-alkylguanidines such as methylguanidine and ethylguanidine, some of the longer-chain n-alkylguanidines such as n-octylguanidine has been found to block the ACh-activated channels in a voltage-dependent manner. Furthermore, an interesting case has been detected and analyzed in which octylguanidine blocks the channels at both closed and open states (Farley et al., 1981; Vogel et al., 1984).

Octylguanidine block of ACh-activated channels

Among the five n-alkylguanidines tested on ACh-activated channels, i.e., methyl-, ethyl-, propyl-, amyl-, and octylguanidine, octylguanidine was most potent with an apparent dissociation constant of 6 μM at membrane potentials of -85 to -95 mV. In the presence of octylguanidine, the falling phase of the EPC became faster than control at all potentials tested (from -90 mV to +50 mV). The decay could be described by a single exponential function as in the control.

344

Octylguanidine block was voltage-dependent. When the membrane potential was changed from -50 mV to -70 mV or -90 mV in the presence of 10 μM octylguanidine, the EPC amplitude decreased slowly with a half-time of block development ranging from 200 to 500 msec with no clear voltage dependence (Fig. 6). However, the steady-state level of block was voltage-dependent as described later. When the membrane was depolarized from -50 mV to +30 mV in the presence of 10 μM octylguanidine, EPC amplitude was restored with a slow time course.

Current-voltage relationship

EPC amplitude was measured during each 2.2-sec potential step from the holding potential of -50 mV, and is plotted as a function of the test potential level (Fig. 7). The control I-V curve is approximately linear regardless of the time at which it is obtained after the beginning of test pulse (open circles). After application of 10 μM octylguanidine, however, the shape of I-V curve is different depending on the time when EPC is evoked after the beginning of test pulse. When measured 5 msec after the beginning of test pulse, a linear I-V relation is obtained (closed circles) although the line is less steep than that of control. When measured 2 sec after the beginning of test pulse, the I-V relationship is highly non-linear (closed triangles).

EPC measured 5 msec after the beginning of test pulse reflects the sum of open channel block associated with each potential step and the close channel block at -50 mV. The amplitude measured at 2 sec after the beginning of potential step reflects the sum of open and closed channel block at each potential step. Therefore, open channel block by octylguanidine is voltage-independent, whereas closed channel block is voltage-dependent.

Closed channel block

Closed channel block found with octylguanidine has also been suggested by other investigators. A cyclic model was proposed for procaine block of ACh-activated channels (Adams, 1977). This model includes both open and

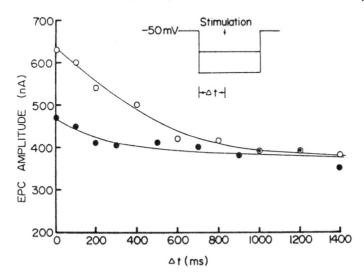

Fig. 6. Time course of development of block by 10 μM octylguanidine. Peak end-plate current amplitude is plotted as a function of time after the beginning of a 2.2 sec voltage step from -50 mV to -70 mV (closed circles) or to -90 mV (open circles). Only one EPC was elicited during each step. From Farley et al. (1981).

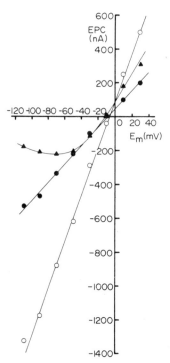

Fig. 7. Current-voltage relationships obtained from the control end-plate (open circles) and in the presence of 10 μM octylguanidine (closed circles and closed triangles). The measurements represented by the closed and open circles were obtained by eliciting a single EPC 5 msec after the beginning of a 2.2 sec voltage step, and the closed triangles by eliciting an EPC 2 sec after the voltage step. From Farley et al. (1981).

closed channel block. The voltage dependence of close channel block was not determined, but it was suggested that it is less than that for block of the open channel. Block of end-plate channel by histrionicotoxin is voltage-dependent and part of the blocking action can occur in the absence of receptor activation (Masukawa and Albuquerque, 1978). TEA has also been shown to have a similar blocking action on the closed channel (Adler et al., 1979).

The lack of voltage dependence of open channel block suggests that the octylguanidine molecule binds to a channel site near the external membrane surface. For closed channel block, however, the molecule must bind to a channel site located deeper from the membrane surface. Therefore, there appears to be two separate sites for octylguanidine. However, since voltage profile across the channel may not necessarily be the same when the channel is closed and when it is open, the possibility of a single site cannot be excluded.

Conductance-voltage curve for octylguanidine

The voltage-dependent closed channel block caused by octylguanidine as described above is not dependent on the direction of current flow. This has been demonstrated by an experiment similar to that shown in Fig. 4 for methylguanidine (Vogel et al., 1984). Decreasing the external sodium concentration to one-half of the normal value caused a shift of the reversal potential by some 20 mV in the direction of hyperpolarization without causing a shift of the conductance-voltage curve toward hyperpolarization. Thus, it is clear that octylguanidine block is not current-dependent but voltage-dependent.

SINGLE CHANNEL EXPERIMENTS

Single channel recording experiments have provided further evidence in support of the current-dependent block of ACh-activated channels by shorter-chain alkylguanidines (Farley et al., 1986). Figure 8 illustrates records of single ACh-activated channel currents at various membrane potentials. Currents flow in inward direction at negative potentials, whereas they flow in outward direction at positive potentials. The reversal potential is 0 mV. Application of 2 mM ethylguanidine to the external membrane surface decreased the amplitudes of inward currents recorded at -50 mV (Fig. 9).

Current-voltage relationships of single channel currents before and after external application of 2 mM ethylguanidine are shown in Fig. 10A. Whereas the control I-V relationship is linear, ethylguanidine caused a considerable rectification, current amplitude becoming smaller at negative potentials. When applied to the internal membrane surface, however, ethylguanidine at 20 mM caused a decrease in current at positive potentials (Fig. 10B). Thus the externally applied ethylguanidine decreased the inward currents only, whereas the internally applied ethylguanidine decreased the outward currents only. The ethylguanidine block is obviously not voltage-dependent, but is dependent upon the direction of current flow.

The single channel current data described above are in accordance with the EPC data described earlier in this chapter in that block caused by shorter-chain alkylguanidines such as methylguanidine and ethylguanidine is dependent upon the direction of current flow. Inward current brings the externally applied guanidine molecule to the intrachannel binding site causing a block. Outward currents sweep the molecule away from the site

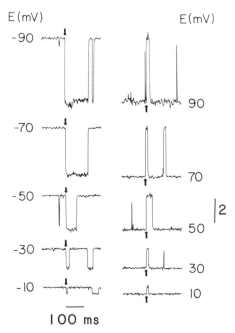

Fig. 8. Current records from single acetylcholine-activated ion channels at various holding membrane potentials (E) indicated in mV. Calibrations, 100 msec and 2 pA. The recordings were made from an inside-out patch with 360 mM CsCl and 250 nM acetylcholine in the pipette and 360 mM CsCl in the bath (internally). The direction of the arrow indicates the direction of channel current.

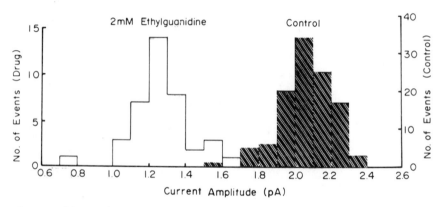

Fig. 9. Amplitude histograms of single acetylcholine-activated ion channel currents before and during external application of 2 mM ethylguanidine. Measurements were made at -50 mV.

causing an unblock, or bring the internally applied molecule to the site causing a block.

SUMMARY AND CONCLUSIONS

Shorter-chain alkylguanidines such as n-methylguanidine and n-ethylguanidine stimulate release of neurotransmitters from nerve terminals and block the acetylcholine-activated ion channels at the end-plate. Block occurs in a manner dependent upon the direction of current flow through the channels, not upon the membrane potential per se. Longer-chain alkylguanidines such as n-octylguanidine do not affect transmitter release, but block the acetylcholine-activated channel with a higher potency than that of shorter-chain alkylguanidines. Octylguanidine blocks the channels at both closed and open states. The open channel block is not voltage-dependent. The closed channel block is voltage-dependent, being intensified with hyperpolarization, and is not current-dependent. Single channel recording experiments have provided additional support for the current-dependent block caused by ethylguanidine. It appears that the shorter-chain alkylguanidine molecule applied externally is swept in the open channel via inward current causing a block. The molecule is trapped inside the channel and can escape with the help of outward currents only when the channel is open. When applied inside, the shorter-chain alkylguanidine molecule is swept in the channel via outward current causing a block.

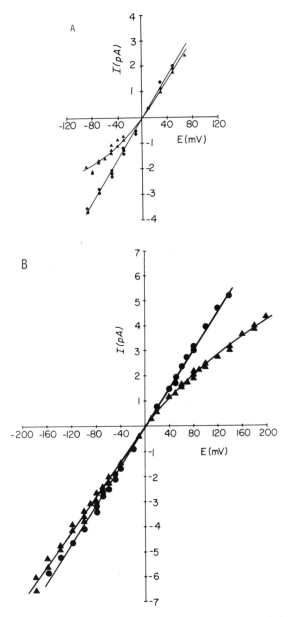

Fig. 10. Current-voltage relationships of single acetylcholine-activated
ion channel currents before and during application of ethylguanidine. A,
I-V relations before (circles) and during application of 2 mM
ethylguanidine externally (triangles). B, I-V relations before (circles)
and during application of 20 mM ethylguanidine internally (triangles).

349

ACKNOWLEDGEMENTS

Our studies quoted in this chapter were supported by NIH grants NS14144 and NS14145. Thanks are due to Sandra Collins and Janet Henderson for secretarial assistance.

REFERENCES

Adams, P. R., 1976, Drug blockade of open end-plate channels, J. Physiol., 260:531-552.
Adams, P. R., 1977, Voltage jump analysis of procaine action at frog end-plate, J. Physiol., 268:291-318.
Adams, P. R. and Sakmann, B., 1978, Decamethonium both opens and blocks end-plate channels, Proc. Nat. Acad. Sci. U.S.A., 75: 2994-2998.
Adler, M., Oliveria, A. C., Eldefrawi, M. E., Eldefrawi, A. T., and Albuquerque, E. X., 1979, Tetraethylammonium; voltage dependent action on end-plate conductance and inhibition of ligand binding to postsynaptic proteins, Proc. Nat. Acad. Sci. U.S.A., 76:531-535.
Armstrong, C. M., 1969, Inactivation of the potassium conductance and related phenomena caused by quaternary ammonium ion injection in squid axons, J. Gen. Physiol., 54:553-575.
Armstrong, C. M., 1971, Interaction of tetraethylammonium ion derivatives with the potassium channels of giant axons, J. Gen. Physiol., 58:413-437.
Cahalan, M. D., 1978, Local anesthetic block of sodium channels in normal and pronase-treated squid giant axons, Biophys. J., 23:285-311.
Courtney, K. R., 1975, Mechanism of frequency dependent inhibition of sodium currents in frog myelinated nerve by the lidocaine derivative GEA 968, J. Pharmacol. Exp. Ther., 195:225-236.
Deguchi, T., and Narahashi, T., 1971, Effects of procaine on ionic conductances of end-plate membranes, J. Pharmacol. Exp. Ther., 176:423-433.
del Castillo, J., and de Motta, G. E., 1977, Influence of succinic anhydride on the decay of end plate currents evoked by high frequency stimulation, Soc. Neurosci. Abstr., 3:371.
Farley, J. M., Yeh, J. Z., Watanabe S., and Narahashi, T., 1981, Endplate channel block by guanidine derivatives, J. Gen. Physiol., 77:273-293.
Farley, J. M., Narahashi, T., and Vogel, S. M., 1986, Block of single acetylcholine-activated channels in chick myotubes by alkylguanidines, Pflügers Arch., 406:629-635.
Giovannetti, S., Biagini, M., Balestri, P. L., Navalesi, R., Giagnoni, P., de Matteio, A., Ferro-Milone, P., and Corfetti, C., 1969, Uremialike syndrome in dogs chronically intoxicated with methylguanidine and creatinine, Clin. Sci. (Oxf.), 36:445-452.
Hamill, O. P., Marty, A., Neher, E., Sakmann, B., and Sigworth, F. J., 1981, Improved patch-clamp techniques for high-resolution current recording from cells and cell-free membrane patches, Pflügers Arch., 391:85-100.
Hille, B., 1975, The receptor for tetrodotoxin and saxitoxin. A structural hypothesis, Biophys. J., 15:615-619.
Hille, B., 1977, Local anesthetic: hydrophilic and hyrdophobic pathways for the drug-receptor reaction, J. Gen. Physiol., 69:497-515.
Kusano, K., 1970, Effect of guanidine on the squid giant synapse, J. Neurobiol., 1:459-469.
Masukawa, L. A., and Albuquerque, E. X., 1978, Voltage- and time-dependent action of histrionicotoxin on the endplate current of the frog muscle, J. Gen. Physiol., 72:351-367.
Neher, E., and Steinbach, J. H., 1978, Local anaesthetics transiently block currents through single acetylcholine-receptor channels, J. Physiol., 277:153-176.

Otsuka, M., and Endo, M., 1960, The effects of guanidine on neuromuscular transmission, J. Pharmacol. Exp. Ther., 128:273-282.

Ritchie, J. M., and Rogart, R. B., 1977, The binding of saxitoxin and tetrodotoxin to excitable tissue, Rev. Physiol. Biochem. Pharmacol., 79:1-50.

Ruff, R. L., 1977, A quantitative analysis of local anaesthetic alteration of miniature end-plate currents and end-plate current fluctuations, J. Physiol., 264:89 -124.

Seyama, I., Wu, C. H., and Narahashi, T., 1980, Current-dependent block of nerve membrane sodium channels by paragracine, Biophys. J., 29:531-537.

Strichartz, G. R., 1973, The inhibition of sodium currents in myelinated nerve by quarternary derivatives of lidocaine, J. Gen. Physiol., 62:37-57.

Takeuchi, A., and Takeuchi, N., 1959, Active phase of frog's end-plate potential, J. Neurophysiol., 22:395-411.

Teravainen, H., and Larsen, A., 1975, Effects of guanidine on quantal release of acetylcholine in mammalian myoneural junction, Exp. Neurol., 48:601-609.

Vogel, S. M., Watanabe, S., Yeh, J. Z., Farley, J. M., and Narahashi, T., 1984, Current-dependent block of endplate channels by guanidine derivatives, J. Gen. Physiol., 83:901-918.

Watanabe, S., and Narahashi, T., 1979, Cation selectivity of acetylcholine-activated ionic channel of frog endplate, J. Gen. Physiol., 74:615-628.

Yeh, J. Z., 1978, Sodium inactivation mechanism modulates QX-314 block of sodium channels in squid axons, Biophys. J., 24:569-574.

Yeh, J. Z., 1979, Dynamics of 9-aminoacridine block of sodium channels in squid axons, J. Gen. Physiol., 73:1-21.

FUNCTIONAL ASPECTS OF CHOLINERGIC SYSTEM

RECEPTOR-RECEPTOR INTERACTIONS IN THE MODULATION OF NICOTINIC RECEPTORS IN ADRENAL MEDULLA *

E. Costa, I. Hanbauer[+], and A. Guidotti

Fidia-Georgetown Institute for the Neurosciences
900 Reservoir Road, Washington, D.C. 20007
[+]Hypertension, Endocrine Branch, NHLBI
National Institute of Health
Bethesda, Maryland 20892

INTRODUCTION

Many important studies directed to clarify the molecular nature of nicotinic receptor function were carried out using chromaffin cells of adrenal medulla as a model. Such a selection was motivated by the convenience of evaluating nicotinic receptor function through a simple measurement of the catecholamines that are released from either perfused adrenal gland or primary cultures of bovine chromaffin cells. For many years, the background rationale for all these studies included the tacit assumption that the release of catecholamines from chromaffin cells was exclusively regulated by acetylcholine (ACh) which was believed to be the only chemical signal released from splanchnic nerves that acts on nicotinic receptors of adrenal chromaffin cells. Moreover, it was believed that the exclusive function of chromaffin cells was the synthesis, storage and secretion of catecholamines. This simple model has been challenged by the discovery in adrenal chromaffin tissues and in their afferent neurons of a number of additional neuromodulators, including γ-aminobutyric acid (GABA) (Kataoka et al., 1984, Alho et al., 1985), substance P (Mizobe et al., 1979), enkephalins (Schultzberg et al., 1978, Yang et al., 1980) and NPY (Majane et al., 1985). The aim of the present paper is to reevaluate many of the literature's tenets on nicotinic receptor function that resulted from an oversimplistic model of cholinergic transmission. The coexistence and corelease in chromaffin cells of more than one neurotransmitter promote the chromaffin cell as a useful model to elucidate how multiple chemical signals modulate nicotinic receptor function.

Recent technological advances made it possible to study the molecular mechanisms whereby transmitter receptors located in the membrane of chromaffin cells modulate the permeability of Na^+, K^+,

---

* Because the use of synaptic transmission modulation as a major focus in drug development is a new research trend, we have dedicated this presentation to Professor A. Karczmar, who was a pioneer in a number of new trends of neuropharmacological research.

355

Ca^{2+} and Cl^- through ion channels. Ion channels are intramembrane protein structures that function as gated pores and allow ions to diffuse across the membrane of neurons. Depending on the type of channel, the gating mechanism may be sensitive to voltage changes across the membrane, to the activation of neurotransmitter receptors, to the presence of various modulators (Ca^{2+} and cotransmitters) or to any combination of the above. Hence, by using the voltage clamping technology, the study of signal transduction at nicotinic receptors of chromaffin cells may determine whether recognition sites for neuropeptides and other transmitters participate in regulating cholinergic receptor function. For example, allosteric modulation of nicotinic recognition sites changes the permeability of specific ions and modifies the ACh-elicited secretion of catecholamines and of other neuromodulators that coexist with catecholamines in chromaffin granules. The present contribution summarizes the information that was obtained with the technology of patch clamping in the whole cell or in the membrane mode on ion channel currents and illustrates the efforts made in our laboratory to understand how multiple chemical signals regulate nicotinic synaptic transmission in adrenal medulla.

Our interest in this matter has general implications which exceed our concern to clarify the molecular nature of a transmitter receptor modulation in adrenal medulla. Ultimately our efforts are directed to reach a better understanding of the similarities and differences existing between the mechanisms that are operative in man-made computers and in brain. An important difference among these two systems resides in the characteristics of the brain transistors (ion channels) which are self-modifiable in a function-dependent manner, whereas the hardware of man-made computers is virtually constant and function-independent. For the sake of this comparison, and using computer terms, the hardware properties of a neuron can be defined by the characteristics of the receptor-modulated transistors, which are the ion channels located in postsynaptic membranes of synaptic junctions. The performance of these transistors can be modified chemically by the release of specific chemical signals causing long term changes of channel structure in postsynaptic receptor related channels. One of the mechanisms for transmitter receptor modification is protein phosphorylation which can be mediated by one of four kinds of protein kinases each specifically activated by cyclic AMP, cyclic GMP or Ca^{2+} both in a calmodulin or diacylglycerol dependent manner. Once a modulatory protein of the receptor is phosphorylated, the transistor function of that receptor is altered. For instance, it may be activated less frequently by its own transmitter or once activated it may stay activated longer. The time constant of the phosphorylation depends both on the turnover of the regulatory protein that is phosphorylated or on the activity of specific phosphoprotein phosphatases. Thus, the characteristics of the change brought about by phosphorylation depends on the microenvironment, the present and past receptor interactions and the genetic background. All these factors and others contribute to the variability of individual brain performance.

TRANSMITTERS AND COTRANSMITTERS

Multiple chemical signals participate in synaptic transmission. Cotransmitters are released from neurons together with a primary transmitter such as ACh and act on various sites of the postsynaptic receptors for the primary transmitter. Cotransmitters are a new entity that differ from the primary transmitters because they modulate the action of a primary transmitter and require its presence to express their action. The presence of cotransmitters helps us to understand the variability of brain function which appears to be virtually infinite. Although the regulation of cotransmitter release is not completely understood, it can be assumed that they may act tonically or phasically. Cotransmitters may modulate specific receptor functions of primary transmitters, promote changes in receptor phosphorylation and thereby may determine the level of receptor responsiveness and performance in health and disease. This complexity in the operation of synaptic communication is becoming a major focus of attention for research strategies directed to produce the new generation of safer neuroactive drugs that our society needs. Since the cotransmitter represents a mechanism of physiological modulation of synaptic transmission, it is clear that a focus on cotransmitter receptors is the way that we should go to rennovate the pharmacology of synaptic communication. In fact, this presentation intends to analyze the current understanding of the endogenous modulation of signal transduction at the nicotinic receptors of chromaffin cells. In this analysis we will take into consideration substance P, GABA, enkephalins and neuropeptide Y (NPY). These neuromodulatcrs are either present in afferent axons to the chromaffin cells or stored in a population of chromaffin cells that regulate directly or indirectly nicotinic receptors. We are aware that additional chemical signals may be pertinent to this analysis, but since their role is still under study, we have limited our focus to those that are better understood.

Before going further, it seems appropriate to give some guidelines as to the scheme that operationally will be followed in classifying the multiple chemical signals operative in the synaptic communication at nicotinic receptors. Provisionally, we distingish two classes of synaptic signals: the transmitters and the cotransmitters. A transmitter: 1) is synthesized and stored in a neuron, alone or in association with other neuromodulators; 2) is released extraneuronally by depolarization; 3) mimics the responses elicited by stimulation of the cell that stores the transmitter; and 4) activates the same signal transduction mechanism by acting on the specific recognition site that mediates physiologically elicited responses. Conversely, a cotransmitter: 1) is synthesized and stored with other cotransmitters and/or primary transmitter(s); 2) is released extraneuronally by depolarization; 3) fails to mimic responses elicited by the stimulation of the neurons where it is stored but; 4) amplifies or reduces the responses and the signal transduction elicited by physiological responses. In a given synapse, pertinent transmitter(s) and cotransmitter(s) act on contiguous recognition sites which often are part of the same functional supramolecular structure. The transmitter receptor includes a recognition site for transmitter and cotransmitter, a coupling device (GTP-binding proteins and others) and a transducer (an ion channel or an enzyme). While the transmitter recognition site is directly coupled with the transducer, the cotransmitter recognition site functions as an allosteric modulatory site for the transmitter recognition site or for the device coupling the transmitter recognition site with the transducer.

SUBSTANCE P

This undecapeptide was first detected in brain and intestine but it is now known to be present in sensory spinal ganglia and in many other brain structures (Pernow, 1983). Substance P possesses excitatory and inhibitory influences on neurons. When applied on chromaffin cells it reduces catecholamine secretion elicited by ACh (Mizobe et al., 1979, Role et al., 1981) because it desensitizes ACh induced ion currents (Stallup and Patrick, 1980). Studies by Clapham and Neher (1984), conducted on chromaffin cells under whole-cell voltage clamp conditions, have shown that substance P by itself fails to act on any kind of transducer mechanism generating ion currents. In contrast, ACh applied to chromaffin cells causes an inward current that diminishes in the continued presence of ACh. This desensitization increases as a simple exponential process with a time constant of 8 to 10 sec. In the presence of substance P the desensitization of the ACh response could be fitted by the sum of two exponentials with time constants of 0.6 and 5 sec, respectively. The recovery time of the ACh desensitization is not affected by the presence or absence of substance P. Detailed studies of the desensitization process indicate that the conductance of individual channels is not changed by substance P, but the mean open time of single channels is shortened. Actually the inverse mean open time is linearly related to the substance P concentration. Interestingly, a similar interaction between ACh and substance P has been reported at the nicotinic receptor of chicken sympathetic ganglion neurons (Role, 1984). Two molecular mechanisms have been invoked to explain such a behavior: channel block by substance P or modification of kinetic constants of the desensitization process. Channel block might be excluded because desensitization is much faster than the inverse process for return to normality. In contrast, if the desensitization is due to a covalent modification of the channel, it is possible that substance P facilitates this process (phosphorylation?) without modifying the process that brings about the return to normality; for instance, dephosphorylation by phosphoprotein phosphatase, if the covalent modification were to be phosphorylation.

This evidence taken together indicates that substance P acts on nicotinic receptors as a putative cotransmitter, in fact, it operates only in the presence of ACh by modifying the ion channel functioning as the nicotinic receptor transducer. Substance P fails to directly activate ion channel or ion permeation, but blocks channel activation by ACh and promotes a transition to a transiently silent state. This silent state could be a "blocked state" similar to that elicited by local anesthetics. The effector of this modulation could be substance P released from the chromaffin cell storage by secretory stimuli. The molecular mechanism triggering the secretion of this modulator is not yet understood, nor it is known whether substance P operates tonically or phasically in the cholinergic transmission of adrenal medulla.

γ-AMINOBUTYRIC ACID (GABA)

In the central nervous system, the amino acid GABA binds to specific recognition sites of a complex receptorial system that includes Cl^- channels located on synaptic membranes. The binding of this inhibitory neurotransmitter to two distinct recognition sites ($GABA_A$ and $GABA_B$) activates a variety of transducer mechanisms including specific permeation of Cl^- ($GABA_A$) or K^+ ($GABA_B$) (Bowery, 1984) and/or reduction of adenylate cyclase catalytic activity ($GABA_B$) (Wojcik and Neff, 1984). The $GABA_A$ recognition sites are specifically activated by muscimol but are insensitive to the action of beta-p-chlorophenyl GABA (baclofen) which specifically activates muscimol-insensitive (Bowery, 1984) $GABA_B$ recognition sites.

Bicuculline is a specific agonist of $GABA_A$ recognition sites, while specific antagonists of $GABA_B$ recognition sites have not been described, yet. The supramolecular organization of $GABA_A$ receptors includes, in addition to a GABA recognition site and a transducer (Cl^- channel), two important regulatory domains. One for the allosteric modulation of the expression of $GABA_A$ recognition sites which is usually referred to as benzodiazepine (BZD)-beta-carboline (BC) recognition site (Costa and Guidotti, 1979, Costa et al., 1983, Haring et al., 1985) and is probably coupled to a specific basic protein termed GABA modulin (Guidotti et al., 1983); and the other one for the modulation of the Cl^- channel opening time which usually is referred to as the picrotoxin or butylbicyclophosphorothionate recognition site (Olsen, 1982; Stephenson et al., 1986). These variabilities in GABA receptor function may have both a physiological and a pharmacological significance. For instance, the GABA receptors of adrenal medullary chromaffin cells appear to have a low binding capacity for beta-carbolines, while they bind benzodiazepines with much greater capacity (Kataoka et al., 1984). Moreover, the binding of the latter ligands is modulated by GABA (Kataoka et al., 1984). The level of interaction between the allosteric modulatory sites and the GABA recognition sites is quite broad: not only is the affinity of the allosteric domain regulating the specific agonists modulated by GABA but also the occupancy of the GABA recognition site by an agonist changes the characteristics of the allosteric modulation of Cl^- channel function. Similar interactions occur at the specific binding sites for barbiturates and picrotoxin.

Alcohol appears to act by facilitating endogenous modulation of GABA induced Cl^- fluxes (Suzdak et al., 1986). Possibly alcoholism increases the endogenous modulator of GABA binding. The increase in Cl^- conductance elicited by GABA causes Cl^- to flow across the neuronal membrane depending on the concentration gradient. When the Cl^- concentration is higher in the extracellular space, GABA opening of Cl^- channels causes Cl^- influx and hyperpolarization of the cell membrane ensues. Conversely, if the gradient is in the opposite direction, the action of GABA cause Cl^- ions to leave the neuron and depolarization ensues. The latter condition occurs in the GABA-induced depolarization of the primary afferents to the posterior horn of the spinal cord; these afferent axons are depolarized by the release of GABA on the receptors of axo-axonic synapses located on these afferents. This Cl^- mediated depolarization is increased by benzodiazepines (Polc and Haefely, 1976). Independently from the Cl^- flux direction elicited by GABA, the ultimate consequence of this transmitter action is a reduction of neuronal excitability. Hence, the activation of $GABA_A$ receptors mediates inhibition of excitability by burst opening of Cl^- channels (Bormann and Chapman, 1985).

For many years it was thought that GABA was not a transmitter operative in the peripheral nervous system. It was in fact believed that in periphery, neuronal inhibition was elicited by catecholamines acting on specific adrenoceptors. But in adrenal medulla it was never possible to show that catecholamine receptors mediate an inhibition of the nicotinic receptors which were activated by ACh released from the splanchnic nerve. In addition, Kataoka et al. (1984) reported that a population of chromaffin cells of bovine adrenal medulla can synthesize, store and release GABA (Table 1). Moreover, about 40% of chromaffin cells contain $GABA_A$ receptors with high affinity recognition sites for GABA, muscimol, butylbicyclophosphorothionate, bicuculline, and benzodiazepines (Table 2). These $GABA_A$ receptors

TABLE 1

CHARACTERISTICS OF INTRINSIC GABAERGIC SYSTEM IN CULTURE OF
BOVINE CHROMAFFIN CELLS.*

GABA content	68 pmole/10^6 cells
GAD activity	769 pmole/10^6 cells
GAD immunoreactivity	+++(40% of cells)
GABA-T immunoreactivity	+++(70% of cells)
^{3}H-GABA uptake	Na^+ dependent
^{3}H-GABA release	increased by Nicotine
GABA/BZD/Cl$^-$ channel complex	Similar to brain
Cl$^-$ channel	GABA activated**

*Data from Kataoka et al. (1984)
**Data from Bormann et al. (1985)

can be differentiated from the GABA$_A$ receptors described in brain by
their low capacity to bind beta-carbolines. This difference may serve
to differentiate two type of GABA$_A$ receptors. According to this
classification, GABA$_{A2}$ receptors differ from GABA$_{A1}$ receptors
because they contain a low affinity beta-carboline recognition site.
In addition, Bormann and Chapham (1985) using the whole cell
patch-clamp technique demonstrated that these GABA receptors, like
classic GABA$_A$ receptors of brain, are Cl$^-$ selective, are blocked by
the GABA receptor antagonist bicuculline and are reversibly
desensitized by high concentrations of GABA. In chromaffin cells, the
Hill plot of the dose response curve of Cl$^-$ channel activation by
GABA has a slope of 2, indicating that a bimolecular binding of GABA to
the specific recognition site is required to open Cl$^-$ channels. GABA
applied to the chromaffin cell membrane activates single channel
currents which display multiple conductance states. Moreover, the
gating properties of GABA activated Cl$^-$ channels located in

TABLE 2

GABA RECEPTOR MARKERS IN COW ADRENAL MEDULLA

LIGAND	BINDING PARAMETERS	
	K_D (nM)	Bmax (fmol/mg prot)
^{3}H-Muscimol	1.8	30
^{3}H-Flunitrazepam	12	68
^{35}S-t-butylbicyclophosphorothionate	38	26
^{3}H-Ro5-4864	nd	nd

The binding constants of various ligands to crude P$_2$ membranes of
adrenal medulla were measured by Standard Techniques - When
^{3}H-muscimol binding was studied the P$_2$ fraction was treated for 1
hr at 37° with 0.05% Triton x 100; nd = not detectable.

Data from Kataoka et al. (1984)

chromaffin cells are similar to the gating properties of Cl⁻ channels located in brain neurons with regard to their potentiation by diazepam but whether beta-carbolines reduce GABA induced Cl⁻ currents was not ascertained.

The results listed in Table 1 and 2 and the recording of GABA activated Cl⁻ channel, failed to prove whether GABA plays a physiological role in the regulation of the chromaffin cell activation elicited by ACh released from splanchnic nerve. In canine adrenal glands, specific immunostaining revealed the presence of glutamic acid decarboxylase (GAD) in chromaffin cells and in fibers located at the border between medulla and the zona reticulata of cortex (Alho et al., 1985). Hence, GABA receptors in adrenal chromaffin cells can be activated by GABA released from either GABA-containing axons or GAD-containing chromaffin cells. These two sources of GABA are not interdependent and their indifferent existence can be documented in monolaterally denervated canine adrenal glands. In this tissue chromaffin cells continue to synthesize and store GABA although GABAergic neuronal fibers are practically nonexistent.

The action of $GABA_A$ receptor stimulation on the release of endogenous neuromodulators from adrenal medulla, caused by drugs or nerve stimulation, was studied by perfusing the adrenal glands of dogs according to Hilton (Hilton et al., 1958). When 4,5,6,7-tetra-hydroisoxazolo [5,4-c] pyridin-3-ol (THIP) was used as the $GABA_A$ receptor agonist, the resting outflow of catecholamines from adrenal gland was increased, but the catecholamine release elicited by splanchnic nerve stimulation was inhibited (Table 3). While GABA and muscimol (two other $GABA_A$ receptor agonists) function like THIP, baclofen (a $GABA_B$ receptor agonist) was inactive. Since denervation of the adrenal gland failed to prevent the THIP induced release of catecholamines, this drug appears to act directly on $GABA_A$ receptors located on adrenal medulla, presumably on chromaffin cell membranes.

TABLE 3

THIP REDUCES ADRENAL CATECHOLAMINE RELEASE INDUCED BY
SPLANCHNIC NERVE STIMULATION IN DOG

| | Catecholamine Release (nmol/ml plasma) | | % Change |
	Basal	Stimulated[a]	Stimulated/Basal
Saline	1.8 ± 0.24	8.2 ± 1.2[*$]	+ 356
THIP[b] (20 mg/ia)	5.0 ± 0.75[*]	4.1 ± 0.82[*]	- 18

a) Splanchnic nerve stimulation (10 v, 6HZ)

b) THIP was injected intraarterially (i.a.) 15 min before splanchnic nerve stimulation. Dogs (20 kg b/w) were prepared according to the technique of Hilton et al (1958). Each value is the mean ± SE of three experiments.

*P<0.01 when compared with basal levels of catecholamines in saline treated dogs.

$P<0.01 when compared with basal levels of catecholamines in saline and THIP treated dogs.

The action of THIP involves exclusively GABA$_A$ receptors because it is blocked by bicuculline but unchanged by hexamethonium or naloxone (Alho et al., 1985; Kataoka et al., 1986). Since THIP facilitates the spontaneous release of catecholamines from adrenal medulla and inhibits the release of adrenal catecholamines elicited by nerve stimulation in a manner that is inhibited by bicuculline, both actions must depend on the stimulation of GABA$_A$ receptors. If both actions are mediated by GABA$_A$ receptors, these two opposite actions must be triggered by the binding of GABA to identical receptors located in different cells. In adrenal medulla, because of a peculiar compartmentation of Cl$^-$ ions, THIP might cause a mild depolarization of chromaffin cell membranes thereby facilitating the spontaneous release of catecholamines. When this depolarization persists, due to the continuous occupancy of GABA$_A$ recognition site, the function of the chromaffin cell is inhibited while the cells remain depolarized. This persistent depolarization reduces the amount of catecholamines released by the ACh liberated by electrical stimulation of splanchnic nerve. THIP also changed, in a similar manner, the release of opioid peptides from adrenal elicited by electrical stimulation of splanchnic nerve (Fujimoto et al., in preparation). These results taken together allow to infer that GABA produced and stored in chromaffin cells is released and acts on GABA$_{A2}$ receptors located on either afferent axons or chromaffin cells. Perhaps the Cl$^-$ ion equilibrium existing in the extracellular space of the adrenal medulla at the Cl$^-$ steady state is such that the opening of Cl$^-$ channels elicited by GABA causes an efflux of Cl$^-$ ion from both chromaffin cells and axons. The ensuing depolarization of chromaffin cells increases the basal rate of spontaneous release of neuromodulators from the chromaffin cells, but at the same time the depolarization of the axons reduces the release of ACh from nerve terminals brought about by electrical stimulation.

In the interest of development of new drugs one can propose that quaternary analogs of THIP or muscimol may lower the intensity of adrenal medullary participation to splanchic nerve activation during stress responses. Since the secretion of catecholamines, enkephalins and other modulators from adrenal medulla probably participates in a number of physiological mechanisms, including the regulation of cardio-vascular responses to catecholamines, one could attempt to regulate selectively catecholamine secretion from adrenal glands using quaternary agonists that act on GABA$_{A2}$ receptors of medulla. Similarly, enkephalins reaching the circulation may play a role in modulating immunoresponses; therefore, quaternary GABA mimetics may be studied as agents that can change modulation of immunological responses during stress.

ENKEPHALINS

Opiate peptides (Schultzbert et al., 1978; Yang et al., 1980) and opiate receptors (Chavkin et al., 1979; Saiani and Guidotti, 1982) are present in chromaffin cells of adrenal medulla. The activation of these receptors by beta-endorphin and enkephalins reduces the action of nicotine on specific membrane ion permeation by decreasing the number of available receptors for this cholinomimetic; thereby, decreasing its potency to release catecholamines (Table 4). Since this action is non-competitive, (Kumakura et al., 1980) it may well be indirect and involve an allosteric modulation of the ACh recognition sites of nicotinic receptors. In addition to being present in chromaffin cells, opiate peptides are also located in splanchnic nerves (Pannula et al.,

TABLE 4

RELATIONSHIP BETWEEN THE POTENCY OF A NUMBER OF OPIATE AGONISTS
IN DISPLACING ^{3}H-ETORPHINE BINDING FROM BOVINE ADRENAL MEDULLA
MEMBRANES AND IN INHIBITING THE ACETYCHOLINE (ACH)-INDUCED
CATECHOLAMINE (CA) RELEASE FROM ADRENAL CHROMAFFIN CELLS IN
PRIMARY CULTURE

Opiate	Inhibition ^{3}H Etorphine Binding (K_inM)	Inhibition of ACh-elicited CA release (IC_{30}; uM)
Etorphine	1	0.1
Beta-endorphine	10	0.2
FK 33-824	15	0.25
Met-enk-[Arg^6-Phe^7]	16	0.65
SKF 10, 047	45	7.0
Levorphanol	50	7.5
Ethylketazocine	100	90
Morphine	300	100
D-Ala^2-D-leu^5-enkephalin	400	200

Data from Saiani and Guidotti 1982.

1984). In both cell types these peptides may coexist with a primary
transmitter: GABA, catecholamines, or ACh, and with one or more
cotransmitters.

It would be important to know whether opioid peptides interact with
nicotinic receptors on chromaffin cells and/or with cholinergic
autoreceptors of splanchnic nerves. Ultimately, one would like to know
whether such an interaction may function as a feedback regulation of
ACh, GABA, catecholamines or enkephalin secretion from adrenal
chromaffin cells. It is important to note that primary cultures of
chromaffin cells prepared from bovine adrenal medulla contain mostly
high molecular weight forms of enkephalin-like peptides. In contrast,
extracts of bovine adrenal medulla or of chromaffin granules contain
both low and high molecular weight opiate peptides (Yang et al.,
1980). One cannot avoid wondering whether a high percentage of the low
molecular weight forms are simply artifacts due to homogenization or
whether only high molecular weight forms are released by nerve
stimulation and have physiological importance. In the dog, high
molecular weight forms of enkephalin-like peptides are secreted
spontaneously from in situ blood-perfused adrenal glands. This
secretion is increased by electrical stimulation of splanchnic nerves
(Hexum et al., 1980; Govoni et al., 1981). The latter procedure also
elicits a voltage-dependent increase of low molecular weight
met^5-enkephalin-like peptides. Since this experimental procedure
involves in situ perfusion of the adrenal gland with blood, it is not

possible to rule out the formation of small molecular weight met[5]-enkephalin-like peptides during the preparation and extraction of plasma. Analysis of met[5]-enkephalin-immunoreactive material by gel filtration followed by high pressure liquid chromatography indicated the presence of authentic met[5]-enkephalin in the blood plasma extract. The content of this peptide was increased by electrical stimulation of the peripheral stump of a splanchnic nerve severed at its exit from the diaphragm. The increased release of opioid peptides was attenuated by hexamethonium suggesting that in vivo the release of these peptides is mediated through the activation of nicotinic receptors (Govoni et al., 1981). This notion was further substantiated with studies on the release of opioid peptides elicited by ACh receptor agonists injected in dogs whose splanchnic nerves were transected at the time of the experiment or two weeks before. In both cases the injection of the cholinomimetics released opioid peptides into the circulation. The involvement of opiate receptors in the release of met[5]-enkephalin immunoreactivity from adrenal gland was also studied (Govoni et al., 1981). Injection of morphine elicited a pronounced increase of met[5]-enkephalin immunoreactivity in the effluent adrenal blood. This increase required an intact splanchnic nerve, and was blocked by naloxone or hexamethonium but not by methylatropine. These findings indicate that morphine may act centrally to trigger an increased activity of the splanchnic nerve which in turn facilitates the secretion of opioid peptides from adrenal medulla. This is in keeping with the notion that morphine increases the tone of central cholinergic efferents. Thus, it is clear that opioid peptides can influence nicotinic receptor function at three major sites: by acting on the adrenal chromaffin cells they reduce the release of opioid peptides and catecholamines from adrenal medulla; by acting on the CNS they can facilitate the neuronally induced release of peptides and catecholamines from adrenal gland; by acting on the catecholamine target organs they may modulate the action of catecholamines on specific receptors. The latter mechanism is still highly speculative for it is not certain whether opioid peptides act on several catecholamine receptors or selectively affect a class of adrenoceptors. Another open question is whether adrenal opioid peptides act on immunocellular mechanisms, such as killer cell activity, thereby modulating immunoresponses. Thus, if this were the case, medullary opioid peptides could participate in neuroimmuno-modulation.

NEUROPEPTIDE Y

In 1982, Tatemoto isolated and sequenced neuropeptide Y (NPY) from extracts of pig brain. NPY is a 36 amino acid peptide which has a considerable sequence homology with the pancreatic polypeptides and peptide YY (PYY). NPY and its chemical analogues were named YY and Y because their carboxy terminus is an amide of tyrosine (Y=tyrosine). It is now certain that NPY is the only member of this class of peptides that is present in brain. The coding sequence of NPY includes 291 bases; the presence of two proteolytic cleavage sites suggests that there might be a 28 amino acid fragment of NPY in addition to the 36 amino acid NPY and the 30 amino acid C flanking peptide of NPY called CPON. CPON is present in the adrenal gland, heart and central nervous system, the hypothalamus content of CPON is very high (Allen et al., 1983; Gray and Morely, 1986). NPY appears to play an important role in the regulation of peripheral and central noncholinergic neurons. In the periphery, NPY is found in the adrenal gland and in the fine nerves of the autonomic nervous system where it is often closely associated with or co-stored in catecholaminergic nerves (Majane et al., 1985). Immunohistochemical studies suggest that in the adrenal medulla, NPY is present in the majority of the norepinephrine secretory granules and probably also colocalizes with met[5]-enkephalin. Furthermore, NPY was shown to be present in varicose nerve fibres which pass through the zona retricularis and penetrate the subcapsular cortical layer. NPY was demonstrated in adrenal medulla of mice, rats, guinea pig, cat, dog, ox and horse (Gray and Morely, 1986). In bovine adrenal gland there are multiple molecular forms of NPY including NPY itself (Kataoka et al., 1985). In primary cultures of bovine chromaffin cells, the cell content of NPY was found to be stable for 4 days in culture. When these cells were transferred from the culture medium to the Locke's solution, NPY immunoreactive material was released spontaneously. The addition of K^+ (45 mM) resulted in a 3-fold increase in the rate of NPY release in a Ca^{2+} dependent manner. Also, the other molecular forms of NPY were released by 45 mM K^+.

The peripheral effects of NPY are: 1) vasoconstriction of cerebral vessels; 2) positive chronotropic and inotropic effects on the heart; 3) hypertension; 4) hypoglycemia following a stimulation of insulin secretion; and 5) hyperthyroidism by enhancing thyroid hormone secretion.

Though the adrenal content of NPY is greater than that of other neuropeptides, its physiological role is still a matter of current investigation. NPY inhibits the nicotine-induced release of catecholamines from primary cultures of bovine chromaffin cells. Chromaffin cells contain a specific binding site for NPY (Higuchi et al., 1986). The NPY potency in blocking nicotine release is greater than that of substance P or enkephalins. The ID_{50} value to block noncompetitively the secretion of catecholamines from chromaffin cells elicited by nicotine is 1.8×10^{-9}M. NPY is much less effective in inhibiting the secretion of catecholamines elecited by K^+ depolarization (Higuchi et al., 1986). The structurally related peptides PYY and APP had little or no effect on catecholamine secretion (Table 5). The importance of NPY in medullary function is indirectly suggested by the extraordinary increase of medullary NPY content with aging. In rats from 3.0 ± 0.4 pmol/g tissue at six weeks of age goes to 1510 ± 580 pmol/g tissue at 69 weeks of age. This increase is tissue specific and unrelated to sex (Higuchi et al., 1986). The molecular mechanism of NPY action is not known; studies of the interaction of NPY with nicotine at the channel level or with Ca^{2+} ionophores have not yet been published.

DISCUSSION

We have discussed the interactions of substance P, opioid peptides, NPY and GABA with nicotinic receptors of adrenal glands. These four neuromodulators coexist in chromaffin cells with catecholamines and are coreleased following depolarization. While the three peptides do not appear to act on specific ion channels located in chromaffin cells or in intrinsic adrenal axons, GABA acts on specific Cl^- channels located in chromaffin cells and presumably in intrinsic axons of adrenal gland. Hence, according to the operative definition given in this paper, GABA is a primary transmitter and modifies the results of the activation of nicotinic receptors by an action on an independent transducer (Cl^- channels modulated by $GABA_{A2}$ recognition sites).

TABLE 5

INHIBITION BY NPY AND OTHER RELATED PEPTIDES
OF THE CATECHOLAMINE (CA) RELEASE ELICITED BY
NICOTINE (3×10^{-6}M) FROM BOVINE ADRENAL CHROMAFFIN
CELLS IN PRIMARY CULTURE

PEPTIDE	INHIBITION OF NICOTINE-ELICITED CA RELEASE (IC_{30}; M)
NPY	1.8×10^{-9}
HPP	2×10^{-8}
PYY	$>2 \times 10^{-6}$
APP	$>2 \times 10^{-6}$

NPY = Neuropeptide Y; PYY = Peptide YY; APP = Avian pancreatic peptide; HPP = Human pancreatic peptide.

Data from Higuchi et al., 1986.

In contrast, the three peptides do not appear to be transduced into a stimulus by an independent receptor transducer system and therefore should be considered, at least provisionally, to function as cotransmitters. This classification applies definitely to substance P which is a modifier of the action of ACh on ion channels. The studies carried out on the opioid peptides and NPY are less complete and do not allow definite conclusions. In the case of the NPY an action on Ca^{2+} channels cannot be ruled out at the present time.

Indeed, membranes of adrenal chromaffin cells contain specific recognition sites for NPY and opioid peptides. However, no evidence is yet available that these sites are connected to a specific ion channel or to phosphatidylinositol hydrolytic enzymes or to a cyclase for the biosynthesis of either cyclic AMP or cyclic GMP. It is possible to suggest that the three peptides modulate ion channel activated by ACh via a receptor-receptor interaction. Studies are now in order to investigate whether NPY and opioid peptides, like substance P, modulate nicotinic receptor activated ion channels.

REFERENCES

Allen, Y.S., Adrian, T.E., Allen, J.M., Tatemoto, K., Crow, T.J., Bloom, S.R. and Polak, J.M., 1983, Neuropeptide Y distribution in the rat brain, Science 221:877-879.

Alho, H., Fujimoto, M., Guidotti, A., Hanbauer, I., Kataoka, Y. and Costa, E, 1985, Gamma aminobutyric acid (GABA) in the adrenal medulla: location, pharmacology and applications, in: Neurology and Neurobiology, ed., Pannula, Pavarinta, Soinila, Vol. 16, pp. 453-464, Alaskan, New York.

Bormann, J. and Clapham, D.E., 1985, γ-aminobutyric acid receptor channels in adrenal chromaffin cells: A patch clamp study, Proc. Natl. Acad. Sci. 82:2168-2172.

Bowery, N.G., Price, G.W., Hudson, A.L., Hill, D.R., Wilkin, G.P. and Turnbull, M.J., 1984, GABA receptor multiplicity: visualization of different receptor types in the mammalian CNS, Neuropharmacology 23:219-231.

Chavkin, C., Cox, B.M. and Goldstein, A., 1979, Stereospecific opiate binding in bovine adrenal medulla, Mol. Pharmacol. 15:751-753.

Clapham, D.E. and Neher, E., 1984, Substance P reduces acetylcholine-induced currents in isolated bovine chromaffin cells, J. Physiol. 347:255-277.

Costa, E., Corda, M.G. and Guidotti, A., 1983, On a brain polypeptide functioning as a putative effector for the recognition sites of benzodiazepine and beta-carboline derivatives, Neuropharmacology 27:1481-1492.

Costa, E. and Guidotti, A., 1979, Molecular mechanisms in the receptor action of benzodiazepine, Ann. Rev. Pharmacol. Toxiol. 19:531-545.

Govoni, S., Hanbauer, I., Hexum, T.D., Yang, H-Y.T., Kelly, G.D. and Costa E, 1981, In vivo characteristics of the mechanisms that secrete enkephalin like peptides stored in dog adrenal medulla, Neuropharmacology 20:639-645.

Gray, T.S. and Morely, J.E., 1986, Neuropeptide Y: Anatomical distribution and possible function in mammalian nervous system, Life Sci. 38:389-401.

Guidotti, A., Corda, M.G., Wise, B.C., Vaccarino, F. and Costa, E., 1983, GABAergic synapses, Neuropharmacology 22:1471-1479.

Haring, Stahli, C., Schoch, B., Takacs, B., Staehelin, T. and Mohler, H., 1985, Monoclonal antibodies reveal structural homogeneity of γ-aminobutyric acid/benzodiazepine receptors in different brain areas, Proc. Natl. Acad. Sci. 82: 4837-4841.

Hexum, T.D., Hanbauer, I., Govoni, S., Yang, H-Y.T., Kelly, G.D. and Costa, E., 1980, Secretion of enkephalin-like peptides from canine adrenal gland following splanchnic nerve stimulation, Neuropeptides 1:137-142.

Higuchi, H., Costa, E. and Yang, H-Y.T., 1986, Inhibition of catecholamine release from bovine chromaffin cells by neuropeptide Y and specific binding of N-[pripionyl-^{3}H] neuropeptide Y in bovine adrenal membrane, J. Pharmacol. Exp. Ther., in press.

Higuchi, H., Yang, H-Y.T. and Costa, E., 1986, Age-related change in neuropeptide Y-like immunoreactive peptides in rat adrenal glands, brains and blood, Mol. Pharmacol. 1986, in press.

Hilton, J.G., Weaver, D.C., Muelheims, C., Glaviano, V.V. and Wegria, R., 1958, Perfusion of the isolated adrenals in situ, Am. J. Physiol. 192:525-530.

Kataoka, Y., Gutman, Y., Guidotti, A., Pannula, P., Wroblewski, J., Cosenza-Murphy, D., W.V. J.Y. and Costa, E., 1984, Intrinsic GABAergic system of adrenal chromaffin cells, Proc. Natl. Acad. Sci. 81:3218-3222.

Kataoka, Y., Fujimoto, M., Alho, H., Guidotti, A., Geffard, M., Kelly, G.D. and Hanbauer, I., 1986, Intrinsic GABA receptors modulate the release of catecholamines from canine adrenal gland in situ, J. Pharmacol. Exp. Ther., in press.

Kumakura, K., Karoum, F., Guidotti, A. and Costa, E., 1980, Modulation of nicotinic receptors by opiate receptor agonists in cultured adrenal chromaffin cells, Nature 283:489-492.

Majane, E.A., Alho, H., Kataoka, K., Lee, C.H. and Yang, H-Y.T., 1985, Neuropeptide Y in bovine glands: distribution and characterization, Endocrinology 117:1162-1168.

Mizobe, F., Kozousek, V., Dean, D.M. and Livett, B.G., 1979, Pharmacological characterization of adrenal paraneurons: Substance P and somatostatin as inhibitory modulators of the nicotinic response, Brain Res. 178:555-566.

Olsen, R.W., 1982, Drug interactions at the GABA receptor-ionophore complex, Ann. Rev. Pharmacol. Toxiol. 22:245-277.

Pannula, P., Yang, H-Y.T., Costa, E., 1984, Coexistence of Met[5]-enkephalin-Arg[6]-Phe[7] with Met[5]-enkephalin and the possible role of Met[5]-enkephalin-Arg[6]-Phe[7] in neuronal function, in: Coexistence of Neuroactive substances in Neurons, V. Chan-Palay and S.L. Palay eds., John Wiley and Sons, Inc., pp. 113-126, 1984.

Pernow, B., 1983, Substance P, Pharmacol. Rev. 35: 85-141.

Polc, P. and Haefely, W., 1976, Effects of two benzodiazepines, phenobarbitone and baclofen on synaptic transmission in the cate cuneate nucleus, Naunyn-Schmiedeberg Ach. Pharmacol. 294:121-131.

Role, L.W., Leeman, S.L. and Perlman, R.L., 1981, Somatostatin and substance P inhibit catecholamine secretion from isolated cells of guinea-pig adrenal medulla, Neuroscience 6:1813-1821.

Role, L.W., 1984, Substance P modulation of acetylcholine-induced currents in embryonic chicken sympathetic and ciliary ganglion neurons, Proc. Natl. Acad. Sci. 81:2924-2928.

Saiani, L. and Guidotti, A., 1982, Opiate receptor-mediated inhibition of catecholamine release in primary cultures of bovine adrenal chromaffin cells, J. Neurochem. 39:1669-1676.

Schultzberg, M., Lundberg, J.M., Hokfelt, T., Terenius, L., Brandt, J., Elde, R.P. and Goldstein, M., 1978, Enkephalin-like immuno-reactivity in gland cells and nerve terminals of the adrenal medulla, Neuroscience 3:1169-1186.

Stallcup, W.B. and Patrick, J., 1980, Substance P enhances cholinergic receptor desensitization in a clonal nerve cell line, Proc. Natl. Acad. Sci., 77:634-638.

Stephenson, F.A., Casalotti, O., Mamalaki, C. and Barnard, E.A., 1986, Antibodies recognising the GABA$_A$/Benzodiazepine receptor including its regulatory sites, J. Neurochem. 46:854-861.

Suzdak, P.D., Schwartz, R.D., Skolnick, P. and Paul, S.M., 1986, Ethanol stimulates γ-aminobutyric acid receptor-mediated chloride transport in rat brain synaptoneurosomes, Proc. Natl. Acad. Sci. 83:4071-4075.

Tatemoto, K., 1982, Neuropeptide Y: Complete amino acid sequence of the brain peptide, Proc. Nat. Acad. Sci. 79:5485-5489.

Wojcik, W.J. and Neff, N.H., 1984, Gamma aminobutyric acid B receptors are negatively coupled to adenylate cyclase in brain, and in the cerebellum these receptors may be associated with granule cells, Mol. Pharmacol. 25:24-28.

Yang, H-Y.T., Hexum, T. and Costa, E., 1980, Opioid peptides in adrenal gland, Life Sci. 27:1119-1125.

ASPECTS OF CHOLINERGIC FUNCTION IN AMYOTROPHIC LATERAL SCLEROSIS

S.-M. Aquilonius and P.-G. Gillberg

Department of Neurology, Akademiska sjukhuset, Uppsala University, S-751 85 Uppsala, Sweden

INTRODUCTION

The degenerative changes in amyotrophic lateral sclerosis (ALS) are preferentially restricted to the cortico-spinal tracts and to the lower motor neurons. Based on this mysterious selectivity, numerous theories regarding the etiology have been put forward, but none has so far been conclusively proved. However, irrespective of etiology, progressive neuronal degeneration should be accompanied by a disturbance of neurotransmission at the synapses of the fiber tracts involved.

The aim of the present research program is to evaluate, from post-mortem studies, the pattern of spinal transmitter changes in ALS. So far, emphasis has been placed on cholinergic mechanisms.

ACETYLCHOLINESTERASE (AChE), CHOLINE ACETYLTRANSFERASE (ChAT) AND CHOLINERGIC RECEPTORS IN THE SPINAL CORD OF CONTROLS AND ALS CASES

Ishii and Friede (10) were pioneers in mapping cholinergic representation within the human spinal cord. Using AChE histochemistry, they observed intense staining in the different motor cell groups of the ventral horn and in the substantia gelatinosa of the dorsal horn, while the staining was weak in all fiber tracts of the white matter, except in the ventral root regions.

More recently developed immunohistochemical methods for detecting ChAT are presently used for mapping cholinergic neurons in the CNS, including the spinal cord, of experimental animals (9, 11, 14), but applications in human spinal tissue are complicated by the demand for instant post-mortem fixation. However, by assay of ChAT in small tissue samples dissected from human spinal cryosections by the "punch technique", a relatively detailed distribution pattern could be demonstrated (1). An area of high ChAT activity in the ventrolateral part of the ventral horn was traced into the ventral root region, indicating the relation of this activity to the motor neurons. In the apical part of the dorsal horn of the human cord another area with high activity of ChAT was demarcated. Subcellular studies suggest that this activity is mainly located at nerve terminals.

An abudance of muscarinic binding sites has been demonstrated in both ventral and dorsal gray matter dissected from human spinal cord (15). In this respect the introduction of in vitro autoradiographic techniques offers a new perspective with regard to resolution (5, 19). Using the ligand ^{3}H-quinuclidinylbenzilate (^{3}H-QNB), the highest density of binding sites was found in the apical part of the dorsal horn and in the motor neuron areas. ^{3}H-QNB binding sites were very low within Clarke´s column, but otherwise the distribution pattern was similar at cervical, thoracic and lumbar levels (7, 18). According to Whitehouse and collaborators (19), the muscarinic binding sites within the motor neuron areas are mainly of the "high affinity agonist type" as judged from the finding of carbachol protection of ^{3}H-methylscopolamine binding.

In autoradiographic studies of the human spinal cord it was found that in contrast to the high density of muscarinic binding sites observed in the motor neuron areas, the binding of ^{3}H-α-bungarotoxin (^{3}H-α-Btx) in corresponding areas was low (7). High ^{3}H-α-Btx binding was seen in the apical area of the dorsal horn in all spinal segments analyzed.

When the above-mentioned cholinergic markers were analyzed in spinal cords from ALS cases, relatively characteristic alterations were found (4, 7) and our results are in close agreement with those reported from other laboratories (12, 15). In ALS the distribution pattern of ChAT was partly preserved, whereas the maximal ChAT activity was markedly reduced. The reduction was not restricted solely to the motor neuron areas but was also noted in the dorsal horn.

Pronounced reductions in muscarinic binding sites within the motor neuron areas of cords from ALS cases seem to parallel degeneration of motor neurons (7, 19). It is not known to what extent these binding sites are located on motor neuron somata, in collaterals, and on Renshaw cells. It seem probable that reduction of muscarinic binding sites within motor neuron areas in ALS is mainly confined to those binding sites of a "high affinity" type (19).

It is possible that cholinergic mechanisms in the apical part of the dorsal horn may take part in the regulation of pain (6). Symptoms of sensory impairment are usually not encountered clinically in ALS. However, ChAT, which seems to be mainly located at terminals within the dorsal horn, is markedly reduced in ALS. Moreover, some reduction of muscarinic binding sites within the dorsal horn was found in our ALS studies and in the ALS investigation by Whitehouse and collaborators (19). These changes might be linked to the morphometric findings of some decrease in the number of large afferent neurons in this disease (13).

It is well known from basic neuropharmacological studies in the cat that the Renshaw cell is nicotinoceptive (17). The finding that ^{3}H-α-Btx binding was low in the motor neuron areas of the spinal cords from human control cases is therefore somewhat unexpected if the binding of this ligand reflects cholinergic nicotinic receptor sites. No significant changes in ^{3}H-α-Btx binding were found in cords from ALS cases (7).

SPECIFICITY OF THE INVOLVEMENT OF CHOLINERGIC STRUCTURES IN ALS

When substance P-like immunoreactivity (SPLI) was measured in tissue parts dissected from human spinal cord, we found the highest value in the dorsal horn at all segmental levels (4), which is in accordance with the findings in an earlier detailed immunohistochemical study (3). We found no clear-cut changes in spinal SPLI in ALS. However, in a recent study by Patten and Croft (16), it was demonstrated by immunohistochemistry that ALS cases had fewer SP-containing fibers than normal in the gray commissure, the nucleus proprius, the medial edge of the dorsal horn and around many anterior horn cells.

^{3}H-etorphine binding, which probably mainly reflects binding to opioid receptors of the delta and mu type sites, was preferentially distributed in the substantia gelatinosa and in the tract of Lissauer in the human spinal cord (7). No significant changes in ^{3}H-etorphine binding were observed.

Autoradiographs obtained with ^{3}H-strychnine, which is considered to reflect binding sites for the inhibitory transmitter glycine, showed a fairly uniform distribution of binding in the gray matter (7). We found no changes in ^{3}H-strychnine binding in ALS cases, although reductions have been observed in another autoradiographic study (19) and in studies on spinal tissue homogenates (8). The latter authors found no alterations in spinal cord binding of ^{3}H-spiroperidol, ^{3}H-muscimol and ^{3}H-dihydro-alprenolol in ALS.

The first fragments of knowledge concerning spinal neurotransmitter abnormalities in ALS have been gained in the last few years. Sensitive chromatographic methods for measuring transmitter amines and immuno-histochemical techniques for determinations of peptides and transmitter-related enzymes represent a methodological potential, as yet largely un-used, in post-mortem studies of human spinal cord. At present, however, it seems that spinal cholinergic structures are profoundly but not selec-tively involved in ALS.

THERAPEUTIC TRIALS WITH CHOLINESTERASE INHIBITORS IN ALS

The above-discussed indications of a disturbance of spinal choli-nergic transmission in ALS prompted us to examine the effects of sympto-matic therapy with the tertiary AChE inhibitor physostigmine in patients with this disorder (2). Seven patients with ALS participated in a double-blind cross-over trial of oral physostigmine and neostigmine (10 and 45 mg/day respectively, for three days). Six of the patients were also gi-ven i.v. injections (1 and 1.5 mg respectively) of the drugs in an open trial. Muscle strength was measured by a myometric technique before and 5, 10, 30 and 60 minutes after i.v. injection of the drugs and on the third day of oral medication. Further, a test battery of neurophysio-logical variables (decremental response, H reflex, tonic vibration re-flex, flexion reflex, and somatosensory evoked potentials) that might reflect changes in neuromuscular and spinal transmission was applied be-fore treatment, 10-30 minutes after injection and on the third day of oral medication.

The results of the trial were negative throughout, as no increase in muscle strength or significant changes in the neurophysiological variables were observed. The lack of therapeutic effect may be due to the presence of such a degree of degeneration involving synaptic struc-tures that functional restoration is impossible.

As long as the etiology of this devasting disorder remains completely unknown, new approaches to symptomatic therapy must be derived from increased knowledge about the physiology and pathophysiology of spinal neurotransmission.

ACKNOWLEDGEMENTS

Studies in the laboratory of the authors were supported by the Swedish Medical Research Council (grant No. 4373).

REFERENCES

1.   Aquilonius, S.-M., Eckernäs, S.-Å. and Gillberg, P.-G. (1981): Brain. Res. 211:329-340.
2.   Aquilonius, S.-M., Askmark, H., Eckernäs, S.-Å., Gillberg, P.-G., Hilton-Brown, P., Rydin, E. and Stålberg, E. (1985): To be published.
3.   Cuello, A., Polak, J. and Pearse, A. (1976): Lancet II:1054-1056.
4.   Gillberg, P.-G., Aquilonius, S.-M., Eckernäs, S.-Å., Lundqvist, G. and Winblad, B. (1982): Brain. Res. 250:394-397.
5.   Gillberg, P.-G., Nordberg, A. and Aquilonius, S.-M. (1984): Brain. Res. 300:327-333.
6.   Gillberg, P.-G. (1985): Thesis Acta Universitatis Upsaliensis, Almqvist & Wiksell International, Stockholm, Sweden.
7.   Gillberg, P.-G. and Aquilonius, S.-M. (1985): Accepted Acta Neurol. Scand.
8.   Hayashi, H., Suga, M., Satake, M. and Tsubaki, T. (1981): Ann. Neurol. 9:292-294.
9.   Houser, C.R., Crawford, G.D., Barber, R.P., Salvaterra, P.M. and Vaughn, J.E. (1983): Brain. Res. 266:97-119.
10. Ishii, T. and Friede, R.L. (1967): IN International Review of Neurobiology (eds) C.C. Pfeiffer and J.R. Smythies, Academic Press, New York.
11. Kan, K.S.K., Chao, L.-P. and Eng, L.F. (1978): Brain. Res. 146: 221-229.
12. Kanazawa, I. (1977): Jap. J. Clin. Med. 35:4025-4029.
13. Kawamura, Y., Dyck, P.J., Shimono, M., Okazaki, H., Tateishi, J. and Doi, H. (1981): J. Neuropathol. Exp. Neurol. 40:667-675.
14. Kimura, H., McGeer, P.L., Peng, J.H. and McGeer, F.G. (1981): J. Comp. Neurol. 200:151-200.
15. Nagata, Y., Oluya, M. and Honda, M. (1981): Neurosci. Lett. Suppl 6: S71.
16. Patten, B.M. and Croft, S. (1984): IN Research Progress in Motor Neurone Disease (ed) F. Clifford Rose, Pitman Press, Bath.
17. Phillis, J.W. (1970): The Pharmacology of Synapsis, Pergamon Press, Oxford, pp 152-160.
18. Scatton, B., Dubois, A., Javoy-Agid, F. and Camus, A. (1984): Neurosci. Lett. 49:239-245.
19. Whitehouse, P.J., Wamsley, J.K., Zarbin, M.A., Price, D.L., Tourtellotte, W.W. and Kuhar, M.J. (1983): Ann. Neurol. 14:8-16.

CHOLINERGIC REGULATION OF REM SLEEP: BASIC MECHANISMS

AND CLINICAL IMPLICATIONS FOR AFFECTIVE ILLNESS AND NARCOLEPSY

Priyattam J. Shiromani and J. Christian Gillin

Department of Psychiatry (V-116A), VA Medical Center

and University of California, San Diego, CA 92161

INTRODUCTION

Rapid eye movement (REM) sleep was first discovered with the observation of a wake-like EEG associated with bursts of rapid eye movements during behavioral sleep in man. When subjects were awakened from this state, they were likely to report dreaming. Since then REM sleep has been discovered in virtually all mammals, some birds and, perhaps, in reptiles.

REM sleep is composed of both tonic (occurring throughout the REM sleep episode) and phasic (occurring only sporadically during REM sleep) events. The major tonic events include cortical desynchronization, loss of muscle tone in antigravity musculature, and theta activity in the dorsal hippocampus. The phasic events include monophasic waves in pons, lateral geniculate nucleus and occipital cortex (these waves are called ponto-geniculo-occipital waves, i.e PGO waves) and rapid eye movements. Data from lesion, transection, pharmacological, and single-unit studies indicate that the various tonic and phasic components of REM sleep are partially controlled by discrete reticular formation (RF) nuclei. Each episode of REM sleep is also accompanied by: increased activity of most brain neurons (exceptions include REM sleep "off cells" in dorsal raphe and locus coeruleus); cardio-respiratory irregularities; activity of the vestibular pathway and middle ear muscle contraction; changes in pupil diameter; penile tumescence; and vivid dreaming in humans.

The mechanisms responsible for sleep are not yet fully understood. Deoxyglucose mapping, for example, has failed to identify sleep centers (Nakamura et al, 1983). Such knowledge, especially concerning the mechanisms of REM sleep generation, may contribute to a better interpretation of the pathophysiology of the sleep, mood, and neuroendocrine disorders associated with depression and narcolepsy.

CHOLINERGIC MECHANISMS AND REM SLEEP

As will be reviewed below, considerable evidence implicates cholinergic mechanisms in many facets of REM sleep. In this book honoring Alexander Karczmar we wish, in particular, to recall the classic paper he and his colleagues published in 1970 suggesting that REM sleep is facilitated as the ratio of cholinergic to aminergic neurotransmission increases (Karczmar et al, 1970). They were the first to demonstrate that REM sleep could be induced by systemic administration of physostigmine to intact reserpinized animals. The idea inherent in their paper – namely, REM sleep is induced by cholinergic mechanisms and inhibited by monoaminergic mechanisms – remains a basic assumption of current research.

It is also of more than passing interest that Otto Loewi's discovery of chemical transmission in the nervous system established acetylcholine as the first neurotransmitter (Friedmann, 1971). He had been aware of the idea that impulses could be transmitted through the release of chemicals at nerve terminals for many years prior to his discovery but the crucial experiment which validated this hypothesis occurred to him in a dream on the night before Easter Sunday, 1920. As is so often the case with the ideas which occur in dreams, he could not clearly recall the experiment the next morning. Fortunately, the dream recurred the following night and at 3 AM he rushed to the laboratory to perform the first experiments which would prove the principle of neurotransmission. It thus appears that acetylcholine triggered the dream which led to the discovery of its own role as a neurotransmitter.

In this chapter, we will suggest that a diffusely represented network of cholinergic or cholinoceptive neurons in the pontine reticular formation (PRF) (perhaps less than 25% of PRF cells) primes, initiates and maintains the consolidated state of REM sleep. In addition, cholinergic mechanisms are also intimately involved in the various tonic and phasic components of REM sleep.

(i) Acetylcholine and Cortical Desynchronization

Cortical desynchronization is an important distinguishing tonic feature of REM sleep. Before REM sleep was discovered, cortical desynchronization was used to differentiate waking from sleep. During waking the cortical EEG typically shows low voltage fast activity, whereas orthodox sleep is characterized by the presence of slow (1-3 hz) high amplitude waves. With the discovery of cortical desynchronization during (what we now call REM sleep) behavioral sleep, however, the usefulness of cortical EEG as an indicator of waking began to be questioned.

Moruzzi and Magoun (1949) showed that the mesencephalic reticular formation was important for desynchronizing the cortex. Over the years various RF nuclei, particularly the norepinephrine containing locus coeruleus (LC) were initially implicated in cortical EEG desynchronization (Jouvet, 1972). Data from lesion and single unit studies, however, show that the LC is not necessary for cortical desynchronization during waking and REM sleep (Jones et al, 1977; Robinson et al, 1977; for review see Ramm, 1979; Vertes, 1984).

The cholinergic system, on the other hand, does play an important role. Systemically administered atropine readily produces slow high amplitude waves, even during behavioral waking. Local infusion of cholinergic agonists, such as carbachol, bethanachol, or oxotremorine, into the RF increases cortical desynchronization (Baghdoyan et al, 1984a, b; George et al, 1964; Shiromani and McGinty, 1983; Silberman et al, 1980). Intense behavioral and EEG arousal is noted with carbachol injections into the mesencephalic RF (Baghdoyan et al, 1984a; Baxter, 1969; Shiromani et al, 1985). Single unit studies have shown that mesencephalic RF cells increase discharge during waking and REM sleep compared with slow wave sleep (for review see Steriade et al, 1980).

374

(ii) Acetylcholine and rapid eye movements

Evidence from lesion studies (Morrison and Pompeiano, 1966) suggests that the vestibular nuclei may be involved in the elaboration of rapid eye movements during REM sleep. Evidence in support of this comes from studies which show that phasic changes in firing rates of vestibular neurons occur during REM sleep in intact cats (Bizzi, Pompeiano and Somogyi, 1964), in the decerebrate preparation (Thoden, Magherini and Pompeiano, 1972a, b), and in acute decerebrate animals treated with acetylcholine potentiating agents, such as physostigmine (Thoden et al, 1972a, b). Furthermore, Mergner and Pompeiano (1977) have shown that increased discharge rates of medial vestibular neurons and abducens motor-neurons, which innervate the lateral rectus muscles of the eye, occur 11-15 msec prior to activity in the lateral rectus muscle. Vestibular lesions, however, only abolish bursts of rapid eye movements but do not interfere with isolated, slow eye movements or with REM sleep per se.

The excitation in vestibular and abducens motor-neurons may be generated by nuclei located within the para-median reticular formation (Cohen and Henn, 1972; Henn and Cohen, 1975). Indeed, reticular units do show bursts preceding saccadic eye movements (Cohen and Henn, 1972; Henn and Cohen, 1975; Keller, 1974; Luscher and Fuchs, 1972; Sparks and Travis, 1971). Moreover, cells in the giganto-cellular tegmental field show cyclic changes in discharge rates preceeding rapid eye movements, not only in intact animals (Pivik et al, 1977), but also in decerebrate animals treated with acetylcholine potentiating agents (Hoshino et al, 1976b; Pompeiano, 1980).

(iii) Acetylcholine and PGO waves

Ponto-geniculo-occipital (PGO) waves are slow monophasic waves which occur either singly or in clusters of 3-4 just prior to and during REM sleep. These waves can be recorded from the pons, lateral geniculate nucleus (LGN) and occipital cortex. These are areas which are directly related to the visual system.

The neurons responsible for PGO waves are hypothesized (for review see Sakai, 1980) to be located in and around the brachium conjunctivum (which Sakai (1980) calls the "X" area), the rostral part of the lateral parabrachial nucleus which is just caudal to the "X" area, and the rostral part of the locus coeruleus. Some neurons in these areas have been shown to fire in phasic bursts (3-5 spikes) as much as 5-25 msec before the onset of a PGO wave (McCarley et al, 1978; Sakai, 1980). During wakefulness some of these units also fire in conjunction with eye movements. Electrical stimulation of this area has been shown to induce PGO waves, while electrical ablation abolishes the PGO waves (Sakai, 1980).

The PGO executive neurons appear to be cholinergic or at least cholinoceptive in nature. Atropine significantly reduces PGO bursts (Jacobs et al, 1972), while physostigmine triggers PGO bursts in collicular or pontine transected cats (Magherini et al, 1971). Microinfusions of carbachol in the dorso-lateral pontine tegmentum has been shown to induce PGO activity selectively (Baghdoyan et al, 1984a; Shiromani and McGinty, 1983). A vestibular component also appears to be involved because carbachol microinfusion into the vestibular region evokes PGO waves tightly coupled to stereotyped eye movements (Shiromani, personal observations).

The PGO mechanism is not exclusively under cholinergic control;

noradrenergic and serotonergic inputs from the locus coeruleus and dorsal raphe nucleus (DRN) are hypothesized to inhibit the cholinergic PGO executive neurons (Sakai, 1980). Evidence in support of the inhibitory influence is provided by studies which show that electrical stimulation of DRN inhibits PGO waves (Jacobs et al, 1973), while lesions or cooling of DRN immediately releases PGO activity (Sakai, 1984). Treatments which decrease serotonin or norepinephrine also immediately release PGO activity (Sakai, 1984). Moreover, DRN and LC neurons show complete cessation of activity just prior to and in temporal contiguity with PGO activity (Chu and Bloom, 1974; McGinty and Harper, 1976; Sheu et al, 1974).

The anatomical profile of the PGO neuronal network confirms the electrophysiological and pharmacological evidence. Utilizing retrograde tracer and immunohistochemical studies, Sakai (for review see Sakai, 1984) has shown that neurons in the "X" area project directly to the LGN (from where PGO waves are usually recorded) and stain positively for choline acetyltransferase (CHAT), a specific marker of cholinergic neurons. In turn, the neurons in the "X" area receive norepinephrine and serotonin afferents from the DRN and LC.

(iv) Acetylcholine and atonia

Much evidence supports the hypothesis that the cataplectic episodes of narcoleptic humans and dogs are related to the muscle atonia of normal REM sleep. The inhibition of antigravity musculature is hypothesized (Sakai, 1980) to result from activation of a discrete group of non-monoaminergic cells located ventrally in the locus coeruleus complex. These peri-LC neurons (Sakai, 1980) may exert an excitatory influence on magnocellular (Mc) neurons located in the medullary RF. The Mc neurons correspond to the medullary inhibitory center of Magoun and Rhines (1949) and are postulated (Fung et al, 1982; Glenn et al, 1978; Morales and Chase, 1978; Pompeiano, 1976, 1980) to induce a generalized inhibition of spinal motor-neurons by exciting spinal inhibitory inter-neurons.

Electrical stimulation of the medullary RF, especially the Mc, elicits generalized inhibition of spinal motor-neurons (Sakai, 1980), while bilateral electrical ablation of the peri-LC and medial LC abolishes the atonia during REM sleep (Henley and Morrison, 1974). Moreover, neuronal activity within the peri-LC and the Mc is high during periods of atonia in REM sleep (Kanomori et al, 1980; Sakai, 1980). The dorso-lateral pontine tegmentum, which contains the peri-LC, exhibits intense metabolic activity, as determined by the 2-DG method, during concussion induced behavioral suppression (Hayes et al, 1984). It was suggested (Hayes et al, 1984; Katayama et al, 1984) that a common mechanism underlies the atonia of REM sleep and the behavioral suppression which follows concussion. HRP studies (Sakai et al, 1978, 1979) have shown connections between the peri-LC, the Mc and the spinal cord.

The cholinergic system is implicated because infusion of carbachol into the pontine tegmentum readily induces cataplexy in cats (Baghdoyan et al, 1984 a, b; Katayama et al, 1984; Mitler and Dement, 1974;Shiromani and McGinty, 1983, 1985 a, b; Van Dongen et al, 1978). In acute decerebrate cats (Hoshino et al, 1976), systemic infusion of physostigmine induces cataplexy; such a loss of decerebrate rigidity occurs at regular intervals only in a chronic preparation. In narcoleptic dogs (Baker and Dement, 1984; Delashaw et al, 1979), systemically administered cholinomimetics increase the incidence of cataplectic episodes while muscarinic receptor blockers delay these episodes; nicotinic agents have no effect. Moreover, in narcoleptic dogs, increased muscarinic receptor binding is found in several pontine sites (Baker and Dement, 1984). It is hypothesized (Sakai, 1984) that these effects are due to activation of cholinoceptive peri-LC and Mc neurons. Choline acetyltransferase (ChAT), a specific marker of cholinergic neurons, has been found in these areas (Armstrong et al, 1983; Kimura et al, 1981, 1982).

(v) Acetylcholine and hippocampal theta

Regular 4-12 Hz waves can be obtained from the dorsal hippocampus during waking, REM sleep and surgical anesthesia (Vanderwolf et al, 1978; Winson, 1972). This waveform, termed theta activity, can be further divided into two categories depending upon the behavior of the animal and response to atropine (Vanderwolf et al, 1978). The first type of theta (4-7 Hz) occurs during alert total immobility, inter-twitch intervals of REM sleep, and anesthesia (urethane, ether). It also occurs when the animal exhibits what has been termed Type II behavior, such as face-washing, shivering, chattering the teeth, and tremor. This type of theta is abolished by anti-muscarinic drugs such as atropine, and stimulated by physostigmine. The second type of theta (7-12 Hz) occurs when the animal exhibits Type I behaviors such as walking, running, rearing, shifts of posture, and head movement. It also occurs during REM sleep related phasic twitches and it is not abolished by anti-muscarinic drugs. This type of theta is disrupted by anesthetics (ether, urethane) and morphine.

With respect to the anatomical organization of the systems responsible for generating theta, it may be that theta activity detected in the CA1 and the dentate gyrus formations of the dorsal hippocampus is driven by pacemaker bursting cells located in the medial septal nucleus and the diagonal band of Broca (Petsche et al, 1965; Stumpf et al, 1962). The pacemaker cells in turn depend upon reticular innervation (Vanderwolf et al, 1978; Vertis, 1984). The evidence supporting such a pathway is provided by extensive stimulation (Vanderwolf et al, 1978), lesion (Anschel and Lindsley, 1972) and autoradiographic (Rose et al, 1976) studies.

Since there are two types of theta, one atropine-sensitive and the other atropine-resistant, it may be that two ascending brainstem systems are responsible for driving the septal pacemaker cells and generating theta. It is suggested that the system responsible for atropine-sensitive theta is cholinergic and, in fact, identical to the ascending cholinergic reticular system of Shute and Lewis (Vanderwolf et al, 1978). Indeed the first acetylcholinesterase containing pathway that was proved to be cholinergic was that arising from the medial septal and diagonal band nuclei and supplying the hippocampus and dentate gyrus (Lewis and Shute, 1978). The evidence that the PRF area may be driving the pacemaker burst cells is derived from studies in which stimulation of the PRF in rat (Klemm, 1972; Robinson et al, 1977, 1978) and cat (Macadar et al, 1974) triggers theta. Recently Vertes (1980) has confirmed these observations. Further evidence indicating that PRF neurons may drive theta is indicated by single-unit studies which show that PRF cells discharge maximally whenever theta is present (Vertes, 1979). Direct projections from the PRF to the septum have been demonstrated (Lynch et al, 1973; Robertson et al,1973).

The organization of the atropine-resistant theta system, on the other hand, is puzzling particularly since a major catecholamine input to the hippocampus from the LC is not responsible for generating this type of theta (Kolb and Whishaw, 1977; Monmaur and Delacour, 1978). Morphine (15mg/kg), however, selectively abolishes atropine-resistant theta.

Naloxone is able to reverse morphine's effect (Vanderwolf et al, 1978). Ether and urethane also abolish this type of theta (Vanderwolf et al, 1978). It is not known how these agents alter atropine-resistant theta.

(vi) Acetylcholine and REM sleep generation

While discrete RF nuclei may be responsible for generating the major tonic and phasic components of REM sleep, we suggest that a PRF cholinergic mechanism primes the various RF nuclei. Transection (Jouvet, 1972; Siegel et al, 1983, 1984) and electrical lesion studies (Jouvet, 1972) have made it clear that the machinery needed for REM sleep generation resides within the PRF. Jouvet (for review see 1972) initially postulated that brainstem cholinergic mechanisms played an important role in the generation of REM sleep and there is compelling evidence to support a brainstem cholinergic-REM sleep link. Increased acetylcholine is found during REM sleep in cortex (Celesia and Jasper, 1966; Jasper and Tessier, 1971) and striatum (Gadea-Ciria et al, 1973) of normal cats and in ventricular perfusates of conscious dogs (Haranath et al, 1973). In normal humans (Sitaram et al, 1976, 1977, 1978a, b, 1980), intravenous infusions of physostigmine or arecoline during non-REM decrease the latency to REM sleep, although infusions during or immediately after REM sleep produce arousal. In addition, an orally active muscarinic agonist (RS-86), shortens REM latency in normal volunteers (Spiegel, 1984). In cats and rats (Amatruda et al, 1975; Baghdoyan et al, 1984a, b; George et al. 1964; Gnadt and Pegram, 1985; Hobson et al, 1983; Mitler and Dement, 1974; Shiromani and McGinty, 1983, 1985a, b; Silberman et al, 1980), administration of cholinergic agonists, e.g., carbachol, directly into the PRF readily evokes elements of REM sleep (atonia, PGO waves, rapid eye movements), or complete REM sleep which may be unusually long. Infusions into midbrain or medullary sites fail to induce REM sleep (Baghdoyan et al, 1984 a; Shiromani et al, 1986) while local infusion of scopolamine blocks the cholinomimetic induced REM sleep (Shiromani and McGinty, 1983).

We have begun a series of experiments to determine the role of PRF cholinergic mechanism in the regulation of REM sleep. In the first series of experiments, in rats, a muscarinic agonist (carbachol) or antagonist (scopolamine) were chronically infused into various brainstem regions or the fourth ventricle (Shiromani, 1983; Shiromani and Fishbein, 1985). An Alzet osmotic mini-pump, which provides continuous infusion of pharmacological agents over a 5-day period, was used to deliver the drugs. The results showed that infusions of scopolamine produced a 61.5% REM sleep decrease during the light cycle (i.e., the rats subjective rest period). The REM sleep loss was due to a decrease in both incidence and duration of REM sleep episodes.

Carbachol, on the other hand, increased REM sleep by 63% during the night cycle. The REM sleep augmentation occurred mainly in the pontine reticular formation (PRF) and it was due to increased incidence of REM sleep episodes and not the result of a change in REM sleep duration. There were no changes in total sleep time or non-REM sleep.

The cholinomimetic induced divergent REM sleep alterations provide important clues as to how REM sleep might be generated. It has been suggested (Hobson et al, 1975; McCarley et al, 1975) that REM sleep generation depends upon activation of PRF neurons. It is our hypothesis that the carbachol induced REM sleep augmentation was a result of a muscarinic receptor mediated recurrent priming of PRF neurons. During the light cycle, carbachol was unable to alter REM sleep because at this time muscarinic activation was already at maximum and PRF neurons optimally primed. During the dark cycle, however, there was a gradual

378

reduction in receptor sensitivity which was reversed by carbachol.

The finding that scopolamine shortened the duration of REM sleep episodes in addition to its effects on frequency would suggest that triggered REM sleep episodes were aborted because scopolamine prevented the development of sustained PRF neuronal activity necessary for the continuation of REM sleep.

In the second series of experiments, we examined the PRF neuronal response to carbachol infusion (Shiromani and McGinty, 1985b). Six cats were implanted with standard sleep recording electrodes and two moveable micro-drives which permitted simultaneous infusion of pharmacological agents and recording of extra-cellular unit potentials within and at various distances from the infusion field.

Fifty-six single reticular neurons were recorded. Twenty-two of the 56 reticular units were located ipsilaterally and within one mm of the infusion field, and micro-infusions of carbachol evoked three distinct patterns of effect; 8 cells were excited, 12 cells inhibited and 2 cells showed no change. The excitation or inhibition was even seen when the units were further away from the infusion area. Nineteen cells were located contralateral to the infusion site: 6 cells were excited, 8 cells inhibited, while 5 cells showed no change. The remaining 15 cells were located ipsilaterally, 2-3 mm away from the infusion site: 2 of these cells were excited, 11 cells inhibited while 2 cells increased discharge initially and then showed decreased activity.

In the 16 cells (28.6%) excited by carbachol, the increased unit activity preceded the development of the tonic and phasic components of REM sleep, with peak discharge coinciding with the highest levels of atonia, PGO activity and EEG desynchronization. In the 31 cells (55.4%) that were inhibited by carbachol, the inhibition preceded the emergence of REM sleep and it persisted even during REM sleep; under control condition these cells displayed the increased discharge pattern during REM sleep which is typical of reticular cells. Thus, cells inhibited by carbachol may not be critically involved in REM sleep generation.

The results from the single-unit study support data from acute iontophoretic studies (Bradley et al, 1966; Greene and Carpenter, 1981; Guyenet and Aghajanian, 1977; Olpe et al, 1983) which also found that in the reticular formation, application of cholinomimetics elicited both excitatory and inhibitory responses. We showed for the first time that both excitatory and inhibitory responses were closely time-linked to the stimulation of REM sleep related phenomena. These results provide additional support for the hypothesis that pontine cholinergic mechanisms play an important role in the generation of REM sleep.

We determined that in the freely behaving cat, microinfusions of carbachol produced excitation and inhibition of pontine neurons. We suggest that normal REM sleep generation and the cholinomimetic induced REM sleep are due to a muscarinic receptor mediated neuronal priming effect which, as a result of a slow EPSP (Krnjevic, 1974), lowers the threshold of excitability of neurons, and promotes a neuronal state highly receptive to additional excitatory input. When such a threshold of excitation is exceeded, further depolarization will activate specific neuronal sub-groups responsible for the various tonic and phasic components of REM sleep.

Since we postulate that muscarinic receptor activation is responsible for REM sleep, it should be possible to up-regulate muscarinic receptors and produce a concomitant REM sleep augmentation.

Accordingly, in an on-going study we are seeking to determine if REM sleep augmentation is coupled to muscarinic receptor up-regulation during withdrawal from a 7-day chronic scopolamine treatment. Preliminary findings (Sutin et al, 1985) indicate a significant (53%) REM sleep augmentation during withdrawal from scopolamine. Muscarinic receptor density is also significantly increased in the caudate (+32%) and hippocampus (+24.6%) during withdrawal. There is no significant change in cortex (+ 7.3%), brainstem (+ 1.0%) or cerebellum (+ 19.8%). One possible interpretation of these findings is that while brainstem receptor numbers remain constant, the REM sleep augmentation might be due to altered cellular second messenger system.

CLINICAL IMPLICATIONS

The ideas reviewed above have important implications for clinical disorders characterized by short REM latency (time from the onset of sleep to the onset of the first REM period). The two most prominent of these disorders are major affective disorder and narcolepsy. Does an increased ratio of cholinergic to aminergic central activity account for the short REM latency and for some of the symptoms of depression and narcolepsy?

With regard to depression, complaints of poor sleep have been known in depression since classical times. With the advent of clinical polygraphic sleep studies in the last twenty-five years, however, disorders of sleep maintenance and insomnia have come to be recognized as less important in depression than disorders of REM sleep and Delta sleep (Gillin, 1982; Kupfer, 1976, 1978; McCarley, 1982). Many laboratories throughout the world have now demonstrated that short REM latency is characteristic of most patients with depression, particularly those with endogenous, melancholic, primary, or other forms of major affective disorder of a moderate to severe degree (Ansseau et al, 1984a; Coble et al, 1981; Duncan et al, 1979; Gillin et al, 1979a; Hartmann, 1968; Quitkin et al, 1985; Reynolds et al, 1985; Rush et al, 1982; Schultz et al, 1979;). In addition, both the length of the first REM period and number of eye movements per minute of REM sleep (REM density) are high. Total sleep does tend to be shortened in many patients but about 10% show hypersomnia, often in association with hyperphagia. In addition, loss of the deeper stages of sleep, stages 3 & 4 (Delta sleep), are also common (Borbely et al, 1984; Kupfer et al, 1984a, b).

It is not entirely clear how specific these sleep abnormalities are to depression. Short REM latency has been reported, for example, in certain other psychiatric illnesses, including some patients with schizophrenia, obsessive compulsive disorder and anorexia nervosa (see Gillin, 1982). Moreover, loss of stage 3 & 4 sleep does not seem to be specific to depression. This has been reported in many disorders including insomnia, schizophrenia, and various medical disorders including hypothyroidism and Alzheimer's disease. It is interesting, however, that both REM latency and Delta sleep tend to decrease with age, both in normals and patients with depression (Gillin et al, 1981).

Short REM latency appears to be associated with hypercortisolemia in depression, as manifested either by elevated concentrations of plasma cortisol (Asnis et al, 1983) or with escape on the dexamethasone suppression test (DST) (Ansseau et al, 1984b; Feinberg et al, 1984; Mendlewicz et al, 1984; Rush et al, 1982). Physostigmine appears to elevate plasma ACTH levels to a greater extent in depressed patients than controls (Risch et al, 1980). Moreover, it reverses dexamethasone induced cortisol suppression in normals (Carroll et al, 1980).

Various hypotheses have been proposed to explain short REM latency and other disturbances of sleep in depression (Gillin and Borbely, 1985). These include chronobiological hypotheses, such as the phase advance hypothesis, which postulates that a brain clock or oscillator controlling the circadian rhythm of REM sleep, temperature, and cortisol, is phase advanced in patients with depression (Papousek, 1975; Wehr et al, 1979). Another hypothesis, which incorporates chronobiological considerations, is the two-process hypothesis proposed by Borbely and Wirz-Justice (1982), which postulates that a process which builds up during wakefulness and which is responsible for the Delta activity during sleep is deficient in patients with depression. This accounts for the deficiency of Stage 4 and for the beneficial effects of sleep deprivation in depression.

Other approaches, not necessarily incompatible with the two hypotheses just mentioned, are based on neurochemical implications of our knowledge of the physiology of REM sleep. The hypothesis that short REM latency is controlled by a balance between cholinergic and aminergic influences is quite compatible with the so-called cholinergic-aminergic imbalance hypothesis of affective disorders, originally postulated by Janowsky and associates (1972). In this hypothesis, depression is postulated to result from an increased ratio of cholinergic to aminergic activity.

It has not been possible to directly test this hypothesis. Certain pieces of evidence, however, do seem to be compatible with the notion. First, it is possible to simulate much of the sleep disturbance of depression in normal volunteers by a procedure which apparently upregulates muscarinic receptors (Gillin et al, 1979b). In this study, scopolamine was administered for three consecutive mornings. Since the duration of action of scopolamine is approximately six hours, it was postulated that muscarinic supersensitivity would develop at bedtime during the three-day period of scopolamine administration. As predicted, therefore, REM latency shortened during this treatment period. In addition, other characteristics of sleep in depression were noted, including prolonged sleep latency, reduced total sleep time and sleep efficiency, and increased REM density. In addition, following two days of treatment with scopolamine in the morning, subjects were more sensitive to an IV administration of arecoline, a direct muscarinic agonist, as measured by the time required to induce REM sleep following an injection of arecoline during the second nonREM period (Sitaram et al, 1979). This particuar test with arecoline has come to be known as the cholinergic REM induction test (CRIT) (Gillin et al, 1983).

When the CRIT was applied in patients with affective disorders, it was initially found that bipolar patients [both in a state of clinical remission and while ill], showed a significantly faster REM induction than normal controls (Sitaram et al 1980, 82a,b). This suggests that a state of supersensitivity exists in patients with bipolar illness which is a trait marker. Further studies in identical twins suggested that the response to CRIT might be under partial genetic control (Nurenberger et al, 1983). Since this original study, Sitaram and colleagues have confirmed the general results that patients with an endogenous type depression show a faster cholinergic REM induction on the CRIT (Dube et al, 1985; Jones et al, 1985; Sitaram et al, 1984).

Using another sleep method for assessing cholinergic supersensitivity in depression, Berger et al (1983) found that depressed patients were more likely to awaken to an infusion of physostigmine, administered shortly after sleep onset, than normal controls. Since Sitaram et al (1977) had previously shown time and dose dependent arousal to intravenously administered physostigmine in sleep, this result is consistent with increased responsiveness to physostigmine in depressed patients.

In our own hands, however, recent preliminary data with the CRIT has failed to distinguish endogenous patients from normal controls. Although arecoline (0.5 and 1.0 mg) does appear to produce a dose dependent induction of REM sleep, there is no clear evidence yet in our studies that patients respond differently than normal controls. Furthermore, our preliminary data suggests that the reliability between repeated administrations (0.5mg) is hardly strong enough to be useful in clinical investigations even though it is statistically significant ($r=0.54$, $p<.05$). Further studies are ongoing to further test the reliability.

Studies employing intravenous infusions during sleep are inherently difficult to perform and to interpret. More recently, Berger et al (1985) have studied the effect of an orally administered, long-acting cholinergic agonist (RS-86) on sleep in depressed and normal subjects. The drug shortened REM latency significantly more in patients with endogenous depression than normal controls. This technique permits, therefore, a new method of assessing cholinergic supersensitivity in man.

We have also attempted to test the hypothesis of muscarinic supersensitivity in affective disorders by measurement of muscarinic receptors in skin fibroblasts and brain tissue. First we tried to replicate the work of Nadi et al, (1984) who had claimed that patients with affective disorders had increased number of muscarinic receptors on skin fibroblasts compared with normal controls and with relatives without affective disorders (Kelsoe et al, 1985). We, however, were unable to detect significant numbers of muscarinic receptors on adult skin fibroblasts. Moreover, in the few subjects who did have detectable levels, there is no difference between controls and patients with affective disorders. Secondly, we attempted to measure muscarinic receptors in the brains of patients who had committed suicide (Kaufman et al, 1984). No significant difference in receptor density or affinity was found between patients who had committed suicide and controls.

These two latter results do not disprove the cholinergic-aminergic hypothesis of affective disorders, but they indicate there is a need to develop better techniques for assessing central cholinergic function in humans.

The other disorder characterized by short REM latency is narcolepsy, a chronic disease in humans characterized by excessive daytime sleepiness and attacks of cataplexy (brief episodes of weakness of the major antigravity muscles often preciptated by emotional arousal) (Guilleminault, 1976; Hishikawa and Kaneku, 1965; Rechtschaffen et al., 1963). A characteristic finding of these patients is the rapid onset of REM sleep both during naps and at night. The clinical symptoms of narcolepsy are thought to represent dissociated features of normal REM sleep. For example, cataplexy represents the normal muscle atonia normally seen in REM sleep. Narcolepsy is transmitted on a genetic basis, although the exact mode of transmission is not fully understood at this time. Recent evidence suggests that in humans virtually all patients with narcolepsy have the HLA antigen DR2 (Langdon et al, 1984). Narcolepsy has also been found in certain animals and under the leadership of Dr. William Dement at Stanford University, a colony of narcoleptic dogs have now been bred. Recent evidence suggests that there are increased numbers of muscarinic receptors in the brainstem of these animals (Baker and Dement, 1984). Moreover, there is evidence suggesting an increased turnover of dopamine in these animals. These findings

382

suggest that narcolepsy may be associated with an increased ratio of cholinergic to aminergic (presumably dopaminergic) central activity.

CONCLUSION

A role for cholinergic neurons in control of REM sleep now seems to be firmly established. On the basic science level, the exact details of this role will need to be worked out. This will need to be done in the greater context of mechanisms involved in the general control of sleep and of its relationships to underlying circadian influences. In terms of clinical applications, the knowledge that cholinergic mechanisms are clearly involved in REM sleep may provide clues to the better understanding of pathophysiological mechanisms involved in certain disorders.

REFERENCES

Anschel, M., and Lindsley, D.B. Differentiation of two reticulo-hypothalamic systems regulating hippocampal activity. Electroenceph Clin Neurophysiol 32:209-226, 1972.

Amatruda, T.T., Black, D.A., McKenna, T.M., McCarley, R.W. and Hobson, J.A. Sleep cycle control and cholinergic mechanisms: Differential effects of carbachol at pontine brainstem sites. Brain Res 98:501-515, 1975.

Ansseau, M., Kupfer, D.J., Reynolds, C.F., McEachran, A.B. REM latency distribution in major depression, clinical characteristics associated with sleep onset REM periods. Biol Psychiat 19:1651-66, 1984a.

Ansseau M., Scheyvaerts, M., Donmont, A., Poirrier, R., Legros, J.J., Franck, G. Concurrent use of REM latency and dexamethasone suppression as markers of endogenous depression: a pilot study. Psychiat Res 12:261-72, 1984.

Asnis, G.M., Halbreich, U., Sachar, E., Nathan R.S., Ostrow, L.C., Navacenko, H., Davis, M., Endicott, J., and Puig-Antich, J. Plasma cortisol secretion and REM period latency in adult endogenous depression. Am J Psychiat 140:(6):750-753, 1983.

Armstrong, D.M., Saper, C.B., Levey, A.I., Wainer, B.I. and Terry, R.D. Distribution of cholinergic neurons in the rat brain: Demonstrated by the immunocytochemical localization of choline acetyltransferase. J Comp Neurol 216:53-68, 1983.

Baghdoyan, H.A. Rodrigo-Angula, M.L., McCarley, R.W. and Hobson, J.A. Site-specific enhancement and suppression of desynchronized sleep signs following cholinergic stimulation of three brainstem sites. Brain Res 306:39-52, 1984a.

Baghdoyan, H.A., Monaco, A.P., Rodrigo-Angula, M.L., Assens, F., McCarley, R.W., and Hobson, J.A. Microinjection of neostigmine into the pontine reticular formation of cats enhances desynchronized sleep signs. J Pharmacol Exp Therap 312:173-180, 1984b.

Baker, T.L. and Dement, W.C. Canine narcolepsy-cataplexy syndrome: Evidence for an inherited monoaminergic-cholinergic imbalance. In: Brain Mechanisms of Sleep (eds) D. McGinty, A. Morrison, R.R. Drucker-Colin and P.L. Parmeggiani. New York: Raven Press, In Press, 1984.

Baxter, B.L. Induction of both emotional behavior and a novel form of REM sleep by chemical stimulation applied to cat mesencephalon. Exp Neurol 23:220-30, 1969.

Berger, M., Hochli, D., Zulley, J., Lauer, C., and von Zerssen, D. Cholinomimetic drug RS-86, REM sleep and depression. The Lancet June(1985)1385-1386.

Berger, M., Lund, R., Bronisch, T., von Zerrsen, D. REM latency in

neurotic and endogenous depression and the cholinergic REM induction
test. <u>Psychiat Res</u> 10:113-123, 1983.

Bizzi, E., Pompeiano, O., and Somogyi, I. Spontaneous activity of single
vestibular neurons of unrestrained cats during sleep and
wakefulness. <u>Arch Ital Biol</u> 102:308-320, 1964.

Borbely, A.A., Tobler, I., Loepte, M., Kupfer, D.J., Ulrich, R.F.,
Grochocinski, V., Doman, J., Matthews, G. All night spectral
analysis of the sleep EEG in untreated depressives and normal
controls. <u>Psychiat Res</u> 12:27-33, 1984b.

Borbely, A.A. and Wirz-Justice, A. A two process model of sleep
regulation: II implications for depression. <u>Human Neurobiology</u>
1:205-210, 1982.

Bradley, P.B., Dhavan, B.N. and Wolstencroft, J.H. Pharmacological
properties of cholinergic neurons in the medulla and pons of the
cat. <u>J of Physiology</u> 183:658-674, 1966.

Carroll, B., Greden, J.F., Haskett, R. Neurotransmitter studies of
neuroendocrine pathology in depression. <u>Acta Psychiatr Scand</u>
(Suppl) 280:183-199, 1980.

Celesia, G.G., and Jasper, H.H. Acetylcholine released from cerebral
cortex in relation to state of activation. <u>Neurology (Minneap)</u>
16:1053-1064, 1966.

Chu, N.S. and Bloom, F.E. Norepinephrine containing neurons: changes in
spontaneous discharge patterns during sleeping and waking. <u>Science</u>
179:908-910, 1973.

Chu, N.S. and Bloom, F.E. Activity patterns of catecholamine pontine
neurons in the dorso-lateral tegmentum of unrestrained cat. <u>J
Neurobiol</u> 5:527-544, 1974.

Coble, P., Kupfer, D.J. and Shaw, D.H. Distribution of REM latency in
depression. <u>Biol Psychiatr</u> 16:453-466, 1981.

Cohen, B., and Henn, V. Unit activity in the pontine reticular formation
associated with eye movements. <u>Brain Res</u> 46:403-410, 1972.

Delashaw, J.B., Foutz, A.S., Guilleminault, C. and Dement, W.C.,
Cholinergic mechanisms and cataplexy in dogs. <u>Exp Neurol</u>
66:745-757, 1979.

Dube, S., Kumar, N., Etledgui, E., Pohl, R., Jones, D., Sitaram, N.
Cholinergic REM induction response: separation of anxiety and
depression. <u>Biol Psychiat</u> 20:208-418, 1985.

Duncan, W.C., Pettigrew, K.A., Gillin, J.C. REM architecture changes in
bipolar and unipolar patients. <u>Am J Psychiatry</u> 136:1424-7, 1979.

Feinberg, M. and Carroll, B.J. Biological 'markers' for endogenous
depression. <u>Arch Gen Psychiat</u> 41:1080-5, 1984.

Friedman, A.K. Circumstances influencing Otto Loewi's discovery of
chemical transmission in the nervous system. <u>Pflugers Arch</u>
325:85-86, 1971.

Fung, S., Boxer, P.A., Morales, F. and Chase, M. Hyperpolarizing membrane
responses induced in lumbar motoneurons by stimulation of the
nucleus reticularis pontis oralis during active sleep. <u>Brain Res</u>
248:267-273, 1982.

Gadea-Ciria, M., Stadler, H., Lloyd, K.G. and Bartholini, G.
Acetylcholine release within the cat striatum during the
sleep-wakefulness cycle. <u>Nature</u> 243:518-519, 1973.

George, R., Haslett, W.L. and Jenden, D.J. A cholinergic mechanism in
the brainstem reticular formation: Induction of paradoxical sleep.
<u>Int J Neuropharmacol</u> 3:541-552, 1964.

Gillin, J.C. and Borbely, A. Sleep: a neurobiological window on
affective disorders. <u>Trends in Neurosciences</u> in Press, 1985.

Gillin, J.C., Sitaram, N., Nurnberger, J.I., Gershon, E.S., Cohen, R.,
Murphy, D., Kaye, W., Ebert, M. The cholinergic REM induction test
(CRIT). <u>Psychopharm Bull</u> 19:668-670, 1983.

Gillin, J.C. Sleep studies in affective illness: Diagnostic, therapeutic
and pathophysiological implications. <u>Psychiat Annals</u> 13:367-384,
1982.

Gillin, J.C., Duncan, W.C., Murphy, D.L. Age related changes in sleep in depressed and normal subjects. Psychiat Res 4:73–81, 1981.

Gillin, J.C., Duncan, W.C., Pettigrew, K., Frankel, B.L. and Synder, F. Successful separation of depressed, normal, and insomniac subjects by EEG sleep data. Arch Gen Psychiatr 36:85–90, 1979a.

Gillin, J.C., Sitaram, N. and Duncan, W. Muscarinic supersensitivity: A possible model for the sleep disturbance of primary depression. Psychiat Res 1:17–22, 1979b.

Glenn, L.L., Foutz, A.S. and Dement, W.C. Membrane potential of spinal motoneurons during natural sleep in cats. Sleep 1:199–204, 1978.

Gnadt, J.W. and Pegram, G.V. Cholinergic brainstem mechanisms of REM sleep in the rat. (Personal Communication).

Greene, R.W. and Carpenter, D.O. Biphasic responses to acetylcholine in mammalian reticulospinalneurons. Cellular and Molecular Neurobiology 1:401–405, 1981.

Guilleminault, C. Cataplexy. In: Narcolepsy (eds) C. Guilleminault, W.C. Dement, and P. Passouant. Spectrum, New york, 125–143, 1976.

Guyenet, P.G. and Aghajanian, G.K. Excitation of neurons in the nucleus locus coeruleus by substance P and related peptides. Brain Res 136:178–184, 1977.

Haranath, P.S. and Venkatakrishna-Bhatt, H. Release of acetylcholine from perfused cerebral ventricles in unanesthetized dogs during waking and sleep. Jpn J Physiol 23:241–250, 1973.

Hartmann, E. Longitudinal studies of sleep and dreams in manic-depressive patients. Arch Gen Psychiat 19:312–329, 1968.

Hayes, R.L., Pechura, C.M., Katayama, y., Povlishock, J.T., Giebel, M.L. and Becker, D.P. Activation of pontine cholinergic sites implicated in unconsciousness following cerebral concussion in the cat. Science 223:301–303, 1984.

Henley, K. and Morrison, A.D. A re-evaluation of the effects of lesions of the pontine tegmentum and locus coeruleus on phenomena of paradoxical sleep in the cat. Acta Neurobiol Exp 34:215–232, 1974.

Henn, V. and Cohen, B. Activity in eye muscle motoneurons and brainstem units during eye movements. In: Basic Mechanisms of Ocular Motility and their Clinical Implications (eds) C. Lennestrand and P. Back-y-Rita. Pergamon Press, Oxford, 303–345, 1975.

Hishikawa, Y. and Kaneku, Z. Electroencephalographic study on narcolepsy. Electroencephalogr Clin Neurophysiol 18:249–259, 1965.

Hobson, J.A., Goldberg, M., Vivaldi, E. and Riew, D. Enhancement of desynchronized sleep signs after pontine microinjections of the muscarinic agonist bethanechol. Brain Res 275:127–136, 1983.

Hobson, J.A., McCarley, R.W. and Wyzinski, P.W. Sleep cycle oscillation: Reciprocal discharge by two brainstem neuronal groups. Science 189:55–58, 1975.

Hoshino, K. and Pompeiano, O. Selective discharge of pontine neurons during the postural atonia produced by an anti-cholinesterase in the decerebrate cat. Arch Ital Biol 114:244–277, 1976a.

Hoshino, K., Pompeiano, O., Magherini, P.C. and Mergner, T. Oscillatory activity of pontine neurons related to the regular occurrence of REM bursts in the decerebrate cat. Brain Res 116:125–130, 1976b.

Jacobs, B.L., Asher, R. and Dement, W.C. Electrophysiological and behavioral effects of electrical stimulation of the raphe nuclei in cats. Physiol Behav 11:489–496, 1973.

Jacobs, B.L., Henriksen, S.J. and Dement, W.C. Neurochemical bases of the PGO wave. Brain Res 48:406–411, 1972.

Janowsky, D.C., El-Yousef, M.K. and Dans, J.M. A cholinergic-adrenergic hypothesis of mania and depression. Lancet 2:632–5, 1972.

Jasper, H.H. and Tessier, J. Acetylcholine liberation from cerebral cortex during paradoxical (REM) sleep. Science 172:601–602, 1971.

Jones, B.E., Harper, S.T., and Halaris, A. Effects of locus coeruleus lesions upon cerebral monoamine content, sleep-wakefulness states and the response to amphetamine in the cat. <u>Brain Res</u> 124:473-496, 1977.

Jones, D., Kelwala, S., Bell, J., Dube, S., Jackson, E. and Sitaram, N. Cholinergic REM sleep induction response correlation with endogenous depressive subtype. <u>Psychiat Res</u> 14:99-110, 1985.

Jouvet, M. The role of monoamines and acetylcholine-containing neurons in the regulation of the sleep-waking cycle. <u>Ergebn Physiol</u> 64:166-308, 1972.

Kanamori, N., Sakai, K. and Jouvet, M. Neuronal activity specific to paradoxical sleep in the ventromedial medullary reticular formation of restrained cats. <u>Brain Res</u> 189:251-255, 1980.

Karczmar, A.G., Longo, V.G. and Scotti de Carolis, A. A pharmacological model of paradoxical sleep: The role of cholinergic and monoamine systems. <u>Physiol Behav</u> 5:175-182, 1970.

Katayama, Y., DeWitt, D.S., Becker, D.P. and Hayes, R.L. Behavioral evidence for a cholinoceptive pontine inhibitory area: Descending control of spinal motor output and sensory input. <u>Brain Res</u> 296:241-262, 1984.

Kaufman, C.A., Gillin, J.C., Hill, B., O'Laughlin, T., Phillips, I., Kleinman, J.E. and Wyatt, R.J. Muscarinic binding in suicides. <u>Psychiat Res</u> 12:47-55, 1984.

Keller, E.L. Participation of medial pontine reticular formation in eye movement generation of monkeys. <u>J Neurophysiol</u> 37:316-332, 1974.

Kelsoe, J., Gillin, J.C., Janowsky, D.J. Heller-Brown, J., Risch, S.C. and Lumkin, B. Letter to the Editor, <u>N Eng J Med</u> 312:861-2, 1985.

Kimura, H. and Maeda, T. Aminergic and cholinergic systems in the dorsolateral pontine tegmentum. <u>Brain Res Bull</u> 9:403-499, 1982.

Kimura, H., McGeer, P.L., Peng, J.H. and McGeer, E.G. The central cholinergic system studied by choline acetyltransferase immuno-histochemistry in the cat. <u>J Comp Neurol</u> 200:151-201, 1981.

Klemm, W.R. Effects of electrical stimulation of brainstem reticular formation on hippocampal theta rhythm and muscle activity in unanesthetized cervical and midbrain-transected rats. <u>Brain Res</u> 41:331-344, 1972.

Kolb, B., and Whishaw, I.Q. Effects of brain lesions and atropine on hippocampal and neocortical electroencephalogram in the rat. <u>Exp Neurol</u> 56:1-22, 1977.

Krnjevic, K. Chemical nature of synaptic transmission in vertebrates. <u>Physiological Reviews</u> 54:418-540, 1974.

Kupfer, D.J., Ulrich, R.F., Coble, P.A., Jarnatt, D.B., Grochocinski, V., Doman, J., Matthews, G. and Borbely, A.A. Application of automated REM and slow wave analysis: I normal and depressive subjects. <u>Psychiat Res</u> 13:335-43, 1984b.

Kupfer, D.J. EEG sleep correlates of depression in man. In: <u>Animal Models in Psychiatry and Neurology</u> (eds) I. Hanin and E. Usdin. Pergamon Press, New York, 181-188, 1978.

Kupfer, D.J. REM latency: A psychobiological marker for primary depressive disease. <u>Biol Psychiat</u> 11:159-174, 1976.

Langdon, N., Walsh, K.F., van Dam, M., Vaughan, R. and Parkes, D. Genetic markers in narcolepsy. <u>Lancet</u> ii:1178-1180, 1984.

Lewis, P.R. and Shute, C.C.D. Cholinergic pathways in the CNS. In: <u>Handbook of Psychopharmacology</u> Vol 9, (eds) L.L. Iversen, S.D. Iversen, and S.H. Snyder, Plenum Press, New York, 315-355, 1978.

Luschei, E.S., and Fuchs, A.F. Activity of brain stem neurons during eye movements of alert monkeys. <u>J Neurophysiol</u> 35:445-461, 1972.

Lynch, C., Smith, R.L., and Robertson, R. Direct projections from brainstem to telencephalon. <u>Exp Brain Res</u> 17:221-228, 1973.

Macadar, A.W., Chalupa, L.M. and Lindsley, D.B. Differentiation of brainstem loci which affect hippocampal and neocortical electrical activity. <u>Exp Neurol</u> 43:499-514, 1974.

Magherini, P.C., Pompeiano, O. and Thoden, U. The neurochemical basis of

REM sleep: A cholinergic mechanism responsible for rhythmic activation of the vestibulo-occulomotor system. Brain Res 35:565-569, 1971.

Magoun, H.W. and Rhines, R. An inhibitory mechanism in the bulbar reticular formation. J Neurophysiol 9:165-171, 1946.

Mendlewicz, J., Kerkhots, M., Hoffman, G., Linkowski, P. Dexamethasone suppression test and REM sleep in patients with major depressive disorder. Brit J Psychiat 145:383-8, 1984.

Mergner, T. and Pompeiano, O: Neurons in the vestibular nuclei related to saccadic eye movements in the decerebrate cat. In: Control of Gaze by Brainstem Neurons (eds) R. Baker and A. Bertholz. Elsevier/North-Holland, Amsterdam, pp. 243-252, 1977

McCarley. R.W. REM sleep and depression: common neurobiological control mechanisms. Am J Psychiatry 139:569-570, 1982.

McCarley, R.W., Nelson, J.P., and Hobson, J.A. Ponto-geniculo-occipital (PGO) burst neurons: correlative evidence for neuronal generators of PGO waves. Science 201:269-272, 1978.

McCarley, R.W. and Hobson, J.A. Neuronal excitability modulation over the sleep cycle: A structural and mathematical model. Science 189:58-60, 1975.

McGinty, D.J. and Harper, R.M. Dorsal raphe neurons: Depression of firing during sleep in cats. Brain Res 101:569-575, 1976.

Mitler, M. and Dement, W.C. Cataplectic-like behavior in cats after microinjection of carbachol in pontine reticular formation. Brain Res 68:335-343, 1974.

Monmaur, P. and Delacour, J. Effects de la lesion bilaterale du tegmentum pontique dorsolateral sur l'activite theta hippocampigue au cours du sommeil paradoxal ches le rat. C R Acad Sci 286:761-764, 1978.

Morales, F.R. and Chase, M.K. Intracellular recording of lumbar motoneuron membrane potential during sleep and wakefulness. Exp Neurol 62:821-827, 1978.

Morrison, A.R. and Pompeiano, O. Vestibular influences during sleep. IV. Functional relations between vestibular nuclei and lateral geniculate nucleus during desynchronized sleep Arch Ital Biol 104:425-458,1966.

Moruzzi, G., and Magoun, H. W. Brain stem reticular formation and activation of the EEG. Electroencephalog Clin Neurophysiol 1:455-473, 1949.

Nadi, S. N., Nurnberger, J. N., and Gershon, E. S. Muscarinic cholinergic receptors on skin fibroblasts in familial affective disorder. N Engl J Med 311:225-230, 1984.

Nakamura, R., Kennedy, C., Gillin, J.D., Suda, S., Ito, M., Storch, F.I., Mendelson, W., Sokolof, L., Mishkin, M. Hypnogenic center theory of sleep: no support from metabolic mapping in monkeys. Brain Res 268:372-6, 1983.

Nurnburger, J., Jr., Sitaram, N., Gerson, E.S., Gillin, J.C. A twin study of cholinergic REM induction. Biol Psychiat 18:1161-5, 1983.

Olpe, M.R., Jones, R.S. and Steinmann, M.W. The locus coeruleus: actions of psychoactive drugs. Experientia 39:242-249, 1983.

Papousek, M. Chronobiologiesche aspekete der Zyclothymie. Fortschr Neurol Psychiatr 43:381-440, 1975.

Petsche, H., Gogolak, G., and Van Zweiten, P.A. Rhythmicity of septal cell discharges at various levels of reticular excitation. Electroencephalog Clin Neurophysiol 19:25-33, 1965.

Pivik, R.T., McCarley, R.W., and Hobson, J.A. Eye movement associated discharge in brainstem neurons during desynchronized sleep. Brain Res 121:59-76, 1977.

Pompeiano, O. Mechanisms responsible for spinal inhibition during desynchronized sleep: experimental study. In Narcolepsy edited by C. Guilleminault, W.C. Dement and P. Passouant. Spectrum Publication, New York, 411-449, 1976.

Pompeiano, O. Cholinergic activation of reticular and vestibular mechanisms controlling posture and eye movements. In The Reticular Formation Revisited edited by J. Allan Hobson and Mary Brazier. Raven Press, New York, 1980.

Quitkin, F.M., Rabbin, J.G., Stewart, J.W., McGrath, P.J., Harrison, W., Goetz, R., Puig-Antich, J. Sleep of atypical depressives. J Affect Disorder 8:61-67, 1985.

Ramm, P. The locus coeruleus, catecholamines, and REM sleep: A critical review. Behav Neurol Biol 25:415-448, 1979.

Rechtschaffen, A., Wolpert, W., Dement, W.C., Mitchell, S. and Fisher, C. Nocturnal sleep of narcoleptics. Electroencephalogr Clin Neurophysiol 15:599-609, 1963.

Reynolds, C.F., Soloff, P.H., Kupfer, D.J., Taska, L.S., Restifo, K., Coble, P.A., McNamara, M.E. Depression in borderline patients: a prospective EEG sleep study. Psychiat Res 14:1-15, 1985.

Risch, S.C., Cohen, R.M., Janowsky, D.S., Kalin, N.H., and Murphy, D.L. Plasma beta-endorphin and cortisol elevations accompany the mood and behavioral effects of physostigmine in man. Science, 209:1545-1546, 1980.

Robertson, P.T., Lynch, G.S., and Thompson, R.F. Diencephalic distribution of ascending reticular systems. Brain Res 55, 309-322, 1973.

Robinson, T.E., Vanderwolf, C.H., and Pappas, B.A. Are the dorsal noradrenergic bundle projections from the locus coeruleus important for neocortical or hippocampal activation? Brain Res 138:75-98, 1977.

Robinson, T.T., and Vanderwolf, C.H. Electrical stimulation of the brainstem in freely moving rats. II. Effects on hippocampal and neocortical electrical activity and relations to behavior. Exp Neurol 61:485-515, 1978.

Rose, A.M., Hattori, T., and Fibiger, H.C. Analysis of the septo-hippocampal pathway by light and electron microscopic autoradiography. Brain Res 108:170-174, 1976.

Rush, J., Giles, G.E., Roffwarg, H.P., Parker, C.R. Sleep EEG and dexamethasone suppression test findings in outpatients with unipolar major depressive disorder. Biol Psychiat 17:327=341, 1982.

Sakai, K. Anatomical and physiological basis of paradoxical sleep. In: Brain Mechanisms of Sleep edited by D. McGinty, A. Morrison, R.R. Drucker-Colin and P.L. Parmeggiani. Spectrum, New York, In press, 1984.

Sakai, K. Some anatomical and physiological properties of ponto-mesencephalie-tegmental neurons with special reference to the PGO waves and postural atonia during paradoxical sleep in the cat. In: The Reticular Formation Revisited edited by J.A. Hobson and Mary B. Brazier, Raven Press, New York, 427-447, 1980.

Sakai, K., Sastre, J.P., Salvert, D., Torret, M., Tohyama, M. and Jouvet, M. Tegmento - reticular projections with special reference to the muscular atonia during paradoxical sleep: An HRP study. Brain Res 176:233-254, 1979.

Sakai, K., Touret, M., Salvert, D. and Jouvet, M. Afferents to the cat locus coeruleus as visualized by the horseradish peroxidase technique. In: Interactions between putative neurotransmitters in the brain, edited by S. Garattini, J.P. Pujol and R. Samanin, Raven Press, New York, 319-342, 1978.

Schulz, H., Lund, R., Cording, C., Dirlich, G. Bimodal distribution of REM latencies in depression. Biol Psychiat 14:595-600, 1979.

Sheu, Y.S., Nelson, J.P., and Bloom F.E. Discharge patterns of cat raphe neurons during sleep and waking. Brain Res 73:263-276, 1974.

Shiromani, P. Long-term cholinergic stimulation of pontine nuclei. Effects on paradoxical sleep and memory. Ph.D. Thesis: The City University of New York, 1983.

Shiromani, P. and McGinty, D.J. Pontine sites for cholinergic PGO waves and atonia: Localization and blockade with scopolamine. Soc Neurosci Abstr 9(2):1203, 1983.

Shiromani, P., and McGinty, D. J. Pontine cholinergic mechanisms in the regulation of REM sleep. In: Proceedings of XXIII International Congress of Psychology (ed) J. McGaugh. Elsevier Press, Holland, in press, 1985 a.

Shiromani, P. and McGinty, D. J. Pontine neuronal responses to local cholinergic infusion: Relation to REM sleep. Submitted for publication, 1985 b.

Shiromani, P. J., Siegel, J., Tomaszewski, K., and McGinty, D. J. Alterations in blood pressure and REM sleep after pontine carbachol microinfusion. Exp Neurol 91: In press, 1986

Shiromani, P., and Fishbein, W. Long-term pontine cholinergic microinfusions via mini-pump induces sustained alterations in rapid eye movement sleep. Submitted for publication.

Siegel, J.M., Nienhuis, R. and Tomaszewski, K.S. Rostral brainstem contributes to medullary inhibition of muscletone. Brain Res 268:344-348, 1983.

Siegel, J.M., Nienhuis, R. and Tomaszewski, K.S. REM sleep signs rostral to chronic transections at the pontomedullary junction. Neurosci Lett 45:241-246, 1984.

Silberman, E., Vivaldi, E., Garfield, J., McCarley, R.W. and Hobson, J.A. Carbachol triggering of desynchronized sleep phenomena: Enhancement via small volume infusions. Brain Res 191:215-224, 1980.

Sitaram, N., Dube, S., Jones D., Pohl, R., Gershon, S. Acetylcholine and alpha-1 adrenergic sensitivity in the separation of depression and anxiety. Psychopath Suppl 3, 17:24-39, 1984.

Sitaram, N., Kaye, W.H., Nurnberger, J.I., Ebert, M., Gershon, E.S. and Gillin, J.C. Cholinergic REM sleep induction test: A trait marker of affective illness? In: Biological Markers in Psychiatry and Neurology E. Usdin and I. Hanin (eds), Pergamon Press, New York, 397-404, 1982a.

Sitaram, N., Nurnberger, J.I., Gershon, E.S. and Gillin, J.C. Cholinergic regulation of mood and REM sleep: A potential model and marker for vulnerability to affective disorder. Am J Psychiatry 139:571-576, 1982 b.

Sitaram, N. and Gillin, J.C. Development and use of pharmacological probes of the CNS in man: Evidence for cholinergic abnormality in primary affective illness. Biol Psychiatry 15:925-955, 1980.

Sitaram, N., Moore, A.M. and Gillin, J.C. Scopolamine-induced muscarinic supersensitivity in normal man: changes in sleep. Psychiatry Res 1:9-16, 1979.

Sitaram, N., Moore, A.M. and Gillin, J.C. Experimental acceleration and slowing of REM ultradian rhythm by cholinergic agonist and antagonist. Nature 274:490-492, 1978 a.

Sitaram, N., Moore, A.M. and Gillin, J.C. Induction and resetting of REM sleep rhythm in normal man by arecoline: Blockade by scopolamine. Sleep 1:83-90, 1978 b.

Sitaram, N., Mendelson, W.B., Wyatt, R.J. and Gillin, J.C. Time dependent induction of REM sleep and arousal by physostigmine infusion during normal human sleep. Brain Res 122:565-567, 1977.

Sitaram, N., Wyatt, R.J., Dawson, S. and Gillin, J.C. REM sleep induction by physostigmine infusion during sleep in normal volunteers. Science 191:1281-1283, 1976.

Sparks, D.L, and Travis, R.P. Firing patterns of reticular formation neurons during horizontal eye movements. Brain Res 33:477-481, 1971.

Spiegel, R. Effects of RS-86, an orally active cholinergic agonist, on sleep in man. Psychiat Res 11:1-13, 1984.

Steriade, M., Ropert, N., Kitsikis, A., and Oakson, G. Ascending activating neuronal netwoks in midbrain reticular core and related rostral systems. In: The Reticular Formation Revisited (eds) J.A. Hobson and M.B. Brazier. Raven Press. New York, pp 125–167, 1980.

Stumpf, G. H., Petsche, M., and Gogolak, G. The significance of the rabbit's septum as a relay station between the midbrain and the hippocampus. II. The differential influence of drugs upon the septal firing pattern and the hippocampus theta activity. Electroencephalog Clin Neurophysiol 14:212–219, 1962.

Sutin, E. L., Shiromani, P., Kelsoe, J., Storch, F., and Gillin, J. C. REM sleep and muscarinic receptor binding in rats are augmented during withdrawal following chronic scopolamine treatment. Sleep Res 14:61, 1985.

Thoden, U., Magherini, P.C., and Pompeiano, O. Cholinergic mechanisms related to REM sleep. II. Effects of an anticholinesterase on the discharge of central vestibular neurons in the decerebratecat. Arch Ital Biol 110:260–283, 1972 a.

Thoden, U., Magherini, P.C., and Pompeiano, O. Cholinergic activation of vestibular neurons leading to rapid eye movements in the mesencephalic cat. Biol Opthalmol 82:99–108, 1972 b.

Vanderwolf, C.H., Kramis, R., and Robinson, T.E. Hippocampal electrical activity during waking behavior and sleep: Analysis using centrally acting drugs. In: CIBA Foundation Symposium: Functions of the Septo-Hippocampal System (eds) K. Elliott and J. Whelan, pp 199–221, 1978.

Van Dongen, P.A., Broekamp, L.E., Coola, A.R. Antonia after carbachol microinjections near the locus coeruleus in cats. Pharmacol Biochem Behav 8:527–532, 1978.

Vertes, R.P. Brainstem control of the events of REM sleep. Prog in Neurobiol 22:241–288, 1984.

Vertes, R.P. Brainstem activation of the hippocampus: A role for the magnocellular reticular formation and the MLF. Electroencephalog Clin Neurophysiol 50:48–58, 1980.

Vertes, R.P. Brainstem gigantocellular neurons: patterns of activity during behavior and sleep in the freely moving rat. J Neurophysiol 42:24–228, 1979.

Wehr, T.A., Wirz-Justice A., Goodwin, F.K., Duncan, W., Gillin, J.C. Phase advance of the circadian sleep-wake cycle as an antidepressant. Science 206:210–3, 1979.

Winson, J. Interspecies differences in the occurrence of theta. Behav Biol 7:479–487, 1972.

CHOLINERGIC SYSTEMS IN THE CENTRAL CONTROL OF BODY TEMPERATURE

R. D. Myers

Departments of Psychiatry and Pharmacology and Center for
Alcohol Studies, University of North Carolina School of
Medicine, Chapel Hill, North Carolina 27514

INTRODUCTION

By the mid-1960's, it had become apparent that specific nerve cells in
the anterior hypothalamus (AH) and pre-optic area (POA) are delegated to the
primary physiological mechanisms underlying the control of body temperature
(Boulant, 1980). On the basis of pharmacological studies, it was postulated
in this era that serotonin (5-HT)-containing neurons within the AH/POA released 5-HT in order to activate the neuronal mechanism for heat production
(Feldberg and Myers, 1964). Conversely, noradrenergic neurons within the
same anatomical region were hypothesized to liberate norepinephrine (NE) at
their synapses to activate the functional system for heat dissipation. However, a missing link in this "monoamine theory" centered on the neurohumoral
nature of the anatomical pathways that necessarily mediate the distinct physiological signals emanating from the AH/POA for either the loss or production of body heat (Myers, 1969).

Following the reports of Lomax and colleagues in the late 1960's that
temperature was affected by either oxotremorine or carbamylcholine (carbachol) injected into the POA of the restrained but unanesthetized rat (Lomax
and Jenden, 1966; Kirkpatrick and Lomax, 1970), the possibility was raised
that a cholinergic system could be involved in thermoregulation. Then in
1968, it was reported that in the unrestrained rat, an intracerebroventricular (ICV) injection of acetylcholine (ACh) induces a transient hyperthermic
response (Myers and Yaksh, 1968). Further, eserine injected similarly was
found to produce the same sort of intense rise in core temperature (Myers and
Yaksh, 1968) as would be predicted by the pharmacological property of this
anti-cholinesterase. Interestingly, the higher dose of eserine was less efficacious than an intermediary dose, which suggested at once that the concentration of a drug, which acts on cholinoceptive cells in the hypothalamus, is
one of the critical factors in the manifestation of a change in body temperature.

Two particularly disquieting aspects of these early findings were: (1)
a potential difference between species in terms of the pharmacological response to a cholinomimetic; and (2) that the investigative strategy to the
thermoregulatory question in itself could determine the outcome of the experiment. For example, in the unanesthetized monkey, a solution containing both
ACh and eserine, perfused through the cerebral ventricles of the unanesthetized monkey, produces a dose-dependent hypothermia (Hall and Myers, 1971).

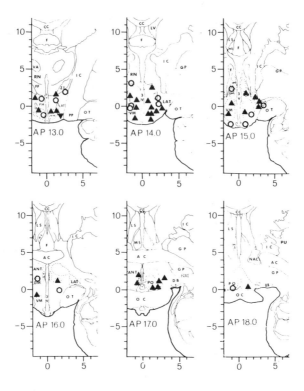

▲ = HYPERTHERMIA
▼ = HYPOTHERMIA
○ = NO RESPONSE

Fig. 1. Anatomical "mapping" at six coronal (AP) levels of sites in
the hypothalamus at which micro-injections of acetylcholine,
acetylcholine-eserine mixture in doses of 2-25 μg produce hyperthermia (▲) or hypothermia (▼). Sites at which these compounds
cause no change in temperature are also indicated (o). (From
Myers and Yaksh, 1969).

Further, an ICV infusion of ACh in the conscious sheep evokes a marked rise
in temperature (Bligh and Maskery, 1969), similar to that seen in the rat
(Myers and Yaksh, 1968), as well as an elevation in both O_2 consumption and
plasma free-fatty acids (Darling et al., 1974). Thus, it was envisaged that
a set of metabolic events could likewise be influenced or perhaps controlled
by central cholinergic synapses.

ANATOMICAL ANALYSIS OF CHOLINERGIC THERMOGENESIS

The first clue to a possible resolution of the inconsistency in the pharmacological action of ACh and other cholinomimetics on body temperature arose
fortuitously in 1969 in a set of anatomical studies on the unanesthetized monkey. When ACh, carbachol or a mixture of ACh and eserine was micro-injected
within sites scattered throughout the hypothalamus, including those "down-

stream" from the thermosensitive zone of the AH/POA, a sharp deflection in
core temperature of the monkey occurred in either direction, hyper- or hypothermia (Myers and Yaksh, 1969). Of special physiological interest was the
intensity of the hyperthermic "spike" and its exceedingly short duration, unlike those produced by any other chemical agent examined neuropharmacologi-
cally in the CNS of a conscious animal (Myers, 1980). Equally notable is the
fact that within the mid-hypothalamic region as well as the caudal hypothalamus (Fig. 1), both 5-HT and NE exerted virtually no effect whatsoever on the
core temperature of the primate.

An anatomical mapping of discrete micro-injection loci (Fig. 1) revealed
that cholinoceptive elements mediate heat production in virtually all areas
throughout the rostral mid- and posterior hypothalamic areas. However, ACh
or carbachol applied to certain sites within the posterior hypothalamus and
its mesencephalic border evoked a transient but significant decline in the
core temperature of the primate (Myers and Yaksh, 1969).

Receptor Characteristics

Anatomical studies undertaken in the unanesthetized monkey are concor-
dant with these initial observations. For example, nicotine micro-injected
into homologous loci in the caudal hypothalamus evokes a sharp hyperthermia
(Hall and Myers, 1982). The rising phase in the primate's temperature which

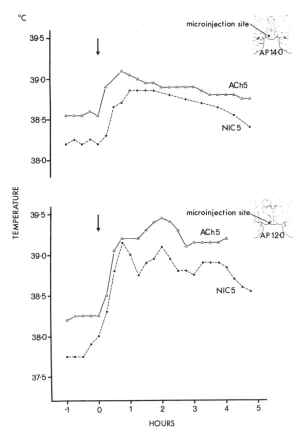

Fig. 2. Body temperature (°C) of monkey after micro-injection of
5 µg of acetylcholine (ACh) or nicotine (NIC) given in a volume
of 1.0 µl. Injections were made at an interval of 48-72 hr;
sites are shown, insets at AP 14.0 (top) and AP 12.0 (bottom)
in two different monkeys (From Hall and Myers, 1972).

occurs immediately after intrahypothalamic nicotine, follows the same time course as that elicited by ACh-eserine or carbachol. These temperature responses are illustrated in Fig. 2, which denotes individual sites identified anatomically within two coronal planes of the monkey's hypothalamus. Again, this finding would support the viewpoint that nicotinic receptors are involved in the specific cholinergic pathways delegated to the maintenance of body heat.

One widely accepted premise in this field is that the muscarinic receptor functionally mediates thermogenesis induced by a drug or an endogenous factor. This idea is based on studies by Hall (see 1973) and others who have shown that atropine applied centrally blocks a physiologically coordinated hyperthermic response irrespective of its origin (Baird and Lang, 1973; Preston, 1974; Tangri et al., 1975). Atropine alone exerts a direct pharmacological action on core temperature of several species when the drug is infused at certain sites in mid- and caudal hypothalamic areas. As presented in Fig. 3, a relatively short-lived decline in the core temperature of the unrestrained rat is produced by the muscarinic receptor antagonist microinjected antero-dorsal to the mammillary bodies (Myers et al., 1976). The similarity

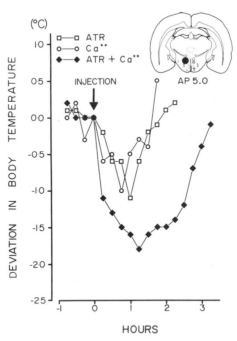

Fig. 3. Hypothermia produced in the same rat by 0.5 μl injections at one week intervals at the site denoted on the histological inset. Atropine alone was 1.0 μg; Ca^{++} alone was 10.4 mM in excess of CSF value; atropine plus Ca^{++} were 0.5 μg and 10.4 mM, respectively (from Myers et al., 1976).

in the characteristics of the fall in temperature evoked by excess Ca^{++} ions applied to the same hypothalamic locus is notable. As based on earlier experiments with cholinergic agonists (Myers, 1974), one could thus deduce that the blockade of muscarinic synapses along the efferent projections subserving heat production would necessarily eventuate in a loss of body heat.

Figure 3 shows also that the simultaneous application of the same concentration of both atropine and excess Ca^{++} ions within the same region of the rat's hypothalamus exacerbates the intensity in the decline of the animal's core temperature in terms of both magnitude and duration. Therefore, it is equally conceivable that cholinergic neurons serve to mediate the output of the physiological "set-point" mechanism, which is hypothesized to be controlled, in part, by cellular Ca^{++} ions within the posterior hypothalamus (review of Myers, 1982).

Overall then, muscarinic as well as nicotinic synapses are believed to comprise a portion of the heat production pathway which originates in the diencephalon and projects caudalward through the neuraxis.

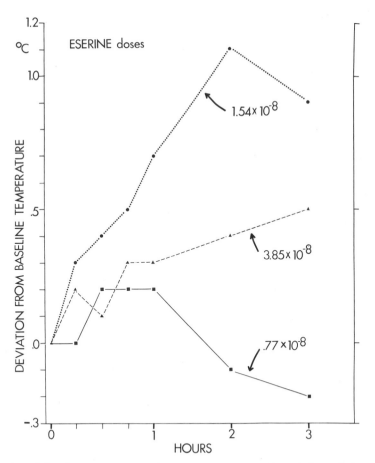

Fig. 4. Colonic temperature in response to eserine injected intraventricularly at 3 doses (moles). Each dose response curve represents the mean deviation from baseline temperature in from 4-7 experiments (from Myers and Yaksh, 1968).

Enzyme Blockade with Anti-Cholinesterases

   As alluded to earlier, further credence to the concept of a cholinergic
heat production system in the brain-stem was provided by an early study using
ICV infusions of an anti-cholinesterase which elevates the endogenous level
of ACh in the brain. As illustrated in Fig. 4, when eserine (physostigmine)
is administered in one of three doses to the unrestrained rat, the highest
dose is less efficacious in producing hyperthermia than the intermediary concentration. Presumably, this could be due to an "overload" of the cholinergic synapses which subsequently serves to block thermogenesis even to the
point of a consequent hypothermic response (Myers, 1974;1980).

   A corollary to the pharmacological issue of dose-efficacy can be seen in
the results of an investigation using a relatively unique anti-cholinesterase,
RX72601. When this compound is administered ICV in the unrestrained cat, the
typical eserine-like hyperthermia ensues (Metcalf et al., 1975). As shown in
Fig. 5, although various doses of this anticholinesterase produce a rise in
temperature of identical slope, differences in magnitude and duration are readily apparent. After the highest dose of 10 μg of RX72601 is infused, the rise
in temperature simply fails to dissipate after the peak is reached (Fig. 5),
but instead persists at an elevated level. In all likelihood, the distinctive
chemical nature of the drug as well as an optimal dose could account for this
result.

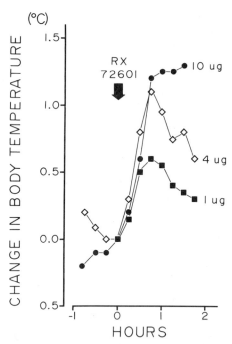

Fig. 5. Hyperthermia induced in a cat by ICV injection (at arrow)
         of 1 (•), 4 (■) or 10 μg (▲) of RX72601 (from Metcalf et al.,
         1975).

A somewhat analogous situation exists in the case of a direct micro-injection of a range of doses of a cholinomimetic in the AH/POA of the cat, also unrestrained. At individual sites located dorsal to the optic chiasm, carbachol produces its typically intense thermogenic effect (Rudy and Wolf, 1972), which is accompanied ordinarily by shivering and vasoconstriction. Once again, however, a high dose of cholinomimetic applied to the same region exerts the opposite effect and produces a fall in the cat's core temperature.

EVOKED RELEASE OF ACh BY THERMAL STIMULUS

It is self-evident that the neuronal activity of an endogenous substance, which is suspected of playing a role as a transmitter of neuronal impulses can be evaluated realistically only if its pre-synaptic release can clearly be physiologically demonstrated (see Myers, 1974). Such a release must be: (1) correlated with a functional response which is evoked pharmacologically by the compound; and (2) coincide anatomically with the physiological system ascribed to the morphologically delimited population of neurons containing the substance. In terms of other regulatory theories involving the hypothalamus, a relatively firm footing for their unique mechanisms was not established until an evoked release of the presumptive neurotransmitter was documented experimentally (e.g., McCaleb et al., 1980).

In experiments with the unanesthetized monkey, the effect of deflecting the ambient temperature of the primate was examined in terms of the resting release of ACh from discrete sites in the brain-stem (Myers and Waller, 1973). Push-pull cannulae were used to perfuse isolated loci extending from the POA through the hypothalamus and mesencephalon. Then during the course of a localized perfusion, the ambient temperature of the monkey's trunk was raised or lowered to ascertain whether the rate of efflux of ACh fluctuates simultaneously with an imposed challenge of warm or cold.

Table 1. Percent of active ACh efflux sites of perfusion in which ACh release was enhanced (↑) or suppressed (↓) by peripheral cooling or warming of the monkey (from Myers and Waller, 1973).

Anatomical Region	ACh Release: Cooling		ACh Release: Warming	
	↑	↓	↑	↓
AH/POA	70%	30%	20%	80%
Mid-Hypothalamus	40%	60%	0%	100%
Posterior Hypothalamus	54%	46%	25%	75%
Mesencephalon	65%	35%	33%	67%

A composite anatomical analysis is presented in Table 1 of the percent of sites of active release in which ACh efflux shifts as the ambient temperature of the monkey is altered. Within the AH/POA as well as the mesencephalon, the sites of release of ACh during cooling of the monkey outnumbers by two to one those in which the output of ACh is evoked by warming. In terms of the suppression of ACh release, this ratio is even more exaggerated in response to warming of the primate. In fact, in all of the mid-hypothalamic sites, warming of the monkey's trunk causes a complete suppression of ACh release.

These observations thus suggest that efferent signals for both heat maintenance and heat dissipation are transmitted by way of distinct cholinergic pathways, with those delegated to thermogenesis predominating over those

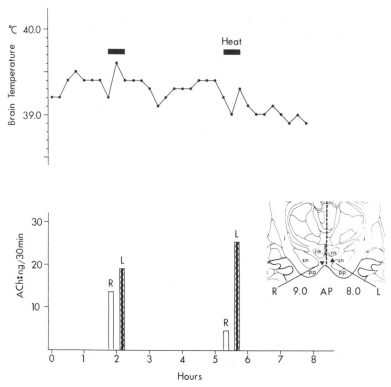

Fig. 6. ACh release in ng/30 min. perfusion interval from two sites
in a single monkey indicated on the anatomical reconstruction in
the inset. The perfusate contained neostigmine, 1.0 μg/ml. The
control perfusion was followed 3 hr. later by a second perfusion
during which the monkey's ambient trunk temperature was elevated
to 45.0° C (From Myers and Waller, 1973).

underlying heat loss. In parallel with this deduction is the finding of Nutik
(1971) who showed that 72% of neurons in the caudal hypothalamus alter their
firing rate in response to cooling of the POA whereas only 28% respond to POA
warming.

To illustrate the characteristics of the simultaneous ACh release at two
mesencephalic sites, Fig. 6 portrays the rate of ACh output during a control
perfusion as well as an experiment performed while the monkey was exposed to
heat. It is clear that a substantial suppression in the rate of ACh output
occurs at one mesencephalic site, whereas the efflux of ACh is elevated con-
currently at the contralateral site.

Monoamine-ACh Interaction

A direct test of the effect on cholinergic activity of monoamines on the
rostral hypothalamus is critical to the ACh-pathway concept. When 5-HT is infused in the AH/POA at the same time that caudal sites in the diencephalon or
mesencephalon are perfused, the typical hyperthermic response to 5-HT is accompanied by an enhancement in the release of ACh at more than half of the
sites of perfusion (Myers and Waller, 1975). On the other hand, NE applied
to the same AH site ordinarily causes a simultaneous reduction in the rate of
ACh efflux as the core temperature of the monkey declines. However, within
several caudal sites, the rate of ACh release is lower during 5-HT hyperthermia but higher during NE hypothermia (Myers and Waller, 1975).

When these findings are integrated with those in which exogenous warming or cooling is used as the thermal stimulus, a cogent interpretation can be based on the concomitant augmentation or inhibition of ACh release. Thus, four categories of cholinergic synapses apparently mediate the thermal effector pathways delegated to the regulation of body temperature. These include synapses that transmit signals for: (1) stimulation of heat production; (2) inhibition of heat production; (3) activation of heat loss; and (4) inhibition of heat loss (Myers, 1980). One could conceive, therefore, that in the primate the respective activity of a population of cholinergic neurons along the efferent pathways of the neuraxis depends entirely on the functional nature of the thermal stimulus, i.e., that either requiring heat gain and a simultaneous inhibition of active heat loss or an excitation of heat loss and consequent inhibition of heat gain.

CONCLUSION

From a neuropharmacological standpoint, it is clear that ACh applied in equimolar doses to circumscribed sites throughout the hypothalamus and parts of the mesencephalon evokes a thermogenesis in two-thirds of the regions examined. Further, the functionally evoked release of the neurotransmitter occurs quite remarkably in a pattern which coincides with the pharmacological results obtained with a cholinomimetic, receptor antagonist and anti-cholinesterase. Taken together, each of these studies provides incontrovertible evidence for the role of ACh in the steady state maintenance of body heat and its conservation as well as in the process of obligatory thermogenesis necessitated by a physiological challenge of cold (Dascombe and Milton, 1981; Simpson and Resch, 1983).

On the other hand, a substantial number of pharmacological and physiological experiments also support the view that endogenous ACh in the brain-stem likewise subserves pathways for heat dissipation and the inhibition of heat production (Myers, 1984). The divergent aspect of this thermolytic component of the cholinergic system originates principally in the caudal hypothalamus and traverses the mesencephalon. From an evolutionary perspective, the 2:1 ratio of cholinergic elements within the brain-stem underlying thermogenesis logically would have arisen in relation to the survival of the organism.

A trenchant interpretation of all of the instances of hypothermia induced by a variety of cholinomimetics, particularly when applied to the AH/POA, is not easily evolved. In evaluating certain of the early experiments, a high dose of a cholinomimetic and a large infusion volume could have been responsible for the loss of body heat in the rat (Avery, 1970). The mechanism could revolve about the well-known functional "tetany" of synapses, as described by Feldberg, when a high dose of ACh applied to autonomic ganglia subsequently blocks transmission of the nerve impulse. As one would expect, the concept of synaptic blockade could be applied in principle to the AH/POA. In fact, this idea could explain the experiments of Lin and colleagues who have infused a cholinomimetic agent ICV, but whose lowest dose (Lin and Chandra, 1981; Chen and Lin, 1980) could still be functionally devastating to the local synapses of neurons within the AH/POA. The resultant pharmacological incapacitation of the mechanism for thermogenesis could be likened to the hypothermia produced by an anesthetic drug applied also to the hypothalamus (Feldberg and Myers, 1965).

Another consideration in the interpretation of results in which a cholinomimetic induces only a hypothermic response concerns the issue of restraint of the test animal. When any animal is studied in an unphysiological state, in a naturalistic sense, one would not necessarily expect to achieve a clear-cut understanding of a complex biological system such as thermoregulation. Since a rat or rabbit is accustomed to a free range of its environment throughout its life, thermoregulation occurs according to a set of functional principles which conceivably may be partially or entirely disrupted when the animal

is constrained in a stock. An emotion-induced perturbation in core temperature, hyperthermia or hypothermia, caused by restraint was documented 30 years
ago (e.g. Grant et al., 1955). Restraint of a rabbit profoundly alters its
resting metabolic rate (McEwen and Heath, 1973), whereas other stressors induce an endorphin-related hyperthermia (Bläsig et al., 1978). Recently, Yano
et al. (1982) demonstrated an increased sensitivity of gastrointestinal structures to ACh in the rat restrained or otherwise exposed to a stressor. Although experiments still done today under the condition of restraint (e.g.,
Lin and Chandra, 1981) may not be invalid, their interpretation may be subject to question, particularly if the obtained results persistently fail to
correspond with data collected in an animal permitted to move about freely.

In conclusion, if all of the results are taken together, the role of diencephalic ACh in thermoregulation is relatively well-documented, at least in
the cat and primate. However, the original reservations raised in the late
1960's about the function of ACh have not been entirely dispelled. That a
species difference may exist is yet a distinct possibility. Moreover, the
use of a restrained experimental animal and over-doses of a cholinomimetic
drug are two methodological issues which will continue to plague the understanding of the part played by cholinergic systems in temperature control.

Perhaps two cogent scientific strategies for future endeavors in this
field would seem to be appropriate: (1) to demonstrate the release of ACh
from AH/POA, posterior hypothalamus and other anatomical areas during the process of temperature regulation; and (2) to identify anatomical sites specific
to the hyper- or hypothermic action of ACh in the specific species being examined (Myers, 1984). Given the sophisticated technology of chromatographic
methods and anatomical tracing, clearcut answers and a resolution to the precise role of ACh in thermoregulation should be ultimately forthcoming in the
years ahead.

SUMMARY

Anatomically distinct cholinergic systems subserving the heat production
and heat loss systems of the body are postulated to originate in the hypothalamus of the cat, primate and other species. When acetylcholine (ACh) or
other cholinomimetic substance is applied by micro-injection to sites throughout the monkey's hypothalamus, an intense rise in the core temperature occurs.
However, within the posterior hypothalamic-mesencephalic interface, a cholinomimetic evokes either a hyper- or hypothermia. Although atropine infused
centrally can block ACh hypothermia, nicotinic agonists also have been found
to elevate body temperature, thus suggesting an involvement of both muscarinic
and nicotinic synapses in the thermoregulatory pathways. Physiological experiments show that when sites in the hypothalamus of the monkey are perfused
by means of push-pull cannulae, the release of ACh is enhanced, suppressed or
unchanged depending upon the ambient temperature of the primate and the locus
of perfusion. Within the AH/POA, ACh release is evoked frequently by peripheral cooling, whereas warming typically reduces the output of the neurotransmitter. In the caudal hypothalamus, ACh release is enhanced at two of
three perfusion sites by cooling of the animal and at one-third of the sites
by peripheral warming. When 5-HT or NE is infused directly into AH/POA, the
hypothalamic release of ACh parallels the amine-induced rise or fall in core
temperature, respectively. Since the primate must defend its set-point temperature of 37°C at an environmental temperature much lower than its own,
the majority of cholinergic synapses thus should be devoted to those functional pathways underlying heat maintenance. This then would explain the 2
to 1 ratio of ACh release as an intrinsic mechanism for survival against a
persistent cold challenge. Overall, the hypothalamic thermoregulatory pathways are characterized by four types of cholinergic synapses which appear to
transmit signals for: (1) activation of heat gain; (2) inhibition of heat
gain; (3) activation of heat loss; and (4) inhibition of heat loss.

The research reported in this chapter has been supported in part by
National Science Foundation Grants BNS78-24491 and BNS84-10663.

REFERENCES

Avery, D. D., 1970, Hyperthermia induced by direct injections of carbachol
in the anterior hypothalamus, Neuropharmacol. 9:175-178.

Baird, J., and Lang, W. J., 1973, Temperature responses in the rat and cat
to cholinomimetic drugs injected into the cerebral ventricles, Eur. J.
Pharmacol. 21:203-211.

Bläsig, J., Höllt, V., Bäuerle, U. and Herz, A., 1978, Involvement of endo-
dorphins in emotional hyperthermia of rats, Life Sci. 23:2525-2532.

Bligh, J., and Maskrey, M., 1969, A possible role of acetylcholine in central
control of body temperature in sheep, J. Physiol. 203:55-57P.

Boulant, J. A., 1980, Hypothalamic control of thermoregulation, in: "Handbook of the Hypothalamus," P. Morgane, J. Panksepp, eds., Marcel Dekker,
New York, pp. 1-82.

Chen, F. F., and Lin, M. T., 1980, Effects of methacholine and acetylcholine
on metabolic, respiratory, vasomotor and body temperature responses in
rabbits, Pharmacol. 21:333-341.

Darling, K. F., Findlay, J. D., and Thompson, G. E., 1974, Effect of intraventricular acetylcholine and eserine on the metabolism of sheep,
Pflügers Arch. Gesamte Physiol., 349:235-245.

Dascombe, M. J., and Milton, A. S., 1981, Dissimilar effects of body temperature in the cat produced by guanosine 3', 5'-monophosphate, acetylcholine
and bacterial endotoxin, Br. J. Pharmac., 74:405-413.

Feldberg, W., and Myers, R. D., 1964, Effects on temperature of amines injected into the cerebral ventricles. A new concept of temperature regulation, J. Physiol., 173:226-237.

Feldberg, W., and Myers, R. D., 1965, Hypothermia produced by chloralose
acting on the hypothalamus, J. Physiol. 179:509-517.

Grant, R., Lewis, J., and Ahrne, I., 1955, Effects of intrahypothalamic injections of pyrogens, Fed. Proc. 14:61.

Hall, G. H., 1973, Effects of nicotine on thermoregulatory systems in the
hypothalamus, in: "The Pharmacology of Thermoregulation," E. Schönbaum
and P. Lomax, eds., Karger, Basel, pp. 244-254.

Hall, G. H., and Myers, R. D., 1971, Hypothermia produced by nicotine perfused through the cerebral ventricles of the unanaesthetized monkey, Neuropharmacol. 10:391-398.

Hall, G. H., and Myers, R. D., 1972, Temperature changes produced by nicotine
injected into the hypothalamus of the conscious monkey, Brain Res. 37:
241-251.

Kirkpatrick, W. E., and Lomax, P., 1970, Temperature changes following iontophoretic injection of acetylcholine into the rostral hypothalamus of the
rat, Neuropharmacol. 9:195-202.

Lin, M. T., and Chandra, A., 1981, Blockade of nicotinic receptors in brain
with d-tubocurarine induces decreased metabolism, cutaneous vasodilation
and hypothermia in rats, Experientia 37:986-988.

Lomax, P., and Jenden, D. J., 1966, Hypothermia following systematic and
intracerebral injection of oxotremorine in the rat, Int. J. Neuropharmacol. 5:353-359.

McCaleb, M. L., Myers, R. D., Singer, G., and Willis, G., 1979, Hypothalamic
norepinephrine in the rat during feeding and push-pull perfusion with
glucose, 2-DG or insuline, Am. J. Physiol. 236:312-321.

McEwen, G. N. Jr., and Heath, J. E., 1973, Resting metabolism and thermoregulation in the unrestrained rabbit, J. Appl. Psych. 35:884-886.

Metcalf, G., Myers, R. D., and Redgrave, P. C., 1975, Temperature and behavioural responses induced in the unanaesthetized cat by the central
administration of RX72601, a new anticholinesterase, Br. J. Pharmacol.
55:9-15.

Myers, R. D., 1969, Temperature regulation: neurochemical systems in the hypothalamus, in: "The Hypothalamus," W. Haymaker, E. Anderson, and W. Nauta, eds., Thomas, Springfield, Ill., pp. 506-523.

Myers, R. D., 1974, Temperature regulation, in: "Handbook of Drug and Chemical Stimulation of the Brain," Von Nostrand-Reinhold, New York, pp. 237-285.

Myers, R. D., 1980, Hypothalamic control of thermoregulation: neurochemical mechanisms, in: "Handbook of the Hypothalamus," P. J. Morgane and J. Panksepp, eds., Marcel Dekker, New York, pp. 83-210.

Myers, R. D., 1982, The role of ions in thermoregulation and fever, in: "Handbook of Experimental Pharmacology," A. S. Milton, ed., Springer-Verlag, New York, pp. 151-186.

Myers, R. D., 1984, Neurochemistry of thermoregulation, The Physiologist 27: 41-46.

Myers, R. D., and Waller, M. B., 1973, Differential release of acetylcholine from the hypothalamus and mesencephalon of the monkey during thermoregulation, J. Physiol. 230:273-293.

Myers, R. D., and Waller, M. B., 1975, 5-HT and norepinephrine-induced release of ACh from the thalamus and mesencephalon of the monkey during thermoregulation, Brain Res. 84:47-61.

Myers, R. D., and Yaksh, T. L., 1968, Feeding and temperature responses in the unrestrained rat after injections of cholinergic and aminergic substances into the cerebral ventricles, Physiol. Behav. 3:917-928.

Myers, R. D., and Yaksh, T. L., 1969, Control of body temperature in the unanaesthetized monkey by cholinergic and aminergic systems in the hypothalamus, J. Physiol. 202:483-500.

Myers, R. D., Melchior, C. L., and Gisolfi, C. V., 1976, Feeding and body temperature in the rat: diencephalic localization of changes produced by excess calcium ions, Brain Res. Bull. 1:33-46.

Nutik, S. L., 1971, Effect of temperature change of the preoptic region and skin on posterior hypothalamic neurons, J. Physiol. (Paris) 63:368-370.

Preston, E., 1974, Central effects of cholinergic-receptor blocking drugs on the conscious rabbit's thermoregulation against body cooling, J. Pharmacol. Exp. Ther. 188:400-409.

Rudy, T. A., and Wolf, H. H., 1972, Effect of intracerebral injections of carbamylcholine and acetylcholine on temperature regulation in the cat, Brain Res. 38:117-130.

Simpson, C. W., and Resch, G. E., 1983, Organization of the central mechanisms triggering thermogenesis in helium-cold hypothermic hamsters, in: "Environment, Drugs and Thermoregulation," P. Lomax, E. Schönbaum, ed., Karger, New York, pp. 26-30.

Tangri, K. K., Bhargava, A. K., and Bhargava, K. P., 1975, Significance of central cholinergic mechanisms in pyrexia induced by bacterial pyrogen in rabbits, in: "Temperature Regulation and Drug Action," J. Lomax, E. Schönbaum, and J. Jacob, eds., Karger, Basel, pp. 65-74.

Yano, S., Matsukura, H., Shibata, M., and Harada, M., 1982, Stress procedures lowering body temperature augment gastric motility by increasing the sensitivity to acetylcholine in rats, J. Pharm. Dyn. 5:582-592.

INFLUENCE OF FRONTAL DECORTICATION ON DRUGS AFFECTING STRIATAL

CHOLINERGIC ACTIVITY AND CATALEPTIC BEHAVIOR: RESTORATION STUDIES

Herbert Ladinsky, Silvana Consolo, Gianluigi Forloni
Francesco Fiorentini and Gilberto Fisone

Istituto di Ricerche Farmacologiche "Mario Negri"
Via Eritrea, 62 - 20157 Milan, Italy

The striatum, and more generally the basal ganglia, stand out as having an extremely rich content of putative neurotransmitters as compared with many other parts of the brain. Acetylcholine (ACh) and GABA are found in cell bodies intrinsic to the area but a number of other transmitters are known to be associated with afferent pathways leading into the striatum. These include dopamine and serotonin localized, respectively, in the nigro-neostriatal neurons and in the afferents from the dorsal raphe nucleus, noradrenaline, associated with the locus coeruleus input, and GABA, associated with the globus pallidus projections[1].

The frontal cortex sends a massive, presumably glutamate-mediated, excitatory input to the striatum. This is one of the major sources of neuronal input to the basal ganglia and on the basis of electron micro-scopic evidence[2], appears to make synaptic contact with the aspiny den-drites of neurons morphologically similar to the presumed striatal cholin-ergic interneurons[3]. That the corticostriatal pathway may regulate cholin-ergic activity in the striatum is indicated by data showing that the synthe-sis rate of ACh[4], as well as the sodium-dependent high affinity uptake of choline[5], are reduced in the striatum following long-term decortication. Furthermore, glutamate enhances the K^+-evoked release of ACh from striatal slices in vitro through NMDA (N-methyl-D-aspartate) type receptors and glutamic acid-preferring receptors possibly localized on the cholinergic cell[6].

Research outlined in the present study shows that a number of agonists pertaining to various drug classes which are capable of depressing cholinergic activity in the striatum through receptor-mediated responses (reflected as an increase in ACh content) lose their activity after degeneration of the corticostriatal pathway. We further show that it is possible to restore the cholinergic action of one or more of the agonists by drugs or lesions thus providing evidence that the cholinergic neurons of decorticated striata are potentially functional. In addition, we have found that frontal decortication (and depressed striatal cholinergic activity) has important implications in behavioral responses to drugs.

METHODS

Female CD-COBS rats of body weight 175-200 g were killed by focussed microwave irradiation to the head (1.3 KW, 2.45 GHz, 4 sec) and then ACh and choline contents of striatum were measured by the radioenzymatic method of Saelens et al.[7] as modified by Ladinsky et al.[8]. The ACh synthesis rate was determined by the method of Racagni et al.[9] after the i.v. infusion of (^{3}H)choline, the ACh precursor[10]. Choline-0-acetyltransferase activity was measured by the method of Fonnum[11] and acetylcholinesterase activity was determined by the method of McCaman et al.[12]. Saturation curves of (^{3}H)dexetimide binding (0.02-1.5 nM) were determined as described by Laduron et al.[13]. Striatal noradrenaline, dopamine and serotonin contents were measured by electrochemical detection coupled with high pressure liquid chromatography[14,15].

Unilateral degeneration of the nigrostriatal dopaminergic pathway was induced by the infusion of 6-hydroxydopamine · HCl (6-OHDA) dissolved in saline containing ascorbic acid (1 mg/ml) at a rate of 1 μl/min for 4 min into the ventral tegmental area. The coordinates used (AP = 3.5, L = 1.1, H = 2) were taken from the König and Klippel atlas of the rat brain[16]. Frontal decortication was produced by undercutting the cortex in etherized rats with a thin glass knife as previously described[17]. The experiments were performed 14 days after the lesion. The uptake of (^{3}H)glutamic acid was estimated by the method of Divac et al.[18]. Drugs, routes, schedules and solvents used are given in the text.

404

The biochemical data were analyzed statistically by ANOVA (2x2) factorial analysis and Tukey's test for unconfounded means. The Mann-Whitney test was used for statistical analysis of cataleptic behaviour.

NEUROCHEMICAL AND NEUROPHARMACOLOGICAL EFFECTS OF FRONTAL DECORTICATION

Transection of the corticostriatal pathway by undercutting the cortex produced a rapid, marked (55%) and persistent decrease in (^{3}H)glutamic acid uptake in the striatum ipsilateral to the lesion indicating extensive damage to the corticostriatal glutamatergic input. At the same time, the contents of noradrenaline, serotonin and its metabolite 5-HIAA, as well as dopamine and its metabolites DOPAC, HVA and 3-MT, were not altered. The content of GABA, on the other hand, was increased in concomitance with a decrease in the turnover rate of this inhibitory neurotransmitter[19].

ACh (68.7±1.7 nmoles/g) and choline (23.0±1.0 nmoles/g) contents were unchanged. The binding of the powerful muscarinic receptor antagonist (^{3}H)dexetimide to specific muscarinic receptors in the striatum of lesioned animals did not reveal changes either in the density (Bmax = 230±10 pmoles/g wet wt) or in the dissociation constant (K_D = 0.34 nM) of the receptors measured on the 3rd, 14th and 120th postlesion day, indicating that muscarinic receptors are not localized presynaptically on fibers of the corticostriatal pathway. Cortical deafferentiation resulted in a small but significant 17% reduction in acetylcholinesterase activity 14 days postlesion. At the same time, the activity of choline acetyltransferase, a selective marker for the cholinergic neuron, was not altered. This provides clear evidence that the cholinergic neurons intrinsic to the striatum remain intact in decorticated rats. Despite this, cholinergic activity is depressed since both the sodium-dependent high affinity uptake of choline[5] and the turnover rate of ACh are reduced by the decortication.

Chronic, unilateral frontal decortication prevented completely the large increase in striatal ACh content induced by several drugs, such as the typical dopaminergic agonists R-apomorphine, the ergot alkaloids

Table 1. Effect of Dopaminergic Agonists on Striatal Acetylcholine Content in Decorticated Rats.

Drug in columns C and D	Striatal ACh (nmoles/g)				
	A Sham	B Decorticated	C Drug	D Drug+decort.	F int.
R-apomorphine	64.4±1.0	64.0±1.8	80.1±2.2*	67.7±2.1	p<0.01
Bromocriptine	68.9±1.7	69.4±2.1	80.2±2.3*	72.0±2.1	p<0.01
Lisuride	65.1±1.8	66.4±1.4	86.6±2.1*	69.9±1.5	p<0.01
Quinpirole	64.8±2.1	63.7±0.5	88.3±2.3*	70.6±1.7	p<0.01

Doses and times: R-apomorphine, 1.5 mg/kg i.p. 30 min; bromocriptine, 4 mg/kg i.p. 90 min; lisuride, 200 µg/kg i.p. 30 min; quinpirole (LY 171555) 90 µg/kg i.p. 30 min. The data are the means ± S.E.M. (n = 6-12). * = p<0.01 vs the sham-operated group; ANOVA (2x2) and Tukey's test.

bromocriptine and lisuride and the selective D_2 dopamine receptor agonist quinpirole (Table 1). In addition, the striatal ACh-increasing effects of the muscarinic agonist oxotremorine, the purinergic drug 2-chloroadenosine (2-CADO), the opiate methadone and the GABA-mimetic muscimol were prevented in decorticated rats (Fig. 1)

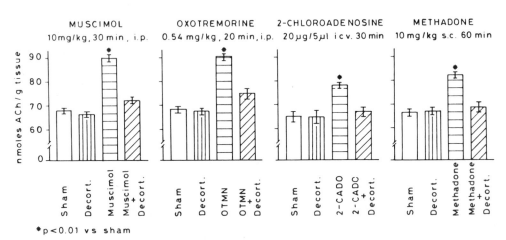

Fig. 1. Effect of muscimol, oxotremorine, 2-chloroadenosine and methadone on striatal acetylcholine content in decorticated rats. The content of striatal ACh is shown on the ordinate. The columns and vertical bars represent the means ± S.E.M. respectively of 6-12 rats.
* = p<0.01 vs the sham-operated group.

Table 2. Effect of R-Apomorphine on the Turnover Rate of
Acetylcholine in Striatum of Decorticated Rats.

Treatment	ACh turnover rate (pmoles/min/mg tissue)
Sham-operated	21.6 ± 1.8
Apomorphine**	—
Decortication	12.5 ± 1.2*
Apomorphine + Decortication	11.8 ± 1.3*

The data are the means ± S.E.M. of 3-6 animals.
*$p<0.01$ vs control group; Duncan's test.
Apomorphine was administered i.p. at the dose of 1.5 mg/kg.
The rats were killed by focussed microwave irradiation to
the head, 30 min after apomorphine and 4 and 6 min after the
i.v. infusion of (methyl-^{3}H)choline. This tracer dose did not
affect either acetylcholine or choline contents.
** ACh turnover rate was not measured because of the .change
in the steady state level of ACh induced by apomorphine at
the doses used.

Table 2 shows that frontal decortication resulted in a marked depression of the ACh turnover rate by 42%. R-apomorphine was not able to further
depress the turnover rate above that produced by decortication alone. This
is in accordance with the loss of the ACh-accumulating effect of apomorphine.
On the other hand, the marked reduction in striatal ACh content induced
by the typical neuroleptic dopamine receptor antagonists, pimozide or haloperidol, and the atypical ones clozapine and L-sulpiride, as well as the
antimuscarinic agent scopolamine, were not influenced by the lesion (Table 3).

The data taken together suggest that in decorticated animals the
cholinergic neurons intrinsic to the striatum, being already depressed by
the loss of the excitatory input can no longer respond to drugs or stimuli
that normally slow down their activity whereas these neurons are still
responsive to agents that activate them.

However, choline chloride, given i.p. at the dose of 250 mg/kg, produced a marked increase in striatal ACh of about 30% and this effect was

Table 3. Effect of Typical and Atypical Neuroleptics and Scolopamine on Striatal Acetylcholine Content in Decorticated Rats.

Drug in columns C and D	Striatal ACh (nmoles/g)				
	A Sham	B Decorticated	C Drug	D Drug+decort.	F int.
Pimozide	66.3±1.4	62.2±3.2	44.7±1.9*	37.8±1.6*	n.s.
Haloperidol	71.1±3.0	67.8±5.2	39.1±2.7*	40.5±1.6*	n.s.
Clozapine	66.5±1.4	62.9±1.8	37.5±1.9*	37.8±1.6*	n.s.
L-Sulpiride	66.8±1.4	64.2±3.2	49.4±2.9*	47.9±2.9*	n.s.
Scopolamine	67.4±3.0	65.4±3.1	42.5±4.3*	46.9±2.8*	n.s.

Doses and times: pimozide, 1 mg/kg i.p. 240 min; haloperidol, 0.25 mg/kg i.p. 30 min; clozapine, 20 mg/kg i.p. 60 min; L-sulpiride, 100 mg/kg i.p. 180 min; scopolamine, 0.5 mg/kg i.p. 30 min. The data are the mean ± S.E.M. (n = 6-12).
*=p<0.01 vs the sham-operated group; ANOVA (2x2) and Tukey's test.

not mitigated by the lesion (Table 4). How choline was still active despite the depressed synthesis rate of ACh and the depressed choline uptake activity in decorticated striata is a matter of speculation at the moment. Choline is known to be a weak muscarinic receptor agonist[20] but oxotremorine, a much more powerful cholinomimetic drug, was blocked by decortication. It is conceivable that choline acted through its property of being the precursor of ACh[21]. Whatever the mechanism whereby choline acts may be, the data show that the cholinergic neuron of the decorticated striatum is capable of a response when a proper stimulus is applied.

Table 4. Effect of Choline on Striatal Acetylcholine Content in Decorticated Rats.

Treatment	Striatal ACh (nmoles/g)
Sham-operated	65.1 ± 2.8
Choline	84.7 ± 3.0*
Decortication	63.0 ± 2.2
Choline + Decort.	85.4 ± 2.6*

Choline chloride was administered i.p. at the dose of 250 mg/kg. The rats were killed 30 min later. The data are the means ± S.E.M. (n = 8).
*=p<0.01 vs the sham-operated group; interaction: n.s. ANOVA (2x2) and Tukey's test.

RESTORATION OF NEUROPHARMACOLOGICAL ACTIONS IN DECORTICATED RATS

When it became apparent from the above results that the cholinergic neurons are potentially functional, we began looking for means to restore the cholinergic action of one or more of the agonists in decorticates. Two such means were successful: 1), pretreatment with choline (100 mg/kg i.p., 10 min); and 2), a short-term (48 h) lesion of the nigrostriatal dopaminergic input.

Choline chloride, at the dose of 100 mg/kg, did not significantly affect striatal ACh in sham-operated rats or in the decorticated animals (data not shown) but, when administered prior to apomorphine, methadone or 2-CADO and in the decorticated rats, it allowed these drugs to express their full inhibitory effects of the cholinergic neuron (Table 5).

Our present working hypothesis is that the cholinergic neuron in-trinsic to the striatum may be maintained in a functional equilibrium state by a balance between the excitatory input from the cortex and an inhibitory input, in this case dopamine from the substantia nigra. Loss of the excita-tory influence shifts the balance in favour of inhibition which may account, in part, or even in whole, for the depression of the cholinergic neuron in

Table 5. Choline Pretreatment Reinstates the Acetylcholine-In-creasing Effects of Apomorphine, Methadone and 2-Chloro-adenosine in Striatum in Decorticated Rats.

Drug	Striatal ACh (nmoles/g)		
	Drug alone	Drug + choline pretreat.	F int.
Saline	66.2 ± 1.6	66.7 ± 2.8	—
R-apomorphine	70.7 ± 2.6	88.9 ± 3.1*	p<0.01
Methadone	69.7 ± 3.3	91.8 ± 6.3*	p<0.01
2-CADO	63.6 ± 4.4	80.5 ± 2.5*	p<0.01

The experiments were performed 14 days after unilateral frontal decortication. Doses and times: R-apomorphine, 0.8 mg/kg i.p. 30 min; methadone, 10 mg/kg s.c. 60 min; 2-chloroadenosine, 25 μg i.c.v. 15 min; choline chloride, 100 mg/kg i.p. 25 min. The data are the means ± S.E.M. (n = 6-12).
*=p<0.01 vs respective control; ANOVA (2x2) and Tukey's test.

Table 6. Effect on Short Term (48 h) Dopaminergic Deafferentation on the
Cholinergic Action of Apomorphine, Methadone and 2-Chloroadeno-
sine in Decorticated Rats.

| Drug | Striatal ACh (nmoles/g) | | F int. |
	Decort. + drug	Combined lesion + drug	
Saline	67.5 ± 1.6	69.7 ± 2.8	—
R-apomorphine	70.7 ± 2.6	80.8 ± 1.8*	p<0.01
Methadone	66.3 ± 2.8	65.1 ± 2.6	n.s.
2-CADO	70.0 ± 2.5	66.9 ± 3.4	n.s.

Dopamine deafferentation was produced by the infusion of 6-OHDA into the
ipsilateral nigrostriatal pathway 12 days after unilateral lesion of the
frontal cortex and the experiments were performed 48 h later. Doses and
times: R-apomorphine, 0.8 mg/kg i.p. 30 min; methadone, 10 mg/kg s.c.
60 min, 2-chloroadenosine, 25 µg/5 µl, i.c.v. 15 min. The data are the
means ± S.E.M. (n = 12).
* = p<0.01 vs respective control; ANOVA (2x2) and Tukey's test.

lesioned animals. To test this, we destroyed the nigroneostriatal dopami-

nergic input ipsilateral to the frontal lesion and examined the action of

apomorphine, methadone and 2-CADO on striatal ACh content. In animals with

the combined lesion, the level of ACh was not significantly different from

the decorticated group (Table 6). The refractoriness of the cholinergic

neurons to R-apomorphine in the decorticated group was completely restored

in the dually-lesioned group. The lesion of the nigroneostriatal pathway

proved to be selective, since it permitted the action of a dopaminergic

drug to be reinstated but did not allow the restoration of methadone or

2-CADO effects. This finding suggests, furthermore, that there may be

different populations of cholinergic neurons in the striatum[22], perhaps

all being under the excitatory control of the cortical (glutamatergic)

neurons, but having different types of inhibitory control.

BEHAVIORAL EFFECTS OF FRONTAL DECORTICATION

Frontal decortication (and depressed striatal cholinergic activity)

has important implications in behavioral responses to drugs (Table 7). It

has long been known that lesions of the corticostriatal pathway enhance the

behavioral effect of amphetamine[23] and apomorphine and abolish the

Table 7. Behavioral Consequences of Decortication.

Increase in spontaneous locomotor activity

Increase in amphetamine-induced locomotor activity

Increase in apomorphine-induced stereotyped behavior

Decrease in haloperidol-induced catalepsy

Enhancement of opioid-induced catalepsy

---

cataleptogenic action of haloperidol[24]. We have found that lesion of the corticostriatal pathway plays an important role not only in those behavioral events connected with changes in dopaminergic transmission but also in the expression of catalepsy induced by opiates.

Catalepsy was scored 14 days after lesion according to the modified method of Dunstan et al.[25]. Four tests (horizontal plane, inclined grid at a 25° angle, 8 cm bar, Buddha position) were used. Animals were given one point for each position held for 10 sec. The degree of catalepsy was expressed as a total score (0-4), obtained by summing the individual scores. The experiments were run in double blind condition.

The cataleptic effect of morphine and methadone was markedly increased in animals with bilateral deafferentiation of the cortex. Minimally effective doses of morphine (8.5 mg/kg,s.c.) or methadone (3.5 mg/kg,s.c.) in normal rats produced marked catalepsy in the lesioned animals (Fig. 2).

The onset of maximum catalepsy occurred, respectively, 30 min and 60 min after injection of methadone (Fig. 2A) and morphine (Fig. 2B) with a duration of action lasting at least 90 min for each drug. Higher doses of methadone (5 and 10 mg/kg,s.c.) which by themselves produced clear cut cataleptic behavior, were not enhanced by decortication. This explains why Lloyd et al.[26] using a high dose of morphine (25 mg/kg) did not find enhancement in decorticated animals.

Naloxone (10 µg/2 µl saline) injected bilaterally into the striata of

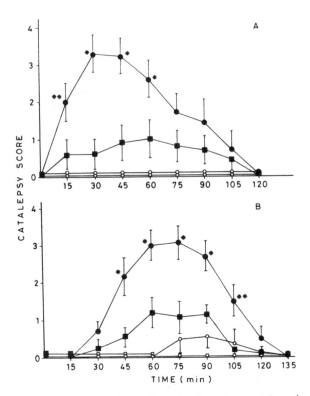

Fig. 2. Enhancement of methadone (Panel A) and morphine (Panel B) induced cataleptic response in bilaterally frontally decorticated rats and the antagonism by naloxone (10 µg/ 2µl), applied bilaterally intrastriatally 5 min before the administration of narcotics. The catalepsy score is shown on the ordinate and the time after methadone (3.5 mg/kg s.c.) or morphine (8.5 mg/kg s.c.) is shown on the abscissa. Each point represents the mean score and S.E.M. of 5-7 rats. Symbols: (■) sham-operated; (●) decorticated; (□) sham-operated + naloxone; (O) decorticated + naloxone. **=p<0.05, *=p<0.01 vs sham-operated and naloxone-treated groups.

alert rats through indwelling cannulae implanted in the areas (coordinates AP = 9.5, L = 2.7, H = 2.1) at least four days before experimentation, completely prevented the behavioral effect of both drugs (Fig. 2A, B), indicating that a site in this area is likely to be an essential link for narcotic cataleptic behavior. It should be noted that the method by Dunstan et al.[25] does not distinguish, in the cataleptic scoring used, which of the two components comprised in the effect of systemically injected narcotics is enhanced by decortication: i.e. catalepsy and/or muscular rigidity.

Table 8. Effects of Oxotremorine and Choline on Methadone
Catalepsy in Decorticated Rats.

Drug	Dose	Methadone catalepsy score
Saline	—	3.27 ± 0.28
Oxotremorine	2.5 µg i.s.	2.45 ± 0.62
	5.0 µg i.s.	1.63 ± 0.84*
	10.0 µg i.s.	1.29 ± 0.37**
Choline	200 mg/kg i.p.	1.22 ± 0.62**

Bilaterally decorticated rats were given bilateral intrastriatal injections of oxotremorine or an intraperitoneal
injection of choline chloride 5 min before the administration of methadone (3.5 mg/kg s.c.). Catalepsy scores
were taken every 15 min over a 120 min period. The scores
referred to in the Table were those taken at 45 min when
the peak score was obtained in the saline-treated group.
In sham-operated controls, the dose of methadone used
produced negligible cataleptic behavior. The data are the
means ± S.E.M. (n=5).
*=$p<0.05$; **=$p<0.01$ vs saline-treated group – Mann-Whitney
test.

Since, an increase in cataleptic response to morphine has also been
observed after lesion of the striatum[27], it appears that the behavioral
changes induced by decortication are mediated through functional modification in the striatum.

Both the bilateral injection of oxotremorine (2.5, 5 and 10 µg) into
the striata and the intraperitoneal administration of choline chloride,
200 mg/kg, were able to reverse the enhanced cataleptic effect of methadone
in decorticated rats (Table 8). It thus follows from these first findings
that cholinergic neurons within the striata are involved in the mechanism(s)
by which frontal decortication influences narcotic behavior. Further studies
are in progress to elucidate the role that the striatal cholinergic system
plays in the expression of the cataleptic behavior.

SUMMARY AND CONCLUSIONS

As a result of the loss of the excitatory corticostriatal afferents: 1), neurochemical markers for cholinergic neurons intrinsic to the striatum are not changed; 2), striatal cholinergic neurons become refractory to many agonists but choline chloride, the precursor of ACh, which also possesses a weak cholinergic agonist property, is still active; 3), striatal cholinergic neurons respond to antagonists; 4), the cholinergic response to agonists in decorticated rats is reinstated selectively either by choline chloride pretreatment or by 6-OHDA lesion of the nigroneostriatal pathway; 5), behavioral changes occur in decorticated animals: haloperidol catalepsy is abolished whereas methadone and morphine catalepsy is enhanced; 6), the relationship of the excitatory corticostriatal pathway with the cholinergic and dopaminergic systems in the striatum reported here may be of relevance to the mode of action of drugs that alleviate the symptoms of neurological and psychiatric disorders and may further suggest new approaches to therapy.

REFERENCES

1. P.C. Emson, ed., Chemical Neuroanatomy. Raven Press, New York (1983).
2. R. Hassler, J.W. Chung, U. Rinne, and A. Wagner, Selective degeneration of two out of the nine types of synapses in cat caudate nucleus after cortical lesions. Exp. Brain Res. 31: 67-80 (1978).
3. H. Kimura, P.L. McGeer, F. Peng, and E.G. McGeer, Choline acetyltransferase-containing neurons in rodent brain demonstrated by immunohistochemistry. Science 208: 1057-1059 (1980).
4. P.L. Wood, F. Moroni, D.L. Cheney, and E. Costa, Cortical lesions modulate turnover rates of acetylcholine and γ-aminobutyric acid. Neurosci. Lett. 12: 349-354 (1979).
5. J.R. Simon, Cortical modulation of cholinergic neurons in the striatum. Life Sci. 31: 1501-1508 (1982).
6. J. Lehmann, and B. Scatton, Characterization of the excitatory amino acid receptor-mediated release of [^{3}H]acetylcholine from rat striatal slices. Brain Res. 252: 77-89 (1982).
7. J.K. Saelens, M.P. Allen, and J.P. Simke, Determination of acetylcholine and choline by an enzymatic assay. Arch. Int. Pharmacodyn. Ther. 186: 279-286 (1970).
8. H. Ladinsky, S. Consolo, S. Bianchi, R. Samanin, and D. Ghezzi, Cholinergic-dopaminergic interaction in the striatum: The effect of 6-hydroxy-dopamine or pimozide treatment on the increased striatal acetylcholine levels induced by apomorphine, piribedil and d-amphetamine. Brain Res. 84: 221-226 (1975).

414

9. G. Racagni, M. Trabucchi, and D.L. Cheney, Steady-state concentrations of choline and acetylcholine in rat brain parts during a constant rate infusion of deuterated choline. Naunyn Schmiedebergs Arch. Pharmacol. 290: 99-105 (1975).

10. A. Vezzani, A. Zatta, H. Ladinsky, S. Caccia, S. Garattini, and S. Consolo, Effect of dimethylamino-2-ethoxyimino-2-adamantane (CM 54903), a non-polar dimethylaminoethanol analog, on brain regional cholinergic neurochemical parameters. Biochem. Pharmacol. 31: 1693-1698 (1982).

11. F. Fonnum, A rapid radiochemical method for the determination of choline acetyltransferase. J. Neurochem. 24: 407-409 (1975).

12. M.W. McCaman, L.R. Tomey, and R.E. McCaman, Radiomimetric assay of acetylcholinesterase activity in submicrogram amounts of tissue. Life Sci. 7: 233-244 (1968).

13. P.M. Laduron, M. Verwimp, and J.E. Leysen, Stereospecific in vitro binding of $[^3H]$dexetimide to brain muscarinic receptors. J. Neurochem. 32: 421-427 (1979).

14. R. Keller, A. Oke, I. Mefford, and R.N. Adams, Liquid chromatographic analysis of catecholamines: Routine assay for regional brain mapping. Life Sci. 19: 995-1004 (1976).

15. F. Ponzio, and G. Jonsson, A rapid and simple method for the determination of picogram levels of serotonin in brain tissue using liquid chromatography with electrochemical detection. J. Neurochem. 32: 129-132 (1979).

16. J.F.R. König, and R.A. Klippel, The Rat Brain. A Stereotaxic Atlas of the Forebrain and Lower Parts of the Brain Stem. Williams & Wilkins, Baltimore (1963).

17. S. Consolo, M. Sieklucka, F. Fiorentini, G. Forloni, and H. Ladinsky, Frontal decortication and adaptive changes in striatal cholinergic neurons in the rat. Brain Res., in press.

18. I. Divac, F. Fonnum, and J. Storm-Mathisen, High affinity uptake of glutamate in terminals of corticostriatal axons. Nature 266: 377-378 (1977).

19. P. Worms, B. Scatton, M.-T. Willigens, A. Oblin, and K.G. Lloyd, Cortical influences on striatal function, in: "Psychopharmacology of the Limbic System", M. Trimble, and E. Zarifian, eds., Oxford University Press, Oxford, pp. 68-75 (1984).

20. H. Ladinsky, S. Consolo, and P. Pugnetti, A possible central muscarinic receptor agonist role for choline in increasing rat striatal acetylcholine content, in: "Nutrition and the Brain, vol. 5 , A. Barbeau, J.H. Growdon, and R.J. Wurtman, eds., Raven Press, New York, pp. 227-241 (1979).

21. I.H. Ulus, R.J. Wurtman, M.C. Scally, and M.J. Hirsch, Effect of choline on cholinergic function, in: "Cholinergic Mechanisms and Psychopharmacology", D.J. Jenden, ed., Plenum Press, New York, pp. 525-538 (1978).

22. A.M. Graybiel, and C.W. Ragsdale Jr., Histochemically distinct compartments in the striatum of human, monkey, and cat demonstrated by acetylthiocholinesterase staining. Proc. Natl. Acad. Sci. USA 75: 5723-5726 (1978).

23. S.D. Iversen, S. Wilkinson, and B. Simpson, Enhanced amphetamine responses after frontal cortex lesions in the rat. Eur. J. Pharmacol. 13: 387-390 (1971).
24. B. Scatton, P. Worms, K.G. Lloyd, and G. Bartholini, Cortical modulation of striatal function. Brain Res. 232: 331-343 (1982).
25. R. Dunstan, C.L. Broekkamp, and K.G. Lloyd, Involvement of caudate nucleus, amygdala or reticular formation in neuroleptic and narcotic catalepsy. Pharmacol. Biochem. Behav. 14: 169-174 (1981).
26. K.G. Lloyd, M.T. Willigens, and P. Worms, Cortical lesions differently affect neuroleptic-and non-neuroleptic induced catalepsy in rats. Br. J. Pharmacol. 74: 821P (1981).
27. B. Costall, and R.J. Naylor, Neuroleptic and non-neuroleptic catalepsy. Arzneimittelforsch. 23: 674-683 (1973).

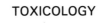

TOXICOLOGY

SUCCINYLCHOLINE - CLINICAL AND TOXICOLOGICAL ASPECTS

Bo Holmstedt[1], Ingrid Nordgren[1,x], Gun Jacobsson[1],
Inga Jäderholm-Ek[2] and Torsten Silander[3]

1. Department of Toxicology, Karolinska Institutet
   Box 60 400, S-104 01 Stockholm, Sweden
2. Department of Anaesthesia, Ersta Hospital
   S-116 35 Stockholm, Sweden
3. Department of Surgery, Ersta Hospital
   S-116 35 Stockholm, Sweden

INTRODUCTION

The history of succinylcholine (SCh) from 1906 up to date has been
well documented by Dorkins (1982). It was introduced as a muscle relaxant
by several groups around 1950. Its short lasting effect made it ideal for
intubation before surgery. For prolonged muscle relaxation it has been
largely superseded by other synthetic compounds. Untoward effects have
been noted, such as prolonged apnea, cardiovascular effects and muscle
fasciculations. In 1954 SCh was introduced in veterinary medicine as a
casting agent for large animals (Hansson and Edlund, 1954; Hansson, 1958).

In recent years SCh has figured in alleged or proven murder cases
(La Du, 1967; MacDonald, 1968; Bailey, 1971; Schoop, 1981; Bowles, 1980
and 1981; Woods, 1982, Eklind, 1983). The first of these cases was the
so-called Coppolino case. At the time when this occurred, evidence was
brought forward with paper chromatography for the occurrence of succinylmonocholine in muscle tissue. More recent cases have prompted the development of a specific and sensitive chemical method to be used forensically
as well as clinically. The method is based upon gas chromatography - mass
spectrometry and deuterium labelled internal standard (Nordgren et al.,
1983). It is now possible to analyze concentrations of SCh as low as
2 ng/g tissue.

In the present paper we report studies on the elimination of SCh
from human plasma in vivo and in vitro, distribution to different tissues
and urinary excretion. We also report studies on tissue distribution and
elimination from plasma in the dog, following doses ranging between 2 and
106 mg/kg i.v. or i.m. The dogs were either kept under artificial respiration or allowed to die from the dose given.

---

[x]To whom correspondence should be sent

MATERIALS AND METHODS

Chemicals

All chemicals were of analytical grade. The reagents were prepared as described by Nordgren et al. (1983).

In vitro Incubations

SCh was added to human plasma in concentrations ranging between 5 and 5000 µg/ml. The plasma was incubated at 37°C. Aliquots were taken for analysis of remaining SCh in a time series during a 30 min period. The samples were collected in tubes containing eserine (final concentration 10^{-4}M), and kept frozen until analyzed.

Patients

Blood, urine and different tissues were taken from 12 patients operated on because of the following diagnosis: cholelithiasis (4), macromastia (2), nephrolithiasis (3), kidney tumour (3), adenocarcinoma of the pancreas (1), laparotomy because of adhesions (1). The patients were premedicated with diazepam and pethidine. All except four received first an epidural block with mepivacaine. An epidural catheter was introduced for refilling and was also used for postoperative painrelief with pethidine. The patients were then kept asleep with thiopental. To obtain relaxation for tracheal intubation, 50-75 mg of succinylcholine was used. The patients were then kept asleep with a mixture of nitrous oxide and oxygen together with enfluran. In most patients only the intubation dose succinylcholine was given. In three patients, however, three repeated doses of SCh were given permitting studies of the rate of elimination. Blood was collected in tubes containing eserine (final concentration 10^{-4}M). The blood samples were centrifuged and the plasma removed. All samples, i.e. plasma, urine and tissue, were immediately frozen and kept frozen until analyzed.

Dog Experiments

Mongrel dogs were anaesthetized with pentobarbital and received SCh in doses ranging between 2-106 mg/kg i.v. or i.m. Two of the dogs were kept under artificial respiration while others were left to die from the dose administered.

In order to study tissue distribution and elimination from plasma, tissues were removed 1-45 min after administration of SCh, and blood was collected by means of an indwelling catheter in heparinized tubes containing eserine (final concentration 10^{-4}M) 0.5-36 min after the SCh injection. In view of embalming in forensic cases, some tissues were injected with and soaked in FAX (Champion Chemical Co., Ontario, Canada), a commercially available glutaraldehyde embalming fluid diluted 1:8 with water. The samples were kept frozen until analyzed.

RESULTS

In vivo Studies in Humans

The elimination of SCh from human plasma in vivo was studied in three patients upon administration of three doses of SCh, 50 mg each, at 15-20 min intervals. This clinical dose of SCh was found to be rapidly eliminated, even after repeated administrations, as demonstrated in Fig. 1.

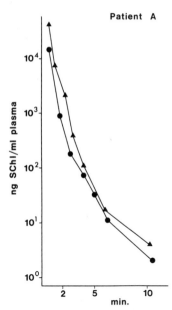

Fig. 1. Elimination of SCh
from plasma in vivo
(patient A). Three
doses of 50 mg SCh
were administered
at 20 min intervals.
● first dose
▲ third dose

The amount of unchanged SCh excreted in urine was studied in five
patients, and was found to range between 4.0-7.1 per cent of the total
amount administered. This is in fair agreement with previous reports
(Koelle, 1975). In two of our cases the SCh could be followed for 12 h
and in the other three for 24 h.

Of the tissues analyzed nothing was found in liver, smooth muscle
from pylorus, pancreas, pancreatic tumour, mammary tissue, bile from
choledochus and gallbladder, striated muscle and adipose tissue. SCh could
be found above the limit of detection only in the kidney. In this organ
the amount of SCh was in the range 230-380 ng per g 0.5-1 h after injection and 80-120 ng per g 1.5-2 h after injection. In kidney tumours
(hypernephroma and cancer), however, the concentration was found to be
much lower, 5-20 ng per g.

Studies in Dogs

The elimination of SCh from plasma in relation to tissue distribution
was studied in dogs administered different doses (2-106 mg/kg i.v. or i.m.)
with and without artificial respiration (Nordgren et al., 1984).

When the dogs were artificially ventilated, the SCh was rapidly
eliminated from the plasma, even after high doses, as illustrated by
Fig. 2.

In cases where the dogs were not kept under artificial respiration,
the decrease in the concentration of SCh in plasma leveled off when the

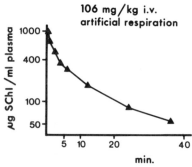

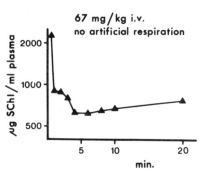

Fig. 2. Elimination of SCh from plasma in a dog kept under artificial respiration. The dog was injected i.v. with 2 mg/kg, 1.5 h later followed by a second dose of 106 mg/kg. The curve demonstrates the elimination after the second dose.

Fig. 3. Elimination of SCh from plasma in a dog that was not artificially ventilated but died from the dose administered (67 mg/kg i.v.).

circulation failed and the animals died as demonstrated in Fig. 3. Cessation of respiration occurred after 30 sec. Drop in blood pressure and cessation of regular heart beats occurred after about 4 min.

The concentrations of SCh found in tissues from one of the dogs are shown in Table 1. The highest amounts were found in the kidney. When comparing dogs administered different doses of SCh, we found the tissue concentration to increase in a dose dependent manner. However, the relative distribution between the organs seemed to be the same irrespective of the dose administered, and with or without artificial respiration. When comparable doses were given the tissue concentrations were higher in the animals that were allowed to die (no artificial ventilation) from the dose of SCh. I.m. injection led to lower tissue levels compared to i.v. administration of the same dose (Nordgren et al., 1984).

Table 1. Levels of SCh in tissues after administration of 2 mg/kg i.v., 1.5 h later followed by a second dose of 106 mg/kg i.v. The dog was kept under artificial respiration. Tissues were removed at times given in table and embalmed with FAX.

	Time after the second dose of SCh (min)	/ug SChI per g
Kidney	13	1175
Kidney	38	803
Liver	43	5
Diaphragm	45	65
Spleen	42	107

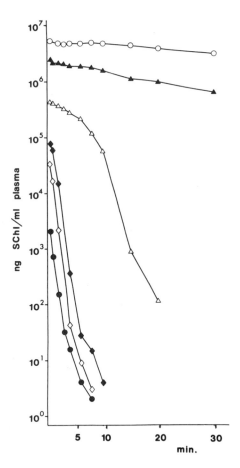

Fig. 4. Elimination of SCh from human
plasma <u>in vitro</u> upon incubation at 37°C.
Initial concentration:
○ 5000 /ug/ml plasma
▲ 2500 /ug/ml plasma
△ 500 /ug/ml plasma
◆ 100 /ug/ml plasma
◇ 50 /ug/ml plasma
● 5 /ug/ml plasma

In vitro Experiment with Human Plasma

The hydrolysis of SCh in human plasma <u>in vitro</u> is demonstrated in
Fig. 4. At low doses, where the initial concentrations are lower than or
comparable to SCh levels found <u>in vivo</u> after administration of clinical
doses, the ester is rapidly eliminated. However, at the two highest concentrations used in this study the time needed for a 50% decrease of the
initial drug concentration is much longer, and the drug levels decline
at an essentially constant rate during the time studied. At an intermediate concentration (500 /ug/ml) the rate of disappearance is initially
low, but increases when the drug level is sufficiently reduced. This
indicates that at high levels of SCh the plasma cholinesterase activity
is rate limiting and the rate of hydrolysis independent of drug concentra-

423

tion. Consequently, the tissue distribution becomes increasingly important at higher SCh doses.

DISCUSSION

It has been pointed out that the lack of a reliable chemical method with sufficient sensitivity for the determination of SCh has made pharmaco-kinetic determinations difficult. Attempts have been made to use nerve block and enzyme determinations as well as radioactively labelled SCh to establish its disappearance rate and excretion. Also the inadequacy of previous methods have hampered the possibilities of comparison between in vitro and in vivo experiments. Dilution of enzyme in in vitro experiments as well as the use of a different substrate for the cholinesterase determinations have been pointed out as disadvantages (Holst-Larsen, 1976; Dorkins, 1982). The present investigation avoids both the dilution effects and the discrepancy in the use of substrate.

It has been proven that SCh in clinical doses is rapidly eliminated from human plasma, reaching the limit of detection in about 10 min. This is consistent with previous knowledge obtained by indirect methods (Dal Santo, 1968). A search for the compound in various organs after clinical administration reveals the presence of SCh only in the kidney. The substance could also be identified and quantitated in the urine. In dog experiments at higher doses the compound could be identified in several tissues, with the highest concentrations in the kidney.

When SCh was incubated in vitro with undiluted human plasma, we found that the time required for an initial drug concentration to decrease by 50% is dose dependent. It increases with increasing drug levels, which in all likelihood means that the system is capacity limited with respect to plasma cholinesterase activity.

In dogs given increasingly high doses (2-106 mg/kg), SCh disappears from plasma continously when under artificial respiration. When dogs were allowed to die from respiratory arrest and circulatory failure the elimination from plasma ceased. This may be explained by the lack of redistribution to tissues, and to the high substrate concentration in plasma. The comparison between in vivo and in vitro in this case is hampered by the fact that the pseudocholinesterase in dogs blood has a very low specific activity (Meyer, 1971).

SCh has contributed to legal as well as medical history. In April 1967, Carl Coppolino, an anaesthetist was convicted of killing his wife with succinylcholine chloride (Bailey, 1971; Helpern, 1977). Respiratory paralysis would occur with a sufficient dose of the drug, and in the absence of artificial ventilation this would, of course, result in death. In retrospect the crime seemed very elegant, for the hydrolysis of the drug would ultimately result in succinate and choline, many grams of which are already present in the body. Functionally, the drug would then seem to disappear without trace. In the early 1960s it was thought impossible to detect this drug in the human body. New tests were stimulated by, and devised for, the trial of the anaesthetist (La Du, 1967). On autopsy an injection track had been found in the left buttock. After appropriate control experiments, the tissue of this area and adjacent areas as well as tissue from the right buttock were extracted and subjected to paper chromatography using two developing agents. The analysis was aimed at detecting succinylmonocholine, and a spot with an R_f value corresponding to this compound was found with the highest intensity in the region of the injection track (estimated amount 30 µg per g tissue).

Unluckily the results have never been published but the testimony makes straightforward reading. The validity of these tests has later been under attack (Gringauz, 1978; Southern Reporter, 1969; Newsweek, 1979). Had the tissue been preserved it could probably have been analyzed for the parent compound succinylcholine by the method described above.

SUMMARY

Tissue distribution and elimination from plasma have been studied in dogs administered 2-106 mg/kg i.v. or i.m., and either kept under artificial respiration or allowed to die from the dose given, as well as in humans given clinical doses during surgery. In addition, in vitro studies with incubated human plasma have been performed.

In man, the elimination of clinical doses from plasma in vivo was very rapid, even after repeated administration. We found about five per cent of the dose administered to be excreted unchanged in urine. It could be followed for 12-24 h. Of the tissues studied, the kidney was the only one where SCh could be detected.

In dogs, the levels of SCh in plasma rapidly decreased when the dogs were kept under artificial respiration, even after high i.v. doses, while the levels of SCh stopped decreasing upon cessation of circulation and death. We also found that SCh is extensively distributed to tissues. Of the organs analyzed, the highest amounts of SCh were found in the kidney. The ratio of distribution between various organs was the same irrespective of the dose.

It has generally been accepted that SCh disappears rapidly from blood and tissues due to hydrolysis by cholinesterases. In vitro studies in human plasma showed that the time required to decrease the initial drug concentration by 50% is dose dependent. In concentrations comparable to clinical doses the elimination was rapid, but increase in concentrations led to a decrease in the rate of disappearance, which probably means that the system is capacity limited with respect to plasma cholinesterase activity. This explains the extensive tissue distribution found after higher doses, and also why SCh can be detected in tissues after circulatory failure.

KEY WORDS

Gas chromatography - mass spectrometry, Muscle relaxation, Succinylcholine, Tissue distribution, Urinary excretion.

ACKNOWLEDGEMENTS

This work was supported by grants from the Swedish Medical Research Council B85-14X-00199 and by the Wallenberg Foundation.

REFERENCES

Bailey, L.F., 1971, "The defence never rests".
Bowles, B., 1980, "The Davis case", Detroit Free Press, Oct. 12.
Bowles, B., 1981, "The Davis case", Detroit Free Press, Jul. 6.
Dal Santo, G., 1968, Kinetics of distribution of radioactive labelled muscle relaxants. III: Investigations with ^{14}C-succinyldicholine and ^{14}C-succinylmonocholine during controlled conditions. Anesthesiology, 29:435.

Dorkins, H.R., 1982, Suxamethonium – The development of a modern drug from 1906 to the present day. Medical History, 26:145.

Eklind, P., 1983, "The Death Shift", Texas Monthly, Aug. 106-197.

Gringauz, A., 1978, "Drugs, how they act and why", C.V. Mosby, ed., Saint Louis.

Hansson, C.H., 1958, Studies on succinylcholine as a muscle relaxing agent in veterinary medicine. Thesis. Stockholm, Sweden.

Hansson, C.H. and Edlund, H., 1954, Nord. Vet. Med., 6:671.

Helpern, M., 1977, "Autopsy", St. Martin Press Inc., N.Y.

Holst-Larsen, H., 1976, The hydrolysis of suxamethonium in human blood. Br. J. Anaesth., 48:887.

Koelle, G.B., 1975, "The Pharmacological Basis of Therapeutics", 5th edn., p. 585, L.S. Goodman and A. Gilman, ed., Macmillan, New York, Toronto, London.

La Du, B., 1967, Testimony in case No 1331, vol. V, pp. 467-587. In the circuit court of the twelfth judicial circuit of Florida and for Collier county.

MacDonald, J.D., 1968, "No Deadly Drug", Ballantine Books.

Meyer, H., 1971, Untersuchungen über Typ und Aktivität der Pseudo-cholinesterase (E.C. 3.1.1.8.) in serum reinrassiger Hunde. Thesis, Berlin.

Newsweek Mag., 1979, "Coppolino hopes for vindication", May 7.

Nordgren, I., Forney, R., Carroll, T., Holmstedt, B., Jäderholm-Ek, I. and Pettersson, B.-M., 1983, Analysis of succinylcholine in tissues and body fluids by ion-pair extraction and gas chromatography – mass spectrometry. Arch. Toxicol., Suppl. 6:339.

Nordgren, I., Baldwin, K. and Forney, R., 1984, Succinylcholine – Tissue distribution and elimination from plasma in the dog. Biochemical Pharmacology, 33(15):2519.

Schoop, H., 1981, 180 Ungeklärte Todesfälle: Pfleger mordete mit Curare, Die Welt, No. 23, p. 16, Jun. 7.

Southern Reporter, 1969, 2nd series, vol. 223, West Publishing, p. 68, St. Paul, Minn.

Woods, M., 1982, "MCO Expert Finds Test for Murder Tool", The Blade, Feb. 10.

PATHOLOGY OF EXPERIMENTAL NERVE AGENT POISONING

Charles G. McLeod, Jr., Henry G. Wall

U. S. Army Medical Research Institute of Chemical Defense
Aberdeen Proving Ground, Maryland   21010-5425

INTRODUCTION

Historically, organophosphorus toxicity has been most frequently associated with delayed peripheral neuropathies (Spencer, 1978; Lotti, 1984). Studies of accidental human exposures to these compounds and numerous animal experiments have shown that the symptomatic and morphologic effects of these toxic substances are related to distal disruptions of motor nerve tracts. The best described of these substances are triorthocresylphosphate (TOCP) and certain of the agricultural insecticides. More recently several investigators have defined an entirely different syndrome caused by two of the organophosphorus chemical warfare agents (Petras, 1981; Lemercier, 1983; McLeod, 1984; Samson, 1984; Martin, 1985; Singer, 1985; Singer, 1985). These highly toxic "nerve agents" are potent acetylcholinesterase inhibitors that have been found to induce severe brain pathology in several experimental animal models. The purpose of this review is to describe the light and electron microscopic pathological changes that are caused by these agents and to propose several possible etiologic mechanisms based on comparisons of observed lesions with other forms of central nervous system injury.

BACKGROUND

Since World War II the chemical warfare nerve agents have been studied extensively in man as well as in animal models (Lohs, 1975). Several recently published reviews have summarized and referenced much of this data, some of which was previously classified or available only in technical reports from military laboratories (Spencer et al, 1982; McLeod, 1985; Vojvodic, 1981; Boskovic, 1981). The United States Army has had a renewed interest in these agents, primarily in the areas of antidote development, mechanisms of action, pathology and behavioral toxicity. This research activity, including extensive contracted research is unclassified, published in the open literature and summarized each year at the Army Bioscience Review sponsored by the lead laboratory in this field, the U. S. Army Medical Research Institute of Chemical Defense at Aberdeen Proving Ground, Maryland. This new interest in the chemical warfare nerve agents by the U. S. Army and its allies has led to many important findings, one of which is that in animals these organophosphorus compounds cause severe permanent brain injury. Much of the current research effort is aimed at defining these changes, determining their etiology and effects of prophylactic and antidotal therapy on lesion development.

Currently, there is no evidence that man will not be susceptible to this severe brain injury. Indeed, significant brain pathology has been observed in several laboratory species following nerve agent poisoning including the rat, guinea pig, cat, and monkey. It should be noted that many of the early studies concerning nerve agents were not designed to detect brain pathology (Harris et al, 1953). Either pathological examination was not performed or animals did not survive long enough to allow development of lesions which could be detected by light microscopy. At least one early investigator (Thornton, 1962) and probably others observed certain forms of brain pathology following nerve agent exposure, but apparently none of these findings were published in the open literature.

Clinical Features of Experimental Nerve Agent Poisoning

The nerve agents soman (pinacolyl methylphosphonofluoridate) or sarin (isopropyl methylphosphonofluoridate) when given by subcutaneous injection cause strong tremors and eventually tetanic convulsions, the onset and duration depending on dosage administered. In a typical LD50 study of either of these agents, most of the high dose animals die within one to four hours. Medium and low dose animals have variable signs, but many have profuse salivation, tearing, cyanosis (as expressed by darkened tongue and eyes in albino rats or guinea pigs), progressively stronger tremors and convulsions. Mortality in experiments of this type can be affected markedly by various environmental factors including handling of the animals, loud noise or type of cages (gang verses single cages). Many of the surviving animals will have had prolonged periods of strong tremors and convulsions, yet begin to take food and water and appear clinically normal except for a slight decrease in activity and a characteristic "ruffled" appearance. When handled some of these animals (rats) may exhibit unusual aggressive behavior and an exaggerated "startle" reaction which is best characterized by their leaping 10-20" vertically as a response to a sharp noise. It is these surviving animals that best exhibit the characteristic brain pathology of nerve agent poisoning.

Gross Pathology

Pathological changes observed in animals examined 24-48 hours post exposure are limited to non-specific agonal changes including focal lung and adrenal hemorrhages. Lung edema is not a prominent feature when animals are examined shortly after death. Occasionally a bloody frothy liquid is observed in the nares, trachea and lung. This is apparently more frequently caused by a tongue laceration during the convulsions than by spontaneous vessel rupture.

Animals examined more than one week after exposure may show poor condition and weight loss as compared to unexposed controls. A few animals may show moderate brain atrophy and dilation of brain ventricles.

Light Microscopic Pathology

Animals examined one to two days following exposure to soman or sarin exhibit acute neuronal degeneration and necrosis which is most pronounced in the cortex, hippocampus, and dorsal thalamus (Figure 1A). Extreme vacuolar change and perivascular hemorrhages are also seen in animals examined during the first three days following poisoning. There are two characteristic patterns of injury

428

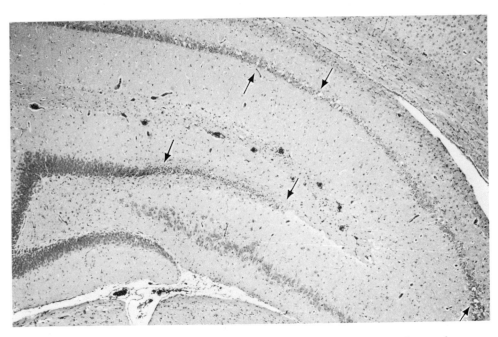

Fig. 1A. Rat hippocampus with acute neuronal degeneration and
necrosis (arrows).

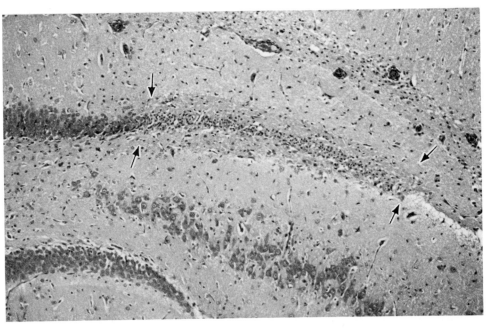

Fig. 1B. The "microinfarction" pattern of brain injury (Enlargement of
Fig. 1A). Arrows demark a well-defined zone of acute necrosis
within the hippocampus of a rat. All neurons and supportive
structures within this zone are necrotic.

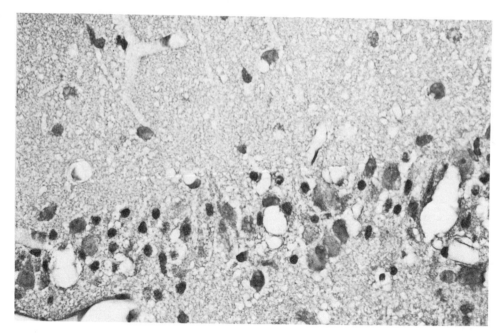

Fig. 2.   The dark contracted nuclei represent the "diffuse" or random
          pattern of necrosis within this hippocampus. Several viable
          cells show swelling. Supportive structures are normal except
          for the vacuolar change which is mostly extracellular.

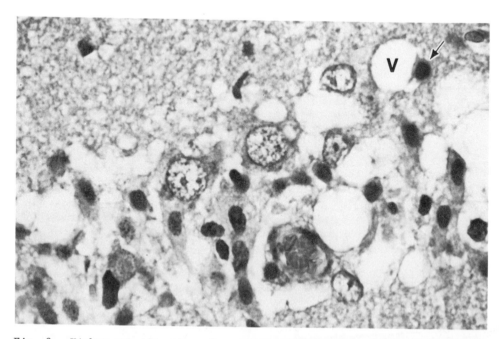

Fig. 3.   Higher magnification of a segment of rat hippocampus affected by
          severe diffuse neuronal necrosis and vacuolar change. Note large
          vacuole (v) adjacent to a necrotic contracted neuron (arrow).

in affected animals. The first is a well defined "microinfarct" which has very distinct boundries between normal and necrotic tissue. Within these lesions all cellular elements and supportive structures are necrotic. This pattern of injury is observed most frequently in the hippocampus and cortex (Figure 1B). The second pattern of injury is "diffuse" and in this case there is a random necrosis that affects neurons of the cortex, hippocampus, amygdaloid nuclei and thalamus. Other cellular components are spared (Figure 2). Vacuolar degeneration is often a striking lesion, affecting large areas within the hippocampus and thalamus (Figure 3).

Animals examined more than one week following exposure exhibit progressive malacia and sometimes mineralization in the more severely affected sites of injury. Mild gliosis and vascular hypertrophy are also seen. Some animals exhibit microscopic features of brain atrophy including reduction of cortical mass, hippocampal shrinkage and ventricular dilation.

The cerebellum is seldom affected by these acute or chronic pathological changes. Likewise, dense myelinated tracts are spared. Special stains for myelinated axons may show disruption, "beading" or loss of these structures; however, this is apparently a secondary or "Wallerian" effect which is observed only in or adjacent to areas that have extensive neuronal loss.

Many animals having severe brain lesions are found by light microscopy to have myocardial fiber degeneration with an associated mild myocarditis (Figure 4). These changes are found randomly within both ventricles. Mild fibrosis is seen as a late consequence of this acute degenerative process.

Electron Microscopic Brain Pathology

The hippocampus is the only structure that has been examined extensively by electron microscopy (Wall, 1985). In rats significant alterations are observed one hour after exposure to a convulsive dose of soman. These changes include swelling of endoplasmic reticulum, the perinuclear space, and mitochondria of neurons (Figure 5) and astrocytes. All of these early ultrastructural alterations apparently reflect changes in cell volume regulation and in extracellular fluid components, as suggested by the light microscopic findings (Figure 2, 3). No significant changes are apparent in cytoskeletal components. Ultrastructural alterations become progressively more severe, and by 24 hours after soman exposure neuron cell bodies, dendrites and axons reveal widespread disintegration of organelles (Figure 6). Mitochondrial cristae loss and mitochondrial rupture is observed along with membranous profiles, condensed and disintegrated polyribosomes and disarrayed cytoskeletal components. Axonal myelin exhibits clefts between lamina. Electron dense granular deposits, suggestive of mineralization, are deposited on and between myelin lamina also. Markedly dilated astrocytes are also readily apparent as cells with electron-lucent cytoplasmic compartments containing few organelles. At 48 to 72 hours after soman exposure rat hippocampi reveal extensive neuronal and neuropil degeneration (Figure 7). However, some cells show early mitochondrial swelling and endoplasmic reticulum dilatation. These findings suggest a delayed injury response. Some degenerated cells are also surrounded by neural and glial processes that show little or no pathologic alteration. This finding suggests that some cells either have resistance to injury or have recovered from sublethal injury.

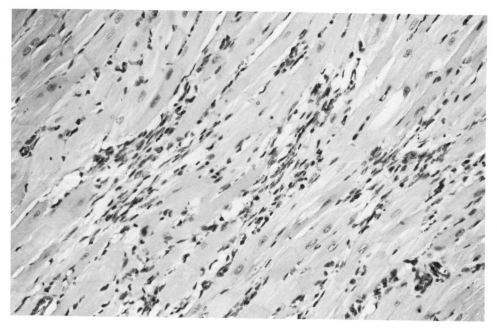

Fig. 4. A section of rat heart exhibits muscle fiber vacuolar change and necrosis. There is a mild inflammatory reaction to this loss of tissue.

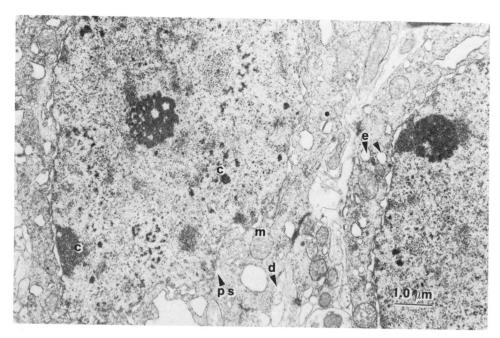

Fig. 5. Two hippocampal pyramidal perikarya and intervening cell processes from a rat that convulsed and was killed one hour after soman exposure. Note dilated perinuclear space (ps), endoplasmic reticulum (er), and dendritic (d) process. Mitochrondria (m) are swollen and nuclear chromatin (c) is condensed.

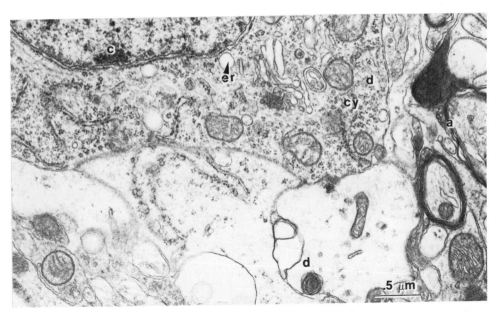

Fig. 6. Hippocampal perikaryon and adjacent cell processes from a rat
that convulsed and was killed 24 hours after soman exposure.
Swollen dendritic (d) processes, membranous profiles, and
axons (a) with early myelin degeneration are adjacent to a
pyramidal cell body that contains dilated endoplasmic
reticulum (er), condensed cytosol (cy), and nuclear chromatin (c).

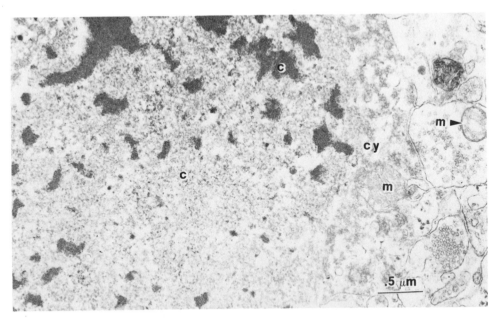

Fig. 7. Hippocampal pyramidal perikaryon from a rat that convulsed
and was killed 72 hours after soman exposure. The nuclear
membrane is absent. Nuclear chromatin (c) is condensed and
fragmented. Amorphous masses suggestive of aggregates of
ribosomes are scattered throughout the cytoplasm (cy).
Swollen dendrites with degenerated mitochondria (m) and
aggregates of vesicles abut the pyrimidal cell.

DISCUSSION

In all morphologic studies conducted recently at the Army Institute of Chemical Defense, there has been a strong but not absolute correlation between convulsions and development of significant brain pathology in animals exposed to nerve agents. Other investigators have had similar findings. Some animals can have tremors, no apparent convulsive episodes and develop brain pathology. In these cases, which have been seen in the rat, guinea pig and cat, lesions have been mild as compared to animals that have prolonged convulsions (Singer, 1985).

Although the guinea pig develops lesions that are similar in appearance and distribution to those in the rat after exposure to nerve agents, the incidence of lesion development is lower in the guinea pig. This difference is apparently caused by a higher rate of acute mortality in the convulsing guinea pigs (Singer, 1985). There are probably many other species differences; however, higher mammals, including cats and primates have been found to develop significant brain lesions after exposure to nerve agents (Petras, 1984).

The ultrastructural lesions found in the hippocampus of soman exposed rats are consistent with those described in the brains of rats (Brown and Brierly, 1972), cats and monkeys (Garcia et al., 1978) that were examined within one hour after experimental anoxic or ischemic injury. The early endoplasmic reticulum and mitochondrial changes, and later progressive organelle degeneration, are also consistent with structural changes described for a wide variety of ischemic non-neural cells (Trump et al., 1980). These similarities do not imply that soman's mechanism of action is solely via hypoxia. Further functional studies are needed to assess the role of brain cell respiration and metabolic activity in lesion development after soman intoxication.

The exact mechanisms causing these light and ultrastructural lesions remain to be defined. However, based on the morphologic features and the fact that anticonvulsants prevent their development (Singer, 1984; Martin, 1985) it is likely that they are caused by cellular energy deficits during the critical time of intense neuronal firing (convulsions). Also, the pattern of discrete segmental necrosis observed in the hippocampus and cortex of some animals suggests that this lesion may have a vascular origin such as focal sustained vasospasm.

References

Boskovic, B., 1981, The treatment of soman poisoning and its perspectives, Fund. & Appl. Tox., 1:203-213.

Brown, A. W., Brierly, J. B., 1972, Anoxic-ischaemic cell change in rat brain. Light microscopic and fine structural observations. J. Neurol. Sci., 16:59-84.

Garcia, J. H., Lossinsky, A. S., Kauffman, F. C., and Conger, K. A., 1978, Neuronal ischemic injury: light microscopy, ultrastructure and biochemistry, Acta. Neuropathol. (Berl), 43:85-95.

Harris, C., Koon, W., Crook, J. W., Christensen, M., and Oberst, F. W., 1953, Do pathological lesions develop in dogs repeatedly exposed to low doses of GB vapor? DTIC Tech. Report #AD3399, Chemical Corps, Medical Labs, Army Chemical Center, Aberdeen Proving Ground, Maryland.

Lemercier, G., Carpenter, P., Sentenac-Romanou, H., and Morelis, P., 1983, Histological and histochemical changes in the central nervous system of the rat poisoned by an irreversible anticholinesterase organophosphorus compound, Acta. Neuropathol. (Berl), 61:123-129.

Lohs, Kh., 1975, Delayed toxic effects of chemical warfare agents, Stockholm: Almqvist & Wiksell, International Peace Research Institute, c1975.

Lotti, M., Becker, C. E., and Aminoff, M. J., 1984, Organophosphate polyneuropathy: Pathogenesis and prevention, Neurol. 34, 658-662.

Martin, L. J., Doebler, J. A., Shih, T. M., and Anthony, A., 1985, Protective effect of diazepam pretreatment on soman-induced brain lesion formation, Brain Res. 325, 287-289.

McLeod, C. G., Jr., Singer, A. W., and Harrington, D. G., 1984, Acute neuropathology in soman poisoned rats, Neurotoxicology, 5:53-58.

McLeod, C. G., Jr., 1985, Pathology of nerve agents: Perspectives on medical management, Accepted for publication, Fund. & Appl. Toxicol.

Petras, J. M., 1981, Soman neurotoxicity, Fund. & Appl. Toxicol., 1:242.

Petras, J. M., 1984, Brain pathology induced by organophosphate poisoning with the nerve agent soman, U. S. Army Medical Research Development Command 4th Annual Chemical Defense Bioscience Review.

Samson, F. E., Pazdernik, T. L., Cross, R. S., Giesler, M. P., Mewes, K., Nelson, S. R., and McDonough, J. H., 1984, Soman induced changes in brain regional glucose use, Fund. Appl. Toxicol., 4:173-183.

Singer, A. W., 1984, Effect of valium and atropine on mortality and pathology in guinea pigs exposed to soman, U. S. Army Medical Research Development Command 4th Annual Chemical Defense Bioscience Review.

Singer, A. W. and McLeod, C. G., Jr., 1985, Effect of diazepam on soman induced neuropathology, Submitted for publication, Neurotoxicology.

Singer, A. W., Graham, J. S., and McLeod, C. G., Jr., 1985, Acute neuropathology and cardiomyopathy in soman and sarin poisoned rats, Submitted for publication, Tox Letters.

Spencer, P. S., Schaumburg, H. H., 1978, Distal axonopathy: One common type of neurotoxic lesion, Environ. Health Perspect. 26:97-105.

Spencer, P. S., Albuquerque, E. X., Dettbarn, W. D., Drachman, D. B., Generoso, W. M., Karczmar, A. G., Koelle, G., and Standaert, F. S., 1982, Chapters 1 (Introduction) and 2 (Anticholinesterases), In: "Possible Long-Term Health Effects of Short-Term Exposure to Chemical Agents," Vol 1, Anticholinesterases and Anticholinergics., Nat. Acad, Press, Washington D.C.

Thorton, K. R., and Brigden, E. G., 1962, Morphological changes in the brain of guinea pigs following VX poisoning, Suffield Technical Paper No. 230.

Trump, B. F., McDowell, E. M., and Arstila, A. U., Cellular reaction to injury, In: "Principles of Pathobiology," ed. LaVia.

Vojvodic, V., 1981, Toxicology of war gases, Belgrade Military Publishing House, Inst for Mil Med Inform and Documentation, Biblioteka Pravila: udzbenici., 5:198-226.

Wall, H. G., McLeod, C. G., Jr., Hutchison, L. S., and Shutz, M., 1985, Development of brain lesions in rats surviving after experiencing soman induced convulsions: Light and electron microscopy, U. S. Army Medical Research Development Command 5th Annual Chemical Defense Bioscience Review.

ORGANOPHOSPHORUS ANTICHOLINESTERASE-INDUCED

EPILEPTIFORM ACTIVITY IN THE HIPPOCAMPUS

Frank J. Lebeda and Paul A. Rutecki

Section of Neurophysiology, Department of Neurology
Epilepsy Research Center, Baylor College of Medicine
Houston, TX 77030

INTRODUCTION

In the study of epileptogenesis, the pharmacological induction of convulsant activity has provided important information regarding the cellular events involved in the production of abnormal electrical discharges. This research approach has benefited from the advent of in vitro central nervous system (CNS) tissue slices and the use of microelectrode recording techniques (Yamamoto, 1972). Synchronous repetitive discharges induced by the drugs examined thus far are the characteristic features of the epileptiform activity recorded in vivo and in vitro. These discharges are considered to be correlated with abnormal interictal electroencephalographic (EEG) recordings (Ayala et al., 1973). The corresponding intracellular event is comprised of a series of action potentials superimposed on an envelope of depolarization. This envelope of depolarization was termed the paroxysmal depolarizing shift (PDS) by Matsumoto and Ajmone Marson (1964) in characterizing penicillin-induced discharges in vivo. Recent studies have shown that the event underlying the drug-induced PDS is a net excitatory response produced by a synchronous synaptic input (Johnston and Brown, 1981; Lebeda et al., 1982).

A number of structurally diverse convulsants produce PDSs. Some convulsant drugs have been considered to exert at least some of their effects by interfering with chloride-dependent synaptic activity mediated by γ-aminobutyric acid (GABA) (Dingledine and Gjerstad, 1980; Schwartzkroin and Prince, 1980) -- a major inhibitory neurotransmitter in supraspinal regions (Krnjevic et al., 1966). Picrotoxin (PTX) is representative of the class of convulsants that produce disinhibition. Other convulsants, however, produce epileptiform activity without abolishing inhibitory neurotransmission, e.g., 4-aminopyridine (4-AP) (Rutecki et al., 1984).

Acetylcholine has also been shown to be capable of promoting epileptiform activity (Bernardo and Prince, 1981). This effect is consistent with the predominantly excitatory effects of cholinergic agonists (Krnjevic et al., 1971; Brown and Adams, 1980; Bernardo and Prince, 1981; Valentino and Dingledine, 1981). In accord with this line of reasoning, it has been suggested that the convulsant effects produced by anticholinesterase (anti-ChE) agents, particularly the organophosphorus (OP) anti-ChEs, are the direct consequence of the accumulation of acetylcholine (ACh) due to the irreversible blockade of ChE in the CNS (Lipp, 1972; Rump et al., 1973).

The anti-ChE hypothesis for OP-induced epileptogenesis has, however, been questioned by numerous investigators (Hampson et al., 1950; Harwood, 1954; Machne and Unna, 1963; Karczmar, 1967; Brimblecombe, 1974; O'Neill, 1981; Ellin, 1982). Since the OPs are irreversible inhibitors of ChE, the anti-ChE hypothesis predicts that the epileptogenic effects of the OPs should also be irreversible. Contrary to this prediction, abnormal EEG activity could be elicited repeatedly by administration of OP anti-ChEs at times when ChE activity was virtually abolished (Van Meter, Karczmar and Fiscus, 1978). This suggests that effects other than the irreversible inhibition of ChE by these OP agents are also important.

The present study characterizes the epileptiform activity induced by two OP anti-ChEs: diisopropyl phosphorofluoridate (DFP) and pinacolyl methylphosphonofluoridate (soman). OP-induced epileptiform activity was examined in the hippocampal slice preparation, using intracellular and extracellular recording techniques.

A primary objective of this study was to test the anti-ChE hypothesis quantitatively by comparing the rate of spontaneously occurring epileptiform discharges with the decrease in ChE activity produced by OP anti-ChE agents in vitro. Other goals were to determine whether the epileptiform events induced by the OP anti-ChEs were associated with a synchronous synaptic input and whether spontaneous inhibitory neurotransmission was compromised.

The experimental findings showed that the OP-induced convulsant effects could be altered by washing out the agent at a time when ChE activity was markedly suppressed. Furthermore, the discharges induced by the OP agents were associated with a synaptically mediated PDS, and spontaneously occurring inhibitory postsynaptic potentials (IPSPs) were not abolished. Our present working hypothesis is that in addition to the irreversible blockade of ChE, other mechanisms are also important in the generation of epileptiform discharges. Since the OP-induced discharges resembled those produced by 4-AP, another mechanism may involve a reduction of one or more of the different types of potassium currents (see Adams, this volume). A preliminary account of this work has appeared elsewhere (Lebeda and Rutecki, 1985).

MATERIALS AND METHODS

The methods used to prepare hippocampal slices were similar to those described previously (Johnston et al., 1980; Johnston, 1981; Lebeda et al., 1982). Experiments were conducted on Sprague-Dawley male rats (100-200 g). Slices were transferred to an interface recording chamber (Haas et al., 1979), where they were continuously superfused with an oxygenated (95% O_2, 5% CO_2) control or drug-containing saline and maintained in a humidified atmosphere at 33-35° C. Extracellular recordings were made in the CA3 subfield with NaCl-filled microelectrodes and a conventional amplifier; intracellular recordings were made with Cs_2SO_4-filled microelectrodes and a 3-kHz switch clamp circuit. In most of the intracellular studies, AC-coupled recordings were made simultaneously with a nearby extracellular electrode. All records shown represent spontaneous epileptiform activity.

ChE activity of single hippocampal slices was assayed using Ellman's method (Ellman et al., 1961). The protein content of single-slice homogenates was determined by the method of Lowry et al. (1951). Following subtraction of the appropriate blank absorbance reading, enzyme activity was determined as the number of μmoles of substrate hydrolyzed per min per mg of protein. Measurements were expressed as values relative to control.

Unless indicated otherwise, the physiological (control) saline had the following composition (in mM): NaCl, 124; KCl, 5; NaH$_2$PO$_4$, 1.25; NaHCO$_3$, 26; CaCl$_2$, 2; MgSO$_4$, 2; glucose, 10.

RESULTS

Interictal-Like Epileptiform Activity

Under control conditions, extracellular recordings from CA3 subfields of rat hippocampal slices displayed occasional unit activity but no spontaneous epileptiform events. Within 30 min of bath application, 10-25 μM DFP or 0.01-0.1 μM soman produced spontaneously occurring, repetitive discharges that resulted from the synchronous firing of a population of neurons within the vicinity of the recording electrode. These extracellular field discharges were operationally defined as being interictal-like and may correspond to the abnormal electrical behavior that occurs between overt seizures (Ayala et al., 1973).

Synaptic Responses During OP-Induced Interictal-Like Activity

Extracellularly recorded interictal-like events were accompanied by intracellular discharges comprised of an envelope of depolarization, that in turn, triggered a number of action potentials (Figure 1). Evidence has been reported previously to support the hypothesis that the PDS generated by both the PTX class of convulsants (Johnston and Brown, 1981; Lebeda et al., 1982) and the 4-AP class (Rutecki et al., 1984) is synaptically mediated. Therefore, the objective of our first series of experiments was to determine whether the OP-induced depolarizing shift was also due to a synaptic response. The results in Figure 1 show that the PDS waveform could be reversed in polarity upon depolarization. The measured reversal potential for DFP-induced PDSs was -21.1 ± 3.0 mV (N = 4 cells; mean ± S.D.). With soman, the measured reversal potential was -38.1 ± 6.6 mV (N = 5). The reversal of the PDS waveform with maintained depolarization suggests that the OP-induced PDS is indeed synaptically mediated.

In contrast, the PDS induced by PTX has a reversal potential near 0 mV (Lebeda et al., 1983; Johnston et al., in press). If the OPs generate epileptiform activity in which an inhibitory synaptic component is still present, the addition of PTX should change the negative reversal potential obtained with an OP to 0 mV. To test this hypothesis, DFP (25 μM) and PTX (10 μM) were co-applied and the resultant PDSs examined. These PDSs had a measured reversal potential of 1.3 ± 3.1 mV (N = 4), suggesting that the negative reversal potential associated with the OP-induced discharges, reflects an inhibitory synaptic input that temporally overlaps the excitatory synaptic event.

Another set of experiments was performed to determine more directly whether the OPs abolished synaptic inhibition. Spontaneous IPSPs were monitored in these experiments by depolarizing neurons to 0 mV. Since 0 mV is the reversal potential for the excitatory postsynaptic potentials (Brown and Johnston, 1983; Johnston and Brown, 1984), and the reversal potential for these inhibitory synaptic events is about -70 mV (Andersen and Langmoen, 1980), only IPSPs should be present at 0 mV. As illustrated in Figure 2, spontaneously occurring IPSPs were observed in the presence of 25 μM DFP. In fact, some IPSPs may have been larger than those occurring in the control saline. A similar sparing of IPSPs was obtained with 100 nM soman (not shown). On the other hand, 10 μM PTX virtually eliminated spontaneously occurring IPSPs. Thus, neither DFP nor soman induced epileptiform activity by abolishing spontaneously occurring inhibitory neurotransmission.

439

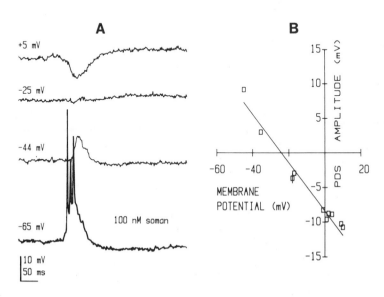

Figure 1. Synaptic basis of soman-induced PDS. A: in this CA3 neuron, at a membrane potential of -65 mV, the spontaneously occurring PDS induced by 100 nM soman consisted of a series of action potentials superimposed on the depolarizing potential. The amplitude of the underlying event was minimal near -25 mV and clearly was reversed in polarity at +5 mV. B: plot of paroxysmal-event amplitude as a function of membrane potential under current-clamp conditions. The amplitudes of the intracellular potential changes were measured when the corresponding amplitude of the extracellular event recorded from an adjacent microelectrode was maximal (extracellular traces not shown). Interpolated reversal potential was -24 mV in this cell. Solid line represents a least-squares fit. Symbols represent mean values from at least three determinations. When present, error bars represent the S.E.M. Action potentials in panel A were attenuated at the sampling frequency used (500 Hz).

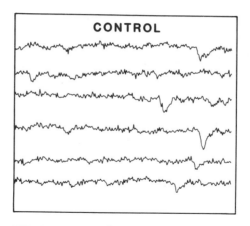

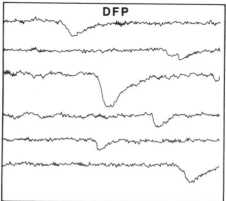

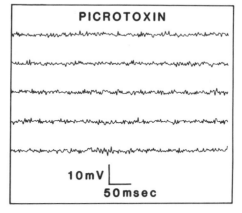

Figure 2. Effects of convulsants on spontaneously occurring IPSPs in three
different neurons. These events were virtually abolished with PTX (10 μM).
DFP (25 μM) did not eliminate spontaneous IPSPs. Recordings made in the
presence of a convulsant were obtained between interictal-like discharges
that were recorded with a nearby extracellular electrode (extracellular
recordings not shown). All of the intracellular recordings were made under
current clamp at a membrane potential of 0 mV (see text).

To characterize the development of epileptiform activity, the frequency of spontaneous, extracellularly recorded discharges was monitored during bath application of the OPs. In these experiments, an on-line computer system was used to determine interdischarge intervals and calculate the mean frequencies in 1- to 2-min time bins. To determine whether these discharges were associated with an irreversible process, sequential bath application and washout of the OP were performed.

As illustrated in Figure 3A, the initial effects of DFP were reversible. The first exposure to 25 µM DFP produced a discharge rate of about 0.18 Hz; subsequent washout abolished these spontaneous discharges. The second exposure to DFP resulted in a higher discharge frequency (about 0.22 Hz). The second washout period, however, did not totally eliminate these events. Following subsequent exposures, the washouts eventually had no effect on discharge frequency. Thus, after an initial reversible phase, a progressively developing irreversible effect was seen to occur with repeated exposures to DFP. Similar development of an irreversible phase was also observed with soman (not illustrated).

To test the hypothesis that the blockade of cholinesterase activity was involved in the transition from a reversible to an irreversible phase, the reaction scheme depicted in the inset of Figure 3B was evaluated (Aldridge, 1953; Main, 1964). The first reaction involved the reversible binding of the inhibitor (I) with the enzyme (E), followed by the irreversible conversion to another drug-bound species (EP). In this model it was assumed that the two drug-bound species were involved in generating discharges. Reversible epileptiform activity could not occur if (EP) was assumed to be the only species involved. By adjusting the rate constants, and assuming a nonlinear relation between ChE inhibition (EI + EP) and the interictal-like discharge frequency, a resonable simulation of the salient experimental results could be obtained (Figure 3B). The value for the irreversible rate constant (k_p), however, had to be made more than three orders of magnitude smaller than Main's (1964) estimate.

One prediction from this model is that the amount of ChE activity (i.e., the concentration of the free enzyme (E)) should increase during the washout periods (Figure 4A). To test this prediction, we measured ChE activities of single hippocampal slices that were subjected to a similar exposure regimen (Figure 4B). In this experiment, the slices were made and maintained in a manner identical to slices in which electrical activity was recorded. In contrast to the model's prediction, the ChE activity did not recover during the washout periods. A quantitatively similar irreversible decrease in ChE activity was also seen with 100 nM soman.

These results are not surprising in view of the established experimental evidence that DFP and soman are irreversible ChE inhibitors. Nevertheless, the same kinetic reaction scheme as shown in Figure 3B could still be used to simulate the block of ChE activity if the rate constants were changed to values consistent with the biochemical literature (Main, 1964). This simulation result is shown as the dotted line in Figure 4B.

Another approach was also used to demonstrate a reversible effect with soman. In this experiment, slices were exposed to 100 nM soman for 60 min--a period sufficient to render the washouts ineffective in reducing the discharge frequency. As shown in Figure 5, after switching the bathing solution from soman to one containing 50 nM atropine, the discharges were abolished. The reintroduction of soman in the presence of atropine restored the epileptiform activity. Repeating this sequence of solution changes produced comparable results. Atropine apparently blocked the

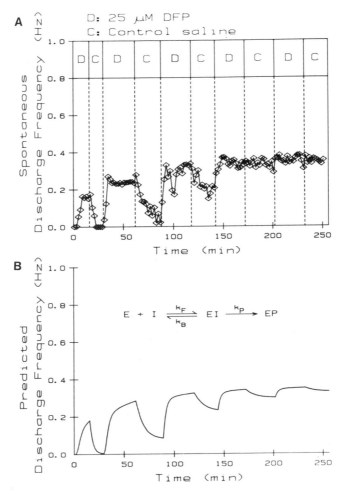

Figure 3. Progressive loss of reversible epileptogenic effects produced by 25 μM DFP. A: the initial washout of DFP eliminated the spontaneously occurring interictal-like events; later washouts became progressively less effective in changing the discharge frequency. B: the kinetic model (inset) simulated the changes in frequency of discharge with repetitive washouts. Solid curve represents the predicted discharge frequency as a function of time during simulated washins and washouts of DFP. S.E.M.s for data in panel A and for those in Figure 5 were typically equal to or smaller than the symbols.

Parameters: $k_F = 10^4 \text{ M}^{-1}\text{min}^{-1}$; $k_B = 0.1 \text{ min}^{-1}$; $k_P = .025 \text{ min}^{-1}$

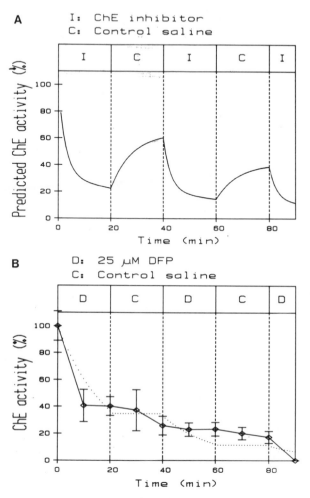

Figure 4. Predicted and experimentally determined ChE activity. A: the kinetic model shown in Figure 3 predicted that ChE should partially recover during washout of DFP. B: normalized ChE activity measured in single slices. Three slices were removed from the interface recording chamber every 10 min. Contrary to the model's prediction in panel A, the ChE activity did not recover during the washout periods. Each symbol represents the mean ± S.E.M. Dotted curve obtained from the same model using different rate constants.

Parameters: k_F = 2000 $M^{-1}min^{-1}$; k_B = .02 min^{-1}; k_P = 30 min^{-1}

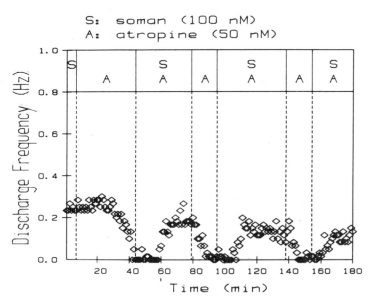

Figure 5. Unmasking a reversible effect of soman in the presence of
atropine. Prior to collecting these data, the preparation was exposed to
100 nM soman for 1 hr, which was sufficient time to make the washouts
ineffective in changing the frequency of extracellularly recorded
discharges. The application of 50 nM atropine eventually blocked these
discharges. When atropine was present, discharges returned during subsequent re-applications of soman but were abolished upon its washout.

effects of ACh accumulation produced by soman's anti-ChE effect, yet
atropine at this concentration, did not block all of the soman-induced
discharges. It is important to note that this experiment is analogous to
the in vivo studies of Van Meter et al. (1978), who found that following
the virtually complete block of brain ChE activity, repeated exposures to
sarin or DFP could elicit seizure activity in the EEG pattern.

Ictal-Like and Irregular Discharge Patterns

In addition to the interictal-like discharges induced by DFP and
soman, other patterns of abnormal electrical activity could be generated by
both agents. The discharges depicted in Figure 6A and C are episodes which
typically were more than 1 sec in duration, occurred at relatively low
frequencies (once every 20-30 sec), were composed of individual discharges
occurring at rates above 2 Hz, and were followed by variable periods of
relative inactivity. Based on these characteristics, the events were
operationally defined as being ictal-like in nature and may be related to
the abnormal electrical activity that occurs during a seizure in vivo.
Furthermore, in the experimental results shown, these events were
eliminated during washout and thus represent another type of reversible
discharge pattern generated by an OP. Under identical experimental conditions, PTX did not produce this type of pattern.

In several experiments with DFP or soman, the interictal-like activity
tended to occur at irregular intervals. This irregular behavior was seen
most dramatically with high concentrations of soman (10 μM; Figure 7A).
Paradoxically, washout produced an enhancement of the discharge frequency.
Prolonged washouts (2 hr) did not alter this frequency. This irregular
discharge frequency may reflect a desynchronized state of the neurons
within this region of the hippocampus, since small, unit-like discharges
emerging from the baseline noise were present during the apparent silent
periods between the large population discharges. Again, the irregular
discharge pattern represents a reversible OP-induced epileptiform effect,
and one that is not commonly observed with the PTX class of convulsants.

DISCUSSION

Using an in vitro CNS preparation, this study has enabled us to
characterize, for the first time, spontaneously occurring epileptiform
activity produced by two OP anti-ChEs: DFP and soman. Both agents produced
a wide spectrum of epileptiform events, ranging from brief (25-150 msec)
interictal-like discharges to ictal-like episodes lasting 1-10 sec. The
existence of these episodes can be exploited in this experimental system to
provide more information concerning the mechanisms responsible for the
development of more sustained epileptiform activity.

The suggestion that a large excitatory synaptic response was the event
underlying the penicillin-induced PDS (Ayala et al., 1973) has received
considerable support from direct measurements of synaptic current and
conductance (Johnston and Brown, 1981). The basis for the interictal-like
discharges produced by both OPs examined was shown to be a postsynaptic
potential consisting of both excitatory and inhibitory components. Similar
conclusions have been drawn concerning discharges induced by 4-AP or by
solutions containing high levels of potassium (Rutecki et al., 1984 and in
press).

Two groups of observations suggest that these OPs act in a manner
distinct from convulsants such as PTX in producing the interictal-like
response. First, both OP agents induced PDSs having substantially more

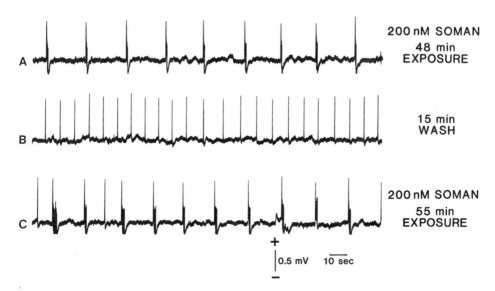

Figure 6. Induction of ictal-like discharges by soman. A: in the presence
of 200 nM soman, these episodes were 2-3 sec in duration, occurred at
relatively slow rates (ca. 1/20 sec), and were associated with intra-
discharge frequencies greater than 2 Hz. B: during washout, these episodes
were eliminated. Note that the interictal-like discharges were still
present during this washout. C: ictal-like discharges returned with re-
exposure to soman.

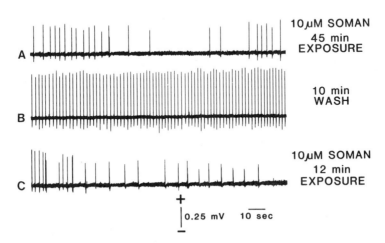

Figure 7. Irregularly occurring discharges induced by a high concentration
of soman. A and C: 10 μM soman induced irregular spontaneous extracellular
activity. B: during washout of soman, the discharge frequency increased
and became more regular.

negative reversal potentials than the PTX class of convulsants. This difference in measured values was eliminated when PTX was co-applied with DFP, a finding strongly suggesting that inhibitory synaptic transmission was present during exposure to the OP alone. Second, neither DFP nor soman abolished spontaneously occurring IPSPs. Whether these agents exert any consistent effect on inhibitory synaptic transmission and whether the difference in measured reversal potentials associated with DFP and soman is significant remain to be determined. The cellular mechanisms generating the longer lasting events (Figure 6) may also involve a synaptic component (Rutecki, unpublished observation).

The extracellular recordings demonstrated that some of the OP-induced epileptiform activity was affected by washouts of the agent used. The sequential kinetic scheme, based on its failure to predict the progressive, irreversible decline in ChE activity, cannot account for the initially reversible phase of OP-induced epileptiform activity. The existence of these time-dependent, reversible components of epileptiform activity produced by DFP and soman suggests that in addition to the irreversible blockade of ChE and the presumed accumulation of ACh, direct, reversible effects of these agents may be important in generating the observed epileptiform responses (Kuba et al., 1974).

Previous experiments by our group have demonstrated that a similar variety of abnormal electrical discharges can be elicited by drugs that are known to block one or more different types of potassium channels, e.g., 4-AP and tetraethylammonium. It has been suggested that ACh mediates excitatory activity in the hippocampus by reducing a steady potassium current (Krnjevic et al., 1971; Bernardo and Prince, 1981; Halliwell and Adams, 1982; Cole and Nicoll, 1983). Based on these earlier studies, we developed the hypothesis that the OPs, in addition to their well-known anti-ChE mechanism, produce some of their reversible convulsant effects by blocking one or more of these types of potassium channels. Further testing of this hypothesis is now being conducted.

ACKNOWLEDGMENTS

The authors thank Judy Walker, who conducted the biochemical analyses and provided skillful artwork, and Hau Ton for his technical assistance. This work was supported by USAMRDC DAMD-17-82-C-2254, the Grass Foundation, and NIH grant NS11535.

REFERENCES

Aldridge, W. N., 1953, The inhibition of erythrocyte cholinesterase by tri-esters of phosphoric acid. 3. The nature of the inhibitory process, Biochem. J., 54:442-448.

Andersen, P., and Langmoen, I. A., 1980, Intracellular studies on transmitter effects on neurones in isolated brain slices, Q. Rev. Biophys., 13:1-18.

Ayala, G. F., Dichter, M., Gumnit, R. J., Matsumoto, H., and Spencer, W. A., 1973, Genesis of epileptic interictal spikes. New knowledge of cortical feedback systems suggests a neurophysiological explanation of brief paroxysms, Brain Res., 52:1-17.

Bernardo, L. S., and Prince, D. A., 1981, Acetylcholine induced modulation of hippocampal pyramidal neurons, Brain Res., 211:227-234.

Brimblecombe, R. W., 1974, "Drug Actions on Cholinergic Systems," University Park Press, Baltimore.

Brown, D. A., and Adams, P. R., 1980, Muscarinic suppression of a novel voltage-sensitive K^+ current in a vertebrate neurone, Nature, 283:673-676.

Brown, T. H., and Johnston, D., 1983, Voltage-clamp analysis of mossy fiber synaptic input to hippocampal neurons, J. Neurophysiol., 50:487-507.

Cole, A. E., and Nicoll, R. A., 1983, Acetylcholine mediates a slow synaptic potential in hippocampal pyramidal cells, Science, 221:1299-1301.

Dingledine, R., and Gjerstad, L., 1980, Reduced inhibition during epileptiform activity in the in vitro hippocampal slice, J. Physiol. (Lond.), 305:297-313.

Ellin, R. I., 1982, Anomalies in theories and therapy of intoxication by potent organophosphorus anticholinesterase compounds, Gen. Pharmacol., 13:457-466.

Ellman, G. L., Courtney, K. D., Andres, V., and Featherstone, R. M., 1961, A new and rapid colorimetric determination of acetylcholinesterase activity, Biochem. Pharmacol., 7:88-95.

Haas, H. L., Schaerer, B., and Vosmansky, M., 1979, A simple perfusion chamber for the study of nervous tissue slices in vitro, J. Neurosci. Meth., 1:323-325.

Halliwell, J. V., and Adams, P. R., 1982, Voltage-clamp analysis of muscarinic excitation in hippocampal neurons, Brain Res., 250:71-92.

Hampson, J. L., Essig, C. F., McCauley, A., and Himwich, H. E., 1950, Effects of di-isopropyl fluorophosphate (DFP) on electroencephalogram and cholinesterase activity, Electroencephalogr. Clin. Neurophysiol., 2:41-48.

Harwood, C. T., 1954, Cholinesterase activity and electroencephalograms during circling induced by the intracarotid injection of di-isopropyl fluorophosphate (DFP), Amer. J. Physiol., 177:171-174.

Johnston, D., 1981, Passive cable properties of hippocampal CA3 neurons, Cell. Mol. Neurobiol., 1:45-55.

Johnston, D., and Brown, T. H., 1981, Giant synaptic potential hypothesis for epileptiform activity, Science, 211:294-297.

Johnston, D., and Brown, T. H., 1984, Biophysics and microphysiology of synaptic transmission in hippocampus, in: "Brain Slices," R. Dingledine, ed., Plenum, New York.

Johnston, D., Hablitz, J. J., and Wilson, W. A., 1980, Voltage clamp discloses slow inward current in hippocampal burst-firing neurones, Nature, 286:391-393.

Johnston, D., Rutecki, P. A., and Lebeda, F. J., Synaptic events underlying spontaneous and evoked paroxysmal discharges in hippocampal neurons, Plenum, New York, (in press).

Karczmar, A. G., 1967, Pharmacologic, toxicologic, and therapeutic properties of anticholinesterase agents, in: "Physiological Pharmacology," W. C. Root, and F. G. Hoffman, eds., Part C, Vol. 3, Academic Press, New York.

Krnjevic, K., Pumain, R., and Renaud, L., 1971, The mechanism of excitation by acetylcholine in the cerebral cortex, J. Physiol. (Lond.), 215:247-268.

Krnjevic, K., Randic, M., and Straughan, D. W., 1966, Pharmacology of cortical inhibition, J. Physiol. (Lond.), 184:78-105.

Kuba, K., Albuquerque, E. X., Daly, J., and Barnard, E. A., 1974, A study of the irreversible cholinesterase inhibitor, diisopropylfluorophosphate, on time course of endplate currents in frog sartorius muscle, J. Pharmacol. Exp. Ther., 189:499-512.

Lebeda, F. J., Hablitz, J. J., and Johnston, D., 1982, Antagonism of GABA-induced responses by d-tubocurarine in hippocampal neurons, J. Neurophysiol., 48:622-632.

Lebeda, F. J., Rutecki, P. A., and Johnston, D., 1983, Synaptic mechanisms action of convulsion-producing anticholinesterases, Def. Tech. Info. Center, DA-300017, Alexandria, Virginia.

Lebeda, F. J., and Rutecki, P. A, 1985, Characterization of spontaneous epileptiform discharges induced by organophosphorus anticholinesterases in the in vitro rat hippocampus, Proc. West. Pharmacol. Soc., 28:187-190.

Lipp, J. A., 1972, Effect of diazepam upon soman-induced seizure activity and convulsions, Electroencephalogr. Clin. Neurophysiol., 32:557-560.

Lowry, O. H., Rosebrough, N. J., Farr, A. L., and Randall, R. J., 1951, Protein measurement with Folin phenol reagent, J. Biol. Chem., 193:265-275.

Machne, X., and Unna, K. R. W., 1963, Actions at the central nervous system, in: "Cholinesterases and Anticholinesterases," G.B. Koelle, ed., (Handbuch der Experimentellen Pharmakologie, Vol. 15), Springer-Verlag, Berlin.

Main, A. R., 1964, Affinity and phosphorylation constants for the inhibition of esterases by organophosphates, Science, 144:992-993.

Matsumoto, H., and Ajmone Marsan, C., 1964, Cortical cellular phenomena in experimental epilepsy: interictal manifestations, Exp. Neurol., 9:286-304.

O'Neill, J. J., 1981, Non-cholinesterase effects of anticholinesterases, Fundam. Appl. Pharmacol., 1:154-160.

Rump, S., Grudzinska, E., and Edelwejn, Z., 1973, Effects of diazepam on epileptiform patterns of bioelectrical activity of the rabbit's brain induced by fluostigmine, Neuropharmacology, 12:813-817.

Rutecki, P. A., Lebeda, F. J., and Johnston, D., 1984, Elevated extracellular potassium- and 4-aminopyridine-induced epileptiform activity in CA3 hippocampal neurons, Soc. Neurosci. Abstr., 10:1.

Rutecki, P. A., Lebeda, F. J., and Johnston, D., Epileptiform activity induced by changes in extracellular potassium in the hippocampus, J. Neurophysiol. (in press).

Schwartzkroin, P. A., and Prince, D. A., 1980, Changes in excitatory and inhibitory synaptic potentials leading to epileptogenic activity, Brain Res., 183:61-73.

Valentino, R. J., and Dingledine, R., 1981, Presynaptic inhibitory effect of acetylcholine in the hippocampus, J. Neurosci., 1:784-792.

Van Meter, W. G., Karczmar, A. G., and Fiscus, R. R., 1978, CNS effects of anti-cholinesterases in the presence of inhibited cholinesterases, Arch. Int. Pharmacodyn., 231:249-260.

Yamamoto, C., 1972, Intracellular study of seizure-like afterdischarges elicited in thin hippocampal sections in vitro, Exp. Neurol., 35:154-164.

MIPAFOX - INHIBITOR OF CHOLINESTERASE, NEUROTOXIC ESTERASE, AND DFP-ASE:

IS THERE A "MIPAFOX-ASE"?

Francis C.G. Hoskin,[a] Elwyn T. Reese,[b] and William J. Smith[b]

Biology Department[a]
Illinois Institute of Technology
Chicago, IL 60616
      and
Science and Advanced Technology Laboratory[b]
U.S. Army Natick Research and Development Center
Natick, MA 01760

INTRODUCTION

In 1946 there was published both the synthesis of the archetypal organophosphorus cholinesterase inhibitor, DFP,[1] and the finding of an enzyme that hydrolyzes and thus detoxifies this compound.[2] In 1963, in the same landmark volume to which Karczmar contributed two chapters on particular aspects of the acetylcholine system often elucidated by the use of DFP,[3,4] Mounter[5] reviewed the subject that has come to be known as "DFPase". While a relationship of a compound that is an inhibitor of cholinesterase to an enzyme that hydrolyzes that compound will be self-

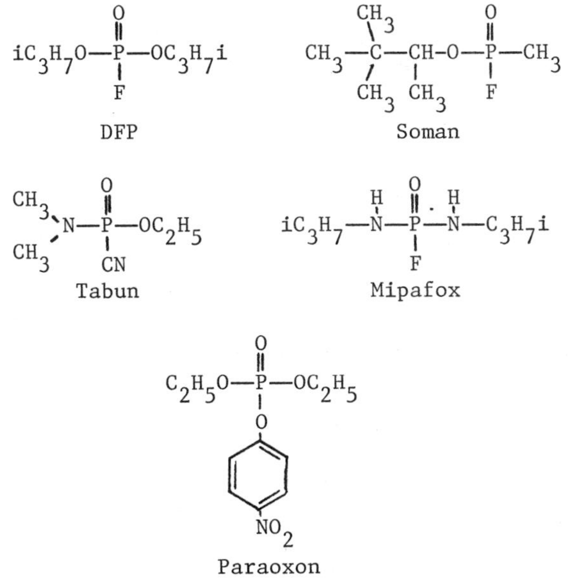

$$iC_3H_7O-\underset{\underset{F}{|}}{\overset{\overset{O}{\|}}{P}}-OC_3H_7i$$

DFP

$$CH_3-\underset{\underset{CH_3}{|}}{\overset{\overset{CH_3}{\diagdown}}{C}}-\underset{\underset{CH_3}{|}}{CH}-O-\underset{\underset{F}{|}}{\overset{\overset{O}{\|}}{P}}-CH_3$$

Soman

$$\underset{CH_3}{\overset{CH_3}{\diagup}}N-\underset{\underset{CN}{|}}{\overset{\overset{O}{\|}}{P}}-OC_2H_5$$

Tabun

$$iC_3H_7-\underset{\overset{H}{|}}{N}-\underset{\underset{F}{|}}{\overset{\overset{O}{\|}}{P}}-\underset{\overset{H}{|}}{N}-C_3H_7i$$

Mipafox

$$C_2H_5O-\underset{\underset{O}{|}}{\overset{\overset{O}{\|}}{P}}-OC_2H_5$$

Paraoxon

Fig. 1. Compounds referred to in text.

evident, every imaginable aspect of the one enzyme is either understood or under study, whereas the other enzyme, seemingly without natural substrate or physiological role, may require some introduction.

To encapsulate what was known in this latter area to about 1963, there is a so-called DFPase that also hydrolyzes the P-F bond of some phosphate and phosphonate structural analogues, and even the P-CN bond of Tabun (see Fig. 1). The enzyme displays a degree of stereospecificity with appropriate substrates. It is widely distributed, but in somewhat better than average levels in mammalian kidney and in certain microorganisms. The DFPase from these various sources is rather unstable, especially in ammonium sulfate, thus requiring for purification an initial cold ethanol precipitation. The enzymatic activity is stimulated several-fold by Mn^{++} at about 10^{-3} M. Finally, although the significance would not be appreciated for another decade, a comparison of data from several sources would have shown that this DFPase, despite the name, hydrolyzes Tabun much faster than DFP (for practical reasons, now Soman much faster than DFP). This is the enzyme that we have now begun to term "Mazur type DFPase"[6] in recognition of its discoverer.[2]

While DFPase has been studied in several laboratories since the 1963 review,[5] 1966 marked the quite unexpected finding of a high level of DFPase in the axoplasm of the squid giant axon.[7] The subsequent use of Tabun for neurophysiological reasons,[8] and the finding of a much higher rate of hydrolysis of DFP than of Tabun by the squid enzyme,[8,9] although again not appreciated at the time, eventually suggested two distinctly different DFPases. The results of another decade of work were recently reviewed,[6] and are further condensed and presented here.

In addition to the Mazur type DFPase, there is also a "squid type DFPase", as we have termed this enzyme for some time now. It hydrolyzes DFP much faster than Soman (originally Tabun, but changed for practical reasons), is indifferent to or even slightly inhibited by Mn^{++}, is narrowly distributed in cephalopod nerve, hepatopancreas, and saliva,[10] and is absent from or masked by the Mazur type DFPase in other vertebrate and invertebrate tissues, even including other squid tissues.[11] Squid type DFPase is extremely stable, is easily purified by ammonium sulfate precipitation and subsequent column procedures, and has a molecular weight of 26,600 in contrast to Mazur type DFPase, variously reported between 45,000 and 65,000.

Now recently a new criterion has emerged for distinguishing between Mazur type and squid type DFPase - one that must reflect fundamental differences in the active sites of these two enzymes. Mipafox, a phosphordiamide (Fig. 1) markedly inhibits the enzymatic hydrolysis of DFP or Soman by Mazur type DFPase, but is without effect on squid type DFPase[12] (see Fig. 2), this despite the more rapid hydrolysis of Tabun, a phosphormonoamide, by Mazur type DFPase than by the squid enzyme.[9] Mipafox is not hydrolyzed by either enzyme, as can also be seen in Fig. 2. By way of background, Mipafox is also a cholinesterase inhibitor[13] of a degree and specificity to have recommended it as an insecticide. Unfortunately, from its earliest (and thus limited) use for that purpose, Mipafox was also implicated in a more slowly developing nerve degeneration[14] attributable to its interaction with "neurotoxic esterase", an enzyme characterized analytically by its hydrolysis of phenyl phenylacetate or phenyl valerate, its resistance to inhibition by paraoxon, and its inhibition by Mipafox.[15]

With these various properties, especially the inhibition of cholinesterase by DFP and the inhibition of DFPase by Mipafox, it is not surprising that a marked increase in toxicity over what might have been expected on an additive basis has been found for combinations of these two.[16] At a

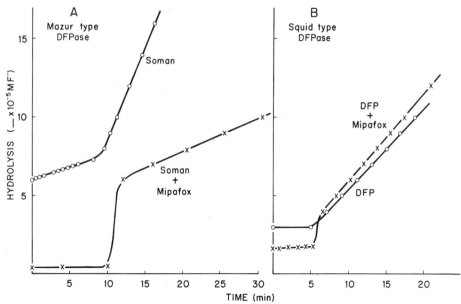

Fig. 2. Effect of Mipafox on the enzymatic hydrolysis of DFP and Soman.
(A) Soman, 0.003 M; Mipafox, 0.001 M; 0.1 ml enzyme purified about
15-fold from hog kidney. Order of addition: (o), Soman, enzyme;
(x), Mipafox, enzyme, Soman. (B) DFP, 0.003 M; Mipafox, 0.003 M;
0.1 ml enzyme purified about 500-fold from squid optic ganglion.
Order of addition: (o), DFP, enzyme; (x), Mipafox, enzyme, DFP.
Final volumes throughout, 5.0 ml; temperature, 23°C. Note that
activities in (A) or (B) are comparable, but not between (A) and
(B). With the permission of Pergamon Press; see ref. 12.

practical level, our finding now of a Mipafox-hydrolyzing enzyme suggests
a means of relief from this potential environmental hazard. However, this
was not the result of a direct search, but rather due to the lack of any
data on possible fungal sources of DFPase, the discovery of a somewhat
unusual phosphodiesterase and a DFPase-like activity in a preparation from
Penicillium funiculosum,[17] and our attempts to characterize this activity
by using Mipafox. The purpose of this introduction has been to review
briefly recent progress on the enzymatic detoxication of cholinesterase
inhibitors. The results to be presented now for the first time describe
the enzymatic detoxication of a DFPase inhibitor, Mipafox, and possible
applications of these findings to the question of a natural substrate and
physiological role for the DFPases.

MATERIALS AND METHODS

The growth of Penicillium funiculosum, purification of the phosphodiesterase and its assay by the use of bis-(p-nitrophenyl) phosphate
(Bis4NPP), assay of DFPase activity by the use of the fluoride-sensitive
electrode, and sources of compounds, either have been described in previous
publications, or are available from our laboratories.[17,18] In order to
make determinations at the lower pH's, one modification has been introduced. The usual DFPase buffer - 400 mM KCl, 50 mM NaCl, 5 mM 1,3-bis-
(tris[hydroxymethyl]methylamino)propane (bis-tris-propane) - was also made
5 mM in acetate, permitting a useful pH range, after adjusting with HCl or
NaOH, of approximately 4 to 7.5 or higher.

RESULTS

The phosphodiesterase preparation (Bis4NPP-hydrolyzing) from <u>Penicil-lium funiculosum</u> hydrolyzed DFP, but not Soman (Fig. 3). This DFPase activity was not Mn^{++} stimulated. Thus, because for the first time there appeared to be a squid type DFPase not of cephalopodic origin, the hydrolysis of DFP was tested in the presence of Mipafox, with an unexpectedly large increase in fluoride release. Thereupon, the phosphodiesterase preparation was tested for its ability to hydrolyze Mipafox. The rate of hydrolysis of Mipafox was much greater than that of DFP, as is also shown in Fig. 3. Both of these activities were heat labile.

In view of the pH optimum of approximately 4 being found for the phosphodiesterase activity[17], this property was determined for the enzymatic hydrolysis of Mipafox and DFP by the <u>Penicillium</u> preparation. The optimum for both substrates was about pH 4 (Fig. 4). The kinetic parameters, K_M and V_{max}, with respect to Mipafox, DFP, and Bis4NPP are presented in Table 1. These values for DFP are approximate because, in view of the high concentrations of this extremely toxic compound that would otherwise have been required, all of the determinations were made at DFP concentrations below the K_M.

Phosphate inhibited the hydrolysis of DFP and of Mipafox (data not shown), as it does also of Bis4NPP,[17] suggesting that the same enzyme hydrolyzes all three compounds. Hydrolysis rates of DFP, of Mipafox, and combinations of the two gave consistent but ambiguous results (neither sums nor averages) probably due to the 10- to 20-fold difference in the K_M's for

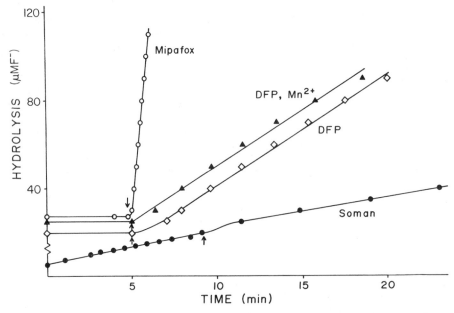

Fig. 3. Release of F^- from Mipafox, DFP, and Soman after addition of a <u>Penicillium funiculosum</u> preparation. Substrate concs., $0.003 \underline{M}$; Mn^{++}, where present, $0.001 \underline{M}$. Reaction volume, 5.0 ml; pH 7.2; 23°C. Arrows show time at which enzyme was added. For clarity, the Soman curve has been displaced downward (see, e.g., Fig. 2). For accuracy of measurement, one-tenth the amount of enzyme preparation was used with Mipafox, but the slope was normalized to reflect the same amount of enzyme in each determination. DFP slope represents 18.7 μmoles DFP hydrolyzed per min and per g protein.

Table 1. Kinetic Constants for the Hydrolytic Action of a <u>Penicillium</u>
<u>funiculosum</u> Preparation on Three Substrates

Substrate	Conditions (pH/°C)	K_M ($\underline{M}$)	V_{max} (μmoles min^{-1} g protein^{-1})
Bis4NPP	4.0/40	1.3×10^{-4}	10,000
Mipafox	4.5/23	1.5×10^{-3}	1,000
DFP	4.5/23	$> 10^{-2}$[a]	< 600[a]

[a]See paragraph 2 of RESULTS for causes of uncertainty.

these two. However, fluoride ion release from DFP and from Mipafox in the
presence or absence of Bis4NPP measures only the hydrolysis of DFP or Mipafox, and similarly the spectrophotometric measurement of p-nitrophenol re-

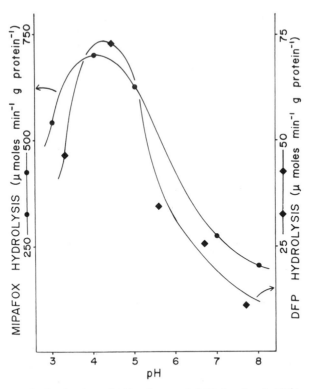

Fig. 4. Enzymatic hydrolysis of Mipafox and DFP by <u>Penicillium funiculosum</u>
preparation as a function of pH. The modification of the usual
bis-tris-propane buffer to accomodate the pH range is described in
MATERIALS AND METHODS. Substrate concs., 0.003 $\underline{M}$. Reaction volume, 5.0 ml; 23°C. Reactions linear over the F$^-$ production range,
$2 \times 10^{-5}\,\underline{M}$ to $12 \times 10^{-5}\,\underline{M}$.

Table 2. Hydrolysis of Mipafox and Bis-(p-Nitrophenyl) Phosphate (Bis4NPP) by a <u>Penicillium funiculosum</u> Preparation[a]

Mipafox (m$\underline{M}$)	Bis4NPP (m$\underline{M}$)	F$^-$ Released	p-Nitrophenol Released
		(μmoles min^{-1} g protein^{-1})	
3	0	500 (500)[b]	
3	1	254 (140)	
3	3	201 (58)	
0	0.43		480 (480)
0.43	0.43		290 (452)
1.67	0.43		250 (386)

[a] Conditions: pH 4.5, 23°C.
[b] Values in parentheses were calculated using K_M's in Table 1 and a simple substrate competition model.[20]

Table 3. Hydrolysis of DFP and Bis-(p-Nitrophenyl) Phosphate (Bis4NPP) by <u>Penicillium funiculosum</u> Preparation[a]

DFP (m$\underline{M}$)	Bis4NPP (m$\underline{M}$)	F$^-$ Released	p-Nitrophenol Released
		(μmoles min^{-1} g protein^{-1})	
3	0	50 (50)[b]	
3	1	16 (7)	
3	3	7 (2)	
0	0.43		480 (480)
0.43	0.43		433 (477)
1.67	0.43		429 (471)
0	0.32		376 (444)
1.25	0.32		331 (437)
2.5	0.32		322 (429)

[a,b] See Table 2.

lease from Bis4NPP in the presence of DFP or Mipafox measures only the hydrolysis of Bis4NPP. The results of these two types of experiments, shown in Tables 2 and 3, while not producing hydrolysis rates exactly as predicted using a simple model,[20] nevertheless are consistent with substrate competition for a single active site.

DISCUSSION

The DFPase activity reported here in <u>Penicillium funiculosum</u> is the first to be found associated with another enzyme, namely, a phosphodiesterase. Although its preferential hydrolysis of DFP relative to Soman, and indifference to Mn^{++}, are characteristic of squid type DFPase, the 10-fold higher rate of hydrolysis of Mipafox than of DFP at equivalent substrate concentrations, the markedly lower pH optimum (compare Fig. 4 and ref. 19), and the 10-fold difference in K_M's seem to suggest yet a different DFPase. The similarity of the pH optima of the Penicillium preparation for all three substrates (Fig. 4 and ref. 17), and especially the reduced rates of hydrolysis of DFP and Bis4NPP, or Mipafox and Bis4NPP, each in the presence of the other (Tables 2 and 3), indicate that the DFP-hydrolyzing and Mipafox-hydrolyzing activities of this Penicillium preparation are due to the phosphodiesterase. Thus the answer to the question originally posed is that there is probably not a "Mipafox-ase".

An additional question may be asked, whether these results have a bearing on squid type or Mazur type DFPase. The differences already cited suggest not. Nevertheless, the still rather poorly understood taxonomic position of the cephalopods, and the finding of what we term Mazur type DFPase in such disparate sources as mammalian kidney and E. coli[6], should encourage a re-examination of these enzymes and the possibility of associated phosphodiesterases with special properties.

While enzymes that degrade toxic organophosphorus compounds may have important practical applications, inhibitors of such enzymes should provide insights into their physiological significance. For example, the role of physostigmine in the elucidation of the neurobiology of acetylcholine is too well known to require citation. In the volume in which Karczmar's contributions have already been noted[3,4] the neurotoxic effects of Mipafox were also well documented,[21] but another decade was required before the relation to the "neurotoxic esterase" was proposed.[14] Now the possibility is raised of using Mipafox to explore the natural function of DFPase. The probable impediments to such an approach have been considered[12]; chief among them is that Mipafox inhibits the ubiquitous Mazur enzyme, whereas an inhibitor of the DFPase present in high levels in that classic neurobiological preparation, the squid giant axon, is not yet available.

ACKNOWLEDGEMENT

This work was partially supported by U.S. Army Research Office grant DAAG29-82-K-0060.

REFERENCES

1. H. McCombie and B.C. Saunders, Alkyl fluorophosphonates: Preparation and physiological properties, Nature (London) 157:287 (1946).
2. A. Mazur, An enzyme in animal tissue capable of hydrolyzing the phosphorus-fluorine bond of alkyl fluorophosphates, J. Biol. Chem. 164: 271 (1946).
3. A.G. Karczmar, Ontogenesis of cholinesterases, in: "Handbuch der Experimentellen Pharmakologie: Cholinesterases and Anticholinesterase Agents", G.B. Koelle, ed., Springer-Verlag, Berlin (1963).
4. A.G. Karczmar, Ontogenetic effects, in: "Handbuch der Experimentellen Pharmakologie: Cholinesterases and Anticholinesterase Agents", G.B. Koelle, ed., Springer-Verlag, Berlin (1963).
5. L.A. Mounter, Metabolism of organophosphorus agents, in: "Handbuch der Experimentellen Pharmakologie: Cholinesterases and Anticholinesterase Agents", G.B. Koelle, ed., Springer-Verlag, Berlin (1963).
6. F.C.G. Hoskin, M.A. Kirkish, and K.E. Steinmann, Two enzymes for the detoxication of organophosphorus compounds - sources, similarities and significance, Fundam. Appl. Toxicol. 4: S165 (1984).
7. F.C.G. Hoskin, P. Rosenberg, and M. Brzin, Re-examination of the effect of DFP on electrical and cholinesterase activity of squid giant axon, Proc. Nat. Acad. Sci. USA 55:1231 (1966).
8. F.C.G. Hoskin, Diisopropylphosphorofluoridate and Tabun: Enzymatic hydrolysis and nerve function, Science 172:1243 (1971).

9. J.M. Garden, S.K. Hause, F.C.G. Hoskin, and A.H. Roush, Comparison of DFP-hydrolyzing enzyme purified from head ganglia and hepatopancreas of squid (Loligo pealei) by means of isoelectric focusing, Comp. Biochem. Physiol. 52C:95 (1975).

10. F.C.G. Hoskin and R.D. Prusch, Characterization of a DFP-hydrolyzing enzyme in squid posterior salivary gland by use of Soman, DFP and manganous ion, Comp. Biochem. Physiol. 75C:17 (1983).

11. F.C.G. Hoskin and K.E. Steinmann, The detoxication of organophosphorus compounds: A tale of two enzymes - or are there more? in "Proceedings of the International Conference on Environmental Hazards of Agrochemicals in Developing Countries", A.H. El Sebae, ed., University of Alexandria, Egypt (1983).

12. F.C.G. Hoskin, Inhibition of a Soman- and diisopropyl phosphorofluoridate (DFP)-detoxifying enzyme by Mipafox, Biochem. Pharmacol. 34:2069 (1985).

13. W.N. Aldridge, The differentiation of true and pseudo cholinesterase by organo-phosphorus compounds, Biochem. J. 53:62 (1953).

14. M.K. Johnson, The primary biochemical lesion leading to the delayed neurotoxic effects of some organophosphorus esters, J. Neurochem. 23:785 (1974).

15. R.J. Richardson, C.S. Davis, and M.K. Johnson, Subcellular distribution of marker enzymes and of neurotoxic esterase in adult hen brain, J. Neurochem. 32:607 (1979).

16. R.C. Gupta and W.-D. Dettbarn, Iso-OMPA and Mipafox induced potentiation of toxicity and prevention of tolerance development to subchronic DFP administration, Fed. Proc. 44:1628, Abstr. No. 7123 (1985).

17. E.T. Reese, J.E. Walker, and D.H. Ball, Extracellular phosphodiesterase of Penicillium funiculosum, ms. submitted, personal communication.

18. F.C.G. Hoskin and A.H. Roush, Hydrolysis of nerve gas by squid-type diisopropyl phosphorofluoridate hydrolyzing enzyme on agarose resin, Science 215:1255 (1982).

19. F.C.G. Hoskin and R.J. Long, Purification of a DFP-hydrolyzing enzyme from squid head ganglion, Arch. Biochem. Biophys. 150:548 (1972).

20. M. Dixon and E.C. Webb, "Enzymes", Academic Press, New York (1979).

21. D.R. Davies, Neurotoxicity of organophosphorus compounds, in: "Handbuch der Experimentellen Pharmakologie: Cholinesterases and Anticholinesterase Agents", G.B. Koelle, ed., Springer-Verlag, Berlin (1963).

22. D.F. Heath, The effects of substituents on the rates of hydrolysis of some organophosphorus compounds. Part I. Rates in alkaline solution, J. Chem. Soc. 3796 (1956).

ADDENDUM

Mipafox synthesized by one of us (F.C.G.H.) by the method of Heath[22], with additional washings and a final vacuum sublimation, has been determined by NMR to be essentially 100% pure. The Mipafox used in the research reported in the body of this paper, purchased from another source[12], appears to be less than 50% pure. With the pure material, we now find no evidence of Mipafox hydrolysis by Penicillium funiculosum at pH 4.3 or 7, but continue to find a DFPase-like activity, i.e., DFP hydrolysis, as shown in Figs. 3 and 4. While the DFPase-like activity continues to parallel that of a phosphodiesterase, the parts of this paper purporting to present new findings involving Mipafox should now be regarded with reservation. The inhibition of Mazur type but not of squid type DFPase[12], also given in Fig. 2, is still found with the high purity material. Details substantiating this addendum, including quantitative corrections of enzyme kinetics, will be submitted for publication in the near future. We hope that the publication of the addendum will help to correct the questionable parts of the oral presentation of this material.

ORGANOPHOSPHATE POISONING AND ITS TREATMENT BY OXIMES

P.G. Waser, C.G. Caratsch, A. Chang Sin-Ren, W.
Hopff, A. Gotheil, E. Kaiser, R. Sammet, and
C. Streichenberg

Institute of Pharmacology, University of Zürich
Gloriastr. 32, CH - 8006 Zürich

In our last report in Oglebay Park (Waser et al., 1983)
we described the poisoning of animals with ^{14}C-labeled
sarin and its kinetics. We demonstrated the low antitoxic
activity of pralidoxime and obidoxime injected 2 - 60 minutes after the poisoning, but causing a marked decrease of
radioactivity when injected 20 minutes before ^{14}C-sarin. We
will report here on the kinetics and distribution of another
organophosphate, ^{32}P-diisopropyl-fluorophosphonate (DFP)
(phosphofluoridic acid bis (1-methylethyl) ester) in mice.
The interaction between sarin and obidoxime or pralidoxime
(2-PAM) will be described, and possible mechanisms of reactivation of the phosphorylated enzyme, or of antagonising
the overflowing acetylcholine will be discussed.

For this purpose we synthesized several labeled and un-
labeled compounds (fig. 1) which are used in this study.

The methods used are wholebody autoradiography (WBA) or
liquid scintillation counting (LSC) of radioactivity in
organ samples. In biochemical experiments the activity of
acetylcholinesterase was measured with the pH-stat method.
The animals used are albino rats and mice of a breeding
institution for specific pathogen free animals (Inst. of
Veterinary Medicine, University of Zürich).

1. Kinetics of ^{14}-C-Sarin

^{14}C-sarin (fig. 1) enters the brain of rats and mice
very rapidly after an intravenous injection (Sammet, 1983;
Waser et al., 1983). After 20 - 30 seconds the whole central
nervous system (CNS), is overflooded with radioactivity,
which later diminishes after 5 - 30 minutes. There is a very
high activity in the kidneys, the adrenal cortex, the lungs
and less in the liver. The peak concentration in most other
organs was reached within a minute. Later all organs within
one hour diminish their radioactivity to one third. Sarin

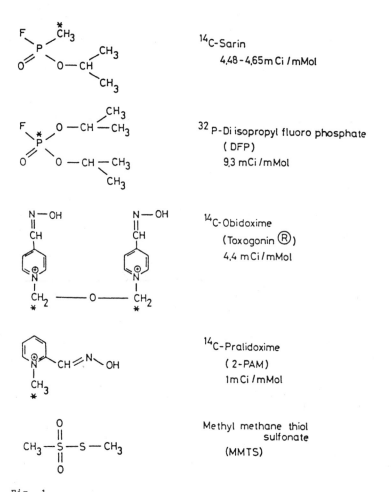

Fig. 1
Structural Formulas of synthesized compounds, asterisk: radioactive atom.

and its metabolites are eliminated mostly through the kidneys and the lungs. The plasma halflife time must be well
over one hour. Liver, bile and elimination into the intestines are not prominent.

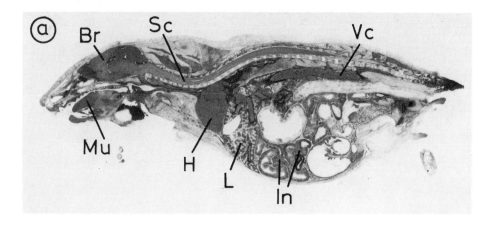

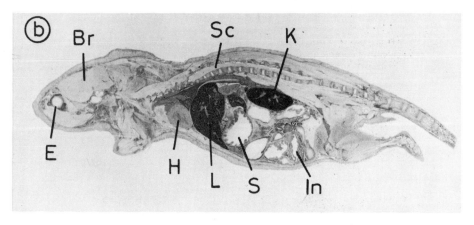

Fig. 2 a
Wholebody autoradiography of mouse section (20 μ), 2 minutes
after i.v. injection of 1.5 mg/kg ^{14}C-sarin: Strong radioactivity in brain, spinal cord, heart, blood, liver (center
of lobules), spleen, intestines, urinary tract.

Fig. 2 b
Mouse with i.v. 1.5 mg/kg ^{14}C-sarin and 1 minute later i.v.
50 mg/kg obidoxime. Evidently less radioactivity in brain
and spinal cord than in Fig. 2 a), more in liver and kidney.

Abbreviations in figures:

A	aorta	L	liver
Ag	adrenal gland	Mu	muscle
Bm	bone marrow	Oe	oesophagus
Br	brain	Sc	spinal cord
E	eye	Sg	salivary gland
H	heart	Sp	spleen
Id	intervertebral discs	St	sternum
In	intestines	Ub	urinary bladder
K	kidney	Vc	vena cava

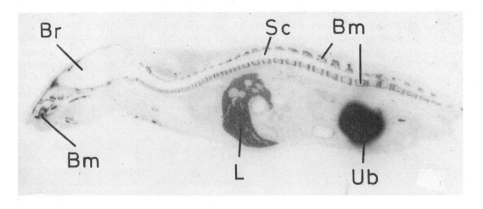

Fig. 3
Autoradiography of mouse section (20 μ) 180 minutes after
i.v. injection of 3.4 mg/kg ^{32}P-DFP. Little radioactivity in
brain and spinal cord, plenty in liver urinary bladder and
some in bone marrow of spine and skull.

2. Distribution of ^{32}P-Diisopropylfluorophosphonate (DFP) in mice

Five minutes after intravenous injection the blood
contains a high radioactivity (Gotheil, 1978). A similar
amount is found in the lungs and cardiac muscle, but a
higher amount in the liver, without any concentration in the
bile or gall bladder. The intestines remain empty over 180
minutes. Urine in kidney pelvis and bladder are strongly,
brain and spinalcord only slightly radioactive (fig. 3). Ten
minutes later the blood and other organs remain unchanged.
Skeletal muscles and especially bones increase their radioactivity within the next 20 minutes. The distribution does
not change much after one to three hours except a slow decrease of general radioactivity in the organs and a further
increase in all bones containing marrow. Even in pregnant
mice the placenta lets radioactivity pass into the fetuses, where it is concentrated again in the spine and
liver.

Elimination is achieved mostly through the kidneys and
the urine and only minimally in the bile.

The interaction of DFP with an oxime and its changes in
distribution were not investigated, as we concentrated our
efforts mainly on sarin-poisoning.

3. Kinetics of ^{14}C-Pralidoxime

The distribution of ^{14}C-pralidoxime (2-PAM) (fig. 1) in
the mouse is very fast (Gotheil, 1978). 5 minutes after the
intravenous injection the blood contains already a low activity compared to the liver and the kidneys. The halflife

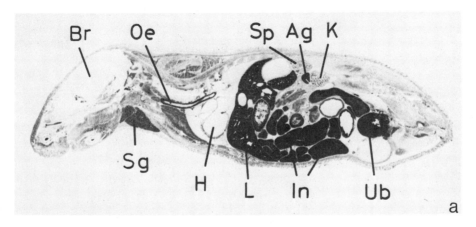

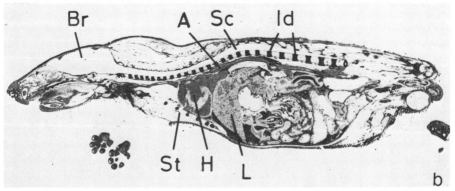

Fig. 4 a
Distribution of 2-PAM in mouse 30 minutes after i.v. injection (75 mg/kg). Brain and spinal cord empty, radioactivity mainly in liver, intestines (bile), urinary bladder and kidney, small amount in salivary gland, no radioactivity in blood (heart) and lungs.

Fig. 4 b
Distribution of ^{14}C-obidoxime in rat 30 minutes after i.v. injection (0.1 g/kg). Brain and spinal cord empty! Radioactivity mainly in heart-blood, intervertebral discs and sternum.

time in the blood plasma was found to be 18 minutes, in the liver 26 minutes (fig. 4 a). Most of the compound is immediately eliminated through the kidneys, but the uptake into the liver points to its metabolic activity and elimination with the bile. The feces in the intestine become increasingly radioactive, and after 1 - 3 hours elimination through kidneys and bile are equal. After 24 hours the radioactive compounds have left the animal body.

4. ^{14}C-Obidoxime distribution and kinetics in rats and mice

^{14}C-obidoxime (fig. 1) 5 - 20 minutes after intravenous injection is concentrated mostly in the kidneys and then eliminated in the urine (Streichenberg, 1984). The plasma concentration diminishes regularly with halflife times of 10 and 60 minutes. A lower concentration is found in the liver and the spleen. A remarkably high concentration is in the intervertebral discs and in the cartilage of skull and bones, as ribs and sternum. Most important is the fact that the CNS remains empty of radioactivity even after 60 minutes (fig. 4b). Obidoxime cannot cross the blood brain barrier, and we found only smallest traces of radioactivity in the cerebrospinal fluid. The metabolism is being investigated now, but as the high water solubility of the bisquaternary molecule causes a rapid elimination through the kidneys only small amounts are entering the liver tissue for degradation, as its relatively low radioactivity predicts.

The placental barrier prevents the transport of obidoxime to the fetuses, but after 90 minutes parallel to an increase in liver activity there is a small concentration in the liver of the fetuses, which might be due to radioactive metabolites.

5. Interaction of Sarin with 2-PAM and Obidoxime

As already demonstrated in Oglebay Park (Waser et al., 1983), obidoxime has a preventive effect on sarin poisoning when given 20 minutes before the injection of the organophosphate. The ^{14}C-concentration of sarin in the brain is lowered 30 seconds after injection of a 20 times overdose, and even more some minutes and up to 60 minutes later. The excretion through the kidneys and liver-bile system is increased, and the concentration in the blood lowered. But the injection of obidoxime one minute after sarin has a much smaller effect, and even less 5 minutes after the sarin injection (Fig. 2). On the other hand the concentration of ^{14}C-obidoxime's in the brain was not changed by sarin injected one minute before. This means that sarin induces no rapid change of the blood-brain barrier, which might be the prerequisite for obidoximes antitoxic action. Again the radioactivity in liver, heart, muscle, and blood was increased, pointing to an interaction outside of the CNS.

When ^{14}C-PAM is injected 5 minutes after the application of sarin, a similar effect is observed (Gotheil, 1978). The radioactivity was increased 10 and 30 minutes later in the liver, lungs, kidneys, cartilage and mucosa of intestines compared to ^{14}C-PAM alone. Lower activities were found in some other organs as the spleen, heart and skelettal muscle and the bile. In the brain and spinal cord there was a slight increase after 10 minutes, and a remarkable doubling of radioactivity after 30 minutes. Main elimination was again through the kidneys and only small amounts with the bile. As ^{14}C-PAM is only slightly demethylated, the tertiary and other metabolites might be entering the brain after half an hour. Sarin might have reacted with 2-PAM giving an unstable phosphorylated oxime with inhibitor activity. The complex might be eliminated more easily through the kidneys removing sarin from the tissues.

6. Effects of Obidoxime on native and Sarin-poisoned frog neuromuscular junctions

The action of obidoxime was studied on single frog neuromuscular junctions (Caratsch and Waser, 1984). The iontophoretic application demonstrated a weak direct depolarizing effect and furthermore a potentiating effect on the acetylcholine-induced depolarization (fig. 5). This effect is only present, when AChE activity of the muscle preparation is normal. When sarin (10^{-6} M) is added to the preparation, the peak in the ACh-induced depolarization is potentiated, but after giving a preceding pulse of obidoxime it is reduced (fig. 6). Obidoxime therefore has a double action. It is a partial agonist of the cholinergic receptor and an antagonist of the AChE. When obidoxime is kept in contact with the synapse for a longer time (300 msec) then the potentiation of the ACh-effect is reversed to an antagonistic effect by reducing the sensitivity of the receptor towards acetylcholine.

Similar results were obtained by investigating the miniature endplate potentials which are produced spontaneously and do not need the interference of other substances to elicit them. These potentials are strongly amplified and prolonged by adding sarin (10^{-6}M) to the bath solution.

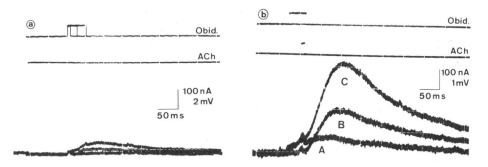

Fig. 5 a
Effect of iontophoretical application of three subsequent obidoxime pulses on a single frog endplate showing a direct depolarization of the cholinergic receptors (Caratsch and Waser, 1984).

Fig. 5 b
Effect of iontophoretical application of acetylcholine and obidoxime on a single endplate. A: effect of obidoxime alone, B: effect of acetylcholine alone, C: combined effect of both substances together.

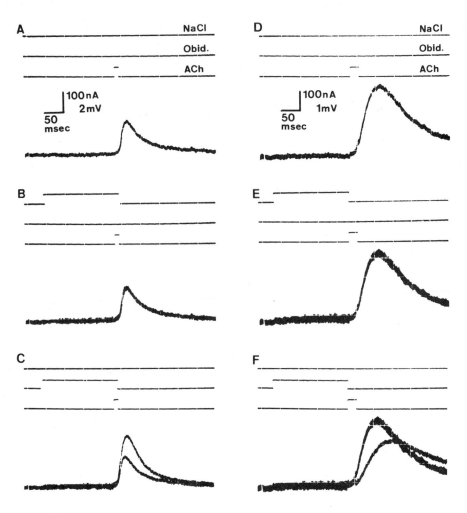

Fig. 6
Effect of acetylcholine, NaCl and obidoxime applied iontophoretically to a single endplate. A to C before adding
sarin to the bath. A: acetylcholine pulse alone (see top
traces), B: preceding NaCl-pulse and ACh pulse with same
response, C: preceding obidoxime pulse with potentiation of
ACh-response; D to F with sarin (10^{-6}M), D and E similar to
A and B but potentiated by blocked acetylcholinesterase, F:
with preceding obidoxime reduction of ACh response by partial antagonism on receptor.

Obidoxime (10^{-5}M) had only a slight action in reducing these
effects, but when injected in concentrated form the antagonist effect was strong for a short time. In conclusion it
seems that obidoxime in the concentration used shows only a
weak reactivation of the poisoned AChE and that a part of
its possible therapeutic effect may be due to its "curare-
like" inhibiton and protection of the cholinergic receptor.

This hypothesis was already put forward by Amitai et al. (1980) and Fossier et al. (1983).

7. Reactivation of Acetylcholinesterase in vitro or antagonism against Sarin-poisoning by Atropine in vivo

Many scientists and clinicians know by own experiences that a reactivation of poisoned AChE by oximes in vivo and in vitro is mostly disappointing. The doubtful effect may be caused by several influences and conditions. The best direct test is probably the in vitro reactivation of AChE, which has been blocked to 100 % by incubation with sarin. For this experiment purified AChE in solution was incubated with sarin and passed through a Sephadex column in order to remove the excess of sarin (Hopff et al., 1984a). After the elution the stoichiometrically blocked enzyme was checked with a pH-stat (Metrohm, CH 9300 Herisau, Switzerland). The enzyme activity was zero. At pH 7.4 autotitration with 0.01 M sodiumhydroxide solution showed that obidoxime added in different concentrations was slow and insufficient for reactivation (table 1). The maximal tolerated i.v. dose for man (250 mg/70 kg) gives a concentration in the total body water corresponding roughly to 5 - 10 μM, the lowest in vitro concentrations. A high concentration (100 μM) can reactivate 20 % of the enzyme, estimated to be necessary for normal physiological activity of the synapses, but only after 3 hours of incubation.

Table 1

Reactivation of AChE inhibited by sarin.

Stoichiometrically inactivated enzyme. At 0-time obidoxime in the adequate dose was added.

Time	5 μM Obidoxime Activity	10 μM Obidoxime Activity	100 μM Obidoxime Activity
0	0	0	0
30 sec	1.1	1.1	4.5
1 min	1.4	2.1	6.1
5 min	1.5	1.6	5.5
15 min	1.4	1.7	7.2
30 min	1.7	1.8	7.8
1 hr	1.9	2.2	9.4
2 hr	2.2	3.1	12.8
3 hr	2.3	3.9	20.0
4 hr	3.1	4.7	23.9
18 hr	5.8	11.7	37.8

The enzyme activity was calculated in % of the non-inhibited starting values.

Table 2

Groups of 6 guinea pigs were injected with sarin s.c. in the neck and obidoxime/atropine or benactyzine i.p. immediately after sarin. All doses in mg/kg.

Sarin	Obidoxime	Atropine	Benactyzine	Lethality
0.075	–	–	–	2/6
0.075	15	15	–	4/6
0.500	–	–	–	6/6
0.500	15	15	–	4/6
0.500	24	8	–	6/6
0.500	24	–	10	2/6
1.000	–	–	–	6/6
1.000	24	15	–	4/6
2.000	24	15	–	6/6
2.000	24	–	10	6/6

As it is apparent from the dosages of 0.5 and 1.0 mg/kg that control animals would have died, the experiments with 2.0 mg/kg were carried out without control animals.

This effect is better in reactivation of insecticide organophosphate-inhibited enzyme, but much worse in soman-treated acetylcholinesterase and animals.

Evidently other mechanisms for antitoxic action in nerve gas poisoning must be found. The use of atropine, the anticholinergic drug occupying muscarinic receptors, is of great importance, but is of no value for blocking the nicotinic receptors. It is interesting, that in animal experiments the combination of obidoxime with atropine has a beneficial protective action against sarin poisoning, which is even increased, when atropine is replaced by benactyzine (table 2). This compound, first used for its tranquilizing action, is approximately one fifth as potent as atropine on muscarinic receptors, but seems to be more selective on central nervous systems in doses producing little peripheral side effects. Its chemical structure furthermore points to a blocking action on nicotinic receptors, which might be an interesting lead for its antitoxic action against nerve gas poisoning. Excessive muscular relaxation in patients has been noted. This effect may be explained by block of the endplates in skeletal muscle, or by inhibition of spinal interneuronal cholinergic synapses. In this context the prophylactic antitoxic action of edrophonium is of interest, as it can be explained again in a protective effect on the AChE and a partial competitive antagonism against ACh on peripheral cholinergic receptors. A convincing strategy against sarin poisoning lies still more in the anticholinergic action of atropine, benactyzine and curarizing compounds, with all the disadvantages of their central actions, muscle relaxation, cardiac effects. etc.

Table 3

Effect of i.p. application of MMTS on rats followed 10 minutes later by sarin applied the same way but on the other side.

Number of animals	MMTS mg/kg	Sarin mg/kg	Death after minutes			Significance
5	6.7	1	3:48	+	0:50	no (p> 0.1)
5	- -	1	3:18	+	0:40	
5	16.7	1	5:48	+	1:18	no (p> 0.1)
5	-- -	1	5:12	+	1:05	
5	33.4	1	11:12	+	4:36	p< 0.05
5	-- -	1	4:36	+	1:40	
10	66.7	2	6:30	+	3:28	p< 0.01
10	-- -	2	3:12	+	0.47	
10	133.5	2	20:55	+	13:16	p< 0.01
10	--- -	2	2:59	+	0.58	

8. Blockade of Acetylcholine Synthesis in Organophosphate Poisoning

As all efforts of antagonizing nerve gas poisoning by reactivating the acetylcholinesterase for immediate hydrolysis of ACh have not been convincing, the limitation of ACh-synthesis is a logical approach to successful treatment. The lethal amount of acetylcholine should be reduced to normal physiological values by blocking its synthesizing enzyme cholineacetyltransferase (CAT) (Hopff et al., 1984b). As a model compound for this purpose we used methylmethane-thiol-sulfonate (MMTS) (fig. 1), which was first used by Mautner (1977). We were aware, that thiol reagents as MMTS have severe side effects which are probably responsible for their lethal effect. Our original aim of finding a tolerable dose of MMTS inhibiting the ACh-synthesis by 80 - 90 % was not attained. But with a higher, for mice already toxic concentration injected intraperitoneally 5 - 15 minutes before sarin, we could demonstrate a significant prolongation of survival time (table 3). The beneficial effect was obtained even when MMTS was injected shortly after sarin. MMTS was protective in the same way against soman poisoning in mice, when injected 10 minutes before. These pilot studies prove the validity of the strategy consisting in limiting the production and output of ACh in nerve gas poisoning. At the moment we are synthesizing new compounds inhibiting CAT and investigating their action on the enzyme both in vivo and vitro. Although some of these inhibitors are less toxic, they are not yet good enough for controling the output of acetylcholine.

9. Conclusions

When critically investigated with pure acetylcholinesterase from Torpedo marmorata, the reactivation of the enzyme by oximes is too small and too late to be used as antitoxic treatment of sarin poisoning in man at normal body temperature and plasma pH. Only when these parameters are manipulated a faster reactivation may be achieved. Soman is even stronger bound to the enzyme by fast ageing, which brings an irreversible situation. Furthermore, obidoxime and pralidoxime do not pass through the blood brain barrier (or placenta) and clearly can act only in the periphery. The best antagonists against the overconcentration of acetylcholine are still atropine and benactyzine, the latter blocking nicotinic receptors as well. Neither an oxime alone, nor a muscarinic antagonist e.g. atropine, benactyzine alone but only in combination showed a beneficial action of antagonizing organophsphate poisoning. A combination with oximes has some small advantages of enhanced antitoxic effect, but higher risks of drug toxicity.

A new strategy of inhibiting the synthesis of acetylcholine by blocking the choline acetyltransferase may bring a new approach to successful treatment.

Acknowledgment

We wish to thank the Swiss Commission for Military Research in Medicine for financial help.

References

Amitai, G., Kloog, Y., Baldeman, D. and Sokolowski, M., 1980, The interaction of bis-pyridinium oximes with mouse brain muscarinic receptor, Biochem. Pharmacology 29: 483-488.

Caratsch, C.G and Waser, P.G., 1984, Effects of obidoxime chloride on native and sarin-poisoned frog neuromuscular junctions, Pflügers Arch. 401: 84-90.

Fossier, P., Baux, G. and Tauc, L., 1983, Direct and indirect effects of an organophosporous acetylcholinesterase inhibitor and of an oxime on a neuro-neuronal synapse, Pflügers Arch. 396: 15-22.

Gotheil, A.M., 1978, Ganztierautoradiographische Untersuchungen über die Verteilung von Pyridin-2-Aldoxim ^{14}C-Methoiodid in Mäusen, allein und unter der Einwirkung von Methylisopropylfluorophosphonat, Dissertation ETH Zürich No. 6220.

Hopff, W.H., Riggio, G. and Waser, P.G., 1984a, Sarin poisoning in Guinea Pigs compared to Reactivation of Acetylcholinesteras "in vitro" as a Basis for Therapy, Acta Pharmacol. et toxicol. 55: 1-5.

Hopff, W.H., Riggio, G. and Waser, P.G., 1984b, Blockade of Acetylcholine Synthesis in Organophosphate Poisoning, Toxicol. and Appl. Pharmacol. 72: 513-518.

Mautner, H., 1977, Choline Acetyltransferase CRC, Crit Rev. Biochem. 4: 341-370.

Sammet, R., 1983, Kinetik von ^{14}C-Sarin and deren Beeinflussung durch Obidoxim - Eine ganztierautoradiographische Untersuchung an der Maus, Dissertation ETH Zürich No. 7288.

Streichenberg, C., 1984, Verteilung und Kinetik von ^{14}C-Obidoxim, Report for diploma of ETH Zürich.

Waser, P.G., Sammet, R., Schönenberger, E. and Chang Sin-Ren, A., 1983, Pharmacodynamics of ^{14}C-Sarin and its Changes by Obidoxime and Pralidoxime, Proceedings of Oglebay Park Meeting.

MUSCARINIC AND NICOTINIC MECHANISMS OF SEIZURES INDUCED BY

CHOLINESTERASE INHIBITORS: OBSERVATIONS ON DIAZEPAM AND

MIDAZOLAM AS ANTAGONISTS[1,2]

Edward F. Domino, Ante Simonic[3], and Halina Krutak-Krol[4]

Department of Pharmacology
University of Michigan
Ann Arbor, MI 48109-0010

Footnotes:

1. A preliminary report was presented at the Second International Meeting on Cholinesterases in Bled, Yugoslavia (Simonic et al., 1983), the American Society for Pharmacology and Experimental Therapeutics, Indianapolis, IN (Krutak-Krol et al., 1984), and at the Fifth Annual Chemical Defense Bioscience Review sponsored by the U.S. Army Medical Research Institute of Chemical Defense, Columbia, MD (Domino et al., 1985).

2. Supported in part by the Psychopharmacology Research Fund (Domino) and the U.S. Army Medical Research and Development Command Contract DAMD17-84-C-4157.

3. Visiting Fulbright Scholar from the Department of Pharmacology, University of Rijeka, Rijeka, Yugoslavia.

4. Present address: Department of Internal Medicine, University of Missouri Medical School, Columbia, MO 64212.

ABSTRACT

The gross behavioral and EEG seizure-inducing effects of various cholinesterase inhibitors (ChEI) were compared to the cholinergic agonists arecoline and nicotine, and the classic convulsants pentylenetetrazol and strychnine in unanesthetized rats. It was also our purpose to determine the possible anticonvulsant activity of potential antagonists. Femoral arterial and venous cannulae, EEG (epidural) and EKG (Lead II) electrodes were surgically implanted under halothane-oxygen anesthesia into adult Sprague-Dawley male rats (200-350 gm). Upon recovery from halothane anesthesia each rat received one of the following: 1) a directly acting cholinergic agonist (arecoline or nicotine); 2) a cholinesterase inhibitor, diethyl-p-nitrophenylphosphate (paraoxon), diisopropylfluorophosphate (DFP), neostigmine, or physostigmine; or 3) a central nervous system convulsant (pentylenetetrazol or strychnine).

Each drug was administered i.v. in logarithmic cumulative doses until the animal exhibited tremors, major motor or cortical EEG seizures, and/or died. All of the cholinergic agonists, including the ChEIs, induced motor tremors. Nicotine produced convulsions, observed in the EEG and gross behavior, while arecoline did not cause cortical EEG or gross behavioral seizures but did produce aberrant body movements. Neostigmine, even in supralethal doses, did not elicit motor or EEG seizures. Physostigmine, in sublethal doses, caused abnormal motor movements with EEG desynchronization. Supralethal doses of physostigmine or the irreversible ChEI paraoxon produced EEG convulsive patterns. Sublethal doses of DFP yielded similar effects. The ChEI seizure activity was partially antagonized by atropine. The nicotinic antagonists mecamylamine, pempidine, or trimethidinium did not alter the ChEI-induced EEG seizure patterns. Pentylenetetrazol produced both gross behavioral and EEG seizures, while strychnine in convulsant doses produced only EEG desynchronization. Supralethal doses of strychnine did induce EEG seizures.

Midazolam was an effective anticonvulsant against all of the convulsants, especially when the induced EEG seizures were recorded in ventilated animals. Nicotine-induced seizures were not only <u>not</u> antagonized by atropine, but were enhanced. Since atropine partially antagonized ChEI induced seizures, it is concluded that both a muscarinic cholinergic as well as a non-cholinergic mechanism is involved.

A comparison was made between diazepam and midazolam given i.m. in antagonizing 2 x LD50 of s.c. paraoxon in the presence of 10 mg/kg atropine. Both benzodiazepines were effective in reducing paraoxon induced seizures and death. However, midazolam was more potent.

INTRODUCTION

It is well known that EEG alterations including seizure activity involve multiple neurotransmitters and receptors. Thus, it is no surprise that central cholinergic mechanisms have been implicated in seizures. A correlation between central cholinergic mechanisms and convulsions was suggested by Pope et al. (1947). Two lines of reasoning support this hypothesis: (1) Direct application of acetylcholine (ACh) to various regions of the brain produces convulsive activity (Eccles, 1964; Krnjevic, 1965) and (2) procedures increasing cerebral excitability cause a rapid decrease in cerebral ACh content and an increase in turnover (Richter and Crossland, 1949; Longoni et al., 1976). Cholinergic agonists including cholinesterase inhibitors (ChEI) induce initial EEG desynchronization and subsequent seizure activity when applied directly to the neocortex and limbic structures, or when given systemically (Cornblath et al., 1976).

Longo (1962) classified various ChEI into two groups based upon their effects on rabbit cerebral electrical activity. Tertiary nitrogen ChEI like physostigmine and the organophosphorous agents caused initial EEG activation upon i.v. administration followed by "electrical grand mal" activity and tonic-clonic motor seizures, especially on intracarotid (i.c.) administration. The second group of ChEI includes neostigmine and other quaternary ammonium compounds which do not readily penetrate the blood-brain barrier. Such ChEI had no effect on cerebral electrical activity, after large i.v. doses. Physostigmine, in large doses given i.v., did not produce electrical seizures in the rabbit but, when given i.c., produced such effects. In contrast, DFP and sarin readily produced EEG seizures when given i.v. Hence, one variable in inducing EEG seizures appears to be the relative ease with which a ChEI passes the blood-brain barrier. We hypothesized that another factor which would alter the seizure-inducing properties of a ChEI was its relative direct muscarinic, nicotinic or non-cholinergic property. It is well known that muscarinic agonists such as arecoline and oxotremorine produce tremor (Bebbington et al., 1966; Brimblecombe, 1974; Szreniawski et al., 1977), while nicotinic agonists like nicotine produce tremor and convulsions (Larson et al., 1961; Silvette et al., 1962; Brimblecombe, 1974).

In this study, the relative gross behavioral and EEG seizure inducing effects of directly acting cholinergic agonists (arecoline, nicotine), ChEI (DFP, neostigmine, paraoxon, physostigmine) and CNS convulsants (pentylenetetrazol, strychnine) were compared in the rat.

METHODS

Male Sprague-Dawley rats weighing 300-400 g usually were divided into groups of 8-10 animals each. All of the animals were anesthetized with a mixture of halothane (1.5-3%) + oxygen (97-98.5%). Polyethylene cannulae were inserted into the femoral artery for recording blood pressure and into the femoral vein for giving i.v. injections. Bipolar EEG electrodes were implanted epidurally above the trunk and forelimb cerebral motor cortex at the following coordinates: anterior 1.5 mm from bregma, left and right 1.5 mm, and vertical 1.0 mm from the skull surface (Pellegrino et al., 1981). The ground electrode was placed on the skull. The electrodes were fixed to the calvarium with acrylic cement. Subsequently, the halothane-oxygen mixture was stopped, all wound edges infiltrated with 1% lidocaine, and the rats were allowed to recover (about 1.5 hr).

Three different studies were undertaken. In Study A, the gross behavior of freely moving conscious animals was observed and correlated with the polygraphic recordings. In Study B, after surgery was completed, including a tracheotomy, the wound edges were infiltrated with 1% lidocaine. Then the animals were given pancuronium (0.5 mg/kg, i.v.) and artificially ventilated with room air under positive pressure. After recovery from halothane anesthesia, during which time the physiological parameters were monitored, various cholinergic agonists were administered i.v. In Study C only gross behavior of normal rats was measured.

The EEG, EKG (Lead II), and arterial blood pressure were recorded on separate channels of a Grass Model 7C polygraph. In both of the polygraphic studies, increasing doses of various cholinergic agonists and antagonists were injected i.v. in a logarithmic manner until the rat had either EEG or major motor seizures or died. All drugs were injected at one min intervals followed by a 0.1 ml 0.9% NaCl flush. Doses of each agent were calculated as mg of free base. The drugs and their sources were: arecoline hydrobromide (Sigma); nicotine tartrate (Sigma); physostigmine salicylate (Sigma); neostigmine bromide and methyl sulfate (K&K Lab); DFP and paraoxon (Sigma); pentylenetetrazol (Knoll); strychnine hydrochloride (British Drug Houses, Ltd.); pancuronium dimethobromide (Organon Inc.); atropine sulfate (Sigma); commercial diazepam solution and midazolam maleate (Hoffmann La Roche); mecamylamine hydrochloride (Merck Sharp & Dohme Research Lab); trimethidinium methosulphate (Wyeth Laboratories); pempidine tartrate (Imperial Chemical Industries Ltd.); and lidocaine hydrochloride (Elkins-Sinn Inc.).

RESULTS

Study A: Polygraph recordings of freely moving rats

Nicotine in small doses (0.1-0.32 mg/kg) produced tremor and EEG desynchronization. Doses of nicotine larger than 1.0 mg/kg induced major motor tonic clonic convulsions. The EEG showed desynchronization followed by electrical seizure activity. Tachyphylaxis to the tremor and tonic clonic convulsions was observed.

Arecoline in a dose of 1.0 mg/kg induced tremor, while a dose of 3.2 mg/kg caused gross motor seizures and death in all animals. However, in doses up to 3.2 mg/kg no changes from the control EEG desynchronization pattern were observed.

Neostigmine in low doses (0.032-0.1 mg/kg) induced tremor and, in larger doses, major motor seizure movements (1.0 mg/kg) and death. Even lethal doses of neostigmine did not influence the EEG.

Physostigmine (0.032-0.32 mg/kg) produced tremor and EEG desynchronization. Larger doses of physostigmine (1.0-3.2 mg/kg) induced motor seizure movements and death. However, in the EEG only desynchronization was seen.

DFP (0.1-1.0 mg/kg) produced tremor and EEG desynchronization (Fig. 1). Larger doses up to 10.0 mg/kg caused tremor in some animals and convulsions in others. In the EEG, desynchronization with or without theta activity was seen. Doses of 10.0 mg/kg always produced both major motor and EEG seizures and death.

Paraoxon (0.1-0.32 mg/kg) produced tremors and EEG desynchronization, while 1.0 mg/kg caused gross behavioral convulsions and death in all animals. Only desynchronization was observed in the EEG in sublethal doses in contrast to DFP. Lethal doses of paraoxon readily produced EEG seizures (Fig. 1).

Pentylenetetrazol (10.0 mg/kg) had a convulsant effect readily seen in both gross behavior and the EEG. Strychnine (0.32-1.0 mg/kg) caused major motor seizures and induced only desynchronization in the EEG.

Study B: Post-halothane paralyzed, locally anesthetized and ventilated rats

Although pancuronium is a neuromuscular blocking agent that is not supposed to penetrate the blood-brain barrier (Kariss and Gossen, 1971), the results of the present study suggest that in large doses in rats it does have a central action. Some of these effects were seen in doses of pancuronium which did not affect systemic blood pressure, but as hypotension was induced by pancuronium the EEG changes were very apparent. These actions of pancuronium probably account for the large doses of various cholinergic agonists needed to induce EEG changes in the paralyzed rat as described below.

Increasing doses of pancuronium were given i.v. approximately every 5 min and the animal ventilated artificially to maintain oxygenation. Large doses of pancuronium produced EEG slowing and a fall in blood pressure. Much larger doses of all of the cholinergic agonists had to be given to alter the EEG, suggesting that pancuronium plus artificial ventilation had significant antagonistic actions. Even supralethal doses of arecoline were not able to produce seizure-like activity in the

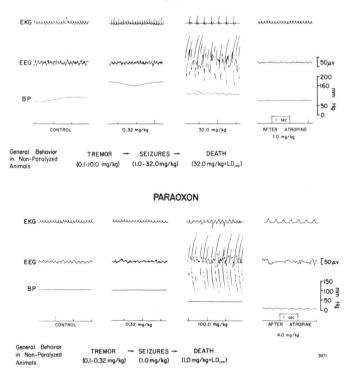

Fig. 1. Effects of accumulative doses of DFP and paraoxon on the EKG, EEG, blood pressure (BP) and gross behavior of the rat.

EEG; only slight desynchronization was seen. Arecoline caused mainly an increase in arterial blood pressure which was followed by bradycardia.

Nicotine (1.0 to 32.0 mg/kg) produced seizure activity in the EEG which was antagonized by midazolam (10.0 mg/kg), but not by trimethidinium (up to 200.0 mg/kg). Sometimes it was very easy to antagonize these EEG seizures (completely and with relatively low doses), but sometimes they were only partially suppressed in the presence of enormous doses of pempidine (60.0-90.0 mg/kg), mecamylamine (20.0-70.0 mg/kg), and/or atropine (1.0-4.0 mg/kg). Generally, nicotine induced hypotension, bradycardia, and arrhythmias.

Neostigmine, even supralethal doses, did not cause any EEG changes. The i.v. injection of neostigmine produced relatively small decreases in arterial blood pressure and heart rate. Administration of physostigmine (0.32-32.0 mg/kg) resulted in a decrease in blood pressure and heart rate. No EEG seizures were observed at these doses. Only supralethal doses of physostigmine (32.0 mg/kg) induced seizures in the EEG. These effects were partially antagonized by atropine (1.0 mg/kg). The EEG convulsant effects of physostigmine were not diminished by pempidine up to 75.0 mg/kg or mecamylamine up to 80.0 mg/kg. Midazolam (10.0 mg/kg) readily antagonized the EEG seizure pattern produced by physostigmine.

DFP (up to 10.0 mg/kg) produced EEG seizures which could be suppressed by atropine (1.0-3.0 mg/kg) and midazolam (10.0 mg/kg).

Mecamylamine up to 80.0 mg/kg and trimethidinium up to 100.0 mg/kg did not antagonize these convulsions. No tachyphylaxis was observed to the EEG convulsions produced by DFP. DFP caused a transient, non-dose dependent increase in arterial blood pressure and bradycardia. Atropine (1.0 mg/kg) prevented this effect (Fig. 1).

Paraoxon in supralethal doses (32.0 or more mg/kg) also induced EEG seizures. No tachyphylaxis was seen to these convulsions. EEG seizures were suppressed by midazolam (10.0 mg/kg) and usually by atropine (1.0-4.0 mg/kg) but not by mecamylamine up to 70.0 mg/kg. Paraoxon produced a marked decrease in blood pressure, bradycardia, and arrhythmia. After 1.0 mg/kg i.v. of atropine, extensive bradycardia and hypotension were still present.

Pentylenetetrazol had marked EEG convulsant effects in doses of 10.0-32.0 mg/kg. Very large doses of 3.2-10.0 mg/kg of strychnine were required to induce EEG seizures, which were antagonized by midazolam (10.0 mg/kg). Both pentylenetetrazol and strychnine increased arterial blood pressure and decreased the heart rate after i.v. injection.

A summary of the results obtained is shown in Table 1.

Study C: Normal naive rats

1. Effects of paraoxon alone

The s.c. administration of low doses (0.032-0.1 mg/kg) of paraoxon to normal rats induced slight gross behavioral changes like grooming, chewing, sniffing, and piloerection. A dose of 0.32 mg/kg caused (within 3-5 min) signs of cholinergic poisoning such as lacrimation, salivation, exophthalmos, fasciculations, tremor and respiratory distress (bradypnea and dyspnea). Thirty percent of the animals developed moderate clonic seizures with a mild tonic component. Sixteen percent of the rats given a dose of 0.32 mg/kg died within 15-20 min. Administration of a larger dose (1.0 mg/kg) produced immediate toxic symptoms: tremor, jerks, and severe respiratory depression. All of these animals developed clonic seizures lasting 2-4 min until they died. Mortality in this group of rats was 100%. The convulsant dose 50 (CD50) of paraoxon was determined to be 0.35 mg/kg with 95% confidence limits of 0.25-0.48. The lethal dose 50 (LD50) calculated from the data was 0.38 mg/kg with 95% confidence limits of 0.27-0.52.

2. Effects of atropine pretreatment on paraoxon toxicity

These results are summarized in Table 2 and Figs. 2 and 3. Rats (8 per group) were pretreated with i.m. atropine in single doses (1.0, 3.2, 10.0, 32.0, and 100.0 mg/kg) 20 min prior to the s.c. administration of paraoxon (0.76 mg/kg = 2 x LD50). Fig. 3 shows that the best protective effect against death was achieved by a 10.0 mg/kg dose of atropine. Therefore, this dose was selected for subsequent experiments. Larger doses of atropine (32.0-100.0 mg/kg) increased mortality slightly compared to the 10.0 mg/kg dose. Treatment with atropine did not prevent paraoxon-induced seizures. However, it decreased salivation, lacrimation, and respiratory distress. Atropine in a dose of 10.0 mg/kg increased the LD50 of paraoxon to 1.18 mg/kg.

3. Effects of midazolam alone

In a separate control series of experiments, naive rats (8 per group) were injected i.m. with midazolam alone in single doses (0.32,

Table 1

Summary of the effects of various drugs on EEG seizures

Convulsant	Possible Antagonist	Effect
Nicotine	Atropine	↑
	Mecamylamine	↓
	Midazolam	↓
	Pempidine	↓?
	Trimethidinium	0
Physostigmine	Atropine	↓?
	Mecamylamine	0
	Midazolam	↓
	Pempidine	0
DFP	Atropine	↓
	Mecamylamine	0
	Midazolam	↓
	Trimethidinium	0
Paraoxon	Atropine	↓?
	Mecamylamine	0
	Midazolam	↓
Pentylenetetrazol	Mecamylamine	0
	Midazolam	↓
	Pempidine	0
	Trimethidinium	0
Strychnine	Atropine	0
	Mecamylamine	0
	Midazolam	↓

0 = No effect   ↓ - Decrease in seizure activity
? = Effect not   ↑ - Increase in seizure activity
    clear

Table 2

Effect of atropine, midazolam, or diazepam alone or in combination on the toxicity of paraoxon[a] in rats

Compound	Dose (mg/kg)	Seizures (3 hr)	Death (24 hr)
0.9% NaCl	1.0 ml/kg	10/10	10/10
Atropine	1.0	8/8	4/8
	3.2	7/8	1/8
	10.0	8/8	0/8
	32.0	8/8	1/8
	100.0	8/8	3/8
40% Propylene Glycol, 10% Ethyl Alcohol in Water	1.0 ml/kg	10/10	10/10
Diazepam (Commercial Solution 5 mg/ml)	0.32	8/8	8/8
	1.0	8/8	8/8
	3.2	6/8	8/8
	10.0	2/11	10/11
	32.0	0/8	8/8
Atropine + Diazepam	10.0		
	0.32	8/8	1/8
	1.0	6/8	1/8
	3.2	13/16	1/16
	10.0	4/8	0/11
	32.0	0/8	0/8
Midazolam	0.32	8/8	8/8
	1.0	6/8	8/8
	3.2	2/8	8/8
	10.0	4/17	13/17
	32.0	0/8	6/8
Atropine + Midazolam	10.0		
	0.32	8/8	0/8
	1.0	5/8	0/8
	3.2	1/8	0/8
	10.0	0/8	0/8
	32.0	0/8	0/8

[a] Atropine, diazepam, and midazolam were given i.m. 20 min before paraoxon 2 x LD50 (0.76 mg/kg, s.c.)

480

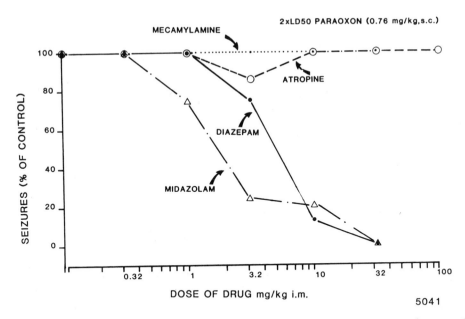

Fig. 2. Comparative effects of atropine, diazepam, mecamylamine, and midazolam alone on paraoxon induced seizures.

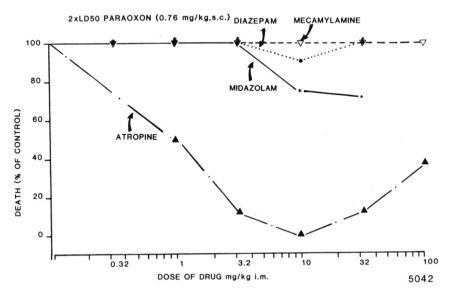

Fig. 3. Comparative effects of atropine, diazepam, mecamylamine, and midazolam alone on paraoxon induced death.

1.0, 3.2, 10.0, and 32.0 mg/kg). Low doses of midazolam produced no obvious effect. With larger doses (3.2-10.0 mg/kg) rapid absorption of midazolam from the i.m. injection was apparent after 2-3 min (i.e., the rats became calm). By 5 min, all of the animals showed skeletal muscle relaxation and some developed ataxia but none fell asleep. A dose of 32.0 mg/kg of midazolam produced an anesthesia-like state.

4. Effects of midazolam pretreatment on paraoxon toxicity

The incidence of paraoxon-induced convulsions was significantly reduced by prior administration of midazolam (Table 2 and Fig. 2). Doses of 3.2-10.0 mg/kg produced 75% protection against seizures produced by 2 x LD50 of paraoxon. However, midazolam alone did not prevent paraoxon-induced respiratory distress and death. Pretreatment with both atropine (10.0 mg/kg) and midazolam (0.32-32.0 mg/kg) produced 100% protection against death. The combination of atropine (10.0 mg/kg) and midazolam (10.0 mg/kg) increased the LD50 of paraoxon to 4.12 mg/kg. This pretreatment regimen provided a protective ratio of 11.0.

5. Effects of diazepam alone

In another separate series of experiments, the effect of diazepam alone in single doses i.m. was tested. Low doses (0.32-3.2 mg/kg) produced no obvious effect. With larger doses (10.0 mg/kg) the animal showed skeletal muscle relaxation and some developed ataxia. A dose of 32.0 mg/kg of diazepam induced an anesthesia-like state. A delay of 10-15 min from injection to occurrence of the first symptoms was seen.

6. Effects of diazepam pretreatment on paraoxon toxicity

In diazepam pretreated animals given paraoxon there was a dose dependent reduction in paraoxon induced convulsions (Table 2 and Fig. 2). Small doses of diazepam (0.32-1.0 mg/kg) had no anticonvulsant activity. A dose of 3.2 mg/kg reduced convulsions by 25%. Doses of diazepam from 10.0-32.0 mg/kg provided 71.8%-100% protection against seizures. However, diazepam alone, even in a very large dose (32.0 mg/kg), did not prevent paraoxon induced respiratory distress and death.

Pretreatment with both atropine (10.0 mg/kg) and diazepam (10.0 mg/kg) provided 100% protection against death. The combination of atropine (10.0 mg/kg) and diazepam (10.0 mg/kg) increased the LD50 of paraoxon to 2.72 (1.73-4.28) mg/kg. This pretreatment regimen provided a protective ratio of 7.16.

7. Effects of mecamylamine pretreatment on paraoxon toxicity

As illustrated in Figs. 2 and 3, mecamylamine in doses up to 100 mg/kg i.m. did not protect against seizures or death due to 2 x LD50 of paraoxon.

DISCUSSION

The results with arecoline are in agreement with previous findings (Domino, 1967) that arecoline produces EEG desynchronization, but not seizure-like activity. We conclude that a) gross motor movements produced by arecoline are not of motor cortical origin, and b) stimulation of muscarinic receptors in the neocortex, even with supralethal doses of arecoline does not produce EEG seizures. One possible explanation is that there are at least two sub-groups of muscarinic receptors in the cerebral cortex. One group (stimulated by arecoline) is not involved in seizure activity. Stimulation of the other subgroup produces EEG seizures. Physostigmine, DFP, and paraoxon can stimulate (either directly or indirectly through ACh accumulation) this subpopulation of muscarinic receptors. Atropine can block both subgroups of muscarinic receptors. Our results are in agreement with _in vitro_ muscarinic receptor binding studies which demonstrate the existence of multiple binding sites for muscarinic agonists and a single uniform population of binding sites for muscarinic antagonists (Hulme et al., 1978; Birdsall et al., 1978a, 1978b, 1979).

It is well known that nicotine produces tremor and, in larger doses, seizures (Larson et al., 1961). Nicotine induced seizures can be suppressed by hexamethonium, caramiphen, mecamylamine, pentolinium, and various central nervous system depressants (Chen and Bohner, 1957; Tarakhovsky, 1957; Spinks et al., 1955; Stone et al., 1958). In our study, mecamylamine and pempidine frequently were able to block EEG seizures produced by nicotine, while trimethidinium was ineffective.

Mecamylamine and pempidine are widely used nicotinic receptor blockers which relatively easily penetrate the blood-brain barrier, in contrast to trimethidinium which cannot (Brimblecombe, 1974). None of these agents is a nicotinic blocker at the neuromuscular junction. Furthermore, in the case of mecamylamine and pempidine, their ganglionic blocking properties are largely non-competitive and presynaptic (Romano and Goldstein, 1980). There are at least five subpopulations of nicotinic receptors in the brain (Romano and Goldstein, 1980; Sloan et al., 1984). There is the possibility that nicotine can stimulate more than one subpopulation of nicotinic receptors, while mecamylamine and pempidine are antagonists at only some nicotinic receptors and that nicotine also has a non-cholinergic action in the brain (Longo, 1962; Abood et al., 1979).

Our results agree with previous observations (Bradley and Elkes, 1953, 1957; Granacher and Baldessarini, 1975; Klemm, 1969) that: a) physostigmine and neostigmine can produce gross motor movements, b) physostigmine, in supralethal doses, can produce EEG seizures which can be antagonized by atropine and, c) neostigmine, a quaternary amine which cannot readily penetrate the blood-brain barrier does not affect the EEG.The cortical and gross behavioral effects of neostigmine and physostigmine are unrelated to the described changes in blood pressure and heart rate which is in agreement with the work of Bradley and Elkes (1953).

The two irreversible ChEI studied readily induce gross motor seizures. In sublethal doses, paraoxon did not act on the cerebral cortex to produce EEG seizures, but did so in supralethal doses. DFP, on the other hand, produced gross motor seizures involving the neo-cortex. The EEG seizures produced by both irreversible ChEI have a muscarinic component (because they can be suppressed by atropine) and a non-nicotinic component (because they cannot be suppressed by mecamyl-amine). It is well known that the behavioral and neurological effects produced by the organophosphorous ChEI cannot be attributed entirely to cholinergic hyperactivity (Lundy and Shih, 1983; Shih, 1982; Sivam et al., 1983; Van Meter et al., 1978). Furthermore, although atropine is a muscarinic antagonist, it can, with large doses, also block nicotinic receptors (Brimblecombe, 1974).

It is well known that pentylenetetrazol produces both gross behavioral tonic-clonic convulsions and EEG seizures (Esplin and Zablocka-Esplin, 1969; Huot et al., 1973; Longo, 1962; Pfeiffer et al., 1957; Preston, 1955). In our experiments, both gross behavioral and EEG seizures were produced by similar doses of pentylenetetrazol. This is in agreement with the literature that pentylenetetrazol produces behavioral seizures primarily at the level of the neocortex (Esplin and Zablocka-Esplin, 1969; Longo, 1962; Preston, 1955).

Strychnine also produces both behavioral motor and EEG seizures (Longo, 1962; Pfeiffer et al., 1957). In our experiments, strychnine produced major motor seizures in low doses (0.32-1.0 mg/kg, i.v.), and EEG desynchronization. Lethal doses above 10.0 mg/kg, i.v. were required to produce EEG seizures. This is in agreement with the results of Longo (1962) and the hypothesis that strychnine acts primarily at the level of the spinal cord (Andersen et al., 1963; Curtis et al., 1971; Evans, 1978; Longo, 1962), but also can act on the neocortex (Biscoe and Curtis, 1967; Curtis et al., 1971; Longo, 1962), and produce cortical epileptiform activity especially after topical application (Feher et al., 1965).

One of the most impressive findings of this reseach was that midazolam (10.0 mg/kg, i.v.) usually completely antagonized the motor and EEG seizure patterns of all of the convulsants tested. Midazolam is a benzodiazepine derivative with a short duration of action (Dundee, 1979), and potent anticonvulsive activity (de Jong and Bonin, 1981; Zbinden and Randall, 1967). It is well known that benzodiazepines block the tremors and convulsive effects of various substances including strychnine, isoniazid, pentylenetetrazol, and organophosphorous ChEI, etc. (Mao et al., 1975; Costa et al., 1975; Guidotti, 1978). This is probably due to their well known effects in enhancing the actions of GABA. It is of interest that there is some evidence of a direct interaction of midazolam with cholinergic receptors (Davies and Polc, 1980). However, in the latter study it was not possible to compare the effects of midazolam with diazepam.

In the present study both benzodiazepines were very effective when combined with atropine in reducing the incidence of paraoxon induced seizures and dramatically reducing the lethality of 2 x LD50 of paraoxon. Midazolam was more potent on a mg/kg basis. When given i.m. to humans, midazolam is better absorbed than is diazepam. Thus, midazolam would be preferred in treating paraoxon poisoning, assuming that the rat data are applicable to humans.

ACKNOWLEDGEMENTS

The authors would like to acknowledge the efforts of Mrs. Krystyna Blusziewicz in these studies.

REFERENCES

Abood, L.G., Lowy, K., Tometsko, A., and MacNeil, M., 1979, Evidence for a noncholinergic site for nicotine's action in brain: psychopharmacological, electrophysiological and receptor binding studies. Arch. Int. Pharmacodyn. Ther. 237:213-229.

Andersen, P., Eccles, J.C., Loyning, Y., and Voorhoeve, P.E., 1963, Strychnine-resistant central inhibition. Nature 200:843-845.

Bebbington, A., Brimblecombe, R.W., and Shakeshaft, D., 1966, The central and peripheral activity of acetylenic amines related to oxotremorine. Br. J. Pharmacol. 26:56-67.

Birdsall, N.J.M., Burgen, A.S.V., and Hulme, E.C., 1978a, Correlation between the binding properties and pharmacological responses of muscarinic receptors. in: Cholinergic Mechanisms and Psychopharmacology, Vol. 24, D.J. Jenden, ed., Plenum Press, New York.

Birdsall, N.J.M., Burgen, A.S.V., and Hulme, E.C., 1978b, The binding of agonists to brain muscarinic receptors. Mol. Pharmacol. 14:723-736.

Birdsall, N.J.M., Burgen, A.S.V., and Hulme, E.C., 1979, Multiple classes of muscarinic receptor binding sites in the brain. in: Receptors: Advances in Pharmacology and Therapeutics: Proceedings of the Seventh International Congress of Pharmacology, Vol. 1, J. Jacob, ed., Pergamon Press, Oxford.

Biscoe, T.J., and Curtis, D.R., 1967, Strychnine and cortical inhibition. Nature 214:914-915.

Bradley, P.B. and Elkes, J., 1953, The effect of atropine, hyoscyamine, physostigmine, and neostigmine on the electrical activity of the brain of the conscious cat. J. Physiol. 120:14P-15P.

Bradley, P.B. and Elkes, J., 1957, The effects of some drugs on the electrical activity of the brain. Brain 80:77-117.

Brimblecombe, R.W., ed., 1974, Drug Actions on Cholinergic Systems, pp. 66-215, University Park Press, Baltimore.

Chen, G. and Bohner, B., 1957, Antagonism of nicotine and some CNS depressants in mice. Fed. Proc. 16:288.

Cornblath, D.R. and Ferguson, J.H., 1976, Distribution of radioactivity from topically applied (H^3) acetylcholine in relation to seizure. Exp. Neurol. 50:495-504.

Costa, E., Guidotti, A., Mao, C.C. and Suria, A., 1975, New concepts on the mechanism of action of benzodiazepines. Life Sci. 17:167-186.

Curtis, D.R., Duggan, A.W., and Johnston, G.A.R., 1971, The specificity of strychnine as a glycine antagonist in the mammalian spinal cord. Exp. Brain Res. 12:547-565.

Davies, J. and Polc, P., 1978, Effect of a water soluble benzodiazepines on the response of spinal neurones to acetylcholine and excitatory amino acid analogues. Neuropharmacol. 17:217-220.

De Jong, R.H. and Bonin, J.D., 1981, Benzodiazepines protect mice from local anesthetic convulsions and death. Anesth. Analg. 60:385-389.

Domino, E.F., 1967, Electroencephalographic and behavioral arousal effects of small doses of nicotine: a neuropsychopharmacological study. Ann. N.Y. Acad. Sci. 142:216-244.

Domino, E.F., Simonic, A., and Krutak-Krol, H., 1985, Comparative muscarinic and nicotinic cholinergic mechamisms involved in seizures induced by cholinesterase inhibitors. Fifth Annual Chemical Defense Bioscience Review, Speakers' Abstract pg. 29, U.S. Army Medical Research Institute of Chemical Defense, Columbia, MD.

Dundee, J.W., 1979, New i.v. anaesthetics. Br. J. Anaesth. 51:641-648.

Eccles, J.C., 1964, The Physiology of Synapses, pp. 1-316, Springer-Verlag, Berlin.

Esplin, D. and Zablocka-Esplin, B., 1969, Mechanism of action of convulsants. in: Basic Mechanisms of Epilepsy, H.H. Jasper, A.A. Ward, and H. Pope, eds., Little Brown and Co., Boston.

Evans, R.H., 1978, Cholinoceptive properties of motoneurones of the immature rat spinal cord maintained in vitro. Neuropharmacol. 17: 277-279.

Feher, O., Halasz, P., and Mechler, F., 1965, The mechanism of origin of cortical convulsive potentials. EEG Clin. Neurophysiol. 19:541-548.

Granacher, R.P. and Baldessarini, R.J., 1975, Physostigmine. Arch. Gen. Psych. 32:375-380.

Guidotti, A., 1978, Synaptic mechanisms in the action of benzodiazepines. in: Psychopharmacology: A Generation of Progress, M.A. Lipton, A. Di Mascio, A., and K.F. DiPalma, eds., Raven Press, New York.

Hulme, E.C., Birdsall, N.J.M., Burgen, A.S.V., and Mehta, P., 1978, The binding of antagonists to brain muscarinic receptors. Mol. Pharmacol. 14:737-750.

Huot, J., Radouco-Thomas, S., and Radouco-Thomas, C., 1973, Qualitative and quantitative evaluation of experimentally induced seizures (pentetrazol induced seizures). in: International Encyclopedia of Pharmacology and Therapeutics, Sec. 19, Vol. I, C. Radouco-Thomas, ed., Pergamon Press, New York.

Karis, J.H. and Gissen, A.J., 1971, Evaluation of new neuromuscular blocking agents. Anesthesiology 35:149-157.

Klemm, W.R., ed., 1969, Animal Electroencephalography, pp. 41-48, Academic Press, New York.

Krnjevic, K., 1965, Cholinergic innervation of the cerebral cortex. in: D.R. Curtis and A.K. McIntyre, eds., Studies in Physiology, Springer Verlag, Berlin.

Krutak-Król, H., Simonić, A., and Domino, E.F., 1984, Comparative muscarinic and nicotinic cholinergic mechanisms in inducing EEG and major motor seizures in the rat. The Pharmacologist 26:118.

Larson, P.S., Haag, H.B., and Silvette, H., eds., 1961, Tobacco Experimental and Clinical Studies, Williams and Wilkins Co., Baltimore.

Longo, V.G., ed., 1962, Electroencephalographic Atlas For Pharmacological Research, Rabbit Brain Research II, Elsevier, Amsterdam.

Longoni, R., Mulas, A., Oderfeld-Novak, B., Marconcini-Pepeu, I., and Pepeu, G., 1976, Effect of single and repeated electroshock applications on brain acetylcholine levels and choline acetyltransferase activity in the rat. Neuropharmacol. 15:283-286.

Lundy, P.M. and Shih, T.M., 1983, Examination of the role of central cholinergic mechanisms in the therapeutic effects of HI-6 in organophosphate poisoning. J. Neurochem. 40:1321-1328.

Mao, C.C., Guidotti, A., and Costa, E., 1975, Evidence for an involvement of GABA in the mediation of the cerebellar cGMP decrease and the anticonvulsant action of diazepam. Naunyn-Schmied. Arch. Pharmacol. 289:369-378.

Pellegrino, L.J., Pellegrino, A.S., and Cushman, A.J., eds., 1979, A Stereotaxic Atlas of the Rat Brain, Plenum Press, New York.

Pfeiffer, C.C., Riopelle, A.J., Smith, R.P., Jenney, E.H., and Williams, H.L., 1957, Comparative study of the effects of meprobamate on the conditioned response, on strychnine and pentylenetetrazol thresholds, on the normal electroencephalogram, and on polysynaptic reflexes. Ann. N.Y. Acad. Sci. 67:734-745.

Pope, A., Morris, A.A., Jasper, H., Eliott, K.A.C., and Penfield, W., 1947, Historical and action potential studies on epileptogenic areas of cerebral cortex in man and the monkey. Res. Publ. Assn. Nerv. Ment. Dis. 26:218-231.

Preston, J.B., 1955, Pentylenetetrazole and thiosemicarbazide: a study of convulsant activity in the isolated cerebral cortex preparation. J. Pharmacol. Exp. Ther. 115:28-38.

Richter, D. and Crossland, J., 1949, Variation in acetylcholine content of the brain with physiological state. Amer. J. Physiol. 159:247-255.

Romano, C. and Goldstein, A., 1980, Stereospecific nicotine receptors on rat brain membranes. Science 210:647-650.

Shih, T.M., 1982, Time course effects of soman on acetylcholine and choline levels in six discrete areas of the rat brain. Psychopharmacology. 78:170-175.

Silvette, H., Hoff, E.C., Larson, P.S., and Haag, H.B., 1962, The actions of nicotine on central nervous system functions. Pharmacol. Rev. 14:137-173.

Simonic, A., Krutak-Król, H., and Domino, E.F., 1983, Muscarinic and nicotinic cholinergic mechanisms involved in seizures induced by cholinesterase inhibitors (ChEI). Second International Meeting on Cholinesterases. Fundamental and Applied Aspects, pp. 159, Bled, Yugoslavia.

Simonić, A., Krutak-Król, H., and Domino, E.F., 1985, Comparative muscarinic and nicotinic cholinergic mechanisms involved in seizures induced by cholinesterase inhibitors. Fifth Annual Chemical Defense Bioscience Review, U.S. Army Research Institute of Chemical Defense, Columbia, MD.

Sivam, S.P., Norris, J.C., Lim D.K., Hoskins, B., and Ho, I.K., 1983, Effect of acute and chronic cholinesterase inhibition with diisopropylfluorophosphate on muscarinic, dopamine and GABA receptors of the rat striatum. J. Neurochem. 40:1414-1422.

Sloan, J.W. and Martin, W.R., 1984, SAR studies of pyridine (P), piperidine (PIP), and pyrrolidine (PY) analogs altering $(\pm)$-[^{3}H]nicotine (Ni) binding in the rat brain P_2 fraction. Fed. Proc. 43:547.

Spinks, A., Young, E.H.P., Farrington, J.A., and Dunlop, D., 1958, The pharmacological actions of pempidine and its ethyl homologue. Br. J. Pharm. 13:501-520.

Stone, C.A., Mecklenberg, K.L., and Torchiana, M.L., 1958, Antagonism of nicotine-induced convulsions by ganglionic blocking agents. Arch. Int. Pharmacodyn. Ther. 117:419-434.

Szreniawski, Z., Kostowski, W., Meszaros, J., Gajewska, S., Faff, J., Bak, W., and Rump, S., 1977, Central anticholinergic effects of N-ethyl-2-pyrrolidylmethyl-cyclopentylphenyl glycollate. Arch. Int. Pharmacodyn. Ther. 226:302-312.

Tarakhovsky, M.L., 1957, Central nicotinolytic action of a new ganglioblocking substance, hexoniate. Pharmacol. & Toxicol. 20:246-250.

Van Meter, W.G., Karczmar, A.G., and Fiscus, R.R., 1978, CNS effects of anticholinesterases in the presence of inhibited cholinesterases. Arch. Int. Pharmacodyn. Ther. 231:249-260.

Zbinden, G. and Randall, L.O., 1967, Pharmacology of benzodiazepines: Laboratory and clinical correlations. Adv. Pharmac. 5:213-291.

THE EFFECTS OF 2,5-HEXANEDIONE ON CHOLINESTERASE IN THE RAT

Barbara F. Bass and Alan M. Goldberg

The Johns Hopkins School of Hygiene and Public Health

615 N. Wolfe Street, Baltimore, Maryland 21205

Acetylcholinesterase (AChE) and butyrylcholinesterase (BChE) are two enzymes that are important because of the role they play in neurotransmission and metabolism of exogenous and endogenous substrates. While both enzymes hydrolyze acetylcholine (ACh), they do so at significantly different rates, AChE being approximately 10X faster (Main, 1976). Both are glycoproteins and exist in homologous sets of six molecular forms, three globular and three asymmetric (Massoulie and Bon, 1982; Vigny et al., 1978). The globular forms consist of the catalytic subunit as a monomer (G_1), a dimer (G_2), and tetramer (G_4). The asymmetric forms are composed of one (A_4), two (A_8), and three (A_{12}) tetramers attached to a collagen tail. The composition of the molecular forms varies from tissue to tissue as well as from species to species.

A significant amount of research has been focused on the cholinesterases in both skeletal muscle and nerve under a number of conditions in which neuromuscular interactions are disturbed. Particular interest has centered on the neurotrophic control of AChE in muscle (Davey and Younkin, 1978; Drachman, 1976; Fernandez et al., 1979; Inestrosa et al., 1977) and to a lesser extent, the distribution and fate of AChE in nerve (Couraud and Di Giamberardino, 1980; Di Giamberardino and Couraud, 1978). Since the discovery of the molecular forms of the enzymes (Hall, 1973), many studies have measured not only changes in total activity levels of the enzymes, but also the changes in the activity levels of the specific molecular forms. It is clear that during neuromuscular disturbances, the molecular forms do not necessarily undergo changes in activity at the exact same time or in the same way (Dettbarn, 1981; Di Giamberardino and Couraud, 1981; McLaughlin and Bosmann, 1976).

Under conditions of denervation in the rat, both AChE and BChE activities in muscle decrease rapidly (Hall, 1973; Ranish et al., 1979). Examination of the molecular forms of AChE has indicated that the activity of endplate and non-endplate specific AChE may decline at different rates, indicating that they are influenced by different factors (Davey and Younkin, 1978; Drachman, 1976). Non-endplate specific AChE is mainly affected by muscle activity, while endplate specific AChE appears to be affected not only by muscle activity, but by an activity-independent factor(s) as well (Davey and Younkin, 1978; Drachman, 1976; Fernandez et al., 1979). Various investigators have suggested that nerve-muscle contact and/or some substance (such as AChE) which undergoes axonal transport and is released at the nerve terminal might be responsible for the activity-independent control of AChE (Davey and Younkin, 1978; Drachman, 1976; Fernandez et al., 1979; Inestrosa et al., 1977).

While much work has been directed at the fate of the cholinesterases in nerve and muscle under a variety of experimental and naturally occurring conditions, little attention has been focused on the changes that may occur in these tissues as a result of exposure to neurotoxic compounds, the hexacarbons (n-hexane, methyl n-butyl ketone, and their metabolites) and acrylamide being two such examples. Both these compounds cause damage in the central and peripheral nervous systems, motor and sensory systems both being affected (Spencer and Schaumburg, 1977). Couraud et al. (1982) have studied the effects of acrylamide exposure on AChE in nerve and muscle of chickens. They found changes in AChE and its molecular forms in the tibialis anterior similar to those seen after denervation. In the sciatic nerve, these investigators observed an increase in the level of the A_{12} form as well as a decrease in the fast axonal transport of the G_4 and A_{12} forms.

The focus of the research presented here was to determine what changes occurred in AChE in the peripheral nervous system and in both AChE and BChE in fast and slow muscle of the rat during hexacarbon intoxication. We chose the tibial nerve for examination based upon work by Spencer and Schaumburg (1978) which indicated that the earliest changes seen in the peripheral nervous system occurred in the branches of the tibial nerve to the calf muscles. The plantaris and soleus muscles were studied because they both are innervated by the same branch of the tibial and because the plantaris is predominantly a fast muscle (84%) (Edgerton et al., 1969) and the soleus, a slow muscle (90%) (Kugelberg, 1976). Spencer and Schaumburg (1977) found that the larger and longer axons appeared to be more sensitive to hexacarbon intoxication. Because fast muscles are innervated predominantly by larger axons and slow ones by smaller axons (Close, 1972; Guth, 1968), we wished to see if the plantaris and soleus muscles were affected differently during hexacarbon exposure.

MATERIALS AND METHODS

Male Sprague-Dawley rats (345 g) were exposed to 0.5% 2,5-hexanedione, a common metabolite of both n-hexane and methyl n-butyl ketone, via their drinking water. The controls were pair-fed in order to accommodate for any weight changes. At weeks 4, 6, 9, and 15 three control and three treated rats were killed. Each rat was anesthetized with sodium pentobarbital (65 mg/kg). In order to limit tissue contamination by AChE and BChE contained in blood, the chest cavity was cut open and the rat was perfused with isotonic saline through the left ventricle until the perfusate ran clear. The plantaris and soleus muscles and the tibial nerves were then removed.

The muscles were cleaned of fat, connective tissue and as much tendon as practical. They were minced with a fine pair of scissors and then homogenized in a high salt extraction buffer containing the following: 10 mM Tris, 1 M NaCl, 1 mM EDTA, 1.0% Triton X-100, 2 mM benzamidine, 5 mM N-ethylmaleimide and 0.7 mM bacitracin (Silman et al., 1979). The latter three compounds, all protease inhibitors, were added to the stock extraction buffer on the day they were to be used. Homogenization was carried out on ice using a Brinkmann Polytron at a setting of 9 for 15 seconds. Samples were then centrifuged on a Beckman J-21 at 20,000rpm (32,000 X g) for 10 minutes at 4°C. The supernatants were stored at -80°C in a Revco freezer until assayed.

The left and right tibial nerves were removed and kept on ice in sodium phosphate buffer pH 7.4. 10 mm nerve segments were cut from nerve with the most distal end point being that at which the last of three branches to the calf muscles appears. The nerve segments were then desheathed, weighed and homogenized in 1 ml Duall homogenizers with the same high salt extraction buffer used with the muscles. Samples were centrifuged in a manner identical to that used with the muscles samples and the resulting supernatants stored at -80°C in a Revco freezer until assayed.

AChE activity was determined based upon the radiometric assay of Johnson and Russell (1975). Total AChE activity was measured by first pre-incubating 10 ul of each sample with 5 ul of tetraisopropyl pyro-phosphoramide (iso-OMPA) (5 X 10^{-5}M final concentration) at room temperature in order to inhibit any BChE present. 5 ul of ^{14}C-ACh (final concentration 1 mM) were then added to the samples and incubation was carried out at either 37°C (muscle and nerve samples) or room temperature (sucrose density gradient samples). The reaction was stopped by the addition of 1.5 ml of 50 mM glycine/HCl buffer, pH 2.5 containing 1 M NaCl. 4.5ml of scintillation cocktail containing 86.4% toluene, 10% n-butanol and 3.6% Liquifluor was then added.

AChE activity in muscle and nerve tissue was expressed per whole muscle or nerve segment. Data was analyzed using a two-way analysis of variance with Duncan's test used for post-hoc analysis.

BChE activity was measured using the same technique to measure AChE activity except that instead of iso-OMPA, BW284C51, at a final concentra-tion of 1 X 10^{-5}M, was used to inhibit AChE.

AChE and BChE molecular forms were separated by velocity sedimentation on 5-20% linear sucrose density gradients made in the extraction buffer already described, but without the protease inhibitors. β-galactosidase (16S) and alkaline phosphatase (6.1S) were added as sedimentation markers. A SW 50.1 rotor was used on a Beckman Model L and spun at 4°C. The centrifuge times and speeds and the various amounts of sample layered on the gradients varied depending on the tissue and were the following:
plantaris -- 150 ul were layered on the gradients which were spun at 35,000rpm (147,000 X g max) for 15 1/3 hours.
soleus -- 75 ul were layered on the gradients which were spun at 37,000rpm (164,000 X g max) for 16 1/6 hours.
tibial -- 150 ul were used and the gradients were spun at 37,000rpm (164,000 X g max) for 15 1/2 hours.

AChE and BChE activities of the gradients were determined as described above. The relative activities of the molecular forms were expressed on a whole muscle or nerve segment basis.

Statistically significant differences between the control and treated groups were determined using two-way analysis of variance (ANOVA) with Duncan's test for post-hoc analysis.

492

The iso-OMPA, BW284C51, benzamidine, bacitracin, N-ethylmaleimide, alkaline phosphatase and β-galactosidase and were purchased from Sigma Chemical Company. The 2,5-hexanedione was purchased from Aldrich Chemical Company and the ^{14}C-ACh and Liquifluor from New England Nuclear.

RESULTS

As a result of 2,5-hexanedione exposure, minimal gait disturbances began to appear in the rats at Week 9. By Week 15, however, all were exhibiting severe signs of the neuropathy, including everted, flat feet, ataxia, and splaying of the hindlimbs.

Both plantaris and soleus muscle wet weights were significantly affected throughout the experiment (Table 1). The plantaris, however, was more severely disturbed, its weight having dropped to 45% of control ($p < .01$) by Week 15.

Total AChE content in the plantaris was significantly elevated to 148% of control ($p < .05$) at Week 4 when the animals displayed no signs of the neuropathy (Fig. 1A). By Week 15, however, when the animals were severely intoxicated, AChE activity had fallen to 36% of control ($p < .01$). BChE levels in the plantaris, while not as significantly altered, showed the same trend with an increase (114%) at Week 4, followed by a decline to 58% ($p < .01$) of control by Week 15 (Fig. 1B).

Analysis of the molecular forms of AChE in the plantaris revealed the presence of three molecular forms, G_1, G_4, and A_{12}. The initial increase in total AChE content was due to increases in the levels of both the G_1 and G_4 forms, A_{12} remaining unchanged (Fig. 2A). By Week 15, however, all

TABLE 1. Muscle Wet Weight

	Week			
	4	6	9	15
Plantaris	95 + 3	92 + 3	78 + 1	45 + 4
Soleus	88 + 5	80 + 1	79 + 6	71 + 2

Weights are expressed as a percentage of control + S.E.M. (n=3)

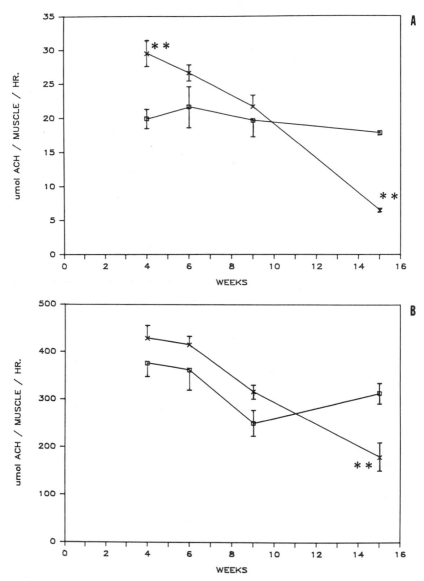

Fig. 1. Cholinesterase activity in the plantaris muscle of control ([ ]--[ ]) and hexacarbon treated (X--X) rats. Each value represents the mean ± S.E.M. (n=3) (* = p<.05; ** = p<.01). A. AChE activity per whole muscle. B. BChE activity per whole muscle.

three forms were depressed below control (Fig. 2B).

In the soleus total AChE activity was consistently depressed below control from Week 4 through Week 15 (Fig. 3A). BChE activity was also similarly decreased throughout the experiment (Fig. 3B). The soleus was

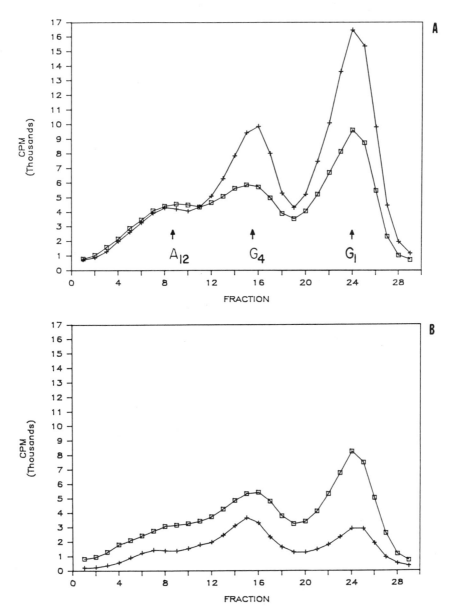

Fig. 2. Velocity sedimentation profiles of AChE molecular forms
in the plantaris muscle of control ([]--[]) and hexacarbon
treated (+--+) rats. Each profile represents the average of the
profiles from three rats and is proportional to AChE activity
per whole muscle. Molecular forms were separated on continuous
5-20% sucrose gradients as described under "Materials and
Methods". The right margin of the profile represents the top of
the gradient. A. Week 4. B. Week 15.

found to contain five molecular forms of AChE, G_1, G_2, G_4, A_8, and A_{12}.
At Week 4 the activity of all forms, except A_{12}, was decreased (Fig. 4A).
It was not until the latter part of the experiment that activity of the A_{12}

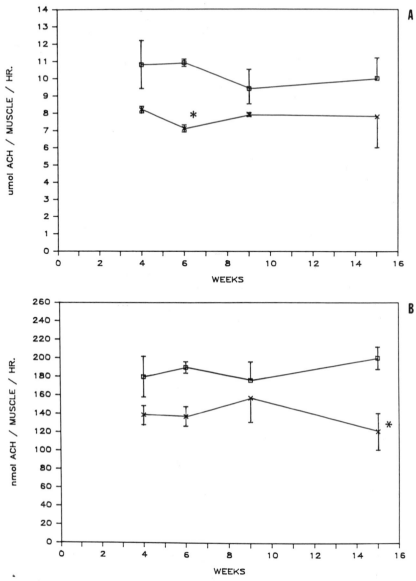

Fig. 3. Cholinesterase activity in the soleus muscle of control
([]--[]) and hexacarbon treated (X--X) rats. Each value
represents the mean ± S.E.M. (n=3) (* = p<.05). A. AChE
activity per whole muscle. B. BChE activity per whole muscle.

form was also decreased (Fig. 4B).

Tibial nerve segment wet weight did not differ from control levels
until the last time point at Week 15 when it was 132% of control and
appeared edematous. Total AChE activity was also increased at this time to
139%. Three molecular forms were extracted from the nerve, G_1, G_2, and
G_4. The increase in total AChE content was due to increases in the G_2 and
G_4 forms, despite a decrease in the G_1 form.

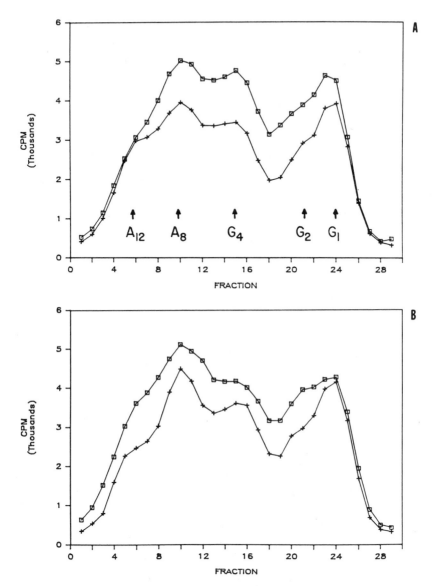

Fig. 4. Velocity sedimentation profiles of AChE molecular forms
in the soleus muscle of control ([]--[]) and hexacarbon treated
(+--+) rats. Each profile represents the average of the
profiles from three rats and is proportional to AChE activity
per whole muscle. Molecular forms were separated on continuous
5-20% sucrose gradients as described under "Materials and
Methods". The right margin of the profile represents the top
of the gradient. A. Week 4. B. Week 15.

DISCUSSION

The tibial nerve was chosen for this study because the earliest morphological changes, as noted by Spencer and Schaumburg (1978), occur in the tibial's branches innervating the calf muscles. The plantaris and the soleus muscles were used because they are both innervated by the same branch of the tibial and because the plantaris is predominantly a fast twitch muscle (Edgerton, 1969) and the soleus, a slow one (Kugelberg, 1976).

The changes seen in the muscle wet weights indicated that both muscles were affected significantly during hexacarbon exposure. The plantaris, however, was the more sensitive of the two, having dropped dramatically to 45% of control by Week 15, when all the animals were exhibiting severe gait disturbances. We assume that the greater susceptibility of the plantaris is a reflection of greater axonal damage in the nerve fibers innervating the plantaris versus those innervating the soleus. This is certainly in keeping with the observations by Spencer and Schaumburg (1977) that larger axons (which usually innervate fast muscle) are more susceptible to damage from hexacarbon exposure.

The first signs of the hexacarbon induced peripheral neuropathy began to appear after 9 weeks of exposure. Disturbances in AChE levels in both muscles, however, were apparent 5 weeks earlier at the first time point taken, Week 4. AChE appears to be a sensitive marker of the hexacarbon neuropathy. It, therefore, would be interesting to see how early, prior to onset of clinical symptoms, AChE activity was affected.

An unusual finding in this study was the increase in total AChE activity in the plantaris during the first part of the experiment. Usually in the rat muscle, AChE activity decreases as a result of neuromuscular disruption (e.g., denervation) (Hall, 1973; Ranish, 1979). It appears likely, however, that this muscle reacts in a different manner to slowly occurring nerve fiber damage than to an abrupt change in neuromuscular functioning, such as that which occurs with denervation.

Soleus AChE activity followed a different course than that seen in the plantaris. It remained constantly depressed throughout the experiment. The fact that the two muscles reacted in different ways to the same trauma is in keeping with observations made by Groswald and Dettbarn (1983), who found differences between fast and slow muscle in the rat during reinnervation after nerve crush.

Total BChE activity in each muscle, while comprising only a small part of total cholinesterase activity, mimicked the pattern of AChE levels in that particular muscle during 2,5-hexanedione exposure. This provides strong evidence for the parallel regulation of the two cholinesterases and supports findings by Silman et al. (1979) that under conditions of denervation and muscular dystrophy, AChE and BChE exhibited similar patterns to each other.

The most unexpected finding in this study was the relative insensitivity of the A_{12} molecular form of AChE to the neuromuscular disturbances caused by exposure to 2,5-hexanedione. The A_{12} form, which is specifically found at the neuromuscular junction in the rat (Fernandez et al., 1979; Hall, 1973; Vigny et al., 1976), is considered to be a sensitive marker of alterations in the relationship between muscle and nerve (Carter and Brimijoin, 1981; Vigny et al., 1976). In our study, however, the A_{12} form was the least sensitive. The activity of all other molecular forms in both the plantaris and the soleus muscles underwent changes at the earliest time point taken, while A_{12} levels were not disturbed until the latter part of exposure, when the animals were exhibiting signs of the neuropathy.

A possible explanation for this phenomenon is based upon the fact that endplate specific AChE (A_{12}) and non-endplate AChE (all other forms) are not regulated in the exact same way (Davey and Younkin, 1978; Drachman, 1976). While both are influenced by muscle activity, the A_{12} form is also regulated by activity-independent factors. There is evidence that the integrity of the neuromuscular junction itself is one of these factors (Drachman, 1972; 1976).

Given the above, if during hexacarbon exposure, neuromuscular transmission were disturbed (thereby disrupting muscular activity) prior to morphological alterations appearing at the neuromuscular junction, one would expect to see, as we did, changes in the activity of the non-endplate forms of AChE before A_{12} activity levels exhibited any changes. Cangioni and his colleagues (1980) have, in fact, found just such disturbances in neuromuscular transmission prior to morphological damage. They observed an increase in the frequency and amplitude of miniature end-plate potentials, reduction of the mean quantal content of the evoked end-plate potentials (epp) and absence of epp's in some muscle fibers, prior to any evidence of neuromuscular pathology. Comparing the alterations in endplate specific AChE to those in non-endplate AChE may prove to be a useful tool in understanding neurotoxicant induced disorders, such as those caused by the hexacarbons.

Total AChE content of the tibial nerve showed no change until the end of the study when the nerve appeared edematous, exhibiting a 32% weight gain. Total AChE activity as well as the molecular forms also were increased only at this time. AChE, therefore, does not appear a sensitive indicator of neural disturbances. This does not rule out, however, that axonal transport of AChE may prove to be a better marker of axonal damage, as evidenced in the chicken by Couraud et al. (1982).

In conclusion, muscle AChE is a good marker of the hexacarbon induced neuropathy, exhibiting significant alterations well in advance of any clinical signs of gait disturbances. Analysis of the molecular forms revealed that non-endplate forms of AChE are far more sensitive to early neural disturbances by 2,5-hexanedione exposure than the endplate specific form, A_{12}. Comparing the distinctions between the two may prove useful in future attempts to understand neuromuscular disorders.

REFERENCES

Cangiano, A., Lutzemberger, L., Rizzuto, N., Simomati, A., Rossi, A., and Toschi, G. (1980) Neurotoxic effects of 2,5-hexanedione in rats: early morphological and functional changes in nerve fibres and neuromuscular junctions. Neurotoxicology 2:25-32.
Carter, J.L., and Brimijoin, S. (1981) Effects of acute and chronic denervation on release of acetylcholinesterase and its molecular forms in rat diaphragms. J. Neurochem. 36:1018-1025.
Close, R. I. (1972) Dynamic properties of mammalian skeletal muscles. Physiol. Rev. 52:129-197.
Couraud, J. Y., and Di Giamberardino, L. (1980) Axonal transport of the molecular forms of acetylcholinesterase in chick sciatic nerve. J. Neurochem. 35:1053-1066.
Couraud, J. Y., Di Giamberardino, L., Chretien, M., Souyri, F., and Fardeau, M. (1982) Acrylamide neuropathy and changes in the axonal transport and muscular content of the molecular forms of acetylcholinesterase. Muscle and Nerve 5:302-312.
Davey, B., and Younkin, S. G. (1978) Effect of nerve stump length on cholinesterase in denervated rat diaphragm. Exp. Neurol. 59: 168-175.
Dettbarn, W. -D. (1981) A distinct difference between slow and fast muscle in acetylcholinesterase recovery after reinnervation in the rat. Exp. Neurol. 74:35-50.
Di Giamberardino, L., and Couraud, J. Y. (1978) Rapid accumulation of high molecular weight acetylcholinesterase in transected sciatic nerve. Nature 271:170-172.
Di Giamberardino, L., and Couraud, J. Y. (1981) Acetylcholinesterase and butyrylcholinesterase: similarities in normal and denervated muscles, differences in axonal transport. In: "Cholinergic Mechanisms". (Eds.) Pepue, G., and Ladinsky, H. Plenum Press, New York, pp. 387-392.

Drachman, D. B. (1972) Neurotrophic regulation of muscle cholinesterase: effects of botulinum toxin and denervation. J. Physiol. 226: 619–627.

Drachman, D. B. (1976) Trophic interactions between nerves and muscles: the role of cholinergic transmission (including usage) and other factors. In: "Biology of Cholinergic Function". (Eds.) Goldberg, A. M., and Hanin, I. Raven Press, New York, pp.161–186.

Edgerton, V. R., Gerchman, L., and Carrow, R. (1969) Histochemical changes in rat skeletal muscle after exercise. Exp. Neurol. 24: 110–123.

Fernandez, H. L., Duell, M. J., and Festoff, B. W. (1979) Neurotrophic control of 16S acetylcholinesterase at the vertebrate neuromuscular junction. J. Neurobiol. 10:441–454.

Groswald, D. E., and Dettbarn, W. –D. (1983) Nerve crush induced change in molecular forms of acetylcholinesterase in soleus and extensor digitorum muscles. Exp. Neurol. 79:519–531.

Guth, L. (1968) "Trophic" influences of nerve on muscle. Physiol. Rev. 48:645–687.

Hall, Z. W. (1973) Multiple forms of acetylcholinesterase and their distribution of endplate and non–endplate regions of rat diaphragm muscle. J. Neurobiol. 4:343–361.

Inestrosa, N. C., Ramirez, B. U., and Fernandez, H. L. (1977) Effect of denervation and of axoplasmic transport blockage on the in vitro release of muscle endplate acetylcholinesterase. J. Neurochem. 28:941–945.

Johnson, C. D., and Russell, R. L. (1975) A rapid, simple radiometric assay for cholinesterase, suitable for multiple determinations. Anal. Biochem. 64:229–238.

Kugelberg, E. (1976) Adaptive transformation of rat soleus motor units during growth. J. Neurol. Sci. 27:269–289.

Main, A. R. (1976) Structure and inhibitors of cholinesterase. In: "Biology of Cholinergic Function". (Eds.) Goldberg, A. M. and Hanin, I. Raven Press, New York, pp. 269–353.

Massoulie, J., and Bon, S. (1982) The molecular forms of cholinesterase and acetylcholinesterase in vertebrates. Ann. Rev. Neurosci. 5: 57–106.

McLaughlin, J., and Bosmann, H. B. (1976) Molecular species in acetyl-cholinesterase in denervated rat skeletal muscle. Exp. Neurol. 52:263–271.

Ranish, N. A., Kiauta, T., and Dettbarn, W. –D. (1979) Axotomy induced changes in cholinergic enzymes in rat nerve and muscles. J. Neurochem. 32:1157–1164.

Silman, I., Di Giamberardino, L., Lyles, J., Couraud, J. Y., and Barnard, E. A. (1979) Parallel regulation of acetylcholinesterase and pseudocholinesterase in normal, denervated and dystrophic chicken skeletal muscle. Nature 280:160–162.

Spencer, P. S., and Schaumburg, H. H. (1977) Ultrastructural studies of the dying-back process. IV. Differential vulnerability of PNS and CNS fibers in experimental central-peripheral distal axonopathies. J. Neuropathol. Exp. Neurol. 36:300–320.

Spencer, P. S., and Schaumburg, H. H. (1978) Pathobiology of neurotoxic axonal degeneration. In: "Physiology and Pathobiology of Axons". (Ed.) Waxman, S. G. Raven Press, New York, pp. 265–282.

Vigny, M., Gisiger, V., and Massoulie, J. (1978) Nonspecific cholin-esterase and acetylcholinesterase in rat tissues: Molecular forms, structural and catalytic properties, and significance of the two enzyme systems. Proc. Natl. Acad. Sci. 75:2588–2592.

Vigny, M., Koenig, J., and Rieger, F. (1976) The motor endplate specific form of acetylcholinesterase: appearance during embryogenesis and reinnervation of rat muscle. J. Neurochem. 27:1347–1353.

ELECTROENCEPHALOGRAPHIC CORRELATES OF NERVE AGENT POISONING

J. F. Glenn, D. J. Hinman and S. B. McMaster

Neurotoxicology Branch
Physiology Division
U.S. Army Medical Research Institute
of Chemical Defense
Aberdeen Proving Ground, MD

INTRODUCTION

Convulsions and seizure activity are major signs of central nervous system (CNS) toxicity induced by organophosphorus (OP) anticholinesterases. Descriptions of the electroencephalographic (EEG) phenomena that accompany anticholinesterase (antiChE) poisoning can be traced back to the early 1940's. Using the then relatively new technique for recording brain activity by electroencephalography, Miller et al. (1940) described the effect of direct application of several cholinergic drugs to cerebral cortex in anesthetized cats and rabbits. Although the EEG techniques utilized might be considered crude by contemporary standards, results from this early EEG study are consistent with our current understanding of the effects of antiChE drugs on the CNS. Three basic classes of EEG waves were described in this study: slow (1.3-10 Hz), fast (11-40 Hz) and "dot" waves (50-100 Hz). The so-called "dot" waves were named because of their appearance as slight discontinuities in the oscilloscope sweeps; apparently the electronic equipment of the time was too slow to accurately follow 50-100 Hz activity. The antiChE agent eserine sulfate (1% solution) produced three major effects on the EEG when applied directly to the cortex: 1) a decrease in amplitude of the slow waves, 2) a decrease in high amplitude fast waves, and 3) an apparent increase in smaller amplitude fast and "dot" wave activities. The description of these effects is generally consistent with the modern-day definition of EEG desynchronization or arousal. Cortically-applied eserine also produced motor signs such as tremor, twitches, and muscle rigidity, indicating stimulation of motor systems; these phenomena occurred contralateral to the side of application. Similar, but weaker, effects were produced by cortical application of acetylcholine (ACh; 0.2-1.0% solution). The effects of ACh were potentiated by pretreatment with the antiChE agent. The combination of eserine and ACh produced large, rapid, rhythmic wave complexes, each complex consisting of two diphasic spikes and smaller waves, at approximately 8-10 complexes per second--probably the first EEG description of antiChE-induced seizure activity. These abnormal waves were accompanied by motor effects. The epileptogenic effects of eserine and/or ACh were prevented by local (0.2%) or systemic (1.18 mg/Kg; i.v.) pretreatment with a cholinergic blocker, atropine sulfate.

Since the early work of Miller et al. (1940), many investigators have described seizures and convulsions, either by EEG or by behavioral techniques, in response to administration of antiChE agents. Although the emphasis of this chapter is on the EEG effects produced by the OP-type antiChE "nerve gases"--primarily soman (GD), sarin (GB) and tabun (GA)-- much more information is available regarding the effects induced by other antiChEs, such as physostigmine (eserine) and DFP. In the following discussion, EEG studies on the effects of various types of antiChEs will be reviewed to present a comprehensive introduction to OP-induced seizures. However, it must be remembered that the effects of OP-type nerve agents may differ both qualitatively and quantitatively from the effects of other antiChE compounds. Thus, particular caution should be exercised when making inferences about mechanisms or neurotoxic effects of the nerve agents based on known effects of other antiChE compounds. In this review, such inferences will be kept to a minimum, and the particular compounds used will be specifically identified. The terms seizures and convulsions are sometimes used interchangeably. Seizures are abnormal neurologic events typified by paroxysmal discharges in EEG recordings and can result in a variety of motor, behavioral and autonomic sequelae. Because the types of sequelae known to follow OP poisoning include some which could be caused by seizures that have no associated convulsive motor signs (see Glenn et al., 1985 for review), in this chapter we will restrict the use of the term convulsion to those seizures that result in overt, discernible motor events.

HISTORICAL SURVEY

Effects of GD and Other Anticholinesterases on EEG Activity

Animal Studies: Acute Effects & Dose-Response. Surprisingly few animal studies have described the effects on EEG activity of the nerve agents GD (Lipp, 1968, 1972, 1973, 1974), GB (Burchfiel et al., 1976; Burchfiel & Duffy, 1982; Karczmar et al., 1966; Longo et al., 1960; Longo, 1962; VanMeter et al., 1978), GA and VX. There is, however, no deficit of information regarding the effects of other antiChEs on the EEG (see Table 1). In general, the effects of antiChEs can be described as a three-stage dose-response curve as shown in Table 1. At low doses (Stage I), antiChEs produce cortical EEG desynchronization or arousal. Although similar in appearance to recordings from awake, alert animals, behaviorally there is no effect in either alert or drowsy subjects. At medium doses (Stage II), subthreshold for convulsions, there is a prominent increase in fast EEG activity which is correlated with alert behavior and motor and autonomic signs of antiChE poisoning. At higher doses (Stage III), the EEG shows generalized synchrony and paroxysmal epileptiform activity (e.g., spikes, spike-and-wave discharges), while behaviorally the animal shows convulsions and occasional signs of limbic or temporal lobe seizures.

Low doses of antiChEs produce a desynchronized EEG pattern suggesting arousal--i.e., an overall decrease in cortical EEG amplitude due to an increase in the ratio of high/low frequency content. In some cases there is an increase in alpha or theta activity, a pattern seen much more consistently in sub-cortical recordings. This pattern has been described in both anesthetized and in unanesthetized animals given either OP-type antiChEs or physostigmine. In unanesthetized, non-paralyzed animals, these low doses produce no effect on overt behavior in either alert or drowsy subjects. The paradoxical lack of behavioral alerting during an EEG "arousal" response in a drowsy/sleeping animal is an example of "EEG-behavioral dissociation" induced by cholinergic drugs (Wikler, 1952). The same pattern of EEG "arousal" is often seen in the initial stages of reaction to higher doses.

Table 1. Profile Of EEG-Behavioral Responses To AntiChEs

Response Category	EEG	Behavior	% AChE Inhibition	Blood Pressure	Selected References	Drug
I	Arousal or Alerting Response cortical desynchronization subcortical synchronization	No effect 'EEG/Behavior Dissociation'	NA	No change	Bokums & Elliott (1968) Bradley & Elkes (1957) Villablanca (1967) Votava et al. (1968)	physostigmine DFP physostigmine physostigmine
II	Arousal or Alerting Response as above with increased high frequency content and increased amplitude	Tremor/Twitches Alert Behavior Peripheral autonomic signs Ataxia	<60%	Increased	Bokums & Elliott (1968) Bradley & Elkes (1957) Freedman & Himwich (1949) Longo et al. (1960) Longo (1962) Miller et al. (1940) Osumi et al. (1975) Rinaldi & Himwich (1955) Traczyk & Sadowski (1962) Yamamoto & Domino (1967)	physostigmine DFP DFP sarin DFP, physostigmine physostigmine chlorfenvinphos DFP physostigmine physostigmine
III	Hypersynchrony Paroxysmal activity Seizures	Convulsions Bizarre behavior aggressive hissing attacking	>60%	Increased preictal/ictal Decreased postictal	Bokums & Elliott (1968) Essig et al. (1950) Freedman & Himwich (1949) Karczmar et al. (1969) Lipp (1968) Longo et al. (1960) De la Manche et al. (1980) Rump et al. (1973) Traczyk & Sadowski (1962) Van Meter et al. (1978)	physostigmine DFP DFP sarin, DFP soman sarin paraoxon DFP physostigmine sarin, DFP

At medium doses, the EEG pattern is characterized by a more marked increase in fast activity, especially the beta activity (13-50 Hz), with maintained decreases in low frequency activity. In spite of great variation in the style and completeness of published descriptions of EEG activity, increased amounts of high frequency activity and higher amplitudes are often reported in studies using doses higher than required to produce desynchronization, but lower than required to evoke seizure activity. The major difference between the effects of low and medium doses, however, is seen in the overt behavioral response. Medium doses are associated with peripheral autonomic (e.g., salivation, meiosis, etc.) and motor signs (e.g., tremors, hyperactivity) of antiChE intoxication, but without overt convulsions. Increased alertness and wakefulness have also been noted (Osumi et al., 1975), indicating a break down in the EEG-behavior dissociation noted at lower dose levels. An increase in blood pressure has been noted at these dose levels (Longo et al., 1960; Longo, 1962).

Seizure inducing doses of antiChEs are associated with generalized EEG synchrony and paroxysmal activity, including epileptiform seizures. The types of paroxysmal activity noted vary greatly among subjects within an experiment as well as between experiments. High-voltage bursts of activity at diverse frequencies, polyspikes, spikes, spike-and-waves, tonic, clonic, "grand-mal," "petit-mal" and status epilepticus are terms that have been used by various investigators to describe antiChE-induced seizure activity. At these doses, brain cholinesterase was inhibited 65-90% by GB or DFP (VanMeter et al., 1978). An estimate of cholinesterase inhibition greater than 60% for the onset of seizures is consistent with that estimated as the threshold for GD-induced behavioral convulsions, 60-70% in mouse (Lundy and Frew, 1984) and 90% in rats (Lundy & Shaw, 1983). Earlier investigators had estimated greater levels of ChE depression at convulsive doses (Hampson et al., 1950; Harwood, 1954); the differences may be attributable to differences in methodological sensitivity. Blood pressure effects of convulsive doses of GB in unanesthetized rabbits were biphasic depending on whether the animal lived or died (Longo et al., 1960). In all animals, blood pressure initially increased and remained elevated during seizures. Animals which ultimately died from the GB showed a decrease in blood pressure, whereas blood pressure remained elevated in surviving animals. These observations were confirmed by Karczmar et al. (1966).

Although division of antiChE-induced EEG, behavioral, biochemical and physiological signs and symptoms into general dose-response categories can be made based on maximum responses within a category, effects characteristic of low and medium doses can be seen with high dose challenges. The time course of the progression of toxic signs appears to depend on the dose, route and rate of administration. Supra-lethal doses can lead to respiratory arrest and cardiovascular collapse without full development of the signs seen at lower doses. It appears obvious that the kinetics of distribution to target sites of action play an important role in the development and characterization of the toxic syndrome. Clues as to the sites of action within the CNS can be found in those EEG studies that measured alterations in activity at multiple cortical and sub-cortical sites, yet difficulties arise in inferring pharmacological sites of action from measurements of changes in EEG activity (see Section II, below).

Human Studies: Acute Effects. Relatively few studies of the acute effects of OPs on EEG activity in humans have been published. Grob and Harvey (1953) summarized the effects of "nerve gas" on the EEG of human volunteers. At doses that produce no symptoms there was no discernible effect on the EEG. At doses that cause "mild" symptoms there was an observable decrement in amplitude. With "moderate" signs and symptoms the EEG tracing was characterized by increased variability in rhythm, increased amplitudes and intermittent slow wave (2-6 Hz) bursts suggestive of interictal patterns recorded in epileptic patients. The epileptiform abnormalities were most marked in the frontal leads and became more prevalent after hyperventilation. Grob and Harvey did not study "more severe" episodes of antiChE poisoning. Although "mild" and "moderate" symptoms are not specifically defined with regard to the EEG studies, these authors state elsewhere in their report that the first effects noted are usually "heartburn" attributable to cardiospasm and "tightness" in the chest attributable to antiChE effects on the respiratory tract. The first CNS effects include tension, anxiety, giddiness, jitteriness and emotional lability. If these symptoms, which would be difficult to detect in animals on the basis of observable signs, are considered to be "mild," then there would appear to be a dose-response category in humans comparable to the low dose category in animals (see Table 1). The EEG effects associated with "moderate" symptoms, obviously sub-convulsive from the descriptions provided, would appear to be comparable to the medium dose-response category. Although tissue cholinesterase levels were not measured, inhibition of red blood cell ChE at the time of first reported symptoms was around 50% following intravascular administration. The threshold ChE level for first symptoms varied greatly (40-90% depression) depending on the route and rate of absorption. Neither onset, severity, nor recovery appeared to correlate highly with the degree of ChE inhibition.

The majority of reports on the EEG effects of OP compounds in humans are clinical studies derived from accidental poisoning in industrial or agricultural settings. Although these data may be more relevant to effects during recovery than during acute toxicity, they are reported here for comparison. One early report summarized clinical experiences with more than 450 individuals accidentally exposed to a variety of OPs, including TEPP, DFP, OMPA, GB and parathion (Holmes & Gaon, 1956). Most of these exposures were by inhalation, although some were cutaneous or oral exposures. In a few cases, EEGs were recorded following either acute or repeated exposure to OPs. Only sparse descriptions of the EEGs were presented. Following acute exposure, there were focal and paroxysmal changes that disappeared with time. In one case of severe poisoning with parathion, EEG changes were observed that persisted for as long as a year. Shortly after the exposure, paroxysmal high-voltage slow waves were recorded; these were generally distributed with some predominance in the posterior leads. In subsequent EEGs, prominent 14 Hz, positive, sharp waves with a comb-like configuration (called "hypothalamic spikes") were recorded. As part of a long-term study of workers occupationally-exposed to accidental GB poisoning, a "triad" of effects attributed to the acute exposure was described (Duffy et al., 1979). These three effects were: 1) increased high frequency activity, 2) decreased low frequency activity, and 3) decreased background voltage.

Finally, EEG findings in severe accidental exposures to insecticides have been reported (Reiger & Okonek, 1975). Three stages of recovery were described. In stage 1, the individuals were comatose and required artificial respiration. The EEG was either flat or of medium amplitude with rhythmic alpha or beta activity. In stage 2, the individuals showed some responsiveness to stimulation, and the EEG showed more synchronization with prominent delta or theta activity. In stages 1 and 2, no plasma cholinesterase was detectable. In stage 3, the level of consciousness improved, and the EEG showed a labile alpha rhythm superimposed upon low frequency activity. In stage 3, cholinesterase activity returned to 20-30% of normal, which was considered a critical level of cholinesterase activity for return of consciousness. The degree to which these effects can be attributed to the direct actions of the antiChE agent rather than to hypoxia or other non-neural toxic effects cannot be determined.

As might be expected from the uncontrolled, clinical origin of much of the data, this review of the human literature indicates much greater variability of EEG response to OPs than the animal studies. Yet, in the only controlled study cited (Grob & Harvey, 1953), the sequence of toxic sequelae for both behavioral and EEG measures is remarkably similar to that reported in animal studies.

Chronic/Repeated Exposure & Persistent/Delayed Effects. Persistent or delayed effects on EEG patterns resulting from either acute or chronic exposure to OP poisoning have been reported. A series of males working in agricultural or industrial occupations and acutely-exposed to OP insecticides was studied (Metcalf & Holmes, 1969). Both low and high dose exposures were included. EEG recordings from untreated subjects made just after the toxic exposure showed slow wave bursts similar to those reported by Grob and Harvey (1953). Even in treated subjects some changes in EEG patterns were seen, particularly an increase in medium-voltage, irregular theta activity that occurred in bursts of from one to five seconds duration. Persistent effects in the EEG, analyzed by autocorrelogram technique, included a less rhythmic EEG with random slowing and increased theta activity. These effects were followed up to a year in one subject. Compared to EEG records from individuals exposed to chlorinated hydrocarbons, OP-exposed individuals had greater background voltages, with more pronounced alpha rhythms. Visual- and auditory-evoked potentials showed a trend toward lower amplitudes and longer peak latencies, although quantitative data were not presented. Changes in sleep patterns were also noted; there was an increased incidence of narcoleptic sleep records based on EEG patterns.

A similar study was conducted using men occupationally-exposed to pesticides (Korsak & Sato, 1977). These subjects had been chronically-exposed to either high or low levels of pesticides and subsequently volunteered to participate in an investigation of EEG effects of such exposures. The EEGs, analyzed by power spectral analysis, showed that the high exposure group had slower dominant alpha frequencies (9-13 Hz) than the low exposure group. Both groups showed augmentation of the theta and beta2 activities (4-7 and 22-25 Hz) respectively. These authors suggested, based on the EEGs and on neuropsychologic testing, that the pesticide exposure was associated with frontal lobe impairment.

In a series of three papers, results from a clinical study of humans exposed occupationally to GB and from an experimental study of monkeys exposed to GB or dieldrin were compared (Burchfiel et al., 1976; Duffy et al., 1979; Burchfiel & Duffy, 1982). The industrial exposure cases, all males, had been exposed to GB levels high enough to produce overt symptoms and to inhibit red cell cholinesterase by at least 75%. The exposures occurred at least one year prior to the study. Unexposed workers, matched for age, sex and socioeconomic status, served as controls. Clinical EEGs and sleep EEGs were recorded. Data from both spectral and visual analysis of the human records were subjected to univariate statistical analysis. Spectral analysis revealed that the exposed subjects had increased high frequency activity (12-30 Hz), while visual inspection showed 3 significant findings: 1) increased low frequency activity (0-8 Hz), 2) decreased amounts of alpha activity (9-12 Hz) and 3) non-specific background abnormalities. There was an additional tendency towards increased amounts of REM sleep in the exposed population. The following groups of monkeys were studied. High dose groups received single doses of GB (5.0 ug/Kg, i.v.) or dieldrin (4.0 mg/Kg, i.v.), which produced severe but non-lethal effects. The monkeys were mechanically ventilated to prevent changes due to hypoxia. Low dose groups received ten weekly doses of GB (1.0 ug/Kg, i.v.) or dieldrin (1.0 mg/Kg, i.v.) , in subclinical but near threshold doses. Vehicle controls were performed. For each animal, awake and sleep EEGs were recorded prior to initial OP administration, 24 hours after the last dose and one year later. In the monkeys given high dose GB, the acute effects included:

1) continuous low-voltage beta activity, 2) high-voltage sharp waves, 3) seizures, and 4) post-ictal depression. Twenty-four hours later, the spikes and slow waves had disappeared, but the fast beta activity persisted. In the one-year recovery recordings, there were modest increases in both beta1 (13-22 Hz) and beta2 (22-50 Hz) activity, especially in the occipito-temporal recording and especially when the monkeys were awake but in a dark room. Similar increases in beta activity were seen with low doses of GB and both dose regimens of dieldrin, although effects in these cases were more consistently seen in frontal-central recordings. No long-lasting effects were seen in any sub-cortical sites (i.e., amygdala, hippocampus, mesencephalic reticular formation, and nucleus centrum medianum of the thalamus).

Pharmacological Mechanisms & Contributing Factors

Anticholinesterases & Acetylcholine. According to accepted theory, antiChEs exert their toxic effects by inhibiting acetylcholinesterase (AChE) to levels which compromise hydrolysis of ACh. An increase in cholinergic activity results from the subsequent accumulation of an excess of ACh at cholinoceptive targets. Whether ACh is considered to be a neurotransmitter or neuromodulator (Krnjevic, 1981), accumulation of excess ACh disrupts critical neural control of target function. Evidence that an excess of endogenous ACh is the driving force behind the toxic syndrome following antiChE poisoning is provided by two major sources: 1) effectiveness of antagonism by cholinergic antagonists (see below), and 2) similarity of effects obtained through administration of exogenous cholinergic agonists, including ACh (see Karczmar, 1976).

The relationship between alterations in cholinergic function and EEG activity is well established. A variety of cholinergic agonists have been shown to produce desynchronizing effects similar to the arousal response either through direct application to neural tissue or through intravascular administration. With the prototypical agonist, ACh itself, nonphysiological concentrations are necessary to evoke this response, although prior "sensitization" through antiChE treatment reduces the amount needed to provoke the response (Miller et al., 1940). Higher concentrations of ACh can induce epileptiform activity similar to that seen after antiChE treatment (Longo, 1962; Miller et al., 1940). Increased levels of endogenous ACh have been measured during EEG arousal (Kanai & Szerb, 1965; Phillis & Chong, 1965; Szerb, 1967) and seizure (Fink, 1966). Several investigators have proposed a role for ACh in the development of epilepsy (Freedman et al., 1949; Tower & McEachern, 1949) and in the control of the sleep-waking cycle (Baghdoyan et al., 1984). Since a full discussion of these topics is beyond the scope of this paper, the reader is referred to the excellent articles by Karczmar (1974, 1976), Laizzo and Longo (1977) and Machne and Unna (1963) for reviews of the pertinent literature on CNS effects of ACh.

Antagonism of AntiChE-Induced Changes in EEG Patterns. Blockade of drug effects by atropine is often used as evidence that a particular drug effect is mediated via cholinergic muscarinic activity. Atropine sulfate has been reported to block the EEG effects of exogenous ACh (Cooke & Sherwood, 1954; Miller et al., 1940) or physostigmine (Bokums & Elliott, 1968; Bradley & Elkes, 1957; Longo, 1962; Miller et al., 1940; Traczyk & Sadowski, 1962). Several investigators have noted that increasing doses of atropine eventually overcome antiChE-induced effects on the EEG (Karczmar et al. 1966; Rinaldi & Himwich, 1955a, 1955b; Wescoe et al., 1948). A mutual antagonism has also been seen in regard to seizure activity (Karczmar et al., 1966; VanMeter et al., 1978). Only two investigators concluded that atropine had no effect on the paroxysmal effects of the antiChEs. The report by Lipp (1972) may be dismissed on the basis of an inadequate dose

(0.1 mg/Kg, i.v.). The report by de la Manche et al. (1980) that paraoxon-induced seizures in rats could not be reversed by atropine at a dose of 5.0 mg/Kg (i.v.) cannot be dismissed on this basis, although differences in species and antiChE between this and all other studies reviewed could have contributed to a discrepancy in results. Although no studies were found that provided a full dose-response relationship, it appears that the antagonism between atropine and antiChE compounds is mutual and dose-dependent.

Many anticonvulsants have been shown to inhibit or reduce the severity of OP-induced seizures. Trimethadione, phenobarbital, pentobarbital or diphenylhydantoin each reversed or prevented DFP-induced seizures in rabbits (Grob & Harvey, 1953; Himwich et al., 1950). Various benzodiazepines were effective against GD-induced seizures in monkeys (Lipp 1972, 1973, 1974) and in rats (Lundy & Shaw, 1983), as well as against DFP-induced seizures in rabbits (Rump et al., 1973). As was the case with atropine, the effects of these anticonvulsants did not always completely restore the EEG to a normal state. The anti-Parkinsonism drug, panparnit, has been found effective in blocking DFP-induced seizures (Essig et al., 1950) and local anesthetics have proven effective in terminating them (Rump & Edelwejn, 1966). Except for panparnit, none of the other anticonvulsants are known to have marked anticholinergic effects. These effects may be due to the non-specific CNS depressant effects of the anticonvulsants, rather than some specific anticholinergic activity.

Systemic Factors. No doubt because of the ubiquitous distribution of AChE and other cholinesterases in the body, as well as because of the potential effects on other neurotransmitter systems (O'Neill, 1983), antiChE agents produce signs and symptoms referable to many sites of action both within the CNS and in the periphery. These signs have been documented repeatedly and include motor, autonomic, neuromuscular and sensory signs, as well as signs indicating effects on complex cerebral functions. Thus, in determining which of these factors contribute to the development of seizures, it is difficult to separate cause, effect, and correlational relationships. Among those factors that have been suggested as contributing to OP-induced seizures are changes in blood pressure, cerebral blood flow, blood glucose, serum electrolytes, and various neurotransmitters or neuromodulators in the CNS. In addition, since convulsive doses of the OPs generally cause respiratory compromise, hypoxia or anoxia must be considered in regard to seizure development.

Convulsive and sub-convulsive doses of OP agents generally cause an increase in systemic blood pressure. This pressor response has been demonstrated with various OPs in humans (Holmes & Gaon, 1956), as well as in experimental animals (GB: Brown, 1960; Longo et al., 1960; DFP: Koppanyi et al., 1947, 1953; Koppanyi & Karczmar, 1951), and by various routes of administration including inhalation. Concomitant with the hypertensive response there is usually some bradycardia (Karczmar et al., 1966). The pressor response may seem paradoxical given the well-documented vasodilatory and hypotensive effects of systemically administered cholinergic agonist drugs. Apparently two mechanisms contribute to the OP-induced pressor response. One mechanism is a peripheral nicotinic pressor action demonstrated in the presence of atropine (Koppanyi et al., 1947, 1953; Koppanyi & Karczmar, 1951). The second mechanism is an atropine-sensitive CNS pressor response demonstrated following intracerebroventricular injection of GD or GB (Brezenoff et al., 1984; Brown, 1960).

The relationship between the pressor response and seizures was investigated in curarized rabbits given GB (Longo et al., 1960). A sub-convulsive dose of GB increased blood pressure (30-40 mm Hg) and produced

EEG arousal. Upon each successive dose of GB, blood pressure was again elevated and remained elevated during seizures. In animals with repeated seizures that died from the effects of GB, a fall in blood pressure occurred during the inter- or post-ictal period. In animals that survived the seizures, the blood pressure remained elevated and no secondary depressor response occurred. These findings are confirmed by other investigators (Karczmar et al., 1966). In humans accidentally-exposed to OPs, increased blood pressure was recorded (Holmes & Gaon, 1956). Systolic blood pressure frequently was as high as 160-170 mm Hg, and as high as 220-240 mm Hg in extreme cases. Lowered blood pressure was recorded only in individuals with respiratory distress.

Cerebral blood flow increases during seizures induced by a variety of convulsant agents (Caspers & Speckmann, 1972; Gibbs, Lennox & Gibbs, 1934; Pinard et al., 1984), as well as antiChE nerve agents (Drewes, 1985; Shipley, personal communication). There has been some speculation that altering the distribution and/or rate of blood flow may modulate the development of OP-induced seizures. Prostaglandin E_2, administered five minutes prior to challenge with a convulsive dose of GD (1.2 LD50, s.c.) in mice, delayed the onset of convulsions (Lundy & Frew, 1984). Similarly, clonidine pretreatment delayed the onset of physostigmine-induced tremors and convulsions (Buccafusco, 1982). Since both prostaglandin E_2 and clonidine modulate cardiovascular function in addition to their direct effects on the CNS, the protective effects may be related to changes in distribution of blood to, and/or flow within, the CNS.

Conflicting results were reported regarding effects of OPs on blood glucose. In humans exposed to various OPs, blood glucose was elevated (Holmes & Gaon, 1956). Likewise, blood glucose was elevated in rats given convulsive doses of GD (McDonough et al., 1983). In contrast, non-significant decreases in both blood glucose and insulin levels occurred in rats given convulsive doses of GD (Clement & Lee, 1980).

There were no changes in serum electrolytes or blood gases correlated with GD-induced convulsions in rats (Clement & Lee, 1980). In that study, blood samples were collected at the onset of overt convulsions to assure that any changes were associated with seizures. Apparently, neither hypoxia nor electrolyte imbalances preceded these convulsions. Furthermore, tissue pO_2 in the brain did not decrease during the development of seizures induced by GD (100-110 ug/Kg, s.c.) in the freely-moving rat (Glenn et al., 1985; Lynch et al., 1985), indicating that tissue hypoxia is not involved in the development of nerve agent-induced seizures. During the initial paroxysmal activity, brain pO_2 actually increased. The increase in pO_2 most likely results from an increase in cerebral blood flow (Caspers & Speckmann, 1972). Consistent with Longo's findings on systemic blood pressure (Longo et al., 1960, Longo, 1962), a secondary fall in pO_2 was seen in the late ictal/ post-ictal period in non-survivors. Serum phosphate was increased and potassium was decreased in humans exposed to OPs (Holmes & Gaon, 1956). In that study, blood samples were collected at various times after OP exposure and were not directly correlated with seizures.

Non-Cholinergic Factors. Although the OPs are recognized to have potent effects on cholinesterase and cholinergic mechanisms, this does not necessarily mean that OP-induced seizures are cholinergically-mediated. In fact, several lines of evidence support the hypothesis that at least some portion of the OP-induced seizure activity is mediated via non-cholinergic mechanisms. The complexity of neuronal and systemic interactions that contribute to seizure activity is consistent with the involvement of multiple transmitters, sites of action and neuronal circuits (Karczmar, 1976).

The OP agents have been shown to cause seizures even after brain cholinesterases were maximally inhibited (VanMeter et al., 1978). Rabbits implanted with cortical and sub-cortical EEG electrodes and pretreated with methylatropine were given three convulsant doses of GB or DFP at fixed intervals. The first dose of GB or DFP produced seizures and inhibited brain AChE by 65-90% (as determined by biochemical assay). Seizures were terminated by atropine sulfate. The second and third doses of the OP, although necessarily higher, reliably produced seizures but did not further inhibit cholinesterase. Thus, the repeat doses of GB or DFP produced seizures independent of cholinesterase inhibition. ChE-independent effects of OP nerve agents have also been shown in autonomic ganglia (Yarowsky et al., 1984) and at the neuromuscular junction (Arcava & Albuquerque, 1985).

Convulsant (lethal) doses of GD significantly increased levels of cyclic GMP (cGMP) in the cerebellum in rats (Lundy & Shaw, 1983). The elevation in cGMP began before the onset of convulsions, but the rate of increase accelerated during and after convulsions. Other brain areas showed no change or a small increase in cGMP. These authors suggested that GD-induced seizures were related to non-cholinergic central excitation because 1) neither atropine nor mecamylamine affected convulsions or the increase in cerebellar cGMP, and 2) the cholinergic innervation of the cerebellum is sparse. Changes in levels of excitatory amino acids in the cerebellum following GD-induced convulsions could not be confirmed, however.

The non-cholinergic mechanism of OP-induced seizures apparently is not mediated via GABA (Lundy et al., 1978). Anticonvulsants known to increase GABAergic activity (amino-oxyacetic acid, diazepam, n-dipropylacetic acid) did decrease GD-induced convulsions in rats. However, GD had no effect on GABA levels in various brain parts or on the activity of either GABA transferase or glutamic acid decarboxylase.

The potential for non-cholinergic involvement in causing the toxic effects of antiChEs has been discussed in detail elsewhere (O'Neill, 1983). Prior to the purification of AChE, a necessary step for AChE assay development, the serine proteases were selected as a parallel enzyme model. This choice was made because of the demonstrated ability of the OP nerve agents to react with this class of enzymes. It was not apparent at that time that this class of enzymes would be shown to be involved in the hydrolysis a new class of neurotransmitters, the biologically active peptides. O'Neill discusses in length the similarity between the EEG effects of opioid peptides and the OPs. The ineffectiveness of phenytoin and phenobarbital in antagonizing peptide-induced seizures indicates that the mechanisms and sites of action may differ from those involved in OP-induced seizures. In addition to possible involvement of opioid peptides, O'Neill discusses similarities between known EEG and behavioral effects of Thyrotropin Releasing Hormone (TRH) and those of the OPs, and cites the recent work of Chubb (1980) on the ability of OPs to prevent hydrolysis of Substance P as evidence for the potential involvement of that putative neurotransmitter in development of the toxic syndrome. Serotonergic sites have also been implicated in the expression of OP toxicity (Valdes et al., 1985).

CNS Sites of Action

The neocortex has been implicated as a site of action for antiChE compounds. In monkeys, exposure to GB produced greater long-term effects on cortical EEG than on sub-cortical EEG (Burchfiel et al., 1976). Lipp (1968) indicated that the EEG effects of GD poisoning were seen earliest and most prominently in the cortical leads, but could not discern a single site of cortical or sub-cortical origin for seizures. Others have concluded that sub-cortical areas are more sensitive to antiChEs. The most frequently

Table 2. Evidence For Sites Of Action Of AntiChE Compounds

PROPOSED SITE OF ACTION	EVIDENCE	REFERENCES
	LESION STUDIES	
Specific Thalamocortical	Spikes blocked in undercut cortex	Chatfield & Dempsey (1942)
Neocortical	Neocortical application induces local EEG changes (Beta)	Chatfield & Dempsey (1942)
Thalamocortical	EEG effects observed in Cerveau sans reticuleé preparation	Desmedt & La Grutta (1955)
Mesodiencephalic RAS	EEG effects observed in Cerveau isolé preparation	Bradley & Elkes (1957)
Mesodiencephalic RAS	EEG effects observed in Cerveau isolé preparation	Longo & Silvestrini (1957)
Rostral Forebrain	EEG effects observed in isolated forebrain preparation	Villablanca (1967)
Neocortex	Epileptiform activity induced in isolated cortical slabs	Krip & Vasquez (1971)
	RESTRICTED DISTRIBUTION STUDIES	
Neocortex	Cortical EEG effects induced by direct application	Miller et al. (1940)
Neocortex	Unilateral EEG effects after carotid injection	Freedman & Himwich (1949)
Diencephalon-Periventricular Gray	Paroxysmal effects after lateral ventricle injections	Cooke & Sherwood (1954)
Hippocampus/Limbic actions independent of neocortex	Spread limited to limbic sites after limbic injections	Baker & Benedict (1968)
Neocortex	Unilateral effects after carotid injection/Cooling of MRF	Gloor et al. (1973)
Neocortex	Unilateral effects after carotid injection	Guberman & Gloor (1974)
Amygdala & Hippocampus	Spread limited to limbic sites after local injections	Smialowski (1976)
Hippocampus (CA3)	Local injections of cholinomimetic produce theta with subsequent seizure spread to limbic & neocortical sites	Turski et al. (1983)
	EVOKED ACTIVITY STUDIES	
Mesodiencephalic RAS	Atropine blocks alerting reaction to electrical stim. of midbrain RAS and administration of ACh and DFP	Rinaldi & Himwich (1955)
Caudatothalamocortical	Effects on caudate recruiting response in Cerveau isolé	Traczyk & Sadowski (1962)

cited areas are limbic system and thalamus, followed closely by reticular formation and basal ganglia. Thus, previous investigations indicate a variety of potential sites of action for the antiChE compounds (see Table 2). Few studies, however, have systematically compared various cortical and sub-cortical sites to determine differential sensitivity to antiChE effects. For purposes of exposition the discussion is broken down into 2 major systems: 1) the mesodiencephalic reticular activating system of Rinaldi & Himwich (1955a), and 2) the limbic system. Because the nervous system contains complex interconnections, care must be taken in inferring an anatomical site of action solely on the basis of EEG changes; the site at which an effect is measured does not necessarily indicate an effective pharmacological site of action. The most relevant evidence presented herein is derived from lesion and local application studies, although more inferential data is provided as well.

Mesodiencephalic Reticular Activating System. Several lines of evidence indicate that the rostral reticular activating system and the diffuse thalamo-cortical projection system are involved in the responses to antiChEs. AntiChEs increase EEG signs of cortical arousal in a dose-dependent manner (see above), thus mimicking stimulation of the reticular activating and thalamo-cortical systems. Rinaldi and Himwich (1955a) postulated that the mesodiencephalic activating system (MDAS), which incorporated both the midbrain reticular formation and diffuse thalamic projection system, was the site of action for the EEG alerting effects of cholinergic compounds. They based their hypothesis on experiments showing that atropine could block EEG alerting effects due to electrical stimulation of the midbrain reticular formation, sensory stimulation, or cholinergic agonists. Their hypothesis was supported in part by studies in cerveau isole preparations that spared the midbrain reticular formation (Bradley & Elkes, 1957; Longo & Silvestrini, 1957; Ilyatchenok, 1962); in these studies the alerting response induced by antiChEs was still present.

513

The requirement for an intact reticular formation has been called into question by other investigators, however. In preparations where the transection removed reticular influences (cerveau sans reticulee), the alerting effect of antiChE compounds was still seen (Desmedt & LaGrutta, 1955; Villablanca, 1967). An intact thalamo-cortical system appears to be sufficient for development of the antiChE effects on the cortical EEG. Of interest in this regard are the earlier findings of Chatfield & Dempsey (1942). These authors separated two antiChE effects on the neocortical EEG. The increase in theta (5-10 Hz) evoked by topical application was attributed to direct, rather than diffuse, thalamo-cortical interconnections because the effect 1) disappeared following undercutting of cortex, and 2) was restricted, rather than diffuse, in distribution. The increase in neocortical high frequency activity persisted after undercutting. The potential importance of the diffuse thalamic projection system was demonstrated by intraventricular injection of ACh and physostigmine in cats (Cooke & Sherwood, 1954). These compounds produced irregular fast activity in several sub-cortical areas in conscious, paralyzed cats or in encephale isole preparations. The activity appeared initially in medial thalamic and periventricular areas, and only secondarily in functionally related areas such as the thalamus, white matter, and cerebral cortex. The EEG effects confirmed the importance of cell groups in the diencephalic periventricular gray matter to the cholinergic response. Furthermore, electrical stimulation of midline thalamic nuclei mimicked the action of intraventricular eserine on the EEG. Thalamo-cortical circuits were invoked as an explanation for the effects of physostigmine and atropine on the cortical EEG and caudate recruiting response (Traczyk & Sadowski, 1962).

There is considerable evidence that antiChEs have direct effects on neocortical EEG responses independent of sub-cortical influences. Topical application of antiChEs or cholinomimetics has been shown to produce local effects that include both arousal responses and seizure activity (Chatfield & Dempsey, 1942; Krip & Vasquez; 1971; Miller et al., 1940). At least some of these effects can be elicited upon undercutting of the affected cortex (Chatfield & Demsey, 1942; Krip & Vasquez, 1971). Based on distribution of blood flow, evidence from intracarotid injections of antiChE compounds may be inferred to be consistent with a neocortical site of action; EEG effects, including seizures, are primarily restricted to the ipsilateral neocortical hemisphere (Freedman & Himwich, 1949; Gloor et al., 1973; Guberman & Gloor, 1974). Similarly, the efficacy of diazepam in treatment of GD poisoning in monkeys was greater in cortical than in sub-cortical areas (Lipp, 1972). Given that diazepam may have a direct effect on cortical processing (Hernandez-Peon et al., 1964), several investigators have inferred a cortical site of action for OP-induced seizures based on the action of diazepam (Lipp, 1972; Rump et al., 1973).

The independent role of the cortex as a primary site of action in the development of antiChE-induced changes in EEG activity should not be surprising in view of its place as the final common path in an ascending cholinergic reticular system (Shute & Lewis, 1963). Cortico-cortical cholinergic pathways have also been identified (Krnjevik & Silver, 1965). Although cholinergic compounds may exert their actions at several points in these pathways, there is sufficient evidence to assume that antiChE compounds can exert a major portion of their actions directly at neocortical sites. The existing literature contains insufficient information to allow conclusions about whether GD or other OPs preferentially affect any one neocortical area more than another. The particular neocortical EEG pattern induced may depend on the balance between local effects and alterations in thalamo-cortical relationships, especially for the development of hypersynchronization and seizures (Chatfield & Dempsey, 1942; Gloor et al., 1973; Guberman & Gloor, 1974).

The effect of antiChEs upon the neuronal circuits normally thought to subserve the arousal response, and the ability of antiChEs to promote seizure activity, are consistent with some recent theories on relationships between arousal mechanisms and etiology of seizures in drug-induced and idiopathic epilepsy. Neidermeyer (1982), Halasz (1982) and Hess et al. (1982) have discussed the promoting influence of phasic shifts in arousal, whether due to stimuli of external or internal origin, on development of epileptiform activity in the EEG. Increased numbers of hypersynchronous events, such as spindles and activation complexes (e.g., K-Complex, "V potentials," etc.), are seen as the onset of seizures approaches. Gloor, Kostopoulos and co-workers (Avoli et al., 1981; Kostopoulos et al., 1981a and b, Kostopoulos & Gloor, 1982; McLachlan, Avoli & Gloor, 1984) have shown a transition between neocortical spindles and spike-wave complexes in the inter-ictal period of penicillin-induced epilepsy. These investigators interpret the transformation from spindles to spike-and-wave as a result of alterations in cortical responsiveness to normal afferent input. A unifying hypothesis could be postulated on the basis of decreased effectiveness of neocortical inhibitory circuits normally involved in the regulation of responsiveness to afferent stimulation, a function normally associated with arousal and attention.

Limbic System Sites. Measurement of local cerebral glucose utilization (LCGU) by autoradiographic techniques provides an alternative to EEG techniques in assessing cerebral activity. LCGU was increased more in sub-cortical than in cortical areas following administration of convulsant doses of GD in rats; the areas showing the greatest increases in LCGU were hippocampal structures, lateral septum, hypothalamus and ventral thalamus, although amygdala and limbic cortex also showed increases (McDonough et al., 1983). The results were similar for convulsions induced by intrahippocampal penicillin and bicuculline (Pazdernik et al., 1985). Substantia nigra and basal ganglia structures showed increases in glucose utilization in pentylenetetrazol- and picrotoxin-induced seizures as well, but not in seizures induced by strychnine. These latter structures appear to be more involved in the spread of seizure activity than in its generation.

Several studies indicated that the hippocampus is one of the primary sites of action of antiChEs. Abnormal EEG patterns were identified in several cortical and sub-cortical areas in cats given escalating doses of physostigmine (Bokums & Elliott, 1968). EEG alterations in the hippocampus were recorded at both sub-convulsive and convulsive physostigmine doses; these authors suggested that the hippocampus was the origin of seizure activity while the amygdala was the origin of bizarre behavior suggestive of temporal seizures. As noted above, alterations in EEG activity in the hippocampus were recorded in monkeys given convulsant doses of GD (Lipp, 1972), and utilization of glucose in the hippocampus increased in rats given convulsant doses of GD (McDonough et al., 1983). Further evidence indicates that the effects of antiChEs on hippocampal activity result from direct actions rather than from indirect effects on afferent input to the hippocampus. Direct application of DFP to the hippocampus in anesthetized cats caused epileptiform spike-and-wave activity in the hippocampus which was subsequently transmitted to functionally related areas of the brain (Baker & Benedict, 1968). The actions on limbic structures were postulated to be independent of those on neocortex. Such DFP-induced activity was antagonized by the muscarinic blocker scopolamine, but not by nicotinic blockers (mecamylamine, hexamethonium, dihydro-beta-erythroidine). Direct application of physostigmine to either hippocampus or amygdala caused similar effects in rabbits (Smialowski, 1976). Similar hippocampal sensitivity (CA3 area) and limbic spread of activity has been noted upon injections of muscarinic agonists in rats (Turski et al., 1983). Others have speculated on the similarity between the distinctive pattern of acute brain damage noted subsequent to limbic status epilepticus and that induced by cholinergically-mediated seizures (Olney, 1983).

AntiChE compounds appear to have independent actions at several cholinoceptive sites within the central nervous system and may influence neural processing through non-cholinergic activity. Despite observations using several different antiChEs, dose levels, and species, no conclusions can be made regarding the relative sensitivity of cortical and sub-cortical areas to antiChE-induced alterations in EEG activity. However, none of these studies systematically compared the effects at various sites using quantitative EEG techniques.

SPECTRAL ANALYSIS OF OP-ACTIONS: WORK IN PROGRESS

Several findings from our on-going research program at the US Army Medical Research Institute of Chemical Defense are relevant to the above discussion and are presented below. In these studies computerized spectral analysis and traditional visual inspection techniques were compared for their usefulness in assessing the central neural effects of the OP nerve agent GD. Most previous EEG studies of OP-induced effects used clinical-type EEG recordings analyzed by traditional visual inspection techniques. Burchfiel and co-workers (Burchfiel et al., 1976; Duffy et al.,1979; Burchfiel et al., 1982), as well as Metcalf and Holmes (1969), included spectral analysis and demonstrated the value of this technique for the study of OP actions in the CNS. Other advanced frequency analysis techniques, such as those used in the pharmaco-EEG studies of Itil (1974) and Fink (1974), have not been applied to the study of OP actions in the CNS. These latter techniques have shown much promise for use in analyzing the central effects of various drugs.

Methods

Complete details of the methodology are described elsewhere (Glenn et al., 1985). Cats were surgically prepared under halothane anesthesia (1.5-3% in O_2) that was supplemented with application of lidocaine to incision and pressure points. Preparation included airway intubation, and arterial and venous catheterization (femoral), as well as electrode implantation in a variety of brain sites. The typical recording configuration was differential bipolar within each site. In the 11 animals reported on here, neocortical sites included sensorimotor (SMC), temporal (TPC), posterior-lateral (PLC) and cerebellar cortices (CBC); while depth electrodes were implanted in the dorsal (DHP) and ventral (VHP) hippocampus, mesencephalic reticular formation (MRF), basolateral amygdala (AMG) and medial septum (SEP). Stereotaxic coordinates were calculated from the atlas of Snider and Niemer (1961), as supplemented by the manual of Ursin and Sterman (1981). Neocortical electrodes consisted of stainless steel screws that were placed through the overlying bone so that they contacted the dura. Depth electrodes consisted of commercially available bipolar electrodes with a 1.0 mm tip separation. Placements were histologically verified and only those data from verified sites were subjected to analysis.

Once the subjects had been fully prepared and stabilized, the halothane anesthesia was discontinued, a paralytic agent, either pancuronium (0.02 - 0.05 ug/Kg; i.v.) or gallamine (5.0 mg/Kg; i.v.) was injected and the animal was mechanically ventilated with oxygen. Supplemental muscle relaxant was administered as needed to maintain paralysis. Approximately one hour elapsed between the termination of general anesthesia and testing. At this time the concentration of halothane in expired gases was less than 0.1%, and the subjects had EEG patterns that were reactive to external stimulation. The treatment design called for intravenous injections at one quarter of the of the historical LD50 (1 LD50 = 15.0 ug/Kg) to be repeated at approximately

10 minute intervals until seizures were noted. Determination of whole blood AChE was made using a radiometric method (Siakotis et al., 1965) from samples taken before GD injection and at 5 minute intervals following the first injection.

The EEG records were subjected to two types of analyses: qualitative (visual) and quantitative (spectral analysis and statistical tests). The paper records were analyzed to determine time of initial seizure activity, defined as a sequence of paroxysmal EEG activity (e.g., a run of spikes) lasting for more than 20 seconds. The records were also analyzed to determine patterns of activity changes in various sites. Distinctive patterns, such as desynchronization, synchronization, and periodic complexes, such as spindle activity, were also noted. Spectral analysis was conducted on a VAX 11/780 using the Power Spectral Analysis System Mark II software package developed at USAMRICD. Artifact-containing epochs were identified and excluded from subsequent spectral analyses. The power in each discrete frequency band was calculated as arbitrary units or as percent of control.

Three types of synoptic presentations based on spectral analysis were prepared: 1) Compressed Spectral Array (CSA) (see Bickford, 1977), 2) changes in integrated power in a specified bandwidth over time (Power vs. Time) and 3) t-test comparisons between spectral power values in the Pre-GD control period and various treatment conditions (see Etevenon & Pidoux, 1977; Fink, 1975; Itil, 1975). The compressed spectral array (CSA) (see figures 2-3) proved particularly useful for assessing changes over time in the "background" EEG pattern in an individual animal. The power vs time analysis provided an alternative method of tracking spectral changes induced by the OP agent. Although the calculation and plotting of the 95% confidence limits is not intended to provide a rigorous statistical test, it proved useful in identifying the sequence of EEG changes related to seizure activity. For statistical analysis of pooled data from all subjects, the method of Shapiro and Glasser (1974) was used; raw data were transformed to z-scores and combined across animals. Data for each electrode site were then subjected to a series of t-tests. Four time periods were selected for statistical comparisons (see legend for figure 2). The first period was three minutes of baseline from the Pre-GD period. The second period was the three minute period beginning 30 seconds after the first injection. The third time period (2 min.) was just prior to the start of seizure activity and the fourth was at the time of peak seizure activity. At each discrete frequency component, estimates of power for each group were independently compared using a t-test algorithm that does not assume homogeneity of variance (Dixon, 1983).

Results & Discussion

EEG Responses to GD. The results of both visual and computer analyses were consistent with each other and with the three-stage dose-response pattern described in section I. The initial EEG response to a single injection of 0.25LD50 GD varied among the sites; visual inspection and spectral analysis were consistent, however, in indicating that neocortical and limbic sites differ in their responses to GD administration. These differences are consistent with the EEG pattern expected during an arousal response. Neocortical sites typically responded with desynchronization within the first three to four minutes following the first injection of antiChE, while limbic sites demonstrated a tendency towards synchronization during the same time period. During the period prior to the development of seizure activity there was a trend towards increased high frequency content and amplitude in the neocortical sites, replicating the pattern of responses expected from a progression through the response stages characterized in table 1.

An example of neocortical desynchronization in the time domain is seen in the EEG tracing provided in figure 1, particularly for SMC and TPC. In the spectral domain desynchronization translates to a decrement in total power. The decrease in integrated power results from a reduction in normally high amplitude, low frequency components in the delta-alpha range. The relative contribution of normally low amplitude high frequencies is increased during an arousal response. This typical decrement in total spectral power, which is characteristic of a neocortical arousal response, is clearly discernible in the integrated power vs. time analysis (figure 2). Although individual variations in the degree of desynchronization exist (compare figure 3), the results of spectral t-tests that combine the responses of all animals during the first three minutes post-challenge demonstrate the consistency of this initial decrease in neocortical low frequency content (figure 5). The increased synchronous activity in the theta band, which is typical of limbic arousal, is represented in the spectral domain by increased delta and theta energy (figure 5), and is seen in the CSA example as higher delta-theta spectral peaks which are especially noticeable after 17:32 (GD#2; figure 4).

It was noted earlier that the EEG response to higher doses of antiChE compounds passed through several stages, which have been arbitrarily separated into 3 dose-response categories in the above discussion. Although it was impossible to assess behavioral arousal in the paralyzed preparations, the initial marked desynchronization produced by a 0.25 LD50 injection of GD appears to be consistent with a borderline stage I (low dose) - stage II (medium dose) response since there is an associated increase in blood pressure and a tendency towards increased neocortical high frequency content typical of stage II (figure 5). This tendency towards increased high frequency content becomes more pronounced as the time of initial seizure activity approaches (compare figure 7). This developing pattern of EEG reaction is typical of a stage II response.

Stage II EEG responses are characterized by increasing amplitude and frequency in both neocortical and limbic sites. The examples of CSA provided in figures 3 and 4 illustrate this progressive trend in the pre-seizure period. An emerging pattern of continuous beta "spindling" at higher than normal amplitudes can be seen in the CSA and associated raw EEG tracings for VHP at 17:45. The high frequency (beta2) spectral patterns during this stage are similar to those described during prolonged recovery from OP intoxication (vide supra).

Visual observations during the late pre-seizure period included the superimposition of higher amplitude synchronous events on a high frequency background. During this "preconvulsive phase" of stage III, transient hypersynchronous events often preceded prolonged or generalized epileptiform seizures. Among those events observed were transient low frequency spindles, sharp waves, spikes, polyspikes and waves, bursts of polyspikes, and complexes with morphology similar to those described as "epileptic" K-complexes by Neidermeyer (1982). These findings are consistent with theories postulating a link between arousal mechanisms and seizure activity (vide supra). Cooke and Sherwood (1954) noted a similar increase in spindles following intraventricular injection of ACh.

In terms of stage III responses, further differences in site-selectivity of OP action become obvious, although few conclusions about relative sensitivity can be drawn. The pattern of seizure activity varied greatly among different subjects in the order of involvement of various sites, in the frequency of "spike" activity during ictal periods, and in the number of sites involved in generalized seizure activity. Neocortical sites evidenced more abrupt, intense and short-lasting seizures compared to the more gradually occurring, but persistent, effects seen in the limbic sites.

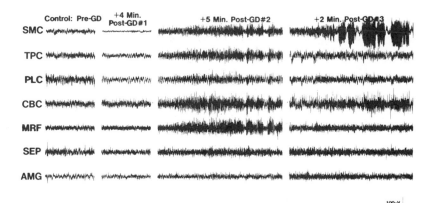

FIGURE 1: EFFECTS OF SOMAN (GD) ON EEG – Sz #3 – First column: EEG activity
in control period prior to first injection of GD; Second column: sample of
EEG activity taken 4 minutes after the first injection of 0.25 LD50 GD
(i.v.); Third column: sample of EEG taken 5 minutes after a second injection
of 0.25 LD50 GD ; Fourth column: sample of EEG taken 2 minutes following a
third injection of 0.25 LD50 GD. Recording sites: SMC – Sensorimotor
cortex; TPC – Temporal cortex; PLC – Posterior-Lateral cortex; CBC –
Cerebellar cortex; MRF – Mesencephalic Reticular Formation; SEP – Medial
Septum; AMG – Amygdala. Time and voltage calibration provided at lower
right.

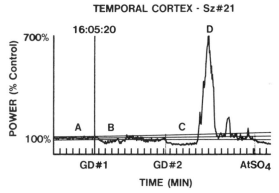

FIGURE 2: EFFECT OF SOMAN (GD) ON EEG POWER – Plot of changes in integrated
EEG power (spectral energy) over time; power within in each sequential 4
second epoch is integrated over the specified frequency band (0.5-50.0 Hz)
and plotted as a function of elapsed time. The ordinate is relative power
and the abscissa is time with tic marks at one minute intervals. The first
injection of GD (GD#1) is indicated by the tall vertical event marker;
subsequent treatment points are indicated by shorter vertical markers and
labeled on the abscissa. The letters A, B, C and D refer to the sampling
periods used in the spectral t-tests (figures 5-10): A – Pre-GD baseline
control; B – Post-GD#1; C – Immediately prior to the initial seizure; D –
Peak of initial seizure activity. Each sample period is 3 minutes in
length. The extrapolated least-squares regression line and 95% confidence
limits of the estimated means were calculated from the power values in
period A.

Table 3. Summary Of Results: Seizure Threshold And Blood Pressure

SUBJECT	SEIZURE THRESHOLD		BLOOD PRESSURE (% OF CONTROL)		
	# Inj.	AChE Levels	Post-GD#1	Pre-Seizure	Post-Seizure
A --	2	NA	139%	160%	83%
B --	2	NA	125%	189%	55%
C --	1	NA	NA	NA	NA
D --	1	NA	109%	112%	52%
E --	2	22%	NA	NA	NA
F --	2	34%	NA	NA	NA
G --	1	36%	149%	134%	57%
H --	2	43%	117%	130%	65%
I --	2	43%	115%	111%	94%
J --	2	24%	140%	170%	117%
K --	3	24%	110%	95%	88%

LEGEND: SEIZURE THRESHOLD: #Inj.= number of 0.25 LD50 doses of GD prior to seizure; AChE levels= percent of control (PRE-GD) whole blood AChE.
BLOOD PRESSURE: Mean femoral arterial readings expressed as percent of control readings taken just before first injection of GD; Post-GD#1= after first injection of GD; Pre-Seizure= prior to start of seizure episode; Post-Seizure= 10 min. after start of seizure episode. NA= Information not available.

This impression is reinforced by examination of the CSA examples provided (figures 3 & 4).

The starting point for seizures was more readily identified in neocortical than in limbic sites. Neocortical seizures typically began with a clearly discernible run of spikes of increasingly higher amplitude. Initial seizure activity in limbic sites differed in character except in those few subjects where there was early generalization of activity between neocortical and limbic sites. Limbic seizure activity often lacked a clear "spike" or "spike-and-wave" pattern; instead, a high amplitude sawtooth pattern progressively developed from a high frequency hypersynchrony in limbic sites, increasing in sharpness at the time of seizure (see EEG tracings contained in figure 4 at 17:45 and 17:55). Although limbic sites appeared less likely to participate in the first seizure episode, the more gradual onset of limbic seizure activity may have contributed to an underestimation of limbic involvement.

Findings from blood pressure and AChE measurements were also consistent with earlier findings (table 3). Increases in blood pressure were usually seen following each 0.25 LD50 injection of GD, and blood pressure normally remained above control readings until after the onset of generalized seizure activity. While no brain tissue measurements of AChE were made, the 57-78% depression in whole blood cholinesterase is consistent with the lower range of brain tissue estimates in earlier work (vide supra). Brain ChE activity is inhibited more than whole blood ChE activity at a given dose of GD (Shih, 1982). Also, convulsive doses of the nerve agents are often assumed to be nearer the LD50 than reported here. The threshold dose for seizures might be lower than that for convulsions, however.

Sensory Motor Cortex

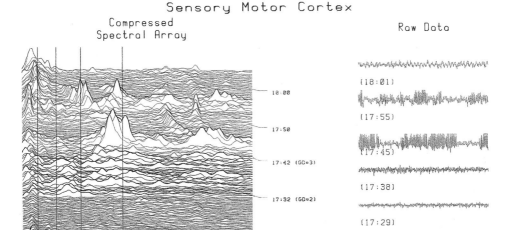

Figure 3

Ventral Hippocampus

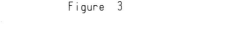
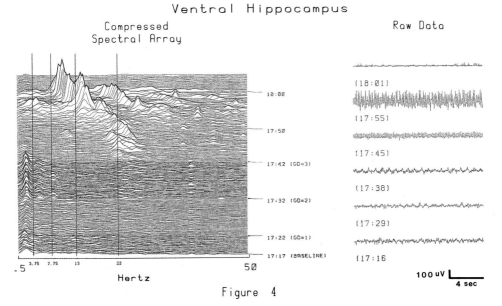

Figure 4

FIGURES 3-4: Left - Compressed Spectral Arrays (CSA): Smoothed average power spectral density functions (power vs. frequency) plotted every 15 seconds. Elapsed time is read from bottom to top as indicated by actual times printed to the right of the CSA. Colors represent drug conditions - black= prior to GD administration; red - subsequent to first injection of GD (3.75 ug/Kg, i.v.); blue - after a cumulative dose of 7.5 ug/Kg; green - cumulative dose equals 11.25 ug/Kg. Y-axis is relative power in arbitrary units; X-axis is frequency in Hertz (0.25 Hz resolution). Red vertical lines separate the traditional EEG frequency bands of Delta (0.5-3.75 Hz), Theta (3.75-7.75 Hz), Alpha (7.75-13.0 Hz), Beta1 (13.0-22 Hz) and Beta2 (22.0-50.0 Hz). **Right** - Samples of EEG tracings (voltage vs. time) selected at times indicated below each trace.

A widely accepted hypothesis holds that antiChEs produce seizures through an increase in cholinergic activity (Martin et al., 1985). Evidence presented here indicates that the EEG effects induced by increasing doses of antiChEs should not be considered monophasic increments on a continuum of cholinergically-mediated arousal. The response is biphasic, at least, with arousal and high-voltage paroxysmal activity being separated by a phase with mixed features of both desynchronization and hypersynchronization. Karczmar (1976) has provided an attractive unifying hypothesis for this apparent dichotomy.

> ...[antiChE] seizures are generally left
> unexplained because it is assumed that they reflect the
> stimulation of cholinergic synapses. Actually, only
> the prodromal desynchrony may relate to this
> stimulation, whereas the cholinergic seizures, i.e.
> hypersynchrony, may in fact be caused by the block of
> cholinergically activated inhibitions resulting from
> blocking effect of accumulated ACh at the pertinent
> synapses. (p.410)

Site-Selectivity of EEG Response to OP Intoxication. The overall conclusion drawn from the various forms of analysis is that there are multiple sites of action, any one of which may serve as a focus for seizure activity. This conclusion is consistent with the literature reviewed above. Based on commonalities of response patterns among subjects revealed by the spectral t-tests, the relative sensitivities of the potential foci may be inferred.

SMC and CBC were the most reliable of the neocortical sites in providing early indication of OP-induced alterations in EEG activity; i.e., the arousal response. These sites were also most likely to show early increases in the amplitude of EEG tracings and to participate in the first seizure episode. Comparing the patterns in EEG spectral alterations along a continuum from anterior to posterior recording sites, a characteristic desynchronization pattern was less likely to be seen in posterior sites (figure 5). The MRF remained relatively unaffected during the initial arousal reaction. As the onset of seizure activity approached, the posterior neocortical sites demonstrated spectral patterns more consistent with an arousal response, while SMC and CBC showed progressive tendencies to increased power across the entire spectrum, especially in the higher frequencies (figure 7).

During the initial post-administration period the distribution of spectral power in limbic sites was relatively unchanged compared to the neocortical sites (figures 5-6). Among limbic sites, only the VHP was a consistent indicator of the arousal response. The limbic spectra during the pre-seizure period (figures 7-8) indicate a relatively greater contribution of high frequency waves in the associated EEG tracings, similar to the pattern seen earlier in neocortical sites.

The spectral pattern during initial seizure activity among various sites is shown in figures 9-10. The smearing of spectral energy across many frequencies due to harmonic distortion introduced by the impulse-like spikes, coupled with variation in the repetition frequency of spike activity among individual subjects, results in a non-specific general increase in spectral power (figure 9). This pattern is seen clearly in SMC, TPC, CBC and MRF, and to a lesser extent in PLC. Of the limbic sites, only the SEP shows a neocortical-like seizure spectra (figure 10). These findings are consistent with the impression gained from visual analysis since SEP was the

FIGURES 5-10: **PAIRED T-TEST COMPARISON** - Individual graphic summaries of significant spectral changes during three experimental time periods; the graph for each site contains the results of 198 separate t-tests pairing spectral values in control and experimental periods. See text and figure 2 for explanation of sample periods. The abscissa of each graph is in Hertz with vertical lines demarcating the EEG bands defined for figures 3-4. Ordinates are in t-values with horizontal lines indicating the associated 99% significance level. Values above the upper horizontal line (P<.005) indicate frequency components in which spectral power significantly increased over control; values below the line indicate significant decreases in spectral power (P<.005).

limbic site most likely to show seizure activity during the initial ictal episode. SMC and CBC are the most reliable sites of initial seizure activity, and the marked increase in these sites is partially attributable to their primacy in determining the sampling period for the initial peak of seizure activity. Similarly, the lesser increase in spectral energy at limbic sites during the time of initial peak seizure activity in neocortical sites is partially due to the more gradual onset of the seizure response in these sites.

The impression imparted by these analyses is that there are direct effects on neocortical sites independent of effects on limbic or reticular structures, especially for stage I and II responses, and that involvement of neocortical sites proceeds fronto-caudally. The identification of a primary focus for seizure activity (stage III) was not identified. While mutual influences between limbic and neocortical sites can be recognized, alterations in limbic activity appear to be largely independent of those in neocortical sites, both in terms of frequency content and time course.

ACKNOWLEDGEMENTS

Dr. Hinman is currently on the staff of NJC Enterprizes, Ltd., New York, NY. A number of individuals made significant contributions to the current study. Two of them, Mr. C.S. Stratton and SP5 A.V. Finger have been with the project since its beginning. Others have participated at various stages of the research. These include Drs. N.K. Marshall and W.G. VanMeter, Mr. N.L. Adams, D.L. Bjork, T.P. Collins, T.M. Grant, B.W. Kuvshinoff, B.G. McHugh, Jr., and M. Nelson. Mr. D. Proper was responsible for computer programming. Secretarial services were provided by Mrs. M. Craven. Special thanks go to the library staff of the Wood Technical Library, especially Diane Zehnpfenning.

The opinions or assertions contained herein are the private views of the authors and are not to be construed as official or as reflecting the views of the U.S. Army or the Department of Defense

In conducting the research described in this report, the investigators adhered to the "Guide for the Care and Use of Laboratory Animals", prepared by the Committee on Care and Use of Laboratory Animals of the Institute of Laboratory Animal Resources, National Research Council.

CTRL vs. FIRST 3 min. POST-GD

SENSORIMOTOR CORTEX

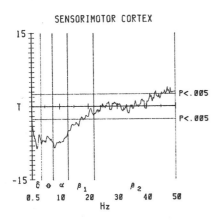

TEMPORAL CORTEX

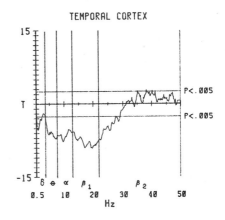

POSTERIOR-LATERAL CORTEX

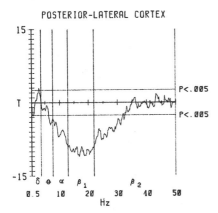

CEREBELLAR CORTEX

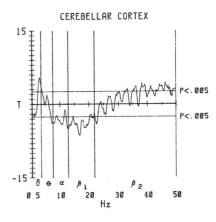

MES. RETICULAR FORMATION

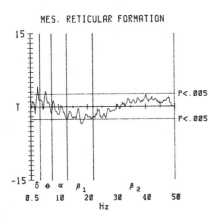

VENTRAL HIPPOCAMPUS

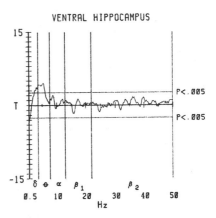

Figure 5

CTRL vs. FIRST 3 min. POST-GD

MEDIAL SEPTUM

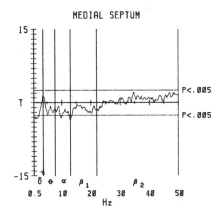

DORSAL HIPPOCAMPUS

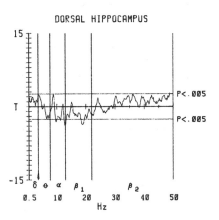

AMYGDALA

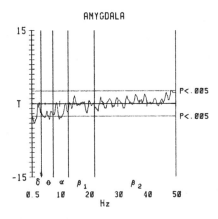

Figure 6

CTRL vs IMMEDIATE PRE-SEIZURE

SENSORIMOTOR CORTEX

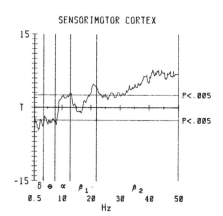

TEMPORAL CORTEX

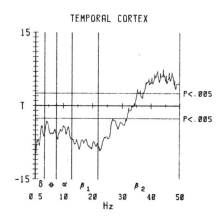

POSTERIOR-LATERAL CORTEX

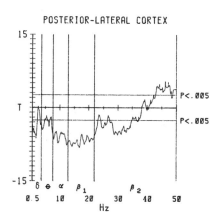

CEREBELLAR CORTEX

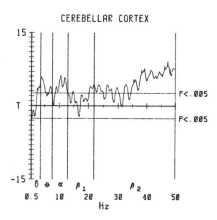

MES. RETICULAR FORMATION

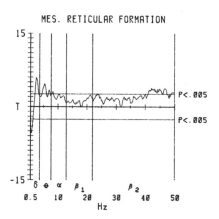

VENTRAL HIPPOCAMPUS

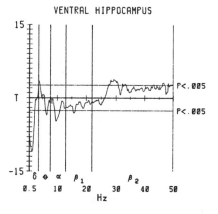

Figure 7

CTRL vs IMMEDIATE PRE-SEIZURE

MEDIAL SEPTUM

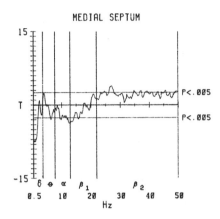

DORSAL HIPPOCAMPUS

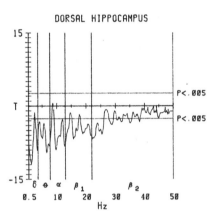

AMYGDALA

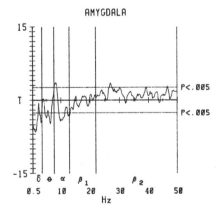

Figure 8

CTRL vs PEAK SEIZURE ACTIVITY

SENSORIMOTOR CORTEX

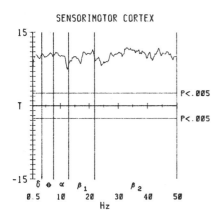

TEMPORAL CORTEX

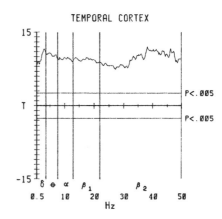

POSTERIOR-LATERAL CORTEX

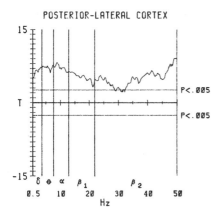

CEREBELLAR CORTEX

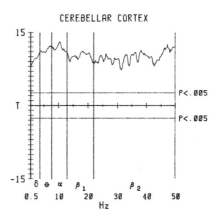

MES. RETICULAR FORMATION

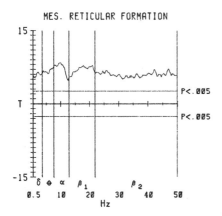

VENTRAL HIPPOCAMPUS

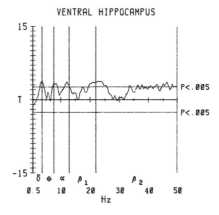

Figure 9

CTRL vs PEAK SEIZURE ACTIVITY

MEDIAL SEPTUM

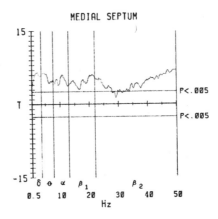

DORSAL HIPPOCAMPUS

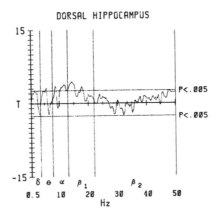

AMYGDALA

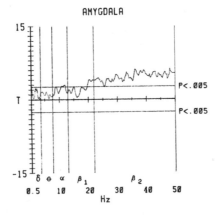

Figure 10

REFERENCES

Arcava, Y. and Albuquerque, E.X., 1985, Direct interactions of reversible and irreversible cholinesterase (ChE) inhibitors with the acetylcholine receptor-ionic channel complex (AChR): Agonist activity and open channel blockade, Soc. Neurosci. Abstr., 11:595.

Avoli, M., Gloor, P., Kostopopulos, G. and Gotman, J., 1981, An analysis of penicillin-induced generalized spike and wave discharges using simultaneous recordings of the cortical and thalamic single neurons, J. Neurophysiol., 50:819-837.

Baghdoyan, H.A., Rodrigo-Angulo, N.L., McCarley, R.W. and Hobson, J.A., 1984, Site-specific enhancement and suppression of desynchronized sleep signs following cholinergic stimulation of three brainstem regions, Brain Res., 306:39-52.

Baker, W. W., and Benedict, F., 1968, Analysis of local discharges induced by intrahippocampal microinjection of carbachol or diisopropylfluorophosphate (DFP), Int. J. Neuropharmacol., 7:135-147.

Bickford, R.G., 1977, Computer analysis of background activity, in: "EEG Informatics," A. Redmond, ed., Elsvier, NY.

Bokums, J.A., and Elliott, H.W., 1968, Effects of physostigmine on electrical activity of the cat brain, Pharmacol., 1:98-110.

Bradley, P.B., and Elkes, J., 1957, The effects of some drugs upon the electrical activity of the brain, Brain, 80:77-117.

Brezenoff, H.E., McGee, J. and Knight, V., 1984, The hypertensive response to soman and its relation to brain acetylcholinesterase inhibition, Acta Pharmacol. et Toxicol., 55:270-277.

Brown, R.V., 1960, The effects of intracisternal sarin and pyridine-2-aldoxime methyl methanesulfonate in anesthetized dogs, Brit. J. Pharmacol., 15:170-174.

Buccafusco, J.J., 1982, Mechanism of the clonidine-induced protection against acetylcholinesterase inhibitor toxicity, J. Pharmacol. Exp. Ther., 222:595-599.

Burchfiel, J.L., Duffy, F.H., and Sim, V.M., 1976, Persistent effects of sarin and dieldrin upon the primate electroencephalogram, Toxicol. Appl. Pharmacol., 35:365-379.

Burchfiel, J.L., and Duffy, F.H., 1982, Organophosphate neurotoxicity: Chronic effects of sarin on the electroencephalogram of monkey and man, Neurobehav. Toxicol. Teratol., 4:767-778.

Caspers, H. and Speckman, E.J., 1972, Cerebral PO2, CO2 and pH: changes during convulsive activity and their significance for spontaneous arrest of seizure, Epilepsia, 13:699-725.

Chatfield, P.O. and Dempsey, E.W., 1942. Some effects of prostigmine and acetylcholine on cortical potentials, Amer. J. Physiol., 135:633-640.

Chubb, I.W., Hodgson, A.J. and White, G.H., 1980, Acetylcholinesterase hydrolyzes substance P, Neurosci., 5:2065-2072.

Clement, J.G., and Lee, M.J., 1980, Soman-induced convulsions: Significance of changes in levels of blood electrolytes, gases, glucose, and insulin, Toxicol. Appl. Pharmacol., 55:203-204

Cooke, P.M., and Sherwood, S.L., 1954, The effect of introduction of some drugs into the cerebral ventricles on the electrical activity of the brain of cats, EEG Clin. Neurophysiol., 6:425-431.

Desmedt, J.E. and LaGrutta, G., 1955, Control of brain potentials by pseudocholinesterase, J. Physiol., 129:46-47P.

Desmedt, J.E. and LaGrutta, G., 1957, The effect of selective inhibition of pseudocholinesterase on the spontaneous and evoked activity of the cat's cerebral cortex, J. Physiol., 136:20-40.

Dixon, W.J., 1983, "BMDP Statistical Software," U. Calif. Press, Berkeley.

Drewes, L.R. and Singh, A.K., 1985, Cerebral metabolism and blood-brain barrier transport: toxicity of organophosphorus compounds, Fifth Ann. Chem. Def. Biosci. Rev., US Army Medical Research and Development Command.

Duffy, F.H., Burchfiel J.L., Bartels, P.H., Gaon, M., and Sim, V.M., 1979, Long-term effects of an organophosphate upon the human electroencephalogram, Toxicol. Appl. Pharmacol., 47:161-176.

Essig, C.F., Hampson, J.L., Bales, P.D., Willis, A. and Himwich, H.E., 1950, Effect of Panparnit on brain wave changes induced by diisopropyl fluorophosphate (DFP), Science, 111:38-39.

Etevenon, P. and Pidoux, B., 1977, From biparametric to multidimensional analysis of EEG, in "EEG Informatics," A. Redmond, ed., Elsvier, NY.

Fink, M., 1966, Cholinergic aspects of convulsive therapy, J. Ment Nerv. Dis., 24:475-484.

Fink, M., 1974, EEG profiles and bioavailability measures of psychotrophic drugs, in "Psychotrophic Drugs and the Human EEG.", T.M. Itil, ed., Modern Prob. Pharmacopsychiatr., 8:76-98, Karger, Basel.

Freedman, A.M., and Himwich, H.E., 1949, DFP: Site of injection and variation in response, Am. J. Physiol., 156:125-128.

Gibbs, F.A., Lennox, W.G. and Gibbs, E.L., 1934, Cerebral blood flow preceding and accompanying epileptic seizures in man, Arch. Neurol. Psychiat., 2:257-292.

Glenn, J.F., Mcmaster, S., Marshall, N.K., Adams, N.L.and Hinman, D., 1985, Electroencephalographic studies of soman's action in the cat, Fifth Ann. Chem. Def. Biosci. Rev., US Army Medical Research and Development Command.

Gloor, P., Testa, G. and Guberman, A., 1973, Brain stem and cortical mechanisms in an animal model of generalized corticoreticular epilepsy, Trans. Am. Neurol. Assoc., 98:203-205.

Grob, D. and Harvey, A.M., 1953, The effects and treatment of nerve gas poisoning, Amer. J. Med., 14:52-63.

Guberman, A. and Gloor, P., 1974, Cholinergic drug studies of generalized penicillin epilepsy in the cat, Brain Res., 78:203-222.

Halasz, P., 1982, Generalized epilepsy with spike-wave pattern (GESW) and intermediate states of sleep, in "Sleep and Epilepsy," M.B. Sterman, M.N. Shouse and P. Passouant, eds., Academic Press, NY.

Hampson, J.L., Essig, C.F., McCauley, A. and Himwich, H.E., 1950, Effects of di-isopropyl fluorophosphate (DFP) on electroencephalogram and cholinesterase activity, EEG Clin. Neurophysiol., 2:41-48.

Harwood, C.T., 1954, Cholinesterase activity and electroencephalograms during circling induced by the intracarotid injection of di-isopropyl fluorophosphate, Am. J. Physiol., 177:171-174.

Hernandez-Peon, R., Rojas-Ramirez, J.A., O'Flaherty, J.J. and Mazzuchelli-O'Flaherty, A.L., 1964, An experimental study of the anticonvulsive and relaxant actions of valium, Int. J. Neuropharmacol., 3:405-412.

Hess, R., Urech, E. and Wieser, H.G., 1982, Arousal patterns in depth recording from epileptics, in "Sleep and Epilepsy," M.B. Sterman, M.N. Shouse and P. Passouant, eds., Academic Press, NY.

Himwich, H.E., Essig, C.F., Hampson, J.L., Bales, P.D., and Freedman, A.M., 1950, Effect of trimethadione (tridione) and other drugs on convulsions caused by diisopropylfluorophosphate (DFP), Am.J. Psychiatry, 106:816-820.

Holmes J.H., and Gaon, M.D., 1956, Observations on acute and multiple exposure to anticholinesterase agents, Trans. Amer. Clin. Climate. Assoc., 68:86-101.

Ilyutchenok, R.I., 1962, The role of cholinergic system of the brain stem reticular formation in the mechanism of central effects of anticholinesterases and cholinolytic drugs, Proc. First Int. Pharmacol. Meeting, 8:211-216.

Itil, T.M., 1974, Quantitative pharmaco-electroencephalography, in "Psychotrophic Drugs and the Human EEG.", T.M. Itil, ed., Modern Prob. Pharmacopsychiatr., 8:43-75, Karger, Basel.

Kanai, T. and Szerb, J.C., 1965, Mesencephalic reticular activating system and cortical acetylcholine output, Nature, 205:80-82.

Karczmar, A.G., 1974, Brain acetylcholine and seizures, in "Psychobiology of

Convulsive Therapy," M. Fink, S. Kety, J. McGaugh and T.W. Williams, eds., V.H. Winston, NY.

Karczmar, A.G., 1976, Central actions of acetylcholine, cholinomimetics, and related drugs, in "Biology of Cholinergic Function," A.M. Goldberg and I. Hanin, eds., Raven Press, NY.

Karczmar, A.G., Kim, K.C., VanMeter, W.G. and Blaber, L.C., 1966, Final report of subcontract #SU630505, in "Treatment for Refractory Anticholinesterases", M.A. Mitz, E. Usdin and J.C. Goan, eds., U.S. Army Contract Report AD#802707, pp.105-225.

Koppanyi, T., Karczmar, A.G., and King, T.O., 1947, The mechanism of action of anticholinesterases, in: "Symp. Milit. Physiol. Milit. Establ. Res. & Develop. Digest Series No. 4", pp 271-285.

Koppanyi, T., Karczmar, A.G., and Sheatz, G.C., 1953, Correlation between pharmacological responses to benzylcholine, methacholine, and acetylcholine and activity of cholinesterases, J. Pharmacol. Exp. Ther., 107:482-500.

Koppanyi, T., and Karczmar, A.G., 1951, Contribution to the study of the mechanism of action of cholinesterase inhibitors, J. Pharmacol. Exp. Ther., 101:327-334.

Korsak, R.J., and Sato, M.M., 1977, Effects of chronic organophosphate pesticide exposure on the central nervous system, Clin. Toxicol., 11:83-95.

Kostopoulos, G. and Gloor, P., 1982, A mechanism for spike-wave discharge in feline penicillin epilepsy and its relationship to spindle generation, in "Sleep and Epilepsy," M.B. Sterman, M.N. Shouse and P. Passouant, eds., Academic Press: NY.

Kostopoulos, G., Gloor, P., Pellegrini, A., and Gotman, J., 1981a, A study of the transition from spindles to spike and wave discharge in feline generalized penicillin epilepsy: microphysiological features, Exp. Neurol., 73:55-77.

Kostopoulos, G., Gloor, Pellegrini, A. and Siatitsas, I., 1981b, A study of the transition from spindles to spike and wave discharge in feline generalized penicillin epilepsy: EEG features, Exp. Neurol., 73:43-54.

Krip, G. and Vazquez, J., 1971. Effects of diphenylhydantoin and cholinergic agents on the neuronally isolated cerebral cortex, EEG Clin. Neurophysiol., 30:391-398.

Krnjevic, K., 1981, Acetylcholine as modulator of amino-acid-mediated synaptic transmission in "The Role of Peptides and Amino Acids as Neurotransmitters", Alan R. Liss, NY.

Krnjevic, K. and Silver, A., 1965, A histochemical study of cholinergic fibres in the cerebral cortex, J. Anat. (London), 99:711-759.

Laizzo, A. and Longo, V.S., 1977, EEG effects of cholinergic and anticholinergic drugs, EEG Clin. Neurophysiol., 7C:7-22.

Lipp, J.A., 1968, Cerebral electrical activity following soman administration, Arch. int. pharmacodyn. Ther., 175:161-169.

Lipp, J.A., 1972, Effect of diazepam upon soman-induced seizure activity and convulsions, EEG Clin. Neurophysiol., 32:557-560.

Lipp, J.A., 1973, Effect of benzodiazepine derivatives on soman-induced seizure activity and convulsions in the monkey, Arch. int. Pharmacodyn., 202:244-251.

Lipp, J.A., 1974, Effect of small doses of clonazepam upon soman-induced seizure activity and convulsions, Arch. int. pharmacodyn., 210:49-54.

Longo, V.G., 1962, "Electroencephalographic Atlas for Pharmacological Research," Elsevier, NY.

Longo, V.G., Nachmansohn, D. and Bovet, D., 1960, Aspects electroencephalographiques de l'antagonisme entre le iodomethylate de 2-pyridine aldoxime (PAM) et le methylflurorophosphate d'isopropyle (sarin), Arch. int. pharmacodyn. 123:282-290.

Longo, V.G. and Silvestrini, 1957, Action of eserine and amphetamine on the electrical activity of the rabbit brain, J. Pharmacol. Exp. Ther., 120:160-170.

Lundy, P.M. and Frew, R., 1984, Evidence of reduced uptake of convulsant in brain following prostaglandin E2, Prostaglandins, 27:725-735.

Lundy, P.M., Magor, G., and Shaw, R.K., 1978, Gamma aminobutyric acid metabolism in different areas of rat brain at the onset of soman-induced convulsions, Arch. int. pharmacodyn., 234:64-73.

Lundy, P.M., and Shaw, R.K., 1983, Modification of cholinergically induced convulsive activity and cyclic GMP levels in the CNS, Neuropharmacol., 22:55-63.

Lynch, T.J., Stratton, C.S. and Glenn, J.F., 1985, Changes in brain po2 during soman-induced seizures in the rat, Soc. Neurosci. Abstr., 11:1262.

Machne, S. and Unna, K.R.W., 1963, Actions at the central nervous system, in "Cholinesterases and Anticholinesterase Agents," Vol. 15, Handbuch der Experimentellen Pharmakologie, Erganzungswk, pp. 679-700. Springer-Verlag, Berlin.

de la Manche, I., Desroches, A., Bouchaud, C., and Laget, P., 1980, Electrocorticogrammes et effets histochimiques accompagnant chez le rat la reactivation des cholinesterases apres action d'un inhibiteur organophosphore, C.R. Acad. Sci. (Paris) (D), 291:401-403.

Martin, L.J., Doebler, J.A., Shih, T-M. and Anthony, A, 1985, Protective effect of diazepam pretreatment on soman-induced brain lesion formation, Brain Res., 325:287-289.

McDonough, J.H., Hackley, B.E., Cross, R., Samson, F., and Nelson, S., 1983, Brain regional glucose use during soman-induced seizures, Neurotoxicol., 4:203-210.

McLachlan, R.S., Avoli, M. and Gloor, P., 1984, Transition form spindles to generalized spike and wave discharges in the cat: simultaneous single-cell recordings in cortex and thalamus, Exp. Neurol., 85:413-425.

Metcalf, D.R. and Holmes, J.H., 1969, EEG, psychological and neurological alterations in humans with organophosphorus exposure, Toxicol. and Physiol., 160:357-365.

Miller, F.R., Stavraky, G.W., and Woonton, G.A., 1940, Effects of eserine, acetylcholine and atropine on the electrocorticogram, J. Neurophysiol., 3:131-138.

Neidermeyer, E., 1982, Petit mal primary generalized epilepsy and sleep, in "Sleep and Epilepsy," M.B. Sterman, M. N. Shouse and P. Passouant, eds., Academic Press:NY.

Olney, J.W., deGubareff, T. and Labruyere, J., 1983, Seizure-related brain damage induced by cholinergic agents, Nature, 301:520-522.

O'Neill, J.J., 1983, Non-cholinesterase effects of anticholinesterases, Prog. Molec. Biol., 8:122-143.

Osumi, Y., Fujiwara, H. , Oishi, R., and Takaori, S., 1975, Central cholinergic activation by chlorfenvinphos, an organophosphate, in the rat, Japan. J. Pharmacol., 25:47-54.

Pazdernik, T.L., Cross, R.S., Giesler, M., Samson, F.E. and Nelson, S.R., 1985, Changes in local cerebral glucose utilization induced by convulsants, Neurosci., 14:823-835.

Phillis, J.W. and Chong, G.C., 1965, Acetylcholine release from the cerebral and cerebellar cortices: its role in cortical arousal, Nature, 207:1253-1255.

Pinard, E., Tremblay, E., Ben-Ari, Y. and Seylaz, J., 1984, Blood flow compensates oxygen demand in the vulnerable CA3 region of the hippocampus during kainate-induced seizures, Neurosci., 13:1039-1049.

Rieger, H, and Okonek, S., 1975, L'E.E.G. dans les intoxations par les inhibiteurs de la cholinesterase (insecticides organo-phosphores), Rev. EEG Clin. Neurophysiol., 5:98-101.

Rinaldi, F. and Himwich, H.E., 1955a, Drugs affecting psychotic behavior and the function of the mesodiencephalic activating system, Dis. Nerv. Sys., 16:133-141.

Rinaldi, F. and Himwich, H.E., 1955b, Alerting response and actions of atropine and cholinergic drugs, AMA Arch. Neurol. Psychi., 73:387–395.

Rump, S. and Edelwejn, Z., 1966, Effects of lignocaine on epileptiform patterns of bioelectrical activity of the rabbit's brain due to diisopropyl phosphorofluoridate (DFP), Int. J. Neuropharmacol., 5:401–403.

Rump, S., Grudzinska, E. and Edelwejn, 1973, Effects of diazepam on epileptiform patterns of bioelectrical activity of the rabbit's brain induced by fluostigmine, Neuropharmacol., 12:813–817.

Shapiro, D.M. and Glasser, M., 1974, Measurement and comparison of EEG–drug effects, in "Psychotrophic Drugs and the Human EEG.", T.M. Itil, ed., Modern Prob. Pharmacopsychiatr., 8:327–349, Basel, Karger.

Shih, T.M., 1982, Time course effects of soman on acetylchoine and choline levels in discrete areas of the rat brain, Psychopharmacol., 78:170–175.

Shute, C.C.D. and Lewis, P.R., 1963, Cholinesterase-containing systems of the brain of the rat, Nature, 199:1160–1164.

Siakotis, A.N., Filbert, M. and Hester, R., 1965, A specific radioisotopic assay for acetylcholinesterase and pseudocholinesterase in brain and plasma, Biochem. Med. 3:1.

Smialowski, A., 1976, The influence of cholinomimetics on bioelectric activity of rabbit's limbic system and behavior, Pol. J. Pharmacol. Pharm., 28:19–26.

Snider, R.S. and Niemer, W.T., 1961, A Stereotaxic Atlas of the Cat Brain, U. Chicago Press, Chicago.

Szerb, J.C., 1967, Cortical acetylcholine release and electroencephalographic arousal, J. Physiol., 192:329–343.

Tower, D.B. and McEachern, D., 1949, Acetylcholine cholinesterase activity in the cerebrospinal fluid of patients with epilepsy, Canad. J. Res.,(E), 27:120–130.

Traczyk, W., and Sadowski, B., 1962, Electrical activity of the "cerveau isole" during caudate nucleus stimulation and its modification by eserine and atropine, Ada. Physiol. Polon., 13:447–457.

Turski, W.A., Cavalheiro, E.A., Turski, L. and Kleinrok, Z., 1983, Intrahippocampal bethanechol in rats: behavioral, electroencephalographic and neuropathological correlates, Behav. Brain Res., 7:361–370.

Ursin, R. and Sterman, M.B., 1981, A Manual for Standardized Scoring of Sleep and Waking States in the Adult Cat, Brain Information Service/Brain Research Service, U. California, Los Angeles

Valdes, J.J., Chester, N.A., Menking, D., Shih, T–M. and Whalley, C., 1985, Regional sensitivity of neuroleptic receptors to sub-acute soman intoxication, Brain Res. Bull., 14:117–121.

VanMeter, W.G., Karczmar, A.G., and Fiscus, R.R., 1978, CNS effects of anticholinesterases in the presence of inhibited cholinesterases, Arch. int. pharmacodyn., 231:249–260.

Wescoe, W.C., Green, R.E., McNamara, B.P. and Krop, S., 1948, The influence of atropine and scopolamine on the central effects of DFP, J. Pharmacol. Exp. Ther., 92:63–72.

Villablanca, H.J., 1967, Effects of atropine, eserine and adrenaline in cats with mesencephalic sections, Arch. Biol. Med. Exp., 3:118–129.

Votava, Z., Benesova, O., Bohdanecky, Z. and Grofova, O., 1968, Influence of atropine, scopolamine and benactyzine on the physostigmine arousal reaction in rabbits, Prog. Brain Res., 28:40–47.

Wikler, A., 1952, Pharmacologic dissociation of behavior and EEG sleep patterns in dogs: Morphine, n-allyl normorphine and atropine, Proc. Soc. Exp. Biol. Med., 79:261–265.

Yamamoto, K., and Domino, E.F., 1967, Cholinergic agonist-antagonist interactions on neocortical and limbic EEG activation, Int. J. Neuropharmacol., 6:357–373.

Yarowsky, P., Fowler, J.C., Taylor, G. and Weinreich, D., 1984, Noncholinesterase actions of an irreversible acetylcholinesterase inhibitor on synaptic transmission and membrane properties in autonomic ganglia, Cell. Molec. Neurobiol., 4:351-366.

DIFFERENTIATION OF MEDULLARY AND NEUROMUSCULAR EFFECTS OF NERVE AGENTS

Daniel L. Rickett[1] and Everette T. Beers

[1]Medical Defense Against Chemical Agents, Headquarters
U.S. Army Medical Research and Development Command
Fort Detrick, Frederick, Maryland 21701
Neurotoxicoloty Branch, Physiology Div. U.S. Army
Medical Research Institute of Chemical Defense
Aberdeen Proving Ground, Maryland 21010-5425

INTRODUCTION

Respiratory insufficiency has long been recognized as the primary
cause of death following acute exposure to lethal doses of
organophosphorus compounds (OP's) (deCandole et al., 1953; Holmes, 1952;
1953a; 1953b; Stewart and Anderson, 1968; Wright, 1954; for review, see
Brimblecombe, 1977). The highly toxic organophosphorus chemical warfare
(CW) nerve agents soman (GD), sarin (GB), tabun (GA), and VX are potent
inhibitors of acetylcholinesterase (AChE) and produce complex and
widespread toxic effects throughout the body. Within the identifiable
confines of the respiratory system alone, the pervasiveness of CW agents'
toxic effects has been noted in a variety of respiratory-related organs
and tissues. Early research established that AChE inhibitors are capable
of either respiratory facilitation or inhibition in a dose-dependent
fashion, that these effects might be attributable to the accumulation of
acetylcholine (ACh), and that their sites of action could be in the
central nervous system (CNS), the periphery, or both.

Because OP's affect many organ systems, research prior to 1950
variously supports contentions that respiratory arrest results from airway
obstruction (Heymans and Jacob, 1947; Verbeke, 1949; Koelle and Gilman,
1949; Holmstedt, 1949), peripheral neuromuscular blockade (MacNamara,
Koelle and Gilman, 1946; Lovatt-Evans, 1951; Douglas and Matthews, 1952),
or central respiratory failure (Modell and Krop, 1946; Modell et al.,
1946; Freedman and Himwich, 1949). This early confusion was instrumental
in leading deCandole and his associates (1953) to examine the lethal
actions of a number of AChE inhibitors in a wide variety of anesthetized
animals, including mice, rats, guinea pigs, rabbits, cats, dogs, sheep,
goats, and monkeys. While the effects of these agents on respiration were
found to vary across species, a general pattern did emerge, which led them
to conclude that central failure, as indicated by decreased phrenic nerve
impulse traffic, seemed "to be the predominant factor in most instances."
That is, to the extent that central failure, bronchospasm and
neuromuscular blockade all contribute to an eventual respiratory arrest,
analyses of the temporal course along which these dysfunctions are
expressed indicated that either onset of central failure preceded and was
more pronounced than other signs of failure or cessation of respiratory
movements was event-locked to a complete loss of central respiratory
drive. Alterations in airway mechanics as manifested by

bronchoconstriction and neuromuscular block were also noted to a varying degree in all species, although these changes only contributed to a relatively depressed level of respiration and were not considered to be the main cause of ventilatory failure; in the monkey, however, central failure appeared to be the sole initiator of respiratory arrest. Research after 1950 generally supports the conclusion that the major actions of nerve agents in producing respiratory failure are mediated through central respiratory mechanisms (Krivoy et al., 1951; Douglas and Matthews, 1952; deCandole et al., 1953; Wright, 1954; Schaumann and Job, 1958; Stewart, 1959; Karczmar et al., 1967; Meeter and Wolthuis, 1968; Stewart and Anderson, 1968; Bay et al., 1973; Muir et al., 1975; Adams et al., 1976; Brimblecombe, 1977; Rickett et al., 1984; Johanson et al., 1985a and 1985b).

While direct evidence supporting peripheral involvement as the primary site of action of OP's is not overwhelming, there is some indirect evidence that appears to lend a degree of credence to such a contention. The major new evidence implicating the periphery is derived from current research into the use of quaternary AChE reactivators, such as pralidoxime, obidoxime, and the H-oximes. Since these quaternary compounds are generally assumed not to readily cross the blood-brain barrier, their efficacy against OP toxicity is believed to originate primarily in the periphery. The use of oximes alone, however, offers little if any significant antidotal benefit (Lundy and Shih, 1983; Shih et al., 1985). When oximes are administered in combination with a tertiary antimuscarinic compound, such as atropine sulfate, which is known to readily penetrate the blood-brain barrier, the protective ratio increased three to ten-fold, depending on species and dosing (Schenk et al., 1976; Gordon et al., 1978; Hauser and Dola, 1980; Maksimovic et al., 1980; Clement, 1981; Wolthuis et al., 1981; Lundy and Shih, 1983; Shih et al., 1985). Quaternary belladonna alkaloids, such as atropine methylnitrate, on the other hand, have been shown to offer no added antidotal effect in OP-intoxicated animals that had been pretreated with oximes (Clement, 1982; Lundy and Shih, 1983; Shih et al., 1985).

The present study was designed to re-investigate the effects of OP's on central and peripheral nervous system components of the respiratory system. Using DIAL (70 mg/kg, IP) anesthetized cats, recordings were made of i) medullary respiratory-related unit activity, ii) phrenic nerve activity, iii) diaphragm electromyographic activity (EMG), iv) contractions of the diaphragm leaflet, v) airflow, vi) femoral arterial pressure, and vii) electrocardiographic activity (ECG). Blood gases and expired CO_2 were monitored also. The agents were infused slowly until cessation of spontaneous respiration; at which time, the phrenic nerve was stimulated supramaximally to test diaphragmatic contraction. Following the diaphragmatic test, infusion of agent was resumed at 3 times the initial concentration in the mechanically ventilated animal, and the diaphragm was tested periodically. For each agent tested, respiratory arrest was preceded by a loss of central drive. Neuromuscular blockade, when not obscured by cardiovascular collapse, required a dose from 5 to 14 times greater than that which produced cessation of respiration.

METHODS

Thirty-five cats of either sex, weighing between 2.5 and 4.0 kg, were used in this study. For at least two weeks prior to the experiment, the cats were housed in the surgical holding area and allowed to acclimate to the technicians; on the day before the study, food was withheld, but the cats were allowed free access to water. On the morning of the study, the animals were anesthetized with intraperitoneal DIAL-urethane (Ciba-Geigy

536

formulation: diallybarbituric acid, 100 mg/ml; urethane, 400 mg/ml; monoethyl urea, 400 mg/ml) at 0.7ml/kg and intubated. Airflow was recorded using a Gould PM15ETC pneumotach attached to the end of the endotracheal tube, which also allowed monitoring of expired CO_2 (IL200 CO_2 Analyzer). Electrocardiograph was recorded from ECG Lead II. Rectal temperature was maintained at approximately $37^{\circ}C$ by a thermostatically controlled water blanket underneath the animal.

Surgical Procedures

Catheters were placed in both femoral arteries: one to record systemic blood pressure (Gould P23 Transducer) and the other to withdraw arterial blood samples for the measurement of blood gases and pH (Corning 165/2 Blood Gas Analyzer). Both femoral veins were cannulated for the infusion of fluids and drugs. Following arterial and venous cannulation, the cat was clamped into the spinal frame at the lower-thoracic, high-lumbar level to stabilize the diaphragmatic region. The diaphragm was accessed through a lateral incision just below the last rib. Two needle electrodes (Grass E2B) for EMG monitoring were carefully threaded into the superficial layer of the diaphragm muscle leaflet innervated by the monitored phrenic nerve. The interelectrode distance was kept to approximately 2 mm. Muscle tension was measured by either stitching or gluing (cyano-acrylic) a silk suture (size 00) to the diaphragm muscle leaflet; the suture was then passed through the incision in PE tubing and the incision loosely closed.

The phrenic nerve was exposed in the neck via a lateral approach. After identifying its emergence at C5-C6, the nerve was carefully desheathed and placed intact into a slit sleeve electrode containing two silver electrodes for differential recording of phrenic nerve activity. The nerve, electrodes and cuff were then covered with warm mineral oil and the incision loosely closed to protect the area.

The offset earbars of the stereotaxic frame were adjusted so that the neck was flexed and the head oriented down at about a 45° angle. This orientation provided ready access to the region of the obex, which was exposed by midline incision and craniectomy from the foramen magnum to the region of the cerebellum. After the dorsal surface of the medulla was exposed, it was kept covered with warm mineral oil. After establishing good phrenic and EMG signals, a BAK stainless steel extracellular electrode (1.0-1.1 Mohm) for recording single extracellular unit activity was placed in the medullary respiratory-related area using a Kopf micromanipulator for lateral and A-P positioning and a Narishige hydraulic micromanipulator for vertical positioning in the respiratory area. Although respiratory-related units were recorded from both the dorsal and ventral respiratory groups, units were usually acquired from the region approximately 2 mm lateral and 2 mm rostral to the obex and 2-5 mm deep.

Recording Procedures

Arterial blood pressure, airflow, ECG Lead II, and diaphragm tension were displayed on a Gould Biophysical Monitor; digital displays allowed direct readout of systolic/diastolic/mean blood pressure, heart rate, respiratory rate, and rectal temperature. Output from the Biophysical Monitor was recorded on a Gould inkwriting polygraph in parallel with a Honeywell 101 FM tape recorder; all electrophysiological signals (diaphragm EMG, phrenic nerve activity and unit activity) were monitored on an oscilloscope prior to recording on the Honeywell 101. Expired CO_2, voice and time were also recorded on the Honeywell 101. The polygraph, biophysical monitor and digital displays allowed real-time analysis of the physiological state of the animal, while the FM tape recorder provided storage of the data for future, detailed analysis.

All electrophysiological signals were filtered and amplified prior to tape recording. Preamplifiers from BAK MD-4 amplifiers were placed within 6 inches of the recording site. The signals were filtered with bandpass filters (Kronhite) set at 100 Hz and 5 KHz; EMG was usually amplified by 1000, while phrenic and unit signals were amplified by 10,000.

Experimental Protocol

The organophosphorus compounds used in this study were the nerve agents soman (GD), sarin (GB), tabun (GA) and VX (Figure 1). All nerve agents were freshly prepared from USAMRICD stocks approximately two hours prior to use. The neat agent was removed from the freezer and allowed to equilibrate for approximately 30 min. Sufficient volumes were withdrawn to make a 100 ml solution of 200 ug/ml in iced saline. This was thoroughly mixed and subsequent dilutions, in iced saline, were made to contain one LD_{50}/15 ml and one LD_{50}/5 ml (agent LD_{50}--soman, 15 ug/kg; sarin, 45 ug/kg; tabun, 47 ug/kg; VX, 5 ug/kg). These solutions were kept on ice until just before use. They were then drawn into 100 ml syringes, allowed to come to room temperature, and infused with an infusion pump at one ml/min. At the conclusion of each experiment, all materials coming into contact with the agent, as well as unused agent, were detoxified by overnight immersion in concentrated NaOH solution (for G agents) or chlorine bleach (for VX).

After completion of surgery and location of a respiratory-related unit, a five minute saline control period was initiated during which normal saline was infused at 1 ml/min, followed by a five minute post-saline control period. After establishing the control periods, agent infusion was begun at 1 ml/min at a concentration of 1 LD_{50} per 15 minutes. Following cessation of spontaneous respiration, diaphragm neuromuscular integrity was tested by stimulation of the phrenic nerve. Stimulation was accomplished by using a Berl Model 220B Stimulator connected to the phrenic nerve electrodes through the stimulating port of the BAK preamplifier. The stimulation parameters employed were 2.0 msec pulses delivered in a 500 msec burst at supramaximal voltage with a frequency of either 10Hz or 100Hz. After phrenic stimulation, mechanical respiration was begun at a rate of 30 breaths per minute and a tidal

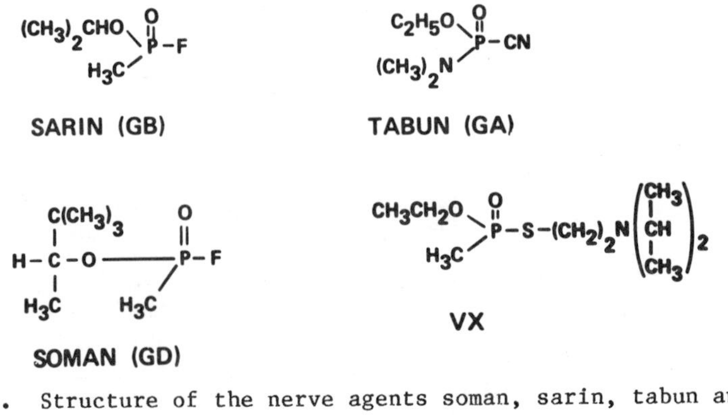

Fig. 1. Structure of the nerve agents soman, sarin, tabun and VX.

volume equivalent to control values; respiratory rate and tidal volume were adjusted to maintain end-tidal expired CO_2 at 4% and to keep blood gases within nominal limits (PCO_2 = 30-40mmHg and PO_2 = 75-90mmHg). Agent infusion was then resumed at 1 ml/min at a concentration of 1 LD_{50} per five minutes (three times the initial concentration) and continued until neuromuscular block was attained or cardiovascular collapse intervened; the diaphragm was tested at frequent intervals by phrenic nerve stimulation. In some animals, rather than infusing more agent after respiratory arrest, the stimulation protocol was tested by phrenic nerve stimulation after blocking the neuromuscular junction with Flaxedil (Davis and Geck).

Data Analysis

The respiratory-related parameters (airflow, diaphragm tension, diaphragm EMG, and phrenic nerve activity) are shown as respiratory cycle-triggered averages, while the unit activity is shown as a frequency histogram of a single unit detected using waveform analysis. Cycle-triggered averaging is a technique that allows the display and comparison of cyclical waveforms independent of frequency changes; for instance, the waveforms for airflow when plotted over two respiratory cycles at respiratory rates of 30 per minute and 15 per minute are displayed over the same horizontal distance, even though the time to complete two cycles at a rate of 15 per minute is twice as long as the time to complete two cycles at 30 per minute. One of the advantages of cycle-triggered averaging is that all time-related parameters are displayed as phase-locked variables during the cycle of interest. Averaging of respiratory parameters from multiple breaths was accomplished by dividing the respiratory cycle into inspiratory and expiratory events with 100 bins in each; inspiration was defined as the period from the beginning of inspiration to peak inspiration, while expiration was defined as the period from peak inspiration to the beginning of the next inspiration (Smolders and Folgering, 1979). Each average contained five respiratory cycles; in some instances, the respiratory rate was so low just prior to respiratory arrest that fewer cycles were included in the average. Thus, all parameters, except unit activity, are shown as cycle-triggered averages of the percent of the peak value at control; unit activity is shown as a cycle-triggered frequency histogram in spikes per second.

The variables in the bargraphs in Figure 7 are depicted as percent of control values at selected points during the infusion period, where 100% infused agent is attained at respiratory arrest. Each bar is the mean + the standard error of the mean (SEM) of the variable at that particular point in the infusion period for all animals tested with that agent. The numbers of animals shown for soman and sarin in the bargraphs is less than in Table 1 because in some of the first experiments with soman and sarin, all the variables were not recorded onto FM tape.

RESULTS

The results are presented in two parts, although the experiments were performed simultaneously. The first part concerns whether or not the agent-induced respiratory arrest results from a block of the diaphragm neuromuscular junction. The second part depicts the progression of the effects of the agents on selected respiratory parameters during the slow (15 minutes per LD_{50}) infusion.

539

Part One: Phrenic Stimulation

The amount of each agent (in LD_{50}'s) required to produce respiratory arrest versus the amount required to block the diaphragm is presented in Table 1. While diaphragm block could be demonstrated consistently in the case of soman, cardiovascular collapse frequently intervened prior to complete block of the diaphragm when the agent administered was sarin, tabun or VX. Consistent with VX's delayed actions, multiple LD_{50}'s were required to produce respiratory arrest; a better strategy may have been to infuse 1.5-2 LD_{50}'s, then wait for effects to develop. When tested by electrical stimulation of the phrenic nerve immediately following cessation of respiration, the diaphragm muscle was able to maintain a tetanic stimulation regardless of the agent administered.

Table 1. Amount of agent required to produce respiratory arrest and neuromuscular block. The data are expressed as multiples of an $LD_{50} \pm$ SEM, infused at 1 LD_{50}/15 min.

AGENT	DOSE TO PRODUCE RESPIRATORY ARREST	DOSE TO PRODUCE NEUROMUSCULAR BLOCK
Soman (n=14)	0.94 ± 0.12	14 ± 2
Sarin (n=13)	0.56 ± 0.05	> 5
Tabun (n=4)	1.25 ± 0.3	> 2
VX (n=4)	14.8 ± 1.1	> 15

Figure 2 depicts the response of the diaphragm to electrical stimulation of the phrenic nerve following respiratory arrest produced by either tabun or VX. This figure clearly shows that electrical stimulation of the phrenic nerve elicits a frequency-following contraction in the diaphragm muscle at a stimulation frequency of 10 Hz and produces a tetanic contraction when the muscle is stimulated at 100 Hz; not only are these contractions seen as increased diaphragm tension, but phrenic stimulation elicits a frequency-following and tetanic response in diaphragm EMG and air flow as well. The responses generated in the diaphragm by phrenic stimulation subsequent to soman or sarin-induced respiratory arrest are substantially the same as those depicted for tabun or VX. For those animals in which Flaxedil was administered prior to phrenic stimulation, diaphragm tension or EMG could not be elicited. The failure to cause a diaphragm contraction in this instance demonstrates that the muscle contractions shown in the figure are being produced as a result of phrenic nerve stimulation and not by direct electrical stimulation of the diaphragm muscle.

Part Two: Responses to Agent Infusion

The progression of the effects of the agents on air flow, diaphragmatic contraction, integrated diaphragm EMG, integrated phrenic nerve activity, and medullary respiratory-related unit activity is seen in Figures 3 to 6. These figures are cycle-triggered averages with the horizontal axis representing two respiratory cycles (one respiratory cycle in the case of soman) rather than time; the respiratory rate (RR) is shown under each histogram. All parameters, except unit activity, are presented as a percent of the control value, where 100% represents the peak value

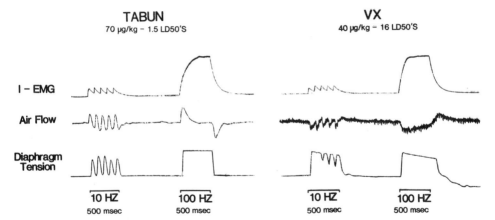

TABUN
70 µg/kg – 1.5 LD50'S

VX
40 µg/kg – 16 LD50'S

I – EMG

Air Flow

Diaphragm
Tension

10 HZ
500 msec

100 HZ
500 msec

10 HZ
500 msec

100 HZ
500 msec

Fig. 2. Response of the diaphragm to phrenic nerve stimulation after
cessation of spontaneous respiration. Stimulation parameters:
2.0 msec pulse, 10 Hz or 100 Hz frequency, 500 msec burst,
supramaximal voltage. Inspiratory airflow is indicated by an
upward deflection of the trace for tabun and by a downward
deflection for VX.

during control; unit activity is shown in spikes per second. The cycle-
triggered analysis allows phase-locked display of the shapes of the
waveforms; however, tidal volume (airflow integrated over time) cannot be
readily inferred from these figures, since time is not a variable here.
Tidal volumes are presented in Figure 7. Each figure is the response of
only one animal for that agent but is representative of the response of
all animals for that particular agent. In each of the figures, cessation
of spontaneous respiration occurred within 1 to 2 minutes following the
last frame.

Of the parameters analyzed in these experiments, medullary
respiratory-related unit activity was the most sensitive to agent
infusion. The figures show that unit activity was affected in a
progressive, dose-dependent fashion, becoming increasingly disrupted until
the neuron ceased activity or began firing randomly. Although some cells
showed an early cessation of activity (as in Figure 4), at other times
either the cells began firing during previously silent periods or there
was a recruitment of previously silent neurons (Figures 3 and 6). Almost
all types of discharges characteristic of a functionally disrupted central
respiratory area were observed, including recruitment of previously silent
neurons, inappropriate firing patterns, cessation of activity, increase in
activity, tonic firing of previously phasic neurons (Figures 3 and 5), and
phase-shifting of the firing pattern of the neuron (Figure 3). Figure 3
shows that a neuron which was previously an inspiratory-related neuron
began firing predominately during expiration. Using spike-triggered
averaging of the phrenic neurogram, it was found that this cell continued
to produce a peak in phrenic activity which was indicative of monosynaptic
delay. Thus, the cell had retained its function although its discharge
had shifted phase.

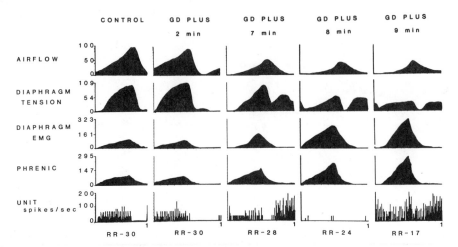

Fig. 3. The dose-dependent actions of soman. Airflow, diaphragm tension, diaphragm EMG and phrenic nerve activity are in percent of control. The single unit activity is expressed as firing frequency over time. The abscissa denotes a single respiratory cycle. RR: respiratory rate.

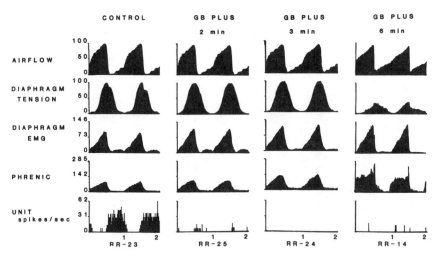

Fig. 4. The dose-dependent actions of sarin. Airflow, diaphragm tension, diaphragm EMG and phrenic nerve activity are in percent of control. The single unit activity is expressed as firing frequency over time. The abscissa denotes two respiratory cycles. RR: respiratory rate.

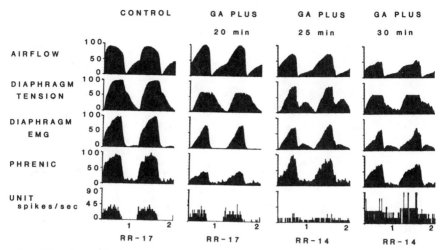

Fig. 5. The dose-dependent actions of tabun. Airflow, diaphragm tension, diaphragm EMG and phrenic nerve activity are in percent of control. The single unit activity is expressed as firing frequency over time. The abscissa denotes two respiratory cycles. RR: respiratory rate.

Inspection of other parameters in Figures 3-6 shows that peak airflow may decrease or remain unchanged even as phrenic and EMG are increasing (Figures 3 and 4), may decrease along with phrenic, EMG and diaphragm tension in a dose-dependent manner (Figure 5), or may increase with increasing phrenic, EMG and diaphragm tension (Figure 6). The last frame of Figure 6 shows that although phrenic and unit activities are becoming desynchronized, the peak firing in the unit activity is phase locked with peaks in phrenic, EMG, and airflow. Since a change in peak airflow is not necessarily indicative of a change in tidal volume, inspiratory tidal volumes are detailed later in Figure 7. A typical response just prior to respiratory arrest was an increase in phrenic activity and EMG, as shown in Figures 3, 4, and 6. Although increased inspiratory effort is appropriate for an animal in respiratory distress, the animals in which blood gas data were obtained at the time of apnea did not show a dramatic change in PCO_2 or PO_2, except for soman-treated animals (all agents, except soman--$PCO_2 < 36mmHg$ and $PO_2 > 80mmHg$; soman--$PCO_2 < 40$ and $PO_2 > 60$). Typically, phrenic activity became increasingly desynchronized, and during the last breaths of the animal, its integrated firing pattern appeared to be inappropriate for adequate ventilatory effort (see Figures 4 and 6). However, at the time of cessation of spontaneous respiration, both phrenic activity and diaphragm EMG were silent, with no central respiratory efforts recorded.

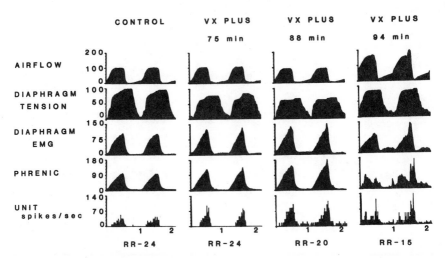

Fig. 6. The dose-dependent actions of VX. Airflow, diaphragm tension,
diaphragm EMG and phrenic nerve activity are in percent of
control. The single unit activity is expressed as firing
frequency over time. The abscissa denotes two respiratory
cycles. RR: respiratory rate.

The bargraphs in Figure 7 represent the percent change from control
values for heart rate, femoral arterial blood pressure, inspiratory tidal
volume, and respiratory rate during the agent infusion period. The time
of infusion for each animal was normalized to the percent of the total
amount of agent infused, such that respiratory arrest represents 100% of
the total agent infused. As pictured in the bargraphs, tidal volume for
the soman, tabun and VX animals increased and remained high until
immediately prior to respiratory arrest, while for the sarin animals,
tidal volume was significantly depressed early in the infusion period.
Since respiratory rate decreased during the agent infusion, the increase
in tidal volume tended to maintain minute ventilation. It is of interest
to note that for all the agents except sarin, there was a more pronounced
decrease in respiratory rate (a centrally mediated parameter) than in
tidal volume; for sarin, the tidal volume decreased to 30% of control
values prior to apnea. Blood pressure was depressed beginning at about
50% of the infusion period for all agents but exhibited a second peak with
tabun and, less obviously, with soman. At respiratory arrest the blood
pressure for soman and tabun was 80% and 70% of control values
respectively, while it was only about 50% of control for sarin and VX. At
the time of respiratory arrest, blood gases were not at critical levels
for those animals in which these data were obtained ($PaCO_2 < 40$ mmHg and
$PaO_2 > 80$ mmHg, except soman--$PO_2 > 60$).

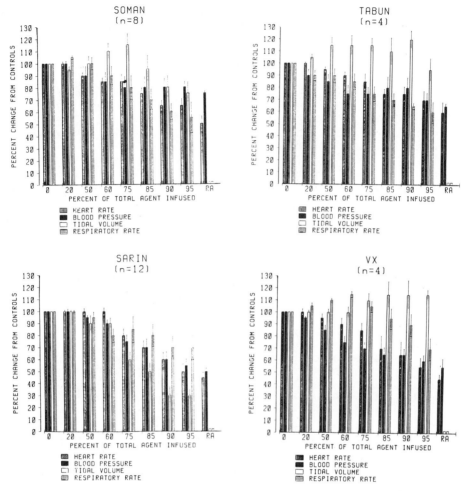

Fig. 7. Response of heart rate, arterial blood pressure, tidal volume and
respiratory rate to the infusion of soman, sarin, tabun or VX at
the rate of 1 LD_{50}/15 min. The amount of agent infused is
normalized to the amount required to produce respiratory arrest
(RA), which represents 100% of the agent infused.

CONCLUSIONS

     Soman, sarin, tabun and VX produce dose-dependent alterations in
medullary respiratory-related unit activity and phrenic nerve activity.
The first appearance of respiratory distress is disruption of the normal
firing pattern of the central respiratory circuits, as evidenced by
alterations in the normal phasic discharge of the respiratory-related
units. This is followed by disruptions in phrenic nerve activity,
diaphragm EMG, airflow and heart rate. Disruption of the normal firing
pattern of these central cells progresses in severity until there is a
complete loss of rhythmic discharge, resulting in the loss of central
respiratory drive. At the time of cessation of spontaneous respiration,
medullary unit activity, phrenic nerve activity, and diaphragm EMG have
ceased; however, the diaphragm muscle still contracts tetanically when
challenged with a 100 Hz train of 2 msec pulses for 500 msec and continues
to contract tetanically when stimulated. At the time of respiratory
arrest blood gases are not critical and blood pressure is from 50% to 80%

of control values. Alterations in, followed by cessation of, central respiratory units at a time when blood gases, arterial blood pressure, and tidal volume are not severely compromised indicates that these changes are mediated within the central nervous system since these other systems are the major peripheral components affecting central respiratory drive.

These findings are in agreement with, and expand upon, the reports by other investigators that, in the anesthetized animal, central respiratory drive is the most sensitive to nerve agent poisoning and that loss of central respiratory drive is the predominate cause of respiratory arrest (e.g., DeCandole et al., 1953; Karczmar et al., 1967; Meeter and Wolthuis, 1968; Adams et al., 1976). Although peripheral effects contribute to the respiratory distress, the preponderance of evidence indicates that these peripheral factors are not a critical component of the toxic syndrome leading to acute lethality. In a series of experiments, Stewart and Anderson (1968) were able to directly demonstrate respiratory arrest in urethanized rabbits by bilateral injections of sarin into medullary respiratory neural substrates. Unilateral injections and injections made distal to these areas were ineffective in producing significant alterations. In addition, they noted that sarin-induced respiratory arrest could be reversed by intravenously administered atropine sulfate. In a recent study in non-human primates, Johanson and his associates (1985) investigated the respiratory depression produced by 2 LD_{50}'s of soman and the relative contributions of central and peripheral mechanisms to that respiratory depression. In 11 of 12 animals, they found the electrical threshold for diaphragm stimulation via the phrenic nerve was unchanged throughout the experiment. There was, however, a large increase in upper airway resistance, an atropine-sensitive drop in blood pressure, and an atropine-sensitive heart block. While diaphragm function was unchanged at the onset of apnea, diaphragm function was reduced during tetanic stimulation at four hours post-exposure after spontaneous return of ventilation had occurred. Johanson concluded that the onset of apnea was due to central respiratory depression rather than to neuromuscular blockade but that the ventilatory depression following the return of spontaneous breathing was due to diaphragm dysfunction rather than to continued depression of central drive.

The increase in phrenic nerve activity and EMG just prior to respiratory arrest may be attributed to the influence of hypercapnia and hypoxia in the case of soman, in which the decrease in respiratory rate (a centrally mediated event) was not sufficiently offset by an increase in tidal volume to maintain minute ventilation; for the other agents, it's possible that the degree of hypoxia and hypercapnia that was observed was sufficient to increase ventilatory efforts prior to the loss of central respiratory drive. Given the apparently low tidal volumes (30% of control values) for the sarin-treated animals just prior to apnea, one would suspect more pronounced changes in blood gases; with respiratory rate at 70-75% of control values, it is possible that minute ventilation was sufficient to maintain blood gases in the nominal range, or that the decrease in tidal volume occurred too quickly to be reflected in the blood gases. However, the fact that blood gases at the time of apnea were not critical for those sarin-treated cats in which blood gas determinations were made requires further investigation.

The depression of tidal volume just prior to respiratory arrest in the present study may have been due to increased lower airway resistance and/or to decreased lung compliance. Abbrecht (1985) has reported a 50% decrease in lung compliance, a ten-fold increase in lung resistance, and decreases in heart rate, cardiac output and arterial blood pressure following soman poisoning in anesthetized dogs; the magnitude of these changes could be significantly attenuated by administration of atropine.

546

In the present study, tidal volumes fell by 50% (70% in sarin-treated animals), and at the onset of apnea arterial blood pressure and heart rate had fallen to approximately 50% to 80% of controls. Except in the case of soman, continued infusion of agent in the ventilated, post-apneic cat resulted in cardiovascular collapse prior to complete blockade of the diaphragm neuromuscular junction.

While this study and others support the contention that the primary acute action of the organophosphorus compounds is depression of central respiratory drive, there is some question as to the cholinosensitivity of medullary respiratory-related neurons. In a direct test of the cholinoceptive properties of medullary respiratory-related neurons, Salmoiraghi and Steiner (1963) found very little evidence that these cells are responsive to iontophoresed ACh. Of 34 respiratory-related units sampled--15 expiratory and 19 inspiratory--32 showed no alteration in discharge as a result of ACh application. The two cells that did respond were both expiratory-related: one increased and one decreased its rate of firing. This dissociation of cellular cholinosensitivity was substantiated by Bradley and his associates (Bradley et al., 1966). More recently, Kirsten et al. (1978) reported that ACh was ineffective in facilitating firing of 72% of respiratory-related units tested. Also, of the three putative neurotransmitters tested (ACh, GABA and glutamate), ACh was the least robust in producing alterations in firing patterns.

The findings of this study support the contention that in the anesthetized cat the central respiratory areas are the most sensitive to agent intoxication. These experiments also show that at the time of acute apnea the phrenic nerve, the medullary unit and the diaphragm EMG have ceased firing, while the diaphragm neuromuscular junction will still contract tetanically when challenged by electrical stimulation of the phrenic nerve. These findings argue in favor of centrally-acting oximes and in support of research directed toward central nervous system respiratory mechanisms in the conscious animal.

ACKNOWLEDGEMENTS AND SUPPORT

The authors wish to acknowledge the help they received from other individuals involved with this research: MAJ John F. Glenn, PhD, who performed some of the experiments and provided invaluable insight during the editing and reviewing of this manuscript; Fred Rybczynski, who wrote the computer programs; and Barbara Perrone, who assisted in the analysis of the data.

The opinions or assertions contained herein are the private views of the authors and are not to be construed as official or as reflecting the views of the Army or the Department of Defense.

In conducting the research described in this report, the investigators adhered to the "Guide for the Care and Use of Laboratory Animals," prepared by the Committee on care and use of Laboratory Animals of the Institute of Laboratory Animal Resources National Research Council.

REFERENCES

Abbrecht, P.H., Bryant, H.J., and Kyle, R., 1985, Cardiopulmonary responses and effects of transtracheal jet ventilation following soman administration in dogs, in: "Abstracts from the Fifth Annual Bioscience Review", Columbia, MD, 29-31 May.

Adams, G.K., Yamamura, H.I. and O'Leary, J.F., 1976, Recovery of central respiratory function following anticholinesterase intoxication, Europ. J. Pharmacol., 38:101-112.

Bay, E., Adams, N.L., von Bredow, J.K.D. and Nelson, J.D., 1973, Respiratory phase shift of pattern in the medullary reticularformation after soman in the cat, Brain Res., 60:526-532.

Bradley, P.B., Dhawan, B.N., and Wolstencroft, J.H., 1966, Pharmacological properties of cholinoceptive neurons in the medulla and pons of the cat, J. Physiol.(London), 183:658-674.

Brimblecombe, R.W., 1977, Drugs acting on central cholinergic mechanisms and affecting respiration, Pharmacol. Ther., 3:65-74.

Clement, J.G., 1981, Toxicology and pharmacology of bis-pyridinium oximes: Insight into the mechanism of action vs soman poisoning in vivo, Fund. Appl. Toxicol., 1:193-202.

Clement, J.G., 1982, HI-6: Reactivation of central and peripheral acetylcholinesterase following inhibition by soman, sarin and tabun in vivo in the rat, Biochem. Pharmacol., 31:1283-1287.

deCandole, C.A., Douglas, W.W., Lovatt-Evans, C., Holmes, R., Spencer, K.E.V., Torrance, R.W. and Wilson, K.M., 1953, The failure of respiration in death by anticholinesterase poisoning, Br. J. Pharmacol. Chemother., 8:466-475.

Douglas, W.W. and Matthews, P.B.C., 1952, Acute tetraethyl pyrophosphate poisoning in cats and its modification by atropine, J. Physiol. (London), 116:202-218.

Freeman, A.M. and Himwich, H.E., 1949, DFP: Site of injection and variation in response, Am. J. Physiol., 156:125-128.

Gordon, J.J., Leadbeater, L. and Maidment, M.P., 1978, The protection of animals against organophosphate poisoning by treatment with a carbamate, Toxicol. Appl. Pharmacol., 43:207-216.

Heymans, C. and Jacob, J., 1947, Sur la pharmacologies du di-isopropyl-fluorophosphonate (DFP) et le role des cholinesterases. Arch. Int. Pharmacodyn. Ther., 233-252.

Holmes, R., 1952, The mechanism of respiratory failure in the rabbit poisoned with GB, personal communication with author.

Holmes, R., 1953a, The effects of GB on the respiration of monkeys, personal communication with author.

Holmes, R., 1953b, The cause of death from acute anticholinesterase poisoning in the rabbit, cat and monkey, personal communication with author.

Holmstedt, B., 1959, Pharmacology of organophosphorus cholinesterase inhibitors, Pharmacol Rev., 11:567-688.

Johanson, W.G., Anzueto, A., Berdine, G.G., Moore, G.T. and White, C.D., 1985, Etiology of respiratory failure in organophosphate intoxication in nonhuman primates, in: "Abstracts from the Fifth Annual Bioscience Review", Columbia, MD, 29-31 May.

Johanson, W.G., Anzueto, A., Berdine, G.G., Moore, G.T. and White, C.D., 1985, Ventilatory support of organophosphate intoxication in nonhuman primates, in: "Abstracts from the Fifth Annual Bioscience Review", Columbia, MD, 29-31 May.

Karczmar, A.G., 1967, Pharmacologic, toxicologic, and therapeutic properties of anticholinesterase agents, Physiol. Pharmacol., 3:163-322.

Kirsten, E.B., Satayavivad, J., St. John, W.M., and Wang, S.C., 1978, Alteration of medullary respiratory unit discharge by iontophoretic application of putative neurotransmitters, Br. J. Pharmacol., 63:275-281.

Koelle, G.B. and Gilman, A., 1949, Anticholinesterase drugs, J. Pharmacol. Exp. Ther., 95:166-216.

Krivoy, W.A., Hart, E.R. and Marrazzi, A.S., 1951, Further analysis of the actions of DFP and curare on the respiratory center, J. Pharmacol. Exp. Ther., 103:351-364.

Lipp, J. and Dola, T., 1980, Comparison of HS-6 versus HI-6 when combined with atropine, pyridostigmine and clonazepam for soman poisoning in the monkey, Arch. Int. Pharmacodyn. Ther., 246:138-148.

Lovatt-Evans, C., 1951, Neuromuscular block by anticholinesterases, J. Physiol.(London), 114:6P.

Lundy. P.M., 1978, The ganglionic blocking properties of the cholinesterase reactivator HS-6, Can. J. Physiol. Pharmacol., 56:857-862.

Lundy, P.M. and Shih, T.-M., 1983, Examination of the role of central cholinergic mechanisms in the therapeutic effects of HI-6 in organophosphate poisoning, J. Neurochem., 40:1321-1328.

Lundy, P.M. and Tremblay, K., 1979, Ganglionic blocking properties of some bispyridinium soman antagonists, Europ. J. Pharmacol., 60:47-53.

Maksimovic, M., Boskovic, B., Radovic, Lj., Tadic, V., Deljac, V. and Binenfeld, Z., 1980, Antidotal effects of bispyridinium-2-mono-oxime carbonyl derivatives in intoxications with highly toxic organophosphorus compounds, Acta Pharm. Jugosl., 30:151-160.

McNamara, B.P., Koelle, G.B. and Gilman, A., 1946, The treatment of di-isopropylfluorophosphate (DFP) poisoning in rabbits, J. Pharmacol. Exp. Ther., 88:27-33.

Meeter, E. and Wolthuis, O.L., 1968, The spontaneous recovery of respiration and neuromuscular transmission in the rat after anticholinesterase poisoning, Europ. J. Pharmacol., 2:377-386.

Modell, W. and Krop, S., 1946, Antidotes to poisoning by di-isopropyl-fluorophosphate in cats, J. Pharmacol. Exp. Ther., 88:34-38.

Modell, W., Krop, S., Hitchcock, P. and Riker, W.F., 1946, General systemic actions of di-isopropylfluorophosphate (DFP) in cats, J. Pharmacol. Exp. Ther., 87:400-413.

Muir, A.W., French, M.C. and Ians, R.H., 1975, Changes in physiological response and cholinesterase level in rabbits poisoned with sarin, soman and a quaternary V agent (T2394), personal communication with author.

Rickett, D.L., Glenn, J.F., Foster, R.E., Traub, R.K. and Beers, E.T., 1984, Differentiation of medullary and neuromuscular actions of nerve agents, in: "Proceedings of the Symposium on Respiratory Care of Chemical Casualties", H.H. Newball, ed., USAMRDC.

Salmoiraghi, G.C. and Steiner, F.A., 1963, Acetylcholine sensitivity of cat's medullary neurons, J. Neurophysiol., 26:581-597.

Schaumann, W. and Job, C., 1958, Differential effects of a quaternary cholinesterase inhibitor, phospholine, and its tertiary analog, compound 217-AO, on central control of respiration and on neuromuscular transmission. The antagonism by 217-AO of respiratory arrest caused by morphine, J. Pharmacol. Exp. Ther., 123:114-120.

Schenk, J., Loffler, W. and Weger, N., 1976, Therapeutic effects of HS-3, HI-6, benactyzine and atropine in soman poisoning of dogs, Arch. Toxicol., 36:71-81.

Shih, T.-M., Whalley, C.E., Valdes, J.J., Lundy, P.M. and Lockwood, P.A., 1985, Cholinergic effects of HI-6 in soman poisoning, in: "Dynamics of Cholinergic Function", I. Hanin, ed., Plenum Press, New York, NY.

Smolders, F.D.J., Folgering, H-Th.M., 1979, Description of the firing pattern of respiratory neurons by frequency modulated interspike interval distributions, Pflugers Archiv, 383:1-8.

Stewart, W.C., 1959, The effects of sarin and atropine on the respiratory center and neuromuscular junctions of the rat, Can. J. Biochem. Physiol., 37:651-660.

Stewart, W.C. and Anderson, E.A., 1968, Effects of a cholinesterase inhibitor when injected into the medulla of the rabbit, J. Pharmacol Exp. Ther., 162:309-318.

Verbeke, R., 1949, Nouvelles contributions a la pharmacologie du diisopropylfluorophosphonate (DFP), <u>Arch. Int. Pharmacodyn. Ther.</u>, 79:1-31.

Wolthuis, O.L., Berends, F. and Meeter, E., 1981, Problems in the therapy of soman poisoning, <u>Fund. Appl. Toxicol.</u>, 1:183-192.

Wolthuis, O.L. and Kepner, L.A., 1978, Successful oxime therapy one hour after soman intoxication in the rat, <u>Europ. J. Pharmacol.</u>, 49:415-425.

Wright, P.G., 1954, An analysis of the central and peripheral components of respiratory failure produced by anticholinesterase poisoning in the rabbit, <u>J. Physiol.(London)</u>, 126:52-70.

ACTIONS OF INTRAVENOUS ESERINE AND PYRIDOSTIGMINE ON CAT SPINAL

CORD RENSHAW CELLS

William G. VanMeter,[1] Karin C. VanMeter, and
Roderick C. Wierwille

College of Veterinary Medicine, Iowa State University
Ames, IA 50011 and United States Medical Research
Institute of Chemical Defense, APG, MD 21010; Dept. of
Pharmacology and Expt'l Therapeutics, School of Medicine
University of Maryland, Baltimore, MD 21201

INTRODUCTION

Protection from irreversible inhibition of cholinesterases (ChE) is
afforded by pretreatment with a carbamate such as physostigmine (Koelle,
1946, 1957). This tertiary drug readily gains access to the CNS, and it
has been shown to raise the LD50 in rats when given prior to toxic doses
of potent, centrally acting irreversible inhibitors of ChE's. Some
protection from exposure to centrally-acting irreversible anticholinesterases (antiChE) also has been reported following pretreatment with
pyridostigmine, a quaternary carbamate (Wolthuis and Vanwersch, 1984).
Using indirect observations, these authors propose a CNS action of
pyridostigmine.

To investigate CNS responses to pyridostigmine, the present study
uses (i) responses of a CNS cholinergic transmitting synapse, i.e., the
spinal motoneuron axon collateral - Renshaw cell interneuron (Eccles et
al, 1954; Eccles et al, 1956; Curtis and Ryall, 1966a and 1966b), to
pharmacologically pertinent drugs and (ii) histochemical analysis of
ChE's (Koelle, 1946, 1957; and Karnovsky and Roots, 1964) in the spinal
cord of cats.

MATERIALS AND METHODS

Adult male cats of mixed breed were anesthetized with DIAL (80
mg/Kg i.p.). After a laminectomy (S1-T13) and transection of the
spinal cord (T13), ipsilateral dorsal and ventral spinal roots (L5-S1)
were separated, cut and placed on platinum stimulating electrodes for
antidromic activation of Renshaw cells. Extracellular unit potentials,
evoked by 1.0 Hz supramaximal stimuli, were identified by latency and
characteristic responses and were recorded by conventional methods from

---

1. Dr. VanMeter is presently on Intergovernmental Personnel Act
   Assignment from Iowa State University to the United States
   Army Medical Research Institute of Chemical Defense, Edgewood,
   MD 21010 where the research was carried out.

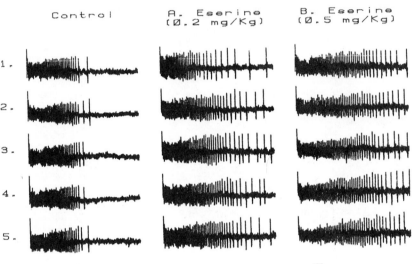

Dose Dependent Increase in
Renshaw Cell Response
to Eserine

Control   A. Eserine   B. Eserine
           (0.2 mg/Kg)   (0.5 mg/Kg)

1.

2.

3.

4.

5.

100 μV

Fig 1: Control-Responses to supramaximal, 1 Hz,
antidromic L7 ventral root stimulation (5 traces in the
left column) typically are a rapidly diminishing high
frequency burst of approximately 100-125 msec. A.
Eserine-Eserine (0.2 mg/Kg i.v.) given 15 minutes
prior, increases frequency and markedly increases the
number of spikes per burst. B. Eserine-Eserine (0.5
mg/Kg i.v.) further enhances the response in the
presence of atropine sulfate (1.0 mg/Kg i.v.). Traces
of raw data in this and following figures are 250 msec.

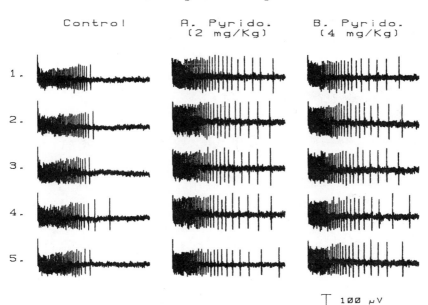

Renshaw Cell Response
to Pyridostigmine

Control   A. Pyrido.   B. Pyrido.
                 (2 mg/Kg)   (4 mg/Kg)

1.

2.

3.

4.

5.

⊥ 100 μV

Fig 2:   Control-Responses above as in Figure 1. A.
Pyridostigmine-Pyridostigmine Br (2.0 mg/Kg i.v.)
given 15 minutes prior, shows an enhancement of
response but less than with eserine (Fig. 1). B.
Pyridostigmine-Pyridostigmine (4.0 mg/Kg i.v.) given
15 minutes prior shows no further enhancement of
response.

Mecamylamine Antagonism of
Eserine Potentiated
Renshaw Cell Response

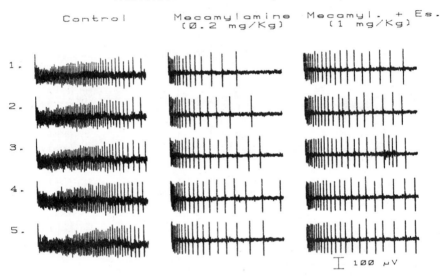

|Control|Mecamylamine (0.2 mg/Kg)|Mecamyl. + Es. (1 mg/Kg)|

Fig 3: Control-Responses as above (fig. 1), but
in the presence of eserine (0.5 mg/Kg i.v.).
Mecamylamine-(0.2 mg/Kg i.v.) given 15 minutes
prior markedly reduces both frequency and duration
of Renshaw cell response. Mecamylamine + Eserine-
Subsequent administration of eserine (1.0 mg/Kg i.v.)
shows an increase in the number of spikes per burst
but not in frequency.

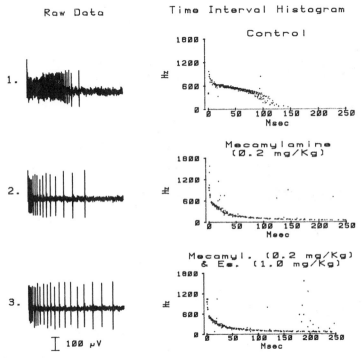

Fig. 4: Raw Data—Samples of raw data from which
TIH's are computed are in the left column. Time
Interval Histograms—The frequency of spikes per
burst for 10 bursts plotted against time (250 msec)
are in the right column. Note the marked depression
after mecamylamine (0.2 mg/Kg i.v.) compared to the
untreated control which is slightly altered by eserine
(1.0 mg/Kg i.v.).

Unit Responses to
Pyridostigmine and Eserine

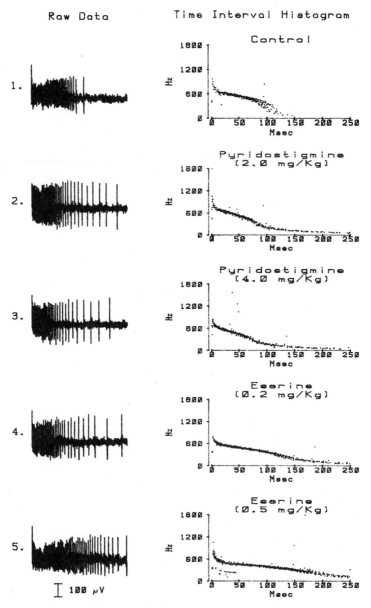

Fig. 5: Raw Data-Samples of raw data for the various
treatments from which TIH's are computed are shown in
the left column. Time Interval Histograms-The
frequency of spikes per burst for 10 bursts plotted
against time (250 msec) are in the right column.
Note the increase in spike frequencies as well as an
increased number of spikes per burst after treatment
with eserine showing a greater effect than
pyridostigmine.

Histochemical Analysis
of Cholinesterases

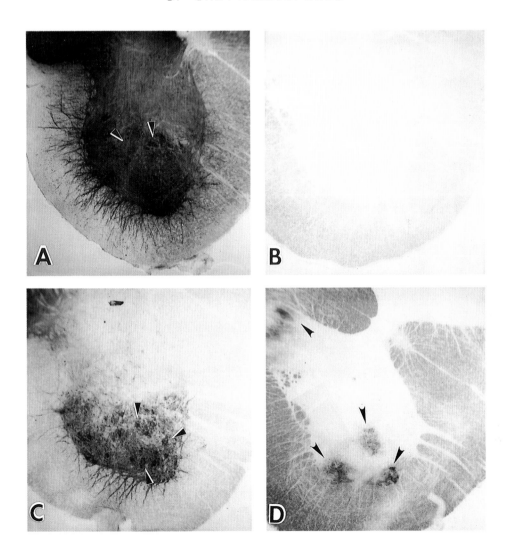

Fig 6: A. Control-Untreated cat spinal cord, the
ventral horn of L7. Note intense stain on motoneuron
cell bodies (arrows). B. Control-Soman (0.02 mg/Kg i.v.)
irreversibly inhibits ChE's. Note the absence of stain.
C. Eserine + Soman-Pretreatment with eserine (0.5 mg/Kg
i.v.) 15 min. prior to soman (0.02 mg/Kg i.v.). Note the
intense stain of motoneurons in lamina IX. D. Pyridostigmine + Soman-Pretreatment with pyridostigmine Br
(2.5 mg/Kg i.v.) 15 min. prior to soman (0.02 mg/Kg
i.v.). Note stain in the dorsal horn and the motoneuron
pools of the ventral horn. Incubation at 37 degrees C.

glass micropipettes (2.7M NaCl, 1-1.5 micron tips) positioned in L7. Responses of these extracellular unit potentials to intravenous administration of atropine sulfate (1.0 mg/Kg), physostigmine salicylate (eserine; 0.2 and 0.5 mg/Kg), pyridostigmine Br (2.0 and 4.0 mg/Kg) and mecamylamine HCl (0.2 mg/Kg) were recorded on analog tape, digitized, and time interval histograms (TIH) computed for 250 msec after stimulus. All cats received atropine methyl nitrate (0.3 mg/Kg) to prevent untoward peripheral cardiovascular responses.

Histochemical analysis of cholinesterase activities was done after in vivo administration of soman (pinacolyl-methylphosphonofluoridate, 0.02 mg/Kg), and soman preceded by either pyridostigmine Br (2.5 mg/Kg i.v.) or eserine (0.5 mg/Kg i.v). The analysis was carried out by the Karnovsky and Roots thiocholine method (1964) modified by 15 minutes preincubation in iso-OMPA (0.2M phosphate buffer, pH 6.8) to inhibit pseudocholinesterases prior to 30 minutes incubation according to the original procedure.

RESULTS

The dose dependent response characteristics of Renshaw cells to eserine (figs. 1 and 5) show a marked increase in duration of response and an increase in unit frequencies. Although the data analyzed are limited to 250 msec., unit responses continued until the next stimulus (i.e., 1 sec.). Pyridostigmine, on the other hand, does not show as definitive a dose dependency (figs. 2 and 5) but does show an increase in the duration of the discharge. These responses seldom exceeded 250 msec. While atropine sulfate fails to antagonize eserine potentiated unit discharges, mecamylamine HCl (figs. 3 and 4) decreases both duration and unit frequencies. The decrease in duration of discharge is antagonized but not reversed by high doses of eserine (1.0 mg/Kg i.v.).

Irreversible inhibition of ChE's after in vivo soman results in an absence of reaction product (fig. 6) during in vitro histochemical analysis. Pretreatment with eserine (0.5 mg/Kg i.v.) followed 15 min later by soman (0.02 mg/Kg i.v.) shows reaction product that indicates the presence of enzyme not irreversibly inhibited. Pretreatment with pyridostigmine (2.5 mg/Kg i.v.) followed by soman with in vitro incubation of tissue sections carried out at 37 degrees shows some protection of ChE's though not as complete as with eserine.

DISCUSSION

In the present study, Renshaw cell discharges are potentiated in the presence of eserine. The prolongation of burst responses to antidromic stimulation of the appropriate ventral spinal roots is an effect attributable to inhibition of cholinesterases (Eccles et al, 1954). Both the spike frequencies and the number of spikes per burst are increased in agreement with the earlier study. These effects are antagonized by mecamylamine, a CNS active antinicotinic drug. However, reversal of this antagonism is weak and requires a significantly greater dose (1.0 mg/Kg i.v.) of eserine. In addition, previous studies have shown that higher doses of mecamylamine (1.0 mg/Kg i.v.) irreversibly block antidromically-induced Renshaw cell discharges (Ueki, Koketsu and Domino, 1961; VanMeter, 1983). Neither DFP nor excess ACh released from repetitive antidromic stimulation is effective in reversing the mecamylamine-induced block (VanMeter, 1984). The latter study concludes that the open channel blocking properties of mecamylamine (Varanda et al, 1985) are a potential mechanism of action. Likewise in the present study, with significantly lower doses of 0.2 mg/Kg i.v. of mecamylamine (cf. 2.0 mg/kg i.v.; VanMeter, 1984), eserine weakly antagonizes the block to increase the number of spikes per burst but has little effect on frequencies.

Pyridostigmine (MW 261.14), a quaternary carbamate, enhances antidromically activated Renshaw cell bursts. However, the response is weak compared to the potentiation of response after eserine (MW 413.5) a tertiary carbamate, given at a significantly lower dose. Also, mecamylamine antagonism is not affected by doses as great as 5.0 mg/Kg i.v. In addition, increases in duration of burst rarely exceed 250 msec at 5.0 mg/Kg i.v. while after eserine (0.200 mg/Kg i.v.) they routinely exceed 1 sec.

The histochemical analysis (in vitro) after in vivo administration of soman shows an absence of stain in the presence of irreversibly inhibited ChE's (Coult et al, 1966). Pretreatment with eserine reversibly inhibits ChE's and "protects" the enzyme from irreversible inhibition by soman given 15 minutes later. The protection is not complete in that the stain is not as intense nor as widely distributed as in control untreated sections. Pyridostigmine given 15 minutes prior to soman also shows some protective effects (at high doses of 2.5 mg/Kg i.v.) against irreversible inhibition. However, pretreatment with this quaternary carbamate results in a stain less intense than with eserine, and it is restricted to areas of motoneuron pools and a few laminae of the posterior horn.

Finally, the data suggest that pyridostigmine, if given in sufficiently large doses as a pretreatment to soman, gains access to the CNS to alter actions of the irreversible inhibitor on a cholinergic transmitting synapse, the motoneuron axon collateral-Renshaw cell interneuron. These data, therefore, give direct evidence for actions of pyridostigmine in the CNS, and thereby support the findings of Wolthuis and Vanwersch (1984).

ACKNOWLEDGEMENTS

The technical assistance of Ms. Janna S. Madren and the computer programming of Mr. Datus L. Proper are gratefully acknowledged.

REFERENCES

Coult, D.B., Marsh, B.D. and Read, G., 1966, Dealkylation studies on inhibited acetylcholinesterase. Biochem. J. 98:869-873.
Curtis, D.R. and Ryall, R.W., 1966a, The excitation of Renshaw cells by cholinomimetics. Exp. Brain Res. 2: 49-65.
Curtis, D.R. and Ryall, R.W., 1966b, The acetylcholine receptor of Renshaw cells. Exp. Brain Res. 2: 66-80.
Eccles, J.C., Fatt, P. and Koketsu, K, 1956, Cholinergic and inhibitory synapses in a pathway from motor-axon collaterals to motoneurons. J. Physiol.(London) 126: 524-562.
Eccles, J.C., Eccles, R.M. and Fatt, P., 1956, Pharmacological investigations on a central synapse operated by acetylcholine, J.Physiol. (London) 131: 154-169.
Karnovsky, M.J. and Roots, L., 1964, A "direct-coloring" thiocholine method for cholinesterases. J. Histochem. Cytochem. 12: 219-221.

Koelle, G. B., 1946, Protection of cholinesterase against irreversible inactivation by di-isopropylfluorophosphate (DFP) in vitro. J. Pharmacol. Exp.Ther. 88: 232-237.

Koelle, G. B., 1957 Histochemical demonstration of reversible anticholinesterase action at selective cellular sites in vivo. J. Pharmacol. Exp. Ther. 120: 488-503.

Ueki,S., Koketsu, K. and Domino, E.F., 1961, Effects of mecamylamine on the golgi recurrent collateral-Renshaw cell synapse in the spinal cord. Exp. Neurol. 3: 141-148.

VanMeter, W. G., 1984, Diisopropylfluorophosphate and tetanic stimulation fail to reverse mecamylamine antagonism of Renshaw cells. Fundam. Appl. Toxicol. 4: S150-S155.

Varanda, W.A., Aracava, Y., Sherby, S.M., VanMeter, W.G., Eldefrawi, M.E. and Albuquerque, E.X., 1985, The acetylcholine receptor of the neuromuscular junction recognizes mecamylamine as a noncompetitive antagonist. Mol. Pharmacol., 28: 128-137.

Wolthuis, O.L. and Vanwersch, R.A.P., 1984, Behavioral changes in rat after low doses of cholinesterase inhibitors, Fundam. Appl. Toxicol. 4: S195-S208.

CONCLUDING REMARKS:

PAST, PRESENT AND FUTURE OF CHOLINERGIC RESEARCH

Alexander G. Karczmar

Loyola University Stritch School of Medicine

Maywood, Illinois   60153, U.S.A.

I.   PROLEGOMENON

First of all, let me state that I am indeed fortunate and lucky: fortunate that so many of my friends were willing to take time for coming to this Meeting and providing Chapters for the book in my honor; lucky to have stayed the course long enough to have at least some excuse for this Meeting being organized for me.

My particular thanks should be extended to Nae Dun, who had the idea in the first place and who worked so hard and successfully organizing the Meeting. Second, my thanks are due to the Department that I had the pleasure to chair for such a long time and particularly to my old friends in the Department such as Joe Davis and Alex Friedman who suffered me for many years and who were eager to help in organizing the Meeting. I should also thank the acting chair, Stan Lorens, for approving Nae Dun's idea and for helping in executing it; a chair may be not particularly desirous to work for the major glory of his predecessor. It is also gratifying that my friend for many years, Israel Hanin, who will be the next chairperson for the Department of Pharmacology and Experimental Therapeutics at Stritch School of Medicine of Loyola University is here and provides both excitment and cooperation. Finally, thanks are due to the current group of the graduate students including my own and probably last graduate student, Lukasz Konopka; they all provided so much logistic and other help for this Meeting.

At a time such as this, I think it is customary for the person honored to expand on how the present times differ from the times of his or her beginnings in Science. Second, it is as customary for the celebrant to pay tribute to those that launched him into a career in whatever his area may be.

I can easily fulfill my first obligation and tell you that there is a far cry from evaluation of acetylcholine via leech or guinea pig muscle to mass spectroscopy-gas chromatography and I am happy to provide the illustration of a set up that Professor Theodore Koppanyi and myself used in the 40's and 50's for acetylcholine evaluation (Fig. 1). It is piquant that this progress contributed to criminology, a subject dear to this eminent student of the Cannon, George Koelle (Koelle, 1959).

Indeed, Bo Holmstedt and Don Jenden pioneered the measurement of picogm. amounts of ACh and related drugs via GC-MS methods, and, at this time, Bo and I. Nordgren described the GC-MS measurement of succinylcholine (SCh) and told us of a crime-detection use of this methodology. Before its advent, small amounts of SCh sufficient for murder would escape detection, particularly if the analysis has to be carried out after exhumation--this is not true anymore. Of course, this methodology has important basic applications as it was applied by Jenden for the measurement of acetylcholine (ACh) turnover, ACh turnover rather than ACh levels being indicative of the state of cholinergic function.

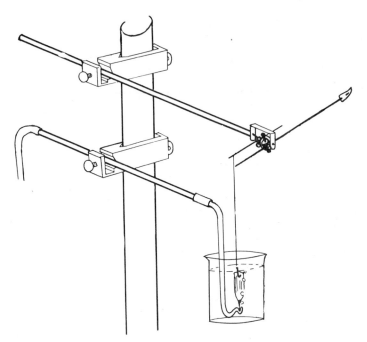

Fig. 1   The legend for this Figure reads as follows in Koppanyi and Karczmar (1955): "The setup for recording...isotonic...responses of the rectus abdominis muscle of a frog to...ACh, physostigmine...and d-tubocurarine. The L-shaped rod to which the muscle is attached, serves at this time as an air or oxygen vent." This setup, used by the late T. Koppanyi since the thirties is essentially identical with Fuhner's (1918) bioassay apparatus which he used to demonstrate physostigmine potentiation of acetylcholine response of smooth muscle and which was used by Loewi (1921) to identify ACh in the heart perfusate (see Karczmar, 1970).

It is as far from ACh bioassays to GC-MS methodology as it is from the evaluation of ganglionic responses via the measurement of the pressor response to i.v. administration of ACh in atropinized mammals to microelectrode study of ACh potentials and elementary events; again, I am glad to show you the former method as employed by myself with Dr. Koppanyi and our early associates such as Teddy King, Jim Dille and Chuck Linegar (Fig. 2). Reviewing this early work another old friend of mine, late Eleanor Zaimis (1963) critized the concept that this method can be used for the measurement of the effects of anticholinesterases (antiChE's) on the sympathetic ganglia as she stated "it is difficult to see how the authors reach such a conclusion". My late friend who was known for her red hair and fiery temperament was not quite fair as it is by now acknowledged that indeed used in this particular way ACh does evoke pressor responses via its ganglionic stimulation; furthermore, what did she want us to do in the 40's to evaluate the phenomena in question?

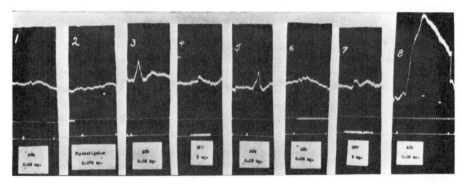

Fig. 2   The legend for this figure reads as follows in Koppanyi and Karczmar (1951): "Antagonism between physostigmine and DFP. Dog, female, weight 8.5 kgm. Sodium pentobarbital anesthesia. Atropine premedication (15 mgm/kgm). All subsequent injections by vein. 1. ACh choline, 0.05 mgm/kgm 2. Five minutes later, physostigmine salicylate, 0.075 mgm/kgm 3. Five minutes later, ACh chloride, 0.05 mgm/kg 4. Fifteen minutes later, DFP, 8 mgm/kgm 5. Five minutes later, ACh chloride, 0.05 mgm/kgm 6. Ten ACh injections, at 30-minute intervals, elicited progressively smaller responses. 7. Six hours after 5, DFP, 8 mgm/kgm 8. Five minutes later, ACh chloride, 0.05 mgm/kgm". These data illustrate in vivo protection afforded by the reversible ChE inhibitor, physostigmine, against the OP antiChE, DFP. This indirect mode of evaluating ACh action via the effector (blood pressure in this case) response was typical for the time in question and analogous to a similar use of the response of the nictitating membrane, also employed by Koppanyi and others. And yet, at the same time, some investigators (not too many) already employed microelectrode for a similar purpose (R.M. Eccles, 1952).

Now as to my early masters and as to how they guided me into pharmacology. My early masters and those that impressed me can be generally characterized as being eccentric but not pharmacologists. In the 30's, some of them did not even know me! For instance, I was very impressed by A. Wojtkiewicz, of Joseph Pidsudski University of Warsaw. He was neither an M.D. nor a Ph.D., as in an early huff he got mad at his preceptors and never worked past the magisterium, however, his contributions were so significant and so well recognized that he became in due time a professor of botany. As there were some two or three thousand students in the first year class that took the course, and as the janitor rather than Prof. Wojtkiewicz signed my course book (which we all needed in those days), he did not know me personally, and he never realized how much I was impressed with his superciliousness and independence. Safely in the USA, I was very taken in the early 40's by Selig Hecht, a prominent Columbia U. biophysicist; his lectures were masterpieces of organization and of the artistry of delivery. Again, there was an elegant and outstanding individual who made me dream that one day I also will be safely superior in front of a blackboard. Oscar Emile Schotte of Amherst College, to whom I was farmed out from Columbia University during the war years to study the effects of nerves on growth and regeneration, again was not a pharmacologist but he was and is a personality. A student of the Nobel Prize Winner Hans Speman, he is, inspite of his name, of Polish-German origin, and he certainly represents well the intellectual superiority of the German pre-Hitler intelligentsia and their, well, superbia: when he could not get the attention of a waiter in an Amherst restaurant he stretched himself flat on the floor till the waiter attended to him--which he did quite fast.

Dr. Theodore Koppanyi whom many of you did know was a copyright eccentric and indeed a pharmacologist, in fact, a father of a number of research areas within the field of pharmacology such as comparative pharmacology, drug metabolism, and behavioral pharmacology. He was a kind, loyal and absent-minded master to me and a devoted friend to my wife and to my late mother-in-law, Dame Bertha Allen. Koppanyi's stories such as "it's toxic", "do you sell shirts here? Are these good shirts?" are well known to all; let me tell at this time that in the caffeteria of Georgetown University Medical School Dr. Koppanyi used to pour coca cola and ketchup on his poached eggs and eat with great gusto this particular concoction. Yet, he made me a pharmacologist and no doubt you may recognize in me certain aspects of his influence as well as the influence exerted on me by the other individuals that I referred to.

II. WHAT IS THIS SYMPOSIUM ABOUT?

Originally, cholinergic transmission, whether at peripheral or central sites, was understood as a simple relay process, released ACh activating postsynaptic receptors which in the case of the Renshaw cell as described here by Sir John Eccles were essentially nicotinic in nature. Subsequently, beginning with the discoveries in the forties of John Eccles, Rosamond Eccles and Benjamin Libet with respect to the ganglia and subsequently with the work on the CNS of such investigators as Chris Krnjevic it was demonstrated that the cholinergic response may be also muscarinic in nature. In addition, it was shown that besides the excitatory cholinergic responses, inhibitory postsynaptic responses can be generated by the cholinergic system in the heart and the ganglia and, in fact, also in the CNS, as proposed in the sixties by Phillis and York (1967) and others. Additional work that was initiated in the thirties by Feng and Li (1941) and followed up in the fifties by George Koelle, Walter and William Riker and Rob Polak concerned nerve terminal sites as they demonstrated that in the peripheral and central nervous system (Polak, 1965; Szerb, 1977) these sites are engaged in the modulation of ACh release.

These findings and concepts that emerged in the thirties through fifties served as the basis for the contemporary research, and this Symposium emphasizes these current aspects of the cholinergic art of which I did not dream of when I first heard of the cholinergic system from Dr. Koppanyi; I will refer to this modern status of cholinergicity. An important aspect of this state of art that was emphasized in the course of this symposium is that there are multiple responses to the cholinergic transmitter, that some of them serve to modulate excitability, and that, conversely, these responses can be subtly modulated so that there is a point to point control of the cholinergic function whether on the cellular and molecular level or on the system level.

Second, several participants of this Symposium correlated this state of art with the use of the animal models and with certain physiological and disease aspects of cholinergic function; I will refer to this subject subsequently. Third, metabolism of ACh relates to its phylogenetic meaning as the latter underlies the role and function of ACh precursors and of their metabolism, and this point was raised here as well.

564

Finally, this Symposium offers an elastic spring-board--a trampoline--with regard to the future development. The early discoverers of the cholinergic system--Fuhner, Loewi, Dale, Feldberg, including also one of the present speakers, Jack Eccles--were no slouchs and their work led to a veritable explosion of the knowledge of the cholinergic system specifically, and of the function of chemical neurotransmitters generally. Today, this explosion proceeds along an exponential curve, the sky seems to be the limit, and it is exciting, extrapolating from the last 100 years or so of the cholinergic lore, to speculate on the future as I will at the end of this paper.

III. STATE OF ART: WHAT IS THE CHOLINERGIC SYSTEM AND WHAT ARE ITS FUNCTIONS AND THOSE OF ITS NEUROTRANSMITTERS?

The Cholinergic system and the CNS. In the thirties thru fifties the knowledge of the cholinergic system focused first of all on the peripheral--autonomic and somatic--sites. Although Dale (1935) clearly proposed central role for the cholinergic system (shortly before his death in 1968, he received a telegram from Don Jenden and Bo Holmstedt, both present here, reporting the first chemical--via MS-GC method--identification of ACh in the CNS), and this concept was further pursued by Feldberg (1945), yet even in the fifties the central geography of the cholinergic system was largely unknown, beyond the cholinergicity of the collateral to the Renshaw cell demonstrated by two members of this audience, Sir John Eccles and President (of Kurume University) Kyozo Koketsu (Eccles, Fatt and Koketsu, 1954). At this meeting, Sir John presented the story of the "extraordinary response of interneurons of the ventral horn". Indeed, the term "Renshaw cell" originated with Eccles (Fig. 3), as he wished to recognize Renshaw's "exciting personality" and link Renshaw's name with the interneuron which was threatened with premature scientific death upon Renshaw's untimely death in 1947 till Eccles, Fatt and Koketsu picked up the story and carried out what were "the most satisfactory investigations of ...Eccles'...life."

Almost 20 years ago, Eccles (1969) in the course of the FASEB Symposium on the Cholinergic System termed as "audacious" the proposal of F.F. Weight that the repetitive spike responses "attributed to the Renshaw cell are generated by repetitive firing of the terminals of motor axon collatorals" rather than by the Renshaw cell that Weight was not sure existed! At that Symposium, Eccles proceeded "strongly" to demolish Weight's evidence (on electrophysiological and anatomical grounds as Thomas and Wilson, 1965, and others since have demonstrated the existance of the Renshaw cell). So, today I am somewhat apprehensive in associating on the same page Dr. Eccles with a younger investigator, except that the rebuttal of Weight by Eccles provided, in my opinion, more celebrity for Weight than would a positive response on Eccles' part. At any rate, my student Bill VanMeter, Karin Sikora-VanMeter and Wierwille contributed at this meeting to Eccles' story as they demonstrated, histochemically, that the facilitatory actions of a number of antiChE's including soman, pyridostigmine and eserine on the Renshaw cell response relate to their inhibition of acetylcholinesterase (AChE), while the block of the Renshaw cell via nicotinolytics may be due to open channel block.

George Koelle, also here, jointly with Lewis and Shute greatly expanded the knowledge of central cholinergicity via George's histo- and cyto-chemical staining of AChE. However, the final words on this matter are being uttered by two of our colleagues here, the McGeers, as based on the method of immunochemical localization of choline-o-acetyltransferase, the enzyme described first as essential for synthesis of ACh by the late David Nachmansohn. In my summary of the 1984 cholinergic meeting in Oglebay, West Virginia, I stated that by virtue of the work of the McGeers "we delineated....with certain degree of finality the important central cholinergic pathways, particularly those emanating from the medial forebrain cholinergic system" (Karczmar, 1986e). It appeared at this meeting that as the matter was presented by the McGeers, Mizukawa Tago and Peng, we may feel almost as confident with respect to the human CNS. In this case, as in that of the cat and the rat, besides the cholinergic networks in and radiations from, the nuclei located in the basal ganglia, cholinergic forebrain nuclei include nucleus basalis, nuclei of the diagonal band and medial septal nucleus, while cholinergic pontine nuclei include nuclei parabrachialis and nucleus cuneiforims; it can be extrapolated from the present and past data of the McGeers that these nuclei radiate to the limbic system including hippocampus and thalamus, and to the cortex.

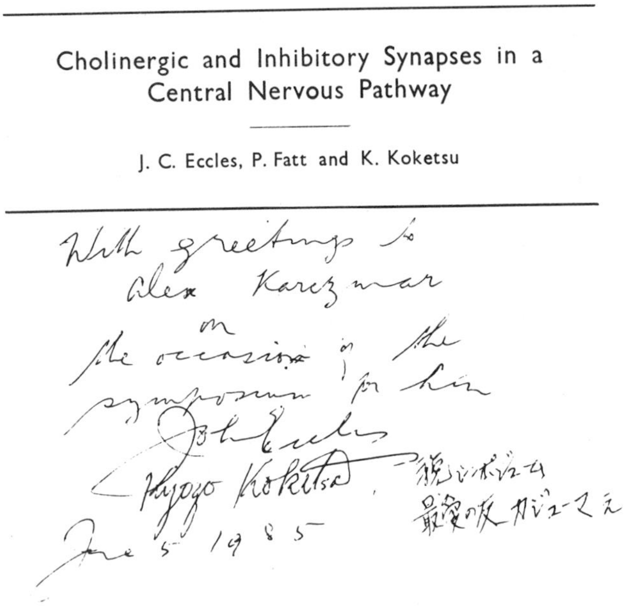

Cholinergic and Inhibitory Synapses in a Central Nervous Pathway

J. C. Eccles, P. Fatt and K. Koketsu

Fig. 3   The cover of a reprint of the 1953 paper by Eccles, Fatt and Koketsu. This little quoted publication in the Australian Journal of Science is the preliminary communication on the Renshaw cell that was followed in 1954 by their classic, full paper which was published (very fast upon the reception of the MS) in the Journal of Physiology.

Behavioral and EEG Actions of Cholinergic Drugs. The knowledge of central and behavioral actions of cholinergic and anticholinergic drugs antedates the demonstration of the central cholinergic synapses and, particularly, the description of central cholinergic pathways. Thus, central actions of atropinics and eserine are known for centuries and, in the thirties, D. Macht spoke of the action of cholinergic drugs on operant behavior and Kremer et al. (1937) of their epileptogenic actions (see also Holmstedt, 1972 and Karczmar, 1970). The demonstration of the EEG actions of these drugs was not far behind (Bradley and Elkes, 1957); pioneering investigations of the late Harold Himwich (Rinaldi and Himwich, 1953), Daniele Bovet and Vincenzo Longo (Bovet et al., 1957) and Ed Domino (1967) should be listed in this context, as these workers emphasized the behavioral and EEG alerting function of the cholinergic system.

Since that time it was demonstrated that not a single overt (including motor or convulsive) "organic" behavior or "non-organic" activity is devoid of cholinergic correlates (o.c.; Karczmar, 1975, 1979 and 1985); discussion of the cholinergic nature of certain mental disease states in this Symposium (see below) is pertinent here.

Among the organic behaviors with cholinergic correlates none are more important than those that underlie the homeostasis of mammalian body temperature, this homeostasis being a component of the energy balance of our body. Bobby Myers initiated, with William Feldberg (1964) the pertinent studies; parenthetically, these studies relate to Feldberg's approach to the study of the brain from its "inner and outer surface" (Feldberg, 1963). At this time, Myers described the role of the cholinergic system of the pre-optic area and the hypothalamus in the temperature control via processes involving both heat gain and heat loss. This system interacts with Ca^{2+} fluxes, indoleamines and catecholamines, and, as shown by Myers elsewhere, it relates teleologically to control of thirst and hunger, altogether constituting the hypothalamico brain stem system concerned with the preservation of body energy.

As already indicated, EEG and behavior are closely related whether with respect to the role of the central cholinergic system in behavior and EEG activity, or to the effects on behavior and EEG of cholinergic drugs. A number of presentations of this Symposium concerns this correlation. Particularly my old friends Enzo Longo, Sra. Scotti de Carolis and their associates contributed to the proof of cholinergicity of EEG activation as they demonstrated that the differential stimulation of nucleus basalis of Meynert (NBM), the source of cholinergic radiation to the cortex, induces EEG alerting similar to that evoked by the stimulation of mesencephalic reticular formation (MRF). Notabene, recruitment, a potential which is characteristically evoked by cholinergic agonists (Longo, 1962) could be evoked by NBM stimulation, but not by MRF stimulation!

Several investigators were concerned with EEG seizures that can be evoked by antiChE's. Ed Domino and his associates returned to Domino's earlier finding of differential EEG actions of muscarinic and nicotinic agonists and demonstrated that muscarinic agonists, including OP antiChE's, induce EEG seizures and/or synergize with convulsive action of nicotinic agonists. Interestingly, they found that while atropine antagonizes partially antiChE-induced seizures, it potentiates the nicotinic seizures suggesting that a "muscarinic component may be seizure-reducing"; data demonstrating this action were adduced some time ago (Karczmar, 1974) and it was proposed that the muscarinic activation antagonizes the hypersynchrony of seizures via its desynchronizing action. In addition, the data obtained by Frank Lebeda and P.A. Rutecki emphasized the significance of hippocampus as a generator of antiChE--induced seizures; some of their findings indicated that these actions are, at least in part, due to presumably direct rather than antiChE actions of soman and DFP. While in their attractive power-spectrum analysis of the action of the drugs my friend Frazier Glenn, my student Don Hinman and S.B. McMaster also obtained evidence as to the generator significance of limbic and reticular structures, they stressed the subcortical sites such as sensorimotor cortex as "the most reliable sites of initial...OP drug-induced...seizure activity"; in agreement with Lebeda they felt that these EEG actions may not depend on AChE inhibition as suggested also by another of my Edgewood Arsenal assocites and students, Bill VanMeter (VanMeter et al., 1978). Parenthetically, OP drugs produce extensive EEG effects in man that range from desynchronizing to seizure activity, and interesting review of this matter is also provided by Glenn, Hinman and McMaster.

Channel-Receptor Macromolecule. The demonstration by Bernard Katz of the elementary events generated by the cholinergic channel led to the concept of a macromolecule that embraces a cholinergic receptor and a cholinergic channel; while the receptor is the primary recognition site for the cholinergic synapses, ACh and cholinergic drugs are capable of both receptor and channel effect. At this meeting, Albuquerque and his associates as well as Rod Parsons dwelt on the actions of organophosphorus (OP) and carbamate, tertiary or quaternary, antiChE's on the macromolecule of the ganglion and the neuromyal junction. They stressed that there are important differences between their actions, as they may either activate the channel, alter ACh-activated channels, or block the channels, this blockade being exerted either in their open or closed conformation; this point was also made by Narahashi in his description of channel action of methylguanidine and related compounds. Vladimir Skok, who worked on several occasions in these laboratories stressed the significance of open channel blockade for ganglionic transmission as he presented data indicating that the non-competitive block of the nicotinic channel in its open conformation by onium compounds correlates better with transmission block than their action on the "recognition center" of the macromolecule; he also feels that besides the ganglionic and neuromyal junctions, other synapses readily react to open channel blockade, both in the case of nicotinic and non-cholinergic (such as glutamate receptors of insect neuromuscular junctions) synapses. Of course, this concept seems to imply that while the receptor may constitute the primary recognition site for the activation of transmission, it may be less important for the block of transmission.

Albuquerque and Parsons raised also the important issue of direct non-antiChE actions of carbamates and OP compounds, whether on the channel or the receptor, a point which has a history dating since the forties (see Karczmar, 1970, 1986c). It is of interest that enzymes such as proteases may also affect the macromolecule, and at this meeting Parsons showed that a protease affects the EPSC decay time which is indicative of the channel action of the protease and Parsons correlated this effect with structural changes. Other related enzymes, such as lipases, seem to generate similar electrophysiological effects at the neuromyal junction (Ohta, Karczmar and Karczmar, 1981); in this case, besides morphological changes, other effects may be involved such as generation of Ca^{2+} carriers (o.c.).

Still another role of the channel was stressed by Adler as his data indicated that both the channel and the receptor participate in the phenomena of desensitization; it should be added in this context that recently Michael Raftery and his associates (1985) provided evidence suggesting that a specific peptide sub-component of the receptor is involved in desensitization.

Second Messengers. Old timers such as myself felt, naively enough that ACh does not need any assist with its action on postsynaptic ionic conductance, particularly as Nishi and Koketsu demonstrated early that ACh accummulates in the synaptic vesicles at high millimolar concentrations and is ejected onto the receptor in these overwhelming concentrations; in fact, at these concentrations ACh causes a burning sensation when applied to the skin. Today, it appears that in many, if not all cases, the permeability changes which underlie the effects of the transmitters require the presence of second messengers as suggested first by Sutherland, expanded by Paul Greengard (1978; Nestler et al., 1984) and emphasized at this meeting by Robert Perlman. The work of Sutherland and Greengard concentrated on the phosphorylating mechanisms initiated by the combination between the cholinergic neurotransmitter and the cyclic nucleotides while the work of Hokin and Hokin (1960) and at this time the studies of Perlman concern phosphatidyl inositol as a second messenger; in fact, as Perlman pointed out a number of links between these two second messenger systems are generated via activation of kinases.

Apparently, the two second messenger systems may interact whenever either is activated by neurotransmitters including acetylcholine; furthermore, a single transmitter may activate both systems. This appears to be true with respect to ACh. While it was considered early Hokin and Hokin (1960) that phosphatidyl inositol system responds to the cholinergic muscarinic activation, cyclic nucleotide involvement in the cholinergic, muscarinic response was also implicated (Greengard, 1978); in this case, cyclic GMP was the responsible nucleotide. At this meeting, Hartzell indicated that in the case of the vertebrate heart the contribution of these two systems to the cholinergic control of contrac- tility and membrane conductance remains unclear; nevertheless, choliner- gic system exerts this control via specific protein phosphorylation. At this meeting, Perlman described some of these phenomena as they occur in mammalian sympathetic ganglia, as he adduced evidence indicating that phosphatidyl inositol is involved not only in muscarinic but also nico- tinic phenomena, possibly via activation of phospholipase C; finally, phosphorylation activity generated by the two second messenger systems regulate catecholaminergic synthesis in the ganglia via an effect on tyrosine hydroxylase

Multiplicity of Cholinergic Post- and Pre-Synaptic Responses. This is another topic of great current interest. Initial studies of John and Rosamond Eccles and Benjamin Libet concerning the variety of postsynap- tic responses to ACh were expanded immeasurably more recently as Sygoro Nishi and Kyozo Koketsu and their successors in these laboratories, Nae Dun, still with us here, and Alan North at this time at MIT but ready to move to Portland, Oregon, differentiated at the ganglia between a number of postsynaptic responses and postsynaptic potentials. In fact, even what appeared originally as a relatively homogeneous response, the slow muscarinic EPSP, can be generated by now to have a number of ionic mechanisms. As stressed at this meeting by Paul Adams (see also Adams, 1986), the muscarinic current which he described originally as the current may actually includes perhaps 7 components; it is not clear today whether each neuron is capable of a variety of muscarinic K responses or different neurons differ as to the ionic mechanisms of their response. It is of great interest that Cole and Roger Nicoll (1984) and Barry Lancaster demonstrated that hippocampal neurons also exhibit K currents of several types. Besides these cholinergic facili- tatory and depolarizing responses, the fast (nicotinic) and the slow (muscarinic) response, there is the third facilitatory mechanism, which is not cholinergic and which was first identified by two of my friends present here, Syogoro Nishi and Kyozo Koketsu (Nishi and Koketsu, 1968). This response was subsequently identified as peptidergic by Nae Dun (see Dun, 1983) and the Jans (1982), the specific peptide depending on species; in some ganglia this response may be serotonergic in nature (Dun et al., 1984).

Finally, there is the ganglionic postsynaptic inhibitory response, the slow IPSP, originally discovered by Jack and Rosamond Eccles (J.C. Eccles, 1935; R.M. Eccles, 1952) and by Libet (Eccles and Libet, 1961). Here, the question is, is the ganglionic IPSP a mono- or di-synaptic phenomenon? The controversy is long and furious (see Karczmar and Dun, 1978 and 1986; and Libet, 1979). At this meeting, the Gallaghers and Hirai, who adduced early the evidence that the IPSP may be monosynapti- cally, muscarinically generated, produced further supportive data with respect to the IPSP of the parasympathetic ganglia. They also adduced evidence that this response depends on calcium-dependent increase in potassium conductance as do the facilitatory muscarinic actions (Adams, 1986).

Now, the question arises as to the significance of these various types of responses. Chris Krnjevic suggested at this meeting that the muscarinic response has a facilitatory function in the case of the CNS; he stressed also that this facilitation includes facilitation of extrinsic "tonic and phasic inhibitory inputs...such as those...mediated by GABA" as well as "enhancement of electrical (ephaptic) interactions particularly prominent in the densely packed hippocampal pyramidal cells". Similarly, at this meeting Paul Adams showed that the slow responses affect cell excitability even when they alter only slightly the membrane potential.

The concept of the multiplicity of cholinergic responses includes, besides postsynaptic responses also the presynaptic sites. The meaning of this site was first stressed in the thirties and forties by Beijing investigators Feng and Li at what was then Peiping Union Medical College, as they demonstrated at the neuromyal junction that it can generate repetitive firing (see, eg. Feng and Li, 1941). Subsequently, Walter Riker, Gerhard Werner and Frank Standaert with respect to the neuromyal junction and William Riker (Riker and Szreniawski, 1959) with respect to the ganglion seemed to consider the nerve terminal as the prime mover of neuromyal transmission, not via release of ACh but in some other fashion (see Standaert and Riker, 1967). An explosive discussion followed when this concept was raised in 1967 at a meeting of New York Academy of Sciences (Karczmar versus Standaert, 1967).

From the cholinergic viewpoint, the primary nerve terminal site is concerned with ACh release and is Ca^{2+} dependent as demonstrated in his Nobel Prize research by Bernard Katz. At this meeting, Gene Silinsky defined calcium as the "naturally occuring full agonist" which opens, via its receptor action, Ca^{2+} channels, inducing a synchronous release of ACh as it needs to activate only small proportion of its receptors for this action. Black widow venom-like, Ca^{2+} provokes an asynchronous discharge of "enormous numbers of ACh packets", while magnesium acts as a Ca^{2+} antagonist.

However, there are additional nerve terminal sites that modulate ACh release. George Koelle described a nicotinic nerve terminal site that acts as a "percussive mechanism" (eg. Koelle, 1963). At this meeting Syogoro Nishi demonstrated that indeed there are nicotinic nerve terminal sites at the cardiac vagus which, when activated, release ACh—this is piquant as earlier Nishi (1970) could not confirm George Koelle's percussive notion at the ganglia. Another illustration of presynaptic facilitation was provided at this meeting by Donald McAfee and his associates as they demonstrated that in the rat superior cervical ganglion synaptic activity augments cyclic AMP in the nerve terminal leading to increased release of ACh and thus to synaptic facilitation. It should be pointed out that analogous presynaptically mediated facilitation may occur in the CNS (see Karczmar, 1986b), and that Libet (1984) describes for several years now cyclic AMP-dependent and/or adrenergically mediated long lasting modulations at ganglionic postsynaptic sites which he feels may constitute a model of memory processes.

Conversely, Polak (1965), Szerb (1977) and others demonstrated the presence at cholinergic including central synapses of a muscarinic nerve terminal receptor, the activation of which blocks ACh release. As shown at this meeting by Chris Krnjevic, ACh-mediated block of release is not confined to ACh, as ACh can block as well the release of other transmitters.

This matter of presynaptic release was pursued at this meeting by Pedata, Pepeu and their associates at the rat cortex and hippocampus, ACh release being facilitated by xanthines and diminished by adenosine and age. Giancarlo Pepeu offers us hope that "drugs...such as phosphatidyl serine...aimed at correcting alteration...due to age...can be envisaged".

What Does the Nerve Terminal Release? Can the cholinergic terminal do more than release ACh? This question has to do with Dale's principle as expanded on a number of occasions, including here, by John Eccles. The Dale principle may be understood as stating that at all the synapses formed by a given neuron the same and single transmitter is released; as stated by the McGeers and Eccles (McGeer et al., 1978), "all synapses made by a motor neuron have ACh as the transmitter, despite great differences in the location (central or peripheral), in the mode of termination, and in the target cells". On the other hand, it may not invalidate Dale's law to state that a neuron may release at all its terminals the same several transmitters or several bioactive substances. In the fifties, I was asked by Bernard B. Brodie this very question-- namely, can a neuron release more than one neurotransmitter? I responded to Steve by saying "well, Steve you ask that because you really are not a pharmacologist" (the Sollman Award Winner Brodie being originally trained as an organic chemist). My answer just shows how young and naive was I and how astute and prophetic Steve Brodie can be. Subsequent to this conversation I and my associates have demonstrated that cholinergic activity generates changes in other neurotransmitter such as serotonin and catecholamines (Glisson, Karczmar and Barnes, 1972). It is true that this finding serves as a demonstration of Feldberg's (Feldberg and Vogt, 1948; Feldberg, 1945) early proposal that cholinergic and non-cholinergic pathways alternate in the CNS, but does not directly relate to Brodie's question. However, Thomas Hokfelt, L.Y. and Y.N. Jan, Kyozo Koketsu and Nae Dun did finally demonstrate that a cholinergic neuron may release, besides ACh, bioactive substances such as ATP and adenosine (it releases also proteoglycans--it is not known as yet whether these are active synaptically), and that, at least at some cholinergic synapses, peptides that may act as neurotransmitters are also released.

Trophic and Morphogenetic Cholinergic Actions. Cholinergic nerves may release bioactive substances that are widely different from neurotransmitters or neuromodulators as they appear to be capable of causing trophic action. Levi-Montalcini's (1964) nerve growth factor (NGF) originally perceived as acting only on ganglion cells and which is generated outside the neurons may be also present in the CNS and taken up by the central neurons. At this meeting, George Koelle presented data indicating that he is near to identifying a substance released from the cholinergic neurons that is involved in the maintenance and in regeneration of AChE. The need for this factor may explain denervation-evoked decrease in postsynaptic ChEs as shown many years ago by Koelle and others. At this meeting Wolff Dettbarn and his associates expanded on this concept as they demonstrated that muscle disuse and use, and particularly weight bearing are also involved in post-reinnervation regeneration of ChEs. Chemical neuropathies which produce denervation-like syndrome also affect ChEs; as shown at this meeting by Alan Goldberg and Barbara Bass, so act hexacarbons that produce central and peripheral neuropathies (resulting in gait and sensory disturbances), and Bass and Goldberg stressed that specific molecular forms of AChE and BuChE may be more sensitive markers of neuropathies than total muscle and/or nerve AChE.

Actually, trophic role of cholinergic neurons must concern more than ChEs. Thus, in the thirties and fourties, Elmer Butler and Oscar

Schotte (1941) and Schotte and I (Schotte and Karczmar, 1944) described the need of innervation for salamander limb regeneration. Later, I found (Karczmar, 1946) that this trophic effect is independent of the type of the nerve and I speculated that any nerve whether cholinergic, adrenergic or peptidergic--the latter term not being used at that time-- releases trophic factors. Subsequently, Edson Albuquerque (Albuquerque et al., 1972) described the trophic effects of cholinergic innervation at the skeletal muscle as he and others tried to dissociate between the possible trophic action of ACh on the one hand and of other substances emanating from the motor nerve terminal on the other. In fact, ACh or other substances generated by the cholinergic nerves may be involved in a wide variety of morphogenetic and developmental actions (cf. Karczmar, 1963a and b; Karczmar et al., 1973). A novel concept pertinent for this morphogenetic action of cholinergic nerves was presented at this meeting by Peng as he proposed that the clustering of cholinergic receptors of the muscle endplate is mediated via activation by the motor nerve of muscle membrane. In his model system the process was mimicked by poly-peptides--could this represent one of the physiological roles of these substances? It must be remembered that in several organisms high levels of AChE and ACh may be present already in the two to four cell stage of development (Karczmar, 1963a). This should be considered in the context of the presence of ACh and/or AChE in non-innervated adult organs such as red blood cells or ephemeral organs such as placenta, as well as in non-motile, aneuronal organisms (o.c.). All this may relate to still another concept: ACh being involved not only in transmissive but also in trophic and developmental phenomena referred to by Jack Eccles as "meta-botropic" actions of ACh (McGeer, Eccles and McGeer, 1978), appears to be phylogenetically old; indeed, ACh may be only a byproduct of choline and phospholipid metabolism which in the course of phylogenesis eventu-ally became used by the parsimonious nature for synaptic transmission. I shall return to this speculation later.

Conversely, cholinergic substances including antiChE's may exert direct morphopathologic actions on neurons and effector cells, as des-cribed in the past by Dettbarn and Albuquerque, and more recently by Drs. Petra, McLeod, Sikora-VanMeter and VanMeter. This allusion to the work of Drs. McLeod, Petras and the VanMeters gives me a chance of reminiscing of the days when Edgewood Arsenal which seems now to regain its ancient glory served as breeding grounds for a number of prominent cholinergikers and my friends such as Henry Wills, George Koelle, and the late Amadeo Marrazzi and Harold Himwich.

IV. APPLICATIONS AND COROLLARIES OF CURRENT CHOLINERGIC STATE OF ART

Modulations. The concept of modulation may be considered as a corollary of the current state of the cholinergic art. This concept posited clearly at this meeting and elsewhere by Kyo Koketsu (see Koketsu and Karczmar, 1986) defines modulation as a change in respon-siveness and/or release of the neurotransmitter induced by endogenous substances which may be released from either the cholinergic terminal or adjacent non-cholinergic terminals, blood borne, present in the glia or interstitial fluids and/or present extrasynaptically, in the neuron or its membrane and activated during transmission. At this meeting, Costa, Guidotti and Hanbauer presented a related picture of modulation as they introduced the concept of endogenous "cotransmitters" acting on a recog-nition site contiguous with that for the "primary" transmitters; the cotransmitters modulate the response to the latter.

Koketsu differentiated between several mechanisms that subserve modulation presynaptically, ACh itself as well as other transmitters such as GABA being capable of modulating the release of ACh; these presynaptic phenomena were already described. Modulations involve also postsynaptic sites (Koketsu and Karczmar, 1986) as well as effector phenomena, and at this meeting Hartzell adduced an interesting example of interaction between catecholaminergic and cholinergic transmission, phosphorylation phenomena and Ca^{2+} fluxes as this interaction regulates cardiac contractility and cardiac conductance phenomena. Another interesting category of postsynaptic interaction was described at this Meeting by Mimo Costa, Alex Guidotti and Inge Hanbauer. This interaction involves catecholamine synthesis in and release from, chromaffin cells, as the nicotinic release of catecholamines from these cells is modulated via GABAergic intracellular receptors (Kataoka et al., 1984). This interaction, which Costa, Hanbauer and and Guidotti refer to as "cellular interaction" is further modulated via another GABA pool which is present presynaptically in the splachnic cells, and also by a number of peptides such as substance P, enkephalins, etc.

Dynamics and Synthesis of ACh. Again, modern state of cholinergic art leads to new departures from the classical picture of ACh synthesis as a resultant of a single neuronal compartment and the uptake into this compartment of choline generated by ChE-dependent hydrolysis of ACh release from the terminal (see, eg., Nachmanson, 1963); as well known, Nachmanson extended this concept into that of unitary role of ACh in conduction and transmission, these two processes being according to Nachmansohn, essentially identical. It was thought subsequently that dietary choline may also contribute to synthesis of ACh, these two sources of choline sufficing in the absence of any metabolic choline for the synthesis in question. After many years of studies of Ansell (cf. Ansell and Spanner, 1982), Tucek (1983), and Lynn Wecker, a participant in this Meeting, it became clear that phospholipid metabolism generates choline, and that, in turn, choline is involved in the formation of membrane phospholipids (see also Blusztajn and Wurtman, 1983). As already pointed out, this picture relates clearly to the phylogenetic role of choline, phospholipids and ACh metabolism in the generation of the membrane. In fact, it was early pointed out by Wecker (1986) and myself that under normal conditions high choline intake contributes to brain choline rather than brain ACh (Karczmar and Kindel, 1981; Saito et al., 1986). However, the results of Bartus et al. (1980) point out otherwise, and Wecker showed that, when neuronal ACh is depleted, choline may be used preferentially for ACh synthesis. This synthesis may be identical with that which as proposed early by Frank MacIntosh (1959) forms the ready releasable store of ACh. Consistent with this concept, my favorite enfant terrible Brian Collier, who studied for many years now the balance of ACh between its storage and releasable compartment (both compartments including the synaptic vesicles), used the interesting piperidino cyclohexanol, AH5183, which blocks choline uptake (not, hemicholinium-way, into the terminal but into the vesicles), to demonstrate that activity, Ca^{2+}, and AH5183 promote shift of ACh from the storage to the releasable compartment. Consistently with this concept, Don Jenden and his associates showed at this Meeting that, in the case of the guinea-pig longitudinal muscle-myenteric plexus preparation, AH5183 blocks evoked but not resting release of ACh as well as slows its synthesis and choline uptake. Interestingly, there was also an increased choline efflux, this choline probably resulting from phospholipid degradation. Furthermore, at this meeting, Wecker and Reinhardt produced evidence indicating that neuromyal activity and resultant adenosine compounds may channel choline away from phosphorylation and phospholipid biosynthesis to acetylation.

Subtypes of Cholinergic Receptors. The development of cholinergic knowledge usually preceeds that of other transmitters and it did so with respect to receptor subdivisions, as the terms "nicotinic" and "muscarinic" were coined by Dale (1914) and as the distiction between nicotinic and muscarinic responses was made even earlier (cf. Karczmar, 1986c).

Subsequently, we seemed to rest on our laurels while adrenergic, histaminergic and dopaminergic receptology claimed the existence of more and more receptors. However, today we recognized at least M_1 and M_2 muscarinic receptors (Birdsall and Hulme, 1976; Birdsall et al., 1986) and related proposals were made with respect to nicotinic receptors (Dun and Karczmar, 1980; Larsson et al., 1986). M_1 and M_2 receptors may characterize muscarinic ganglionic and CNS receptors, respectively (Vickroy et al., 1984). At this meeting Alan North and his associates confirmed the M_2 characterization of central muscarinic neurons as they demonstrated that in the rat, the locus coeruleus neurons are depolarized and nucleus parabrachialis neurons are hyperpolarized via M_2 mechanisms; on the other hand, the neurons of the two enteric plexuses of the guinea pig responded, similarly to ganglionic neurons, via M_1 mechanisms.

Molecular Constituents of the Cholinergic System. Present state of art of the cholinergic system includes our capacity to isolate and identify its cellular as well as subcellular, molecular components. This work led to structural definition of the nicotinic receptor by Raftery, Changeux and others (Raftery et al., 1985; Boyd and Cohen, 1984; Changeux et al., 1984) and of various forms of AChE that were referred to at this meeting by Barbara Bass and Alan Goldberg (see above). It is interesting in this context that these components may subserve different functions; for example, Raftery et al. (1985) proposed that a specific component of the nicotinic receptor subserved differentially the process of desensitization, rather than the whole receptor being involved in this process as suggested originally by Katz, Thesleff and Rang (see Thesleff, 1955; Rang and Ritter, 1969) and myself (Karczmar and Howard, 1955; Karczmar, 1957).

At this meeting, Victor Whittaker (with Elio Borroni) presented an elegant work concerning components of Torpedo's synaptic vesicles and presynaptic plasma membranes, a proteoglycan and three gangliosides, respectively, which are highly antigenic and capable of generating antisera. In turn, antisera can be used as markers of cholinergic neurons in the mammalian CNS and of recycling of the vesicles; the latter study determined the existence of several pools and molecular species of vesicles (see also Richardson, 1984).

Disease States. If there is a jejune aspect of the cholinergic lore, it is that of its applicability to disease states. Of course, cholinergic and anticholinergic drugs are of some clinical use in a number of diseased states, including glaucoma, myasthenia gravis, parkinsonian disease and ulcer; the exotic employment of atropine in coma therapy of depression may be also mentioned (Karczmar, 1979). However, many of these uses are either obsolete or of minor significance. Does the modern state of art of the cholinergic system—eg., the new understanding of senile dementia of Alzheimer Type (SDAT) as primarily a cholinergic disease—bring up a new situation? With particular reference to SDAT, two communications presented at this meeting are of interest. First, Ezio Giacobini in his "View...of ACh...from the Cerebrospinal Fluid" demonstrated that cholinergic components of the human CSF may be used to evaluate the efficacy of choline and/or physostigmine for augmenting brain ACh and to diagnose SDAT. Second, an appropriate animal model constitutes an important tool for the study of neurological conditions including SDAT; the data demonstrating that AF64A, a cholinotoxin developed by Hanin and Fisher (1980), provides, when given to animals, such a model, was presented by Hanin, as he showed that most components of cholinergic function including CAT, choline uptake and release of ACh are affected by AG64A; however, muscarinic receptor binding is unchanged.

The data of Herb Ladinsky, Silvana Consolo and their associates are pertinent in the context of another disease state. They showed that in animals the excitatory cortico-striatal pathways interact motor behavior-wise, with cholinergic agonists and antagonists and with amphetaminics; decortication enhances amphetamine and apomorphine-induced stereotypy and opioid-induced catalepsy while ACh precursors and/or cholinominetics reverse catalepsy as shown here by Ladinsky and his colleagues and stereotypy as shown elsewhere (cf. Karczmar and Richardson, 1985; Karczmar 1986). Speculatively, these data are consistent with the concept that cholinergic activity may be beneficial in schizophrenia (Singh, 1985) as stereotypy and catalepsy which examplify animal schizoid behavior (Karczmar, 1986d) benefit from cholinergic activation and are linked with deficits in cortico-striatal pathways that may be also implicated in schizophrenia (Singh, o.c.). In a similar vein, Priyattam Shiromani and Chris (John C.) Gillin stressed the cholinergicity of REM sleep--a departure from earlier stress on its noradrenergic nature (Jouvet, 1972)--and related the augmentation of this cholinergic parameter to depression, affective disorders (Janowsky et al., 1985) and narcolepsy. This finding may have a therapeutic implication as Kupfer and Edwards (1978) claimed that manic depressives benefit particularly from antidepressant drugs endowed with high atropinic activity. I should add that cholinergic agonists produce in animals a quasi-narcoleptic, quasi-REM sleep state which I referred to as Cholinergic Alert Non-Mobile Behavior (CANMB; Karczmar, 1979, 1986d).

An entirely novel disease role was proposed for the cholinergic system by Sten Aquilonius as he found in patients suffering from amyotrophic lateral sclerosis (ALS) marked reduction of muscarinic binding sites in motoneuron areas and appearance of extrajunctional receptors in the biceps muscle.

Anticholinesterases--Antidoting and Neuropathology. Several presentations that were already alluded to concerned antiChEs, including both carbamate and OP drugs. For example, Frazier Glenn and Lebeda emphasized the significance of the limbic structures in the generation of EEG seizures, while Ed Domino stressed the interaction of central muscarinic and nicotinic sites in this process (see above). Furthermore, Dan Rickett and Everette Beers expanded on the classical controversy as to whether the CNS, the peripheral sites, or, finally, metabolic and other changes constitute the strategic targets of the antiChE toxicity. Employing, in cats, multirecording procedures, they confirmed the medullary respiratory depression as the crucial phenomenon of OP death. This crucial role of respiratory depression in antiChE poisoning was pointed out, earlier (Karczmar, 1964 and 1967) on the basis of cruder methods than those used by Rickett and Beers. Rickett and Beers pointed out also that medullary neurons which are involved directly in respiratory regulation may be not cholinoceptive. That the cholinergic action on these neurons is exerted via activation of such amino acids as glutamate was speculatively suggested earlier (Karczmar, 1985).

In addition, Peter Waser and Francis Hoskin addressed the question of antidoting the OP drugs. Waser stressed poor CNS penetrability of oximes such as 2-PAM and obidoxime as well as their relatively low reactivation potency; as the oximes decrease the levels of ^{14}C sarin in the brain Waser speculated that oximes may react at the periphery with OP drugs, the complex being eliminated or incapable of CNS entry.

Waser presented results concerning another antidotal maneuver, i.e. treatment with CAT inhibitors. A number of still other strategems are explored besides the standard use of oxime-atropine-anticonvulsant combinations (Karczmar, 1985), and Waser's attempt to detoxify OP drugs prior to their reaching the target constitutes a "sink" method; the "sink" can be an oxime, a cholinesterase or a related OP reactant. Or, the OP drug may be hydrolyzed, and Francis Hoskin works for years now with DFPases, somanases and related enzymes. Hoskin recently began exploring sources that may yield significant amounts of phosphodiesterases, and at this time presented the story of fungi such as penicillium fumiculosum as such a source.

Finally, this is a question of antiChE-induced neuropathy. It was already alluded to in the course of the discussion of the trophic role of cholinergic system that, paradoxically, certain cholinergic agonists exert a converse, anti-trophic action as they induce neuropathy. OP antiChE's are the culprits as they can induce neuronal damage, neuromyal defects, and a special kind of axonal neuropathy (delayed neurotoxicity) and demyelination. Not all OP drugs may exert all of these actions. For instance, axonal neuropathy and demyelination are more likely to occur with certain OP insecticides capable of inhibiting the somewhat "mythical" enzyme, the toxic neuroesterase, which may represent a portion of brain esterase activity (Johnson, 1986; Abou Dona, 1983), the inhibition of this enzyme being the initial event in the neurotoxicity; the actual mechanism was not as yet described.

At this meeting, Charles McLeod and Henry Wall described pathology resulting from convulsive doses of soman and sarin; it included encephalomalacia, ventricular dilatation, and, on cellular level changes in neuronal organelles, dendrites and axons, particularly in the hippocampus. Some of these changes are similar to those reported earlier by Sikora-VanMeter et al. (1985). McLeod suggested that these changes may relate to the deficit in energy metabolism due to initially increased and then depressed glucose utilization and 2-decoxyglucose uptake (Pazdernik et al., 1983) and increased glycolysis (McDonough et al., 1983). It remains to distinguish clearly between effects due to EEG seizures, those due directly to OP drugs, and those that may result from respiratory failure in animals not artificially ventilated, localized infarcts or changes in blood flow.

V.   EPILOGUE WHICH IS ALSO A PROLOGUE

This was a rich and exciting symposium and its wide range of subjects illustrates well the multiple significance of the cholinergic system as the topics ranged from micromolecular aspects that include the chemical and antigenic structure of the receptor, through electrophysiological characterization of cholinergic neurons and their terminals and the problems arising from the toxicity of cholinergic agonists and antagonists, to the behavioral aspects of the cholinergic system. Thus, the cholinergic system which has had so many firsts, such as constituting the first demonstrated chemical transmission system both at periphery and in the central nervous system, continues to be the subject of exciting discoveries and to expand into the new areas; what can be more interesting than to realize the role of the cholinergic system in memory processes and therefore in the all important--particularly for this aging country--geriatric phenomena? And, at another extreme, what may be more exciting than to see the responses of the receptor: channel macromolecule to a few molecules of ACh?

The past and current cholinergic accomplishments lend themselves very well to prognostications and quasi-prophecies, and I can think of the cholinergic future along three lines: the developments that are just around the corner and which may become scientific facts before this book has been published; longer range advances which can be guaranteed to occur; and, finally, dreams of the future.

What is Around the Corner? It can be safely predicted that the few developments which are still needed to understand the geography of the central cholinergic system will be forthcoming; among those there will be the determination of the human cholinergic geography. Not much further in the future is the description of the interaction of the cholinergic system with systems activated by other neurotransmitters. Altogether, in a few years we will be able to map the cholinergic system as it impinges upon and is impinged on, pathways activated by other transmitters including catechol and indoleamines, peptides and amino acids.

Similarly, it will be soon resolved what is the functional significance of the actions of cholinergic agonists and antagonists on the channel versus those on the receptor portion of the macromolecule, as well as the functional meaning of their action on the open versus closed channel conformation. These discoveries will be necessarily related to further elucidation of the multiplicity of the post and presynaptic cholinergic responses including the ionic mechanisms that are involved. Still in the same context, a few years will bring about the definition of the sub-populations of nicotinic and muscarinic receptors; this is particularly important from the applied viewpoint as it will lead to the development of drugs of major clinical significance. The disease states were frequently mentioned in the Symposium and the improvement of the knowledge of the specific pre- and post-synaptic receptors and the development of drugs with specific peripheral versus central effects and with specific effects on strategic brain areas will improve the clinical standing of cholinergic system as these developments will lead to drugs of high clinical importance in SDAT, affective and psychotic behaviors (Karczmar and Richardson, 1985), and in autonomic disease (Karczmar, 1986a). Again, the better knowledge of the sub-division of cholinergic receptors and of the function of cholinergic synapses in interaction with the other synapses should lead within forseeable time to devising better antidotes of antiChE drugs such as war gases and insecticides; this development is highly desirable, not only because in our foolishness we may get into activities involving, besides nuclear bombs, war gases, but also because in the countries such as Australia and Japan the intensive use of OP insecticides leads to frequent cases of toxicity, some of them (see Karczmar, 1985) causing symptomology resembling ALS.

Few Blocks Away. Modulation processes should be mentioned first. It will require quite a bit of research to fully understand facilitations and inhibitions that arise from the modulatory activities of the pre- and post-synaptic cholinergic receptors, and to define the significance of the slow postsynaptic potentials for the responsiveness of cholinergic neurons to non-cholinergic neurotransmitters, such as aminoacids, biogenic amines and peptides. The principles that will arise from this knowledge will be applicable to the modulatory systems that indubitably exist at non-cholinergic synapses. Ultimately, we will need a computer program to define the state of responsiveness of cholinergic and/or non-cholinergic neurons as dependent on these modulatory processes; this then will lead to our understanding of the consequences of interaction between various transmitters and I will return to this point below.

The lore of second messengers is relatively new as it begun only two decades ago with the discoveries of the Hokins (1960) and Sutherland (Sutherland et al., 1968). Several new developments can be expected in this area. First, we need a better understanding of the relation between the phophatidylinositol and cyclic nucleotide systems on the one hand and the nicotinic and muscarinic activation on the other; also, we need a more complete understanding of the specific membrane changes (Greengard, 1978) that are induced. This then will lead to the elucidation of the characteristics of various kinases that are involved. Furthermore, other phenomena may be engendered by the second messenger systems; these include morphogenetic and metabotropic actions that I will refer to below. Ultimately, this better definition of the interaction between the cholinergic system, the second messenger systems and the effectors will have to be expanded with respect to the cholinergic interaction with the other neurotransmitter systems.

The metabotropic actions of the second messenger systems, whether activated by the cholinergic drugs or exerted via other mechanisms relate to the trophic actions of the cholinergic system. Some of these actions were described at this Symposium and I commented above that these phenomena are related to the precocious phylogenetic and ontogenetic appearance of the components of the cholinergic system as compared to the emergence of its synaptotropic function (see Karczmar, 1963a). Sometime in the future it will be possible to define the trophic role of the cholinergic system and identify the trophic substances; we will needed also the clarification of the relationship between the trophic function of the cholinergic system and such known trophic substances as NGF and gangliosides.

The related concept is that of choline metabolism. As ontogenetically and phylogenetically the components of the cholinergic system appear precociously with respect to the synaptic function the metabolism of ACh that includes that of choline must have a role in the metabotropic activities of the cholinergic system; thus, better understanding of choline metabolism is needed, particularly with respect to the metabolism of phospholipids and generation of the membrane. May I be so bold as to suggest also that other metabolic processes may interact with the cholinergic system and that synthesis of polypeptides and proteins is similarly linked with the cholinergic system. In a decade we should be able to resolve these points and locate the phylogenetic and ontogenetic meaning of ACh metabolism within the frame work of phospholipid metabolism and other metabolic and cellular processes. The direct action of cholinergic drugs, particularly antiChEs, that does not depend on their synaptic effects which were referred to at this meeting must be understood in this context.

Far, Far, in the Future. The purification, isolation and chemical and immunobiological characterization of the receptors and their channels and of ChEs is an on-going process.

It may be predicted that in the future the various cholinergic receptors and their functionally different domains will be identified in terms of the amino acids sequence and structural relation to the membrane. This in turn should lead to the appropriate identification and purification of specific messenger RNA's that are involved in the generation and differentiation of these receptors and their domains. From this point it will be just a long leap to characterize the cholinergic genomes needed for the formation of cholinergic components and their organization within the cholinergic circuitry. This in turn should lead to identification of defective genomes and/or specific immunoactive processes; it is perceived today that these two kinds of phenomena underlie such cholinergic disease as myasthenia gravis. In the distant future this phenomenology may be extended to autonomic diseases (see Karczmar, 1986a), SDAT and, perhaps, certain forms of mental disease.

Other long range development concerns the expansion of the concepts of cholinergic modulation to other transmitter systems. Altogether, interaction between neurotransmitter and second messenger systems including also processes of synaptic modulation at both cholinergic and non-cholinergic synapses, will be sufficiently defined to become computerized and programmed; at that time, computer-generated model will be able to trace and predict the meandering of signals in the course of the CNS phenomena.

Even today, we can go some ways tracing the cholinergic function that arises during motor activity and its subtle control via the cerebellum and the non-pyramidal system (see Popper and Eccles, 1977); with additional effort this system may be linked with the sensory transmission on the one hand and the effector responses on the other. Furthermore, we begin to be able to describe the basal nuclei circuitry in terms of cholinergic, glutaminergic, gabaergic and enkephalinergic transmitter systems (Cheramy et al., 1979). But this very example shows us how much further we have to go to understand these processes in detail and translate this understanding into predictives of motor function in health and disease. How much further we have to go to extend the motor model system to other brain systems? How much further we have to go to understand the interaction between these systems as the brain constitutes a continuum, each component interacting with all the other components?

Will we ever successfully complete the next leap? Once we know the organic basis of brain function--and the cholinergic system will be obviously in the forefront of the development of this understanding-- shall we be able to include in our understanding the mental phenomena? Will this lead to Jack Eccles' anathema, the reductionism and monism, versus dualism or what he refers to as "Strong Dualist Interactionism"? Eccles (1984) stated "this is the climax of...story...on the human mystery and here the mystery is furthest from comprehension"; very boldly, may I make a prediction as to this mystery? Sometime ago I commented on "what we know now, we will know in the future, and possibly cannot ever know in neurosciences" (Karczmar, 1972), and I described a way of being neither a monist nor a dualist. As I stated at that time "particularly pertinent here is the theory proven by Godel (1931)...that any not unduly simple logical system couched in symbols that constitute a formal logical language can express true assertions which cannot be deduced from its actions" (Karczmar, 1972).

I stated further that "the corrolaries of this theory are that every formal language contains meaningful sentences that cannot be asserted to be either true or false or indeed tested adequately for this purpose" (o.c.; see also Carnap, 1937). In a similar sense Turing (1937) describes open ended systems, and Hodges (1983) refers to this concept as "Turing's enigma". What this line of thought suggests is that dualism does not necessarily mean what Eccles thinks it means (two independent or parallel systems) and that, on the other hand, reductionism and monism are in the Turing-Carnap-Godel sense an impossibility. The mental phenomena may be indeed the open-ended components of either of the two systems. What can be altogether said without recurring to mathematical formulations is that there is no need to look for either a syllogistic, Euclidian geometry or, on the other hand, "dualist interaction" when trying to explain body-mind relationship.

Altogether, it was exciting to be concerned with the cholinergic system for some forty years; it was fun to be involved over these years, in so many of its aspects and, finally, in the "happening" which is this Symposium.

REFERENCES

1. M.B. Abou-Donia: Toxicokinetics and metabolism of delayed neurotoxic organophosphorus esters. Neurotoxicol. 4:113-130, 1983.
2. P. Adams: Muscarinic excitation of vertebrate neurons. In: "Cellular and Molecular Basis of Cholinergic Function". M.J. Dowdall, ed., Ellis Horwood Publ., Chichester, U.K., 1986 (in press).
3. E.X. Albuquerque, J.E. Warwick, J.R. Tasse and F.M. Samsone: Effects of vinblastine and colchicine on neural regulation of the fast and slow skeletal muscles of the rat. Exp. Neurol. 38:607-634, 1972.
4. G.B. Ansell and S. Spanner: Choline transport and metabolism in the brain. L. Horrocks, G.B. Ansell and G. Porcellati eds., 1:137-144, Raven Press, N.Y., 1982.
5. R.T. Bartus, R.L. Dean, J.A. Goas and S.A. Lippa: Age related changes in passive avoidance retention and modulation with chronic dietary choline. Science 209:301-309, 1980.
6. N.J.M. Birdsall, C.A.M. Curtis, P. Eveleigh, E.C. Hulme, E.K. Pedter, D. Poyner, J.M. Stockton and M. Wheatley: Muscarinic receptor subtypes. In: "Cellular and Molecular Bases of Cholinergic Function". M.J. Dowdall, ed., Ellis Horwood Publishers, Chichester, U.K., 1986 (in press).
7. N.J.M. Birdsall and E.L. Hulme: Biochemical studies on muscarinic acetylcholine receptors. J. Neurochem. 27:7-16, 1976.
8. J.K. Blusztajn and R.J. Wurtman: Choline and cholinergic neurons. Science 221:614-620, 1983.
9. D. Bovet, V.G. Longo and B. Silvestrini: Les methodes d'investigations electrohysiologiques dans l'etude des medicaments tranquillisants. In: "International Symposium on Psychotropic Drugs". S. Garattini and V. Ghetti, eds., pp. 193-206, Elsevier, Amsterdam, 1957.
10. N.P. Boyd and J.B. Cohen: Desensitization of membrane-bound acetylcholine receptor by amine non-competitive antagonists and aliphatic alcohols: studies of [3H] acetylcholine binding and 22 Na$^+$ ion fluxes. Biochem. 23:4023-4033, 1984.
11. P.B. Bradley and J. Elkes: The effects of some drugs on the electrical activity of the brain. Brain 80:77-117, 1957.
12. R. Carnap: The Logical Syntax of Language. Harcourt, N.Y., 1937.
13. J.P. Changeux, A. Devillers-Thiery and P. Chemouilli: Acetylcholine receptor: an allosteric protein. Science 225:1335-1345, 1984.
14. A. Cheramy, V. Leviel, A. Nieoullon and J. Glowinski: Role of various nigral afferences on the activity of nigrostriatal dopaminergic pathways. In: "Neurotransmitters". P. Simon, ed., Adv. Pharmacol. Therap. 2:131-143, Pergamon Press, Oxford, 1979.
15. A.E. Cole and R.A. Nicoll: Characterization of a slow cholinergic postsynaptic potential recorded in vitro from rat hippocampal pyramidal cells. J. Physiol. (Lond.) 352:173-188, 1984.
16. H.H. Dale: The action of certain esters and esters of choline and their relation to muscarine. J. Pharmacol. Exper. Therap. 6:147-190, 1914.
17. H.H. Dale: Pharmacology and nerve endings. Proc. Roy. Soc. Med. 28:319-332, 1935.

18. E.F. Domino: Electroencephalographic and behavioral arousal effects of small doses of nicotine. Ann. N.Y. Acad. Sci. 142:216-244, 1967.

19. N.J. Dun: Peptide hormones and transmission in sympathetic ganglia. In: "Autonomic Ganglia". L.G. Elfvin, ed., pp. 345-366, John Wiley, Chichester, U.K., 1985.

20. N.J. Dun and A.G. Karczmar: Blockade of ACh potentials by alpha-bungarotoxin in rat superior cervical ganglion cells. Brain Res. 196:536-540, 1980.

21. N.J. Dun, M. Kiraly and R.C. Ma: Evidence for a serotonin mediated slow excitatory potential in the guinea-pig coeliac ganglia. J. Physiol. (Lond.) 351:61-76, 1984.

22. J.C. Eccles: Facilitation and inhibition in the superior cervical ganglion. J. Physiol. (Lond.) 85:207-238, 1935.

23. J.C. Eccles: Historical introduction. In: "Symposium on Central Cholinergic Transmission and its Behavioral Aspects". A.G. Karczmar, ed., Fed. Proc. 28:90-94, 1969.

24. J.C. Eccles: The Human Mystery. The Gifford Lectures, U. of Edinburgh, 1977-1978, Routledge and Kegan Panel, London, 1984.

25. J.C. Eccles, P. Fatt and K. Koketsu: Cholinergic and inhibitory synapses in a central nervous pathway. The Australian J. Sci. 16:50-54, 1953.

26. J.C. Eccles, P. Fatt and K. Koketsu: Cholinergic and inhibitory synapses in a pathway from motor-axon collaterals to motoneurones. J. Physiol. (Lond.) 126:524-562, 1954.

27. R.M. Eccles: Responses of isolated curarized sympathetic ganglia. J. Physiol. 117:196-217, 1952.

28. R.M. Eccles and B. Libet: Origin and blockade of the synaptic responses of curarised sympathetic ganglia. J. Physiol. (Lond.) 157:484-503, 1961.

29. W. Feldberg: Present views on the mode of action of acetylcholine in the central nervous system. Physiol. Rev. 25:596-642, 1945.

30. W. Feldberg and M. Vogt: Acetylcholine synthesis in different regions of the central nervous system. J. Physiol. 107:372-381, 1948.

31. W. Feldberg: A Pharmacological Approach to the Brain from its Inner and Outer Surface. Williams and Wilkins, Baltimore, 1963.

32. W. Feldberg and R.D. Myers: Effects on temperature of amines injected into the cerebral ventricles. A new concept of temperature regulation. J. Physiol. (Lond.) 173:226-237, 1964.

33. T.P. Feng and T.H. Li: Studies on the neuromuscular junction. XXIII. A new aspect of the phenomena of eserine potentiation and post-tetanic facilitation in mammalian muscles. Chinese J. Physiol. 16:37-50, 1941.

34. A. Fisher and I. Hanin: Minireview: choline analogs as potential tools in developing selective animal models of central cholinergic hypofunction. Life Sci. 27:1615-1634, 1980.

35. H. Fuhner: Untersuchungen uber die peripherale Wirkung des Physostigmines. Arch. Exp. Path. Pharmakol. 82:205-220, 1918.

36. S.N. Glisson, A.G. Karczmar and L. Barnes: Cholinergic effects on adrenergic neurotransmitters in rabbit brain parts. Neuropharmacol. 11:465-477, 1972.

37. K. Godel: Uber formal unentscheidbare Satze der Principia Mathematica und vervandter Systeme. I. Monatshefte f. Math. Physik 38:173-198, 1931.

38. P. Greengard: Cyclic nucleotides, phosphorylated proteins and neuronal function. Raven Press, N.Y., 1978.

39. A. Hodges: Alan Turing: The Enigma. Touchstone Brooks, N.Y., 1983.

40. M.R. Hokin and L.E. Hokin: The role of phosphatidic acid and phosphoionositide in transmembrane transport elicited by acetylcholine and other humoral agents. Int. Rev. Neurobiol. 2:99-136, 1960.

41. B. Holmstedt: The ordeal bean of old calabar: The pageant of _Physostigma_ Venenosum in medicine. In: "Plants in the Development of Modern Medicine". T. Swain, ed. pp. 303-360, Harvard U. Press, Cambridge, Mass., 1972.

42. M.K. Johnson: Acetylcholinesterase and neuropathy target esterase (NTE) compared and contrasted with the aid of organophosphorus esters. In: "Cellular and Molecular Basis of Cholinergic Function". M.J. Dowdall, ed., Ellis Horwood Publs., Chichester, U.K., 1986 (in press).

43. L.Y. Jan and Y.N. Jan: Peptidergic transmission in sympathetic ganglia of the frog. J. Physiol. (Lond.) 327:219-246, 1982.

44. D.S. Janowsky, S.C. Risch, L.D. Judd, L.Y. Huey and D.C. Parker: Brain cholinergic systems and the pathogenesis of affective disorders. In: "Central Cholinergic Mechanisms and Adaptive Dysfunctions". M.M. Singh, D.M. Warburton and H. Lal, eds., pp. 309-334, Plenum Publ. Corp., N.Y., 1985.

45. M. Jouvet: Some monoaminergic mechanisms controlling sleep and waking. In: "Brain and Human Behavior". A.G. Karczmar and J.C. Eccles, eds., pp. 131-160, 1972, Springer-Verlag, Berlin, 1972.

46. A.G. Karczmar: The role of amputation and nerve resection in the regressing limbs of urodele larvae. J. Exp. Zool. 103:401-427, 1946.

47. A.G. Karczmar: Antagonisms between a bis-quaternary oxamide, WIN 8078, and depolarizing and competitive blocking agents. J. Pharmacol. Exper. Therap. 119:39-47, 1951.

48. A.G. Karczmar: Ontogenetic effects of anticholinesterase agents. In: "Cholinesterases and anticholinesterase agents". G.B. Koelle, ed., Handch. d. Exper. Pharmakol. Erganzungswk. 15:179-186, Springer-Verlag, Berlin, 1963a.

49. A.G. Karczmar: Ontogenesis of cholinesterases. In: "Cholinesterases and anticholinesterase agents". G.B. Koelle, ed., Handbch. d. Exper. Pharmakol., Erganzungswk. 15:799-832, Springer-Verlag, Berlin, 1963b.

50. A.G. Karczmar: Pharmacology and antagonism of four organophosphorus agents. Report No. 2, Subcontract No. SU-630505-64, Melpar Inc., Virginia, 1964 (unpublished).

51. A.G. Karczmar: Pharmacologic, toxicologic and therapeutic properties of anticholinesterase agents. In: "Physiological Pharmacology". W.S. Root and F.G. Hofman, eds., 3:163-322, Academic Press, N.Y., 1967.

52. A.G. Karczmar versus F.G. Standaert: Discussion. Ann. N.Y. Acad. Sci. 144:568-570, 1967.

53. A.G. Karczmar: Introduction: history of the research with anticholinesterase agents. In: "Anticholinesterase Agents". A.G. Karczmar, ed., Intern. Encyclop. Pharmacol. Therap., Section 13, 1:1-44, Pergamon Press, Oxford, 1970.

54. A.G. Karczmar: What we know now, will know in the future, and possibly cannot ever "know" in neurosciences. In: "Brain and Human Behavior". A.G. Karczmar and J.C. Eccles, eds., pp. 63-92, Springer-Verlag, Berlin, 1972.

55. A.G. Karczmar: Brain acetylcholine and seizures. In: "Psychobiology of Convulsive Therapy". M. Fink, S. Kety, J. McGaugh and T.A. Williams, eds., pp. 251-270, V.H. Winston and Sons, Washington, D.C., 1974.

56. A.G. Karczmar: Cholinergic influences on behavior. In: "Cholinergic Mechanisms". P.G. Waser, ed., pp. 501-529, Raven Press, N.Y., 1975.

57. A.G. Karczmar: Overview: Cholinergic drugs and behavior - what effects may be expected from a "cholinergic diet"? In: "Nutrition and the Brain". A. Barbeau, J.H. Growdon and R.J. Wurtman,

eds., <u>5</u>:141-175, Raven Press, N.Y., 1979.

58. A.G. Karczmar: Present and future of the development of anti-OP drugs. Fund. Appl. Toxicol. <u>5</u>:S270-S279, 1985.

59. A.G. Karczmar: Autonomic disease and clinical applications of ganglionic agents. In: "Autonomic and Enteric Ganglia". A.G. Karczmar, K. Koketsu and S. Nishi, eds., pp. 459-475, Plenum Publ. Corp., N.Y., 1986.

60. A.G. Karczmar: Ganglionic transmission as a model for CNS function. In: "Autonomic and Enteric Ganglia". A.G. Karczmar, K. Koketsu and S. Nishi, eds., pp. 477-499, Plenum Publ. Corp., N.Y., 1986b.

61. A.G. Karczmar: Historical and anatomical bases of ganglionic and enteric transmission. In: "Autonomic and Enteric Ganglia". A.G. Karczmar, K. Koketsu and S. Nishi, eds., pp. 3-26, Plenum Publ. Corp., N.Y., 1986c.

62. A.G. Karczmar: Schizophrenia and cholinergic system. In: "Receptors and Ligands in Psychiatry and Neurology". A.K. Sen and T. Lee, eds., Cambridge U. Press, Cambridge, U.K., 1986d (in press).

63. A.G. Karczmar: Conference on dynamics of cholinergic function: Overview and comments. In: "Dynamics of Cholinergic Function". I. Hanin, ed., Plenum Publ. Corp., N.Y., 1986e (in press).

64. A.G. Karczmar: Historical development of concepts of ganglionic transmission. In: "Autonomic and Enteric Ganglia". A.G. Karczmar, K. Koketsu and S. Nishi, eds., pp. 3-26, Plenum Publ. Corp., N.Y., 1986f.

65. A.G. Karczmar and N.J. Dun: Cholinergic synapses: physiological, pharmacological and behavioral considerations. In: "Psychopharmacology: A Generation of Progress". M.A. Lipton, A. DiMascio and K.F. Killam, eds., pp. 293-306, Raven Press, N.Y., 1978.

66. A.G. Karczmar: New roles for cholinergics in CNS disease. Drug Therapy <u>4</u>:31-42, 1979.

67. A.G. Karczmar and N.J. Dun: Pharmacology of synaptic ganglionic transmission and second messengers. In: "Autonomic and Enteric Ganglia". A.G. Karczmar, K. Koketsu and S. Nishi, eds., pp. 297-337, Plenum Publ. Corp., N.Y., 1986.

68. A.G. Karczmar and J.W. Howard: Antagonism of d-tubocurarine and other pharmacological properties of certain bisquaternary salts of basically substituted oxamides (WIN) 8077 and analogs. J. Pharmacol. Exper. Therap. <u>113</u>:30, 1955.

69. A.G. Karczmar and G.H. Kindel: Acetylcholine turnover and aggression in related three strains of mice. Progr. Neuropsychopharmacol. <u>5</u>:35-48, 1981.

70. A.G. Karczmar and D.L. Richardson: Cholinergic mechanisms, schizophrenia and neuropsychiatric adaptive dysfunctions. In: "Central Cholinergic Mechanisms and Adaptive Dysfunctions". M.M. Singh, D.M. Warburton and H. Lal, eds., pp. 193-222, Plenum Publ. Corp., N.Y., 1985.

71. A.G. Karczmar, R. Srinivasan and J. Bernsohn: Cholinergic function in the developing fetus. In: "Fetal Pharmacology". L.O. Boreus, ed., Raven Press, N.Y., pp. 127-177, 1973.

72. Y. Kataoka, Y. Gutman, A. Guidotti, P. Panula, J. Wroblewski, D. Cosenza-Murphy, Y.Z. Wu and E. Costa: Intrinsic GABAergic system of adrenal chromaffin cells. Proc. Natl. Acad. Sci. USA: 3218-3222, 1984.

73. G.B. Koelle: Poisons of the Canon. In: "Leaves from the Copper Beeches", pp. 91-96, Livingston Publ. Co., Narberth, Pa., 1959.

74. G.B. Koelle: Cytological distributions and physiological functions of cholinesterases. In: "Cholinesterases and Anticholinesterase Agents". G.B. Koelle, ed., Handbch. d. Exper. Pharmakol. Erganzungswk. <u>15</u>:187-298, Springer-Verlag, Berlin, 1963.

75. K. Koketsu and A.G. Karczmar: General concepts of ganglionic transmission and modulation. In: "Autonomic and Enteric Ganglia".

A.G. Karczmar, K. Koketsu and S. Nishi, eds., pp. 63-77, Plenum Publ. Corp., N.Y., 1986.

76. T. Koppanyi and A.G. Karczmar: Contribution to the study of the mechanism of action of cholinesterase inhibitors. J. Pharmacol. Exp. Therap. 14:327-343, 1951.

77. T. Koppanyi and A.G. Karczmar: Experimental Pharmacodynamics. Burgess Publ. Co., Minneapolis, 1st Ed., 1955.

78. M. Kremer, H.E.S. Pearson and S. Wright: Action of prostigmine on the spinal cord in man. J. Physiol. (Lond.) 89:21-23P, 1937.

79. D.J. Kupfer and D.J. Edwards: Multitransmitter mechanisms and treatment of affective disease. In: "Neuropsychopharmacology". P. Deniker, C. Radouco-Thomas and A. Villeneuve, eds., 1:609-623, Pergamon Press, Oxford, 1978.

80. C. Larsson, A. Nordberg, G. Wahlstrom, U. Arnelo and L. Nilsson: Effects of choline nicotine treatment on brain acetylcholine receptors. In: "Cellular and Molecular Basis of Cholinergic Function". M.J. Dowdall, ed., Ellis Horwood Publs., Chichester, U.K., 1986 (in press).

81. R. Levi-Montalcini: Growth control of nerve cells by protein factor and its antiserum. Science 143:105-110, 1964.

82. B. Libet: Which postsynaptic action of dopamine is mediated by cyclic AMP? Life Sci. 24:1043-1058, 1979.

83. B. Libet: Heterosynaptic interaction at a sympathetic neuron as a model for induction and storage of a postsynaptic memory trace. In: "Neurobiology of Learning and Memory". G. Lynch, J.L. McGaugh and N.M. Weinberger, eds., pp. 405-430, The Guilford Press, New York, 1984.

84. O. Loewi: Uber humorale Ubertragbarkeit der Herzenwirkung. I Mitteilung. Pflugers Arch. ges. Physiol. 189:239-242, 1921.

85. V.G. Longo: Electroencephalographic Atlas for Pharmacological Research. Elsevier, Amsterdam, 1962.

86. F.C. MacIntosh: Formation, storage and release of acetylcholine at nerve endings. Canad. J. Biochem. 37:343-356, 1959.

87. P.L. McGeer, J.C. Eccles and E.G. McGeer: Molecular Neurobiology of Mammalion Brain. Plenum Publ. Corp., N.Y., 1978.

88. D. Nachmansohn: Actions on axons, and evidence for the role of acetylcholine in axonal conduction. In: "Cholinesterases and Anticholinesterase Agents". G.B. Koelle, ed., pp. 701-740, Handbch. d. Exper. Pharmakol. Erganzungswk. 15:701-740, Springer-Verlag, Berlin, 1963.

89. E.J. Nestler, S.I. Walaas and P. Greengard. Neuronal phospho-proteins: physiological and clinical implications. Science 225:1357-1364, 1984.

90. S. Nishi: Cholinergic and adrenergic receptors at sympathetic ganglionic terminals. Fed. Proc. 29:1950-1965, 1970.

91. S. Nishi and K. Koketsu: Early and late after-discharges of amphibian sympathetic ganglion cells. J. Neurophysiol. 31:109-121, 1968.

92. Y. Ohta, G.S. Karczmar and A.G. Karczmar: Phospholipids and amphibian neuromyal transmission. Eighth International Congr. of Pharmacol., Abstracts, p. 646, Tokyo IUPHAR Publs., 1981.

93. J.W. Phillis and D.H. York: Cholinergic inhibition in the cerebral cortex. Brain Res. 5:517-520, 1967.

94. R.L. Polak: Effect of hyoscine on the output of acetylcholine into perfused cerebral ventricles of cats. J. Physiol. (Lond.) 181:317-323, 1965.

95. K.R. Popper and J.C. Eccles: The self and its brain--an argument for interactionism. Springer International, Berlin, 1977.

96. M.A. Raftery, B.M. Conti-Tronconi and S.M.J. Dunn: Structural and functional aspects of the nicotinic receptor. Fund. Appl. Toxicol. 5:S39-S40, 1985.

97. H.P. Rang and J.M. Ritter: On the mechanism of desensitization at cholinergic receptors. Mol. Pharmacol. 6:394-441, 1969.

98. G.P. Richardson, K. Siddle and J.P. Luzio: Immunoaffinity purification of intact, metabolically active, cholinergic nerve terminals from mammalian brain. Biochem. J. 219:647-654, 1984.

99. W.K. Riker and Z. Szreniawski: The pharmacological reactivity of presynaptic nerve terminals in a sympathetic ganglion. J. Pharmacol. Exp. Therap. 126:233-238, 1959.

100. F. Rinaldi and H.E. Himwich: Alerting responses and actions of atropine and cholinergic drugs. A.M.A. Arch. Neurol. Psychiat. 73:387-395, 1955.

101. M. Saito, G. Kindel, A.G. Karczmar and A. Rosenberg: Metabolism of choline in brain of the aged CBF-1 mouse. J. Neurosci. Res. 15:197-209, 1986.

102. O.E. Schotte and E.G. Butler: Morphological effects of denervation and amputation of limbs in urodele larvae. J. Exp. Zool. 87:279-322, 1941.

103. O.E. Schotte and A.G. Karczmar: Limb parameters and regression rates in denervated amputated limbs of urodele larvae. J. Exp. Zool. 97:43-70, 1944.

104. K. Sikora-VanMeter, T. Ellenberg and W.G. VanMeter: Neurotoxic changes in cat neurohypophysis after single and multiple exposure to DFP and Soman. Fund. Appl. Toxicol. 5:1087-1096, 1985.

105. M.M. Singh: Cholinergic mechanisms, adaptive brain processes and psychopathology. In: "Central Cholinergic Mechanisms and Adaptive Dysfunctions". M.M. Singh, D.M. Warburton and H. Lal, eds., pp. 353-397, Plenum Publ. Corp., N.Y., 1985.

106. F.G. Standaert and W.F. Riker, Jr.: The consequences of cholinergic drug actions on motor nerve terminals. Ann. N.Y. Acad. Sci. 144:517-533, 1967.

107. E.W. Sutherland, G.A. Robinson and R.W. Butcher: Some aspects of the biological role of adenosine 3',5'-monophosphate (cyclic AMP). Circulation 37:279-306, 1968.

108. J.C. Szerb: Characterization of presynaptic muscarinic receptors in central cholinergic neurons. In: "Cholinergic Mechanisms and Psychopharmacology". D.J. Jenden, ed., pp. 49-60, Plenum Publ. Corp., N.Y., 1977.

109. S. Thesleff: The mode of neuromuscular block caused by acetylcholine, nicotine, decamethonium and succinycholine. Acta Physiol. Scand. 34:218-231, 1955.

110. R.C. Thomas and V.J. Wilson: Precise location of Renshaw cells with a new marking technique. Nature 206:211-213, 1965.

111. S. Tucek: The synthesis of acetylcholine. In: "Enzymes in the Nervous System". A. Lajtha, ed. 4:219-428, Plenum Publ. Corp., N.Y., 1983.

112. A.M. Turing: On computable numbers with an application to the Enscheidung-problem. Proc. Lond. Math. Soc., Ser. II, 43:544-546, 1937.

113. W.G. VanMeter, A.G. Karczmar and R.R. Fiscus: CNS effects of anticholinesterases in the presence of inhibited cholinesterases. Int. Arch. Pharmacodyn. Ther. 23:249-260, 1978.

114. T.W. Vickroy, M. Watson, H.I. Yamamura and W.R. Roeske: Agonist binding to multiple muscarinic receptors. Fed. Proc. 43:2785-2790, 1984.

115. L. Wecker: The utilization of supplemental choline by brain. In: "Conference on Dynamics of Cholinergic Function". I. Hanin, ed., Plenum Press Corp., N.Y., 1986 (in press).

116. E. Zaimis: Actions at autonomic sites. In: "Cholinesterases and Anticholinesterase Agents". G.B. Koelle, ed., Handbch. d. exper. Pharmakol. 15:530-569, Springer-Verlag, Berlin, 1963.

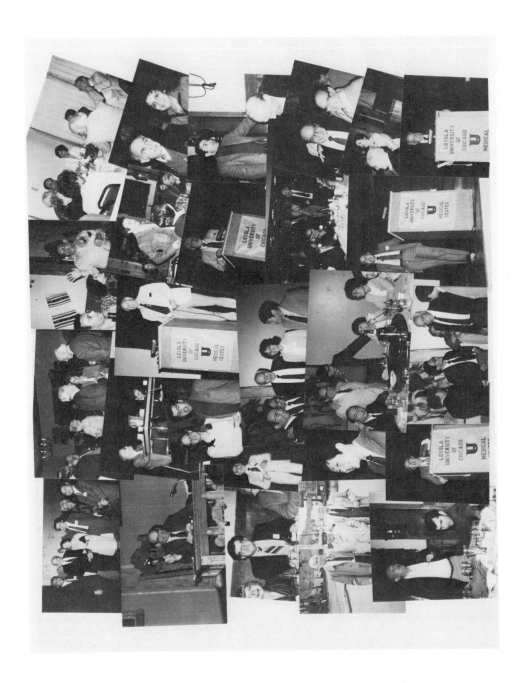

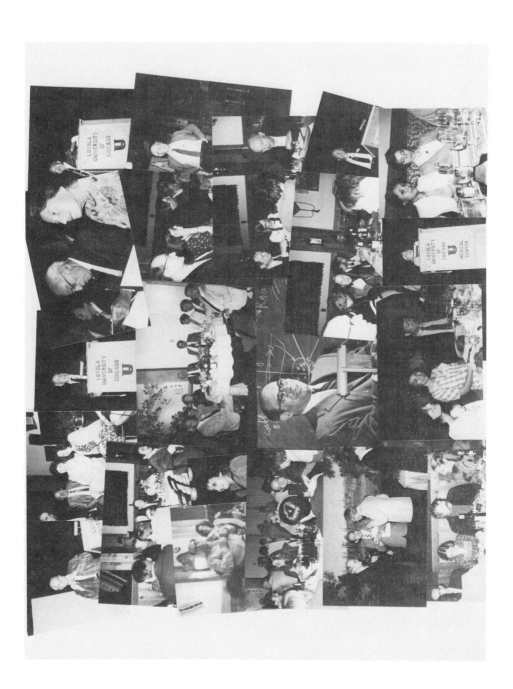

587

INDEX

Acetylcholine, 3, 60–63, 103, 117,
121, 133–143, 191, 192,
218, 219, 251, 437
  action, 227, 271, 275–278
  assay, 180, 561–585
  and atonia, 376–377
  and body temperature, 397–399
  in cortex, cerebral, 271–281
  depolarization, 285–290
  desynchronization, 374, 379
  and EEG, 503, 509–516
  electrophysiology, 329
  exocytosis, 334–335
  ganglionic, 133–143
  in heart, 159–177
  history, 561–585
  and ion channel activation,
    339–351
  methodology, 561–585
  modulation, 179–186, 225–231
  and motoneuron, spinal, 283–293
  and neuron, cortical, 271–278
  neurotransmitter activity
    discovered in *1920*, 374
  pharmacology of ion channel
    activation, 133–143,
    339–351
  pool concept, 136–138
  potential, suppression of, 290
  receptor, 17–25, 195–209, 225,
    573–574
    nicotinic, 195–209, 232, 235,
    242–243
  release, 75–83, 134–140,
    179–186, 219, 225–231,
    239–244, 329–337
  REM, 375
  research trends, past, present,
    future, 561–585
  sensitivity, 231–235
  storage, 133–143
  synthesis, 75–83, 138–141
  translocation, 133
Acetylcholinesterase, 9–10, 47–52,
58, 69, 85–93, 103–110,
121, 122, 369–370, 377,

Acetylcholinesterase, (continued)
467–469, 489, 492, 536
Acrylamide, 490
Actin, 58, 172–173
Activity, epileptiform, 437–450
Adenosine, 150–154, 180–186, 229
Adenosine monophosphate, cyclic,
117, 161, 163
  dibutyryl, 151
Adenosine triphosphatase, 169–172
Adenosine triphosphate, 229, 234
Adenosine triphosphate translocase,
57, 58
Adenylate cyclase, 117, 161
Adrenaline, *see* Epinephrine
AF64A, *see* Ethylcholine aziridinium
Aging, 10, 93–97
AH*5183*, *see* 2-(4-Phenylpiperidine)-
  cyclohexanol
Alkaline earth, cation, 329–337
n-Alkylguanidine, 339
ALS, *see* Amyotrophic lateral sclerosis
Alzheimer's disease, 5, 10, 11, 89,
93, 94, 271
γ-Aminobutyric acid (GABA), 228,
355, 357–362, 437, 512
4-Aminopyridine, 248, 437
Amphetamine, 89
Amylguanidine, 344
Amyotrophic lateral sclerosis,
369–372
Anticholinesterase, 437–450, 503,
512–516
  sites listed, 513
Antigen, plasma membrane-specific,
64–69
Apamin, 205, 249, 250
Aplysia sp., 211
Apomorphine, 405, 407, 409, 410
Arecoline, 381, 382, 473–477, 482
Arrest, respiratory, 535–550
  see Organophosphorus
Artane, 11
Atonia, 376–377
Atrium

DATE DUE